S0-BKE-934

Handbook of Pediatric Nutrition

Second Edition

Patricia Queen Samour, MMSc, RD
Clinical Nutrition Director
Nutrition Services
Beth Israel Deaconess Medical Center
Boston, Massachusetts

Kathy King Helm, RD, LD
Private Practitioner
Publisher
Helm Publishing
Lake Dallas, Texas

Carol E. Lang
Biologist
Office of Pesticide Programs
Health Effects Division
Environmental Protection Agency
Washington, D.C.

JONES AND BARTLETT PUBLISHERS
Sudbury, Massachusetts
BOSTON TORONTO LONDON SINGAPORE

World Headquarters
Jones and Bartlett Publishers
40 Tall Pine Drive
Sudbury, MA 01776
978-443-5000
info@jbpub.com
www.jbpub.com

Jones and Bartlett Publishers
Canada
2406 Nikanna Road
Mississauga, ON L5C 2W6
CANADA

Jones and Bartlett Publishers
International
Barb House, Barb Mews
London W6 7PA
UK

The author has made every effort to ensure the accuracy of information herein. However, appropriate information sources should be consulted, especially for new or unfamiliar procedures. It is the responsibility of every practitioner to evaluate the appropriateness of a particular opinion in the context of actual clinical situations and with due considerations to new developments. The author, editors, and the publisher cannot be held responsible for any typographical or other errors found in this book.

Library of Congress Cataloging-in-Publication Data

Handbook of pediatric nutrition/ [edited by] Patricia Queen Samour,
Kathy King Helm, Carol E. Lang – 2nd ed.
p. cm.
Includes bibliographical references and index.
ISBN 0-7637-3305-9
1. Children—Nutrition Handbooks, manuals, etc. 2. Nutrition disorders in children Handbooks, manuals, etc. 3. Diet therapy for children Handbooks, manuals, etc. I. Samour, Patricia Queen. II. Helm, Kathy King. III. Lang, Carol E. [DNLM: 1. Child Nutrition. 2. Child Nutrition Disorders. 3. Diet Therapy—Child. 4. Diet Therapy—Infant. 5. Infant Nutrition Disorders. 6. Infant Nutrition. 7. Nutrition Disorders—complications—Child.
WS 115 H2363 1999]
RJ206.H23 1999
618.92—dc21
DNLM/DLC
for Library of Congress
99-37336
CIP

Production Credits
Publisher: Michael Brown
Associate Editor: Chambers Moore
Production Manager: Amy Rose
Associate Production Editor: Renée Sekerak
Production Assistant: Jenny L. McIsaac
Associate Marketing Manager: Joy Stark-Vancs
Manufacturing Buyer: Amy Bacus
Printing and Binding: Port City Press
Cover Printing: Port City Press

Printed in the United States of America
07 06 05 04 03 10 9 8 7 6 5 4 3 2 1

Table of Contents

Contributors

Phyllis B. Acosta, Dr PH, RD
Director, Metabolic Diseases
Medical Department
Ross Products Division/Abbott Laboratories, Inc.
Columbus, Ohio

Susan M. Akers, RD, LD
Pediatric Dietitian Specialist
Department of Pediatrics
MetroHealth Medical Center
Cleveland, Ohio

Diane M. Anderson, PhD, RD, CSP, FADA
Associate Professor of Pediatrics
Neonatal Nutritionist
Department of Pediatrics
Medical University of South Carolina
Charleston, South Carolina

Karen V. Barale, MS, RD, CD, FADA
Manager of Food Services
Fred Hutchinson Cancer Research Center
Seattle, Washington

Susan Bessler, MS, RD, CSP
Clinical Dietitian
Department of Gastroenterology and Nutrition
Childrens Hospital Oakland
Oakland, California

Andrea Bull McDonough, MS, RD
Nutrition Therapist and Consultant
Boston, Massachusetts

Karen Hanson Chalmers, MS, RD, CDE
Director
Nutrition Services
Joslin Diabetes Center
Boston, Massachusetts

Paula M. Charuhas, MS, RD, FADA, CD, CNSD
Pediatric Nutrition Specialist
Department of Clinical Nutrition
Fred Hutchinson Cancer Center
Seattle, Washington

Lynn Christie, MS, RD, LD
Nutritionist
Clinical Coordinator
Division of Allergy and Immunology
Department of Pediatrics
Arkansas Children's Hospital
Little Rock, Arkansas

William Cameron Chumlea
Department of Community Health
Department of Pediatrics
School of Medicine
Wright State University
Yellow Springs, Ohio

Harriet Holt Cloud, MS, RD
Owner, Nutrition Matters
Pediatric Nutrition Consultant
Professor Emeritus
University of Alabama, Birmingham
Birmingham, Alabama

Kattia M. Corrales, RD
Pediatric Nutrition Specialist
Combined Program in Pediatric GI/Nutrition
Children's Hospital
Boston, Massachusetts

Carol M. Coughlin, RD
Your Favorite Dietitian
Leicester, Massachusetts

Janice Cox, MS, RD
Neonatal/Pediatric Dietitian
The Children's Hospital at Bronson
Kalamazoo, Michigan

Roseann Cutroni, MS, RD
Clinical Dietitian Specialist
Clinical Nutrition Service
Children's Hospital
Boston, Massachusetts

Lauren R. Furuta, RD, MOE
Clinical Dietitian Specialist
Clinical Nutrition Service
Children's Hospital
Boston, Massachusetts

Michele Morath Gottschlich, PhD, RD, LD, CNSD
Director
Nutrition Services
Shriners Hospitals for Children
Associate Professor
University of Cincinnati
Cincinnati, Ohio

Sharon L. Groh-Wargo, RD, LD, MS
Neonatal Nutritionist
Department of Pediatrics
MetroHealth Medical Center
Cleveland, Ohio

Shumei S. Guo, PhD
Department of Community Health
School of Medicine
Wright State University
Yellow Springs, Ohio

Bridget M. Klawitter, PhD, RD, CD, FADA
Manager
Department of Clinical Dietetics
All Saints Healthcare System, Inc.
Racine, Wisconsin
Nutrition Consultant
Nutrition Management & Consultations
Salem, Wisconsin

Betty Lucas, MPH, RD, CD
Nutritionist
Center on Human Development and Disability
University of Washington
Seattle, Washington

Ingrida Mara Melbardis, RD
Pediatric Dietitian
The Children's Hospital at Bronson
Kalamazoo, Michigan

Myrna Miller, RN, BSN
Nurse Clinician
Gastroenterology
The Children's Medical Center
Dayton, Ohio

Nancy L. Nevin-Folino, MEd, RD, CSP, LD, FADA
Neonatal Nutrition Specialist
Pediatric Specialist
The Children's Medical Center
Dayton, Ohio

Linda Gallagher Olsen, MEd, RD
Clinical Nutrition Manager
Clinical Nutrition Service
Children's Hospital
Boston, Massachusetts

Luz Gómez Pardini, MPH, RD
Director of Public Health Nutrition
Contra Costa Health Services
Martinez, California

Anne Piatek, MS, RD
Nutrition Consultant
St. Louis, Missouri

Nancy S. Spinozzi, RD
Pediatric Dietitian Specialist
Children's Hospital
Clinical Nutrition Service
Boston, Massachusetts

Sherri Utter, MS, RD, CNSD
Pediatric Nutrition Specialist
Combined Program in Pediatric GI/Nutrition
Children's Hospital
Boston, Massachusetts

Karen A. Weaver, MS, RD
Pediatric Dietitian
Department of Clinical Nutrition
Cardinal Glennon Children's Hospital
St. Louis, Missouri

Jacqueline Jones Wessel, MEd, RD, CNSD, CSP, CLE
Nutrition Support Consultant
Pediatric Gastroenterology and Nutrition
Children's Hospital and Medical Center
Cincinnati, Ohio

John Westerdahl, MPH, RD, CNS
Director
Health Promotion Department
Nutritional Services Department
Castle Medical Center
Kailua, Hawaii

Nancy H. Wooldridge, MS, RD, LD
Director of Nutrition
Pediatric Pulmonary Center
Department of Pediatrics
University of Alabama at Birmingham
Birmingham, Alabama

PREFACE

This edition of the *Handbook of Pediatric Nutrition* has many enhanced features over the first edition. Every chapter in the book has been critically reviewed and revised to maintain a state-of-the-art scientific knowledge base of pediatric nutrition. Several new chapters and a detailed appendix were added. The chapter on cardiac disease addresses the specific issues around growth and feeding infants with cardiac conditions, as well as the cardiac treatment and prevention issues of older children. Because more interventions are occurring on an outpatient or ambulatory care setting, rather than the acute care setting, a chapter on nutrition counseling was also added. Counseling techniques for different ages and other suggestions for an effective counseling session are covered in this new chapter.

Due to the ever-increasing use of alternative or complementary medicine in the prevention and/or treatment of diseases such as cancer and AIDS, all chapter authors were asked to address these issues as they pertained to their patient population. As health providers, we must know what our patients are consuming or planning to use, and we must counsel them appropriately with the scientific basis that presently exists. A chapter on botanicals was added to this edition so that pediatric practitioners could have the latest resource on these products, their rationale, and indications for their use.

To facilitate locating key nutrition resource tables, figures, and charts, an expanded appendix was created in this edition. Thus, all growth charts referred to throughout the text can be found easily. Nutritional assessment tools, such as the incremental growth charts, body mass index (BMI) tables and percentiles, triceps skinfold (TSF) and other anthropometric measurements and nomagrams are also included as well as the Tanner stages and laboratory norms of commonly used tests. The Recommended Dietary Allowances (RDAs) and the newer daily recommended intakes (DRIs) are included, as well as general guidelines such as the food guide pyramid, common conversions, and daily values (DVs) for nutrition labeling.

We wish to thank our outside reviewers for their invaluable assistance in working with us on this second edition. We also thank our many authors from both the first and this second edition. They were selected based on their expertise in their particular area(s) of pediatric nutrition practice. This second edition of *Handbook of Pediatric Nutrition* reflects their expertise and their dedication.

Part I

Normal Pediatric Nutrition and Growth

CHAPTER 1

Physical Growth and Development

William Cameron Chumlea and Shumei S. Guo

WHAT IS GROWTH?

Physical growth is the increase in the mass of body tissues as a child changes from an infant to an adult during most of the first two decades of life. This process is complicated because growth is not uniform. Different body tissues in a child grow and mature in set patterns but at different rates or chronologic ages. These differences are magnified among children of the same sex, between the sexes, and among children of different racial backgrounds. Adequate nutrition and exercise are important for the fulfillment of growth and maturation. Normal, healthy children will grow and mature with few, if any, problems. In the United States, however, we are faced with an epidemic of obesity, resulting from overnutrition that affects the growth, current health, and future health of children.[1,2] This chapter provides a general overview of the patterns of normal growth and development, the ages at which growth occurs, and how growth and maturation differ between boys and girls. The growth of the major body tissues, muscle, fat, and bone is discussed, along with how growth is assessed and described for individual children. There is also a brief discussion of the growth of children born with conditions that affect their growth.

HOW IS GROWTH MEASURED?

The most common growth measures of infants and children are recumbent length from birth to 3 years of age, stature after age 3 years, head circumference from birth to age 3 years (Figures 1–1, 1–2, 1–3), and weight at every age.[3] Recumbent length and stature describe the amount of linear growth, which is primarily due to growth of the skeleton. Weight is a measure of the growth in the mass of all body tissues. Weight and length or stature are important measures, but weight standardized for length or stature is descriptive of the level of leanness or adiposity. Recently, the body mass index (BMI) has been introduced as a descriptive measure of the degree of obesity for children and adults.[4] The BMI is calculated as weight divided by stature (or length) squared, with all measures in the metric system ($kg/m^2 \times 10{,}000$). Additional measures to consider in assessing the growth of children are trunk and limb circumference and the thickness of subcutaneous adipose tissue.

GENERAL PERIODS AND PATTERNS OF GROWTH

For convenience of discussion, the growth of a child is divided descriptively into four general periods: infancy—from birth to 2 years of age; the preschool years—from about 2 to 6 years of age; the middle childhood years—from about 7 to 10 years of age; and adolescence—from about 11 to 18 years of age. These growth periods describe differences in the pattern of growth that is occurring and differences in levels of maturation among children.

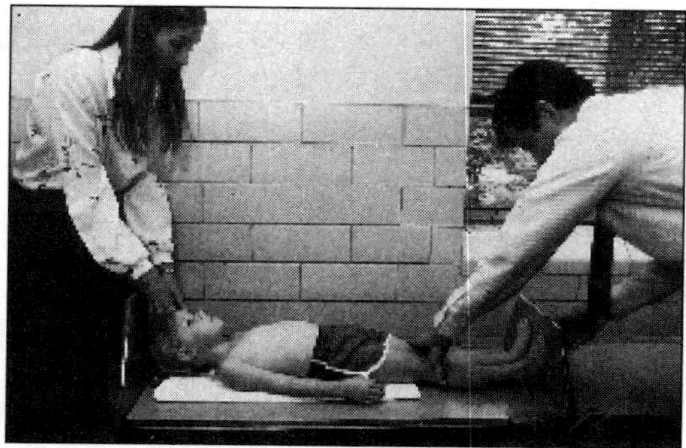

Figure 1-1 Measurement of recumbent length.

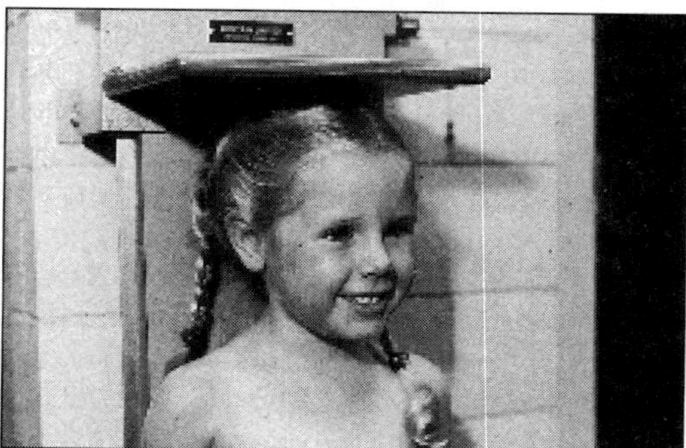

Figure 1-2 Measurement of stature.

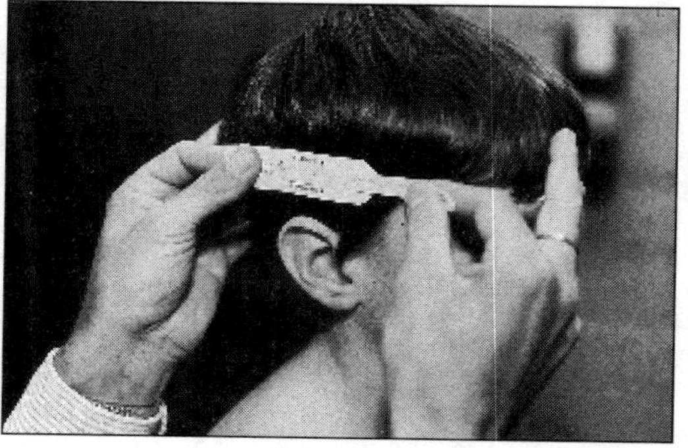

Figure 1-3 Measurement of head circumference.

During infancy, there is a large amount of growth as a child changes from a baby to a very active child. In the next two growth periods, most normal, healthy children grow at a rather steady pace. With adolescence and the onset of puberty, there is a final spurt in growth as a child's body matures into that of an adult. The age divisions of these periods are not distinct because each child is an individual, and there is a range of variation among children in their growth and maturation and the ages at which these occur. At any age, the size of a healthy, well-nourished child will reflect his or her own genetic growth potential, which is some combination of that of the parents. Stature has a strong genetic component, and it is easily recognized that tall parents tend to have tall children and short parents tend to have short children. Weight has a genetic component also and can be used to explain some aspects of obesity, but environmental effects can play a strong role in the development of obesity also. Our understanding of the genetics of growth and maturation will expand considerably over the next decade, as will the effects of nutrition and the environment on growth.

The size of a normal child at a given age is also related to the child's level of maturity. Early-maturing children tend to be taller and heavier than do late-maturing children, but the latter generally finish as taller adults. During the first two decades of life, children grow until they reach adult size, and their body tissues and systems progressively mature until they reach adult levels of function. This is the process of maturation, with maturity as its endpoint. In the body, maturation is a general but interrelated process. However, certain systems or tissues have been studied more closely than others because they provide more information about the level of maturity of a child, relative to that of other children.

Infancy: Birth to Age 2 Years

During the first weeks following birth, an infant adjusts to life on the outside. Numerous physiologic changes occur at birth, or shortly thereafter, to sustain this new life. For example, the lungs start to function, and the stomach and intestines have to process and digest the external food the infant now receives. The very rapid growth that occurred in utero almost stops just before birth, and many full-term infants will lose some weight shortly after birth. If all goes well, by 8–10 days after birth, these infants have regained their birth weight and are growing again.[5]

Infancy is a period of rapid growth in body size. Body dimensions increase at a greater rate than at any other time in postnatal life. Because an infant is small, these proportional increases are not always as obvious as during the adolescent growth spurt. In the first year of life, weight increases 200%, body length 55%, and head circumference 40%. Similar changes occur in the length and breadth of the trunk, arms, and legs. Similar increases and changes occur in body weight. Most normal infants double their birth weight by 5 months of age and triple it by the age of 1 year. Between 1 and 2 years of age, an average child grows about 12 cm in length and gains about 3.5 kg in weight.

Compared with the size of the body, an infant's head is disproportionately large at birth. The diameter of the skull is greater than that of the chest, and the length of the head is about a quarter of the body's total length. At birth, average head circumference is about 35 cm and increases about 12 cm during the first year to a value of about 47 cm. Measuring head circumference during this period is important because it reflects brain growth, and the brain doubles its birth weight by 1 year of age. Obviously, a faltering growth in head circumference can have serious implications for neural growth and maturation, or it could be diagnostic for possible problems of brain growth.

Preschool Years: 2 to 6 Years of Age

During the preschool years, the body's rate of growth slows from its high rate in infancy and stabilizes at a roughly constant rate by about 4–5 years of age. By the age of 4 years, the average annual increase in stature is only about 6–8 cm per year and about 2–4 kg per year in weight. Sex differences in stature and weight during the preschool years are slight, but the pattern of more adipose tissue in girls than boys appears in the values of mean skinfold measurements after the age of 2 years. These mean differences in adipose tissue thickness are distinct by 6 years of age. This period may also be a critical period for the development of increased risk for subsequent obesity later in childhood and adulthood. Children who tend to start their fat development earlier than other children are at an increased risk for obesity and should be monitored closely.[6]

Head circumference continues to be an important measure of growth during the preschool years. From 1 to 2 years of age, the head grows an average of about 5 cm in circumference, but by age 3, the mean annual increase is down to less than 1 cm. The brain more than triples its birth weight by 6 years of age. As in infancy, measurements of head circumference are important during the preschool years because a child with abnormal growth may have abnormal brain growth also. Infancy and the preschool years are the period of most rapid postnatal growth of the brain. The occurrence of adverse conditions at these ages will have the greatest effect on brain growth.

Middle Childhood: 7 to 10 Years of Age

Middle childhood is a period of continued steady growth in body size for most children. These children are also getting ready for the changes that will occur to their bodies during adolescence. On average, boys and girls grow about 5–6 cm per year in stature. Growth in weight of boys is about 2 kg at age 7 years but increases to an average rate of about 4 kg around 10 years of age. The average girl during this period grows slightly more per year in stature and weight than does the average boy, as a function of their increasing maturity over that of boys. This sex difference in growth rate contributes, in part, to the earlier appearance of significant sex differences in the size of girls at the onset of adolescence. At 7 years of age, boys are, on the average, about 2 cm taller than girls of the same age, but there is little difference in weight. By 10 years of age, the average girl is about 1 cm taller than the average boy and about 1 kg heavier. Sex differences in other body areas also start to appear during this period. A particular difference is seen in the thickness of adipose tissue on the body. By 10 years of age, the thickness of subcutaneous adipose tissue in girls is about 25% greater than that of boys at the same age. Middle childhood is also the start of a critical period for increased risk for the development of subsequent obesity in adulthood. Overweight children are at an increased risk for being obese as adults.[2]

The shape and proportions of the body start to change during this period, as a result of differential growth of the skeleton. For example, the legs have a greater rate of growth than does the trunk during middle childhood. The trunk accounts for about 55% of total stature at age 7 years but only about 45% at 10 years of age in White boys and girls. Black children have about the same amount of change in these body proportions as do White children, but in Black children the legs consistently account for about 2% more of the body's stature than in White children at the same ages. These racial and sexual group differences tend to persist throughout life.

Adolescence: 11 to 18 Years of Age

Adolescence is the final frontier before becoming an adult. This is not an easily defined period of life. Adolescence starts before puberty and spans the years until growth and maturation are mostly completed, which is around 16–18 years of age in girls and 18–20 years of age in boys. Puberty is an event. When the reproductive system matures and sexual reproduction becomes possible, puberty has taken place. Puberty is easily identified in girls by the onset of menstruation known as menarche, but there is no similar marker in boys. The average age at menarche for White girls in the United States is 13 years and 12 years for Black girls.

The sex differences in overall body size between girls and boys become larger between 10 and 14 years of age because girls have their growth spurt and reach puberty before boys. On the average, girls reach puberty about 2 years earlier than boys. Within each sex, however, there is a range of ages during which normal children may reach puberty. Normal girls may attain puberty as early as 7.5 years of age or as late as 14.5 years, with boys starting as early as 9.5 years or as late as 15 years of age. The time required for completion of physical and sexual maturity, ie, attainment of adult status, varies also. In general, children who start their pubescent development early pass through the stages quickly; children starting at a later age may take a longer period of time to reach maturity. As a result, late-maturing children have a longer time to grow.

The physical changes that transform a child's body into that of an adult are a final increase in body size and proportions, the development of secondary sex characteristics (growth of pubic hair, genitalia, and the breasts), and development of the ability to reproduce sexually. Between 11 and 14 years of age, most girls have their pubescent growth spurts and are taller than boys of the same age. These girls will also stop growing earlier than boys. Boys, on the average, do not enter their adolescent growth spurts until about 2 years after girls. As a result, boys have an additional 2 years of prepubertal growth in stature. In addition, the adolescent growth spurt lasts for a longer time in boys than in girls, and the amount of growth is larger. In boys, the average peak height velocity—the maximum rate of growth in stature during the adolescent growth spurt—ranges from 9.5 to 10.3 cm per year, though in girls the maximum velocity is 8.4—9.0 cm per year. These sex differences in growth help to produce the average larger body size in men than in women.

The physiologic progression of a child into adulthood is controlled by the central nervous system, which integrates the activities of the endocrine glands. An increase in hormone production from the pituitary, gonads, and adrenal cortex, together with changes in the sensitivity of neuroreceptors, initiate and guide the differentiation of a child's body into its adult form. During childhood, hormone levels are kept low by the active inhibition of the central nervous system. Toward the onset of puberty, there is a progressive decrease in the sensitivity of the inhibition of the nervous system to hormone levels, and the sex hormones appear in the blood in greater concentrations, reaching adult levels at puberty. Testosterone and estrogen influence sexual functions and general body growth and maturation. Boys and girls each produce testosterone and estrogen, but in significantly different amounts. Estrogen accelerates the closure of epiphyseal growth plates in bones and deposition of adipose tissue, but more so in adolescence than in childhood. Testosterone stimulates muscle growth, and, due to its higher levels in boys, more muscle or lean body mass is deposited, particularly during adolescence. Estrogen, testosterone, and several androgenic hormones are also responsible for development of secondary sex characteristics. All hormones must operate together to ensure orderly, coordinated growth of the skeleton, muscles, and internal organs during childhood and adolescence. However, the ages of individual children at the onset and completion of sexual maturation are highly variable.

In boys, the first sign of puberty is enlargement of the testes and scrotum. About a year later, the penis starts to grow, just after the onset of the increased rate of growth in stature. Pubic hair appears shortly after the start of testicular growth. The adult male pattern of pubic hair distribution extends from the genitalia onto the thighs. About 2 years after the appearance of pubic hair, pigmented and coarse hair becomes visible on the face, and axillary hair develops in the armpits. The amount and distribution of hair on the rest of the male body is genetically determined.

Breast buds are the first hint of approaching puberty in young girls. With the beginning of breast development, the uterus and vagina also start to grow. A girl will generally start to menstruate about 2 years after her breasts and uterus start to grow. Pubic hair generally appears in girls with the onset of breast development, although pubic hair may develop before the breasts begin to mature. The distribution of pubic hair on a girl's body is more limited than in boys.

The rate of sexual maturation differs within and between the sexes. For example, two girls of the same chronologic age may have different rates of sexual maturation, and several similar rating systems have been developed to group children into levels of sexual maturity. Most adolescent events, such as attainment of peak height velocity (most rapid growth in stature) or the appearance of pubic hair or its development, occur in girls about a year or two before they occur in boys. However, the time difference between the sexes for mean ages of stages of maturity may be as short as half of a year.

Body size and proportions change as a result of skeletal and muscular growth and differences in the amount and distribution of subcutaneous adipose tissue. During adolescence, boys develop more muscle tissue than do girls, but girls add more total body fat than do boys. Throughout adolescence, secondary sex characteristics (growth of the penis and testicles in boys, breast development in girls, and pubic hair for both) are developing simultaneously with sexual maturation. Concurrent with all this change is an increase in physical ability and performance, though, again, not as much for the average girl as for the average boy.[7]

GROWTH OF BODY TISSUES

Muscle, adipose tissue, and bone are the primary body tissues that change the most during growth. These tissues can now be quantified to provide an estimate of lean body mass and total body fat and bone mineral, but children and adults are continuing to increase in weight. There is a variety of methods for measuring body composition from skinfolds to body density or underwater weighing. Dual energy x-ray absorptiometry (DXA) is the easiest method of measuring the total body composition of most children, even as young as infants. There is a growing amount of literature on the body composition of children that did not exist 10 years ago. Marked and significant changes and sex differences in body composition can be distinguished during growth.[8]

GROWTH OF LEAN BODY MASS

Lean body mass is the metabolically active protoplasm of the body, which is primarily muscle tissue, the internal organs, and the skeleton. Lean body mass cannot avoid containing a small amount of structural fat. Growth in lean body mass is primarily due to an increase in muscle mass. Muscle tissue is the largest single tissue component of the body. At birth, 25% of the body's weight is muscle, but at adulthood, muscle mass accounts for about 50% of the body's weight. The major constituent of muscle tissue is body water. Lean body mass is positively associated with stature; ie, a tall child has a greater amount of lean body mass than does a shorter child at the same level of maturity. Lean body mass increases at a similar rate in boys and girls during childhood and is roughly equal between them until about 13–14 years of age. The lean body mass of girls continues to grow into adolescence, but stops around 15 years of age (see Figure 1–4). The lean body mass of boys starts to increase very rapidly after 13 years of

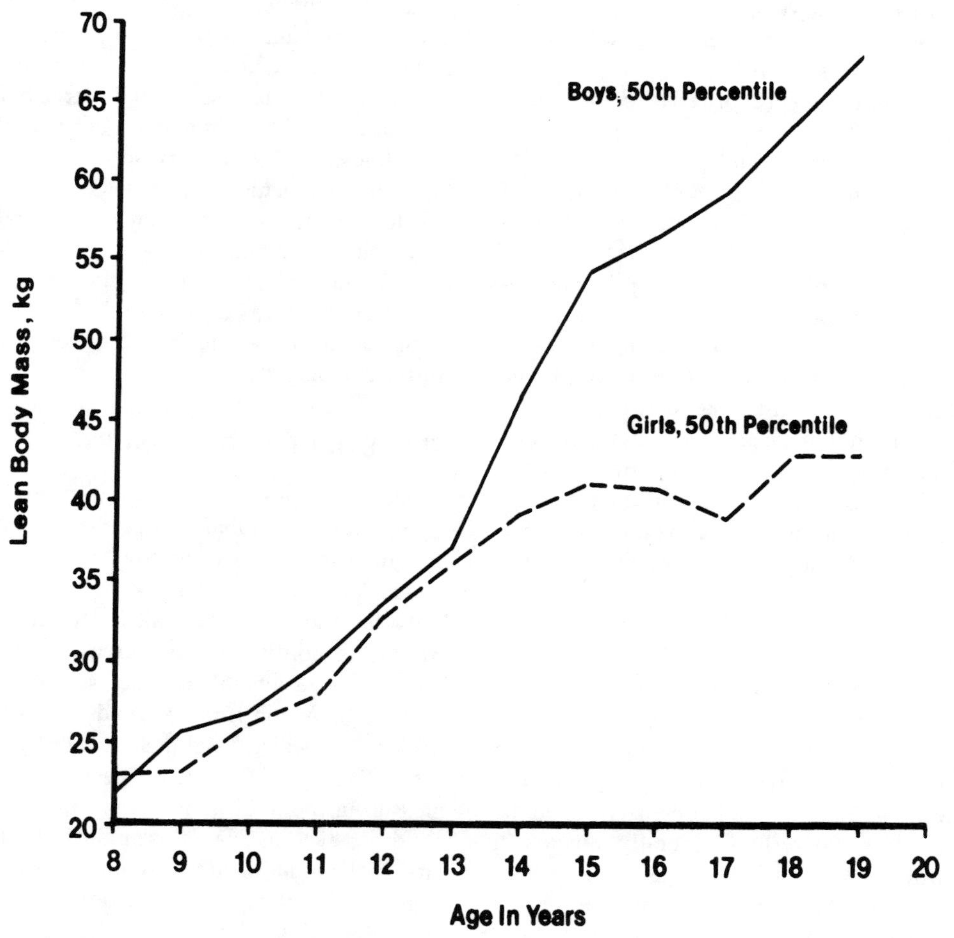

Figure 1-4 Changes in the 50th percentiles of lean body mass (LBM) in boys and girls. *Source:* Forbes GB, Body composition in adolescence, in *Human Growth,* Vol 2 by F Falkner and JM Tanner (eds), 1986, Plenum Press.

age and reaches a maximum rate of increase late in adolescence. The total period of growth in the lean body mass of boys is about twice as long as the same period for girls, and, as a result, lean body mass in boys is several times greater than that of girls. This greater muscle mass in boys is located primarily in the shoulders and arms of the upper body. After puberty, boys have greater absolute amounts of lean body mass than do girls, irrespective of stature.

GROWTH OF TOTAL BODY FAT

Body fat has two important functions: to store energy as adipose tissue and to act as a structural component in cell membranes. Storage fat is primarily subcutaneous adipose tissue, which contains the majority of the body's fat. The remaining adipose tissue is deposited around internal organs and visceral parts of the body. This internal adipose tissue cannot be measured easily. The development of excessive internal adipose tissue occurs predominantly in adulthood. There is significant growth in the adipose tissue of boys and girls. This growth occurs primarily in the subcutaneous or storage compartments of the body. The vast majority of total body fat in children, even among obese children, is subcutaneous. In fact, for American children, the growth in adipose tissue has become an epidemic. Over the past several decades, there has been an increase in the prevalence of obesity for the U.S. population, including children of all ages.[4] Obese children have always been at an increased risk for obesity in adulthood, along with the numerous associated adult health risks, especially diabetes and cardiovascular-related diseases. However, not only are more children obese today than in the past, but they are at greater levels of obesity than were children 10–20 years ago. As a result of this increased obesity and the degree of obesity, many obese children are presenting signs of cardiovascular disease such as hyperlipidemia and athersclerotic plaques, that one would expect to find only in adults.

The distribution and amount of subcutaneous adipose tissue are sex-specific. Girls have significantly more subcutaneous adipose tissue than do boys, and this difference becomes considerable during adolescence. Differences in amounts of adipose tissue between boys and girls reflect actual differences in body composition and are not an artifact of the earlier maturation of girls. Boys and girls also vary in the deposition and patterning of subcutaneous adipose tissue on the arms, legs, and trunk (see Figure1–5). Both sexes deposit adipose tissue on the torso during childhood and adolescence, but in adolescent girls, additional adipose tissue is added to breasts, buttocks, thighs, and across the back of the arms (see Figure 1–6). This additional adipose tissue accentuates the adult sex differences in body shape.

The adipose tissue thickness on the arms and legs of boys increases during childhood but decreases after about 13 years of age because the underlying muscle is growing at a greater rate at this time. During the adolescent growth spurt of boys, muscle grows more rapidly than the fat, causing the subcutaneous adipose tissue on the extremities to be stretched thinner. This differential tissue growth accounts for the fall in the skinfold thickness measures of subcutaneous adipose tissue on the arms and legs. A decreasing triceps skinfold measure in boys may not indicate a loss of body fat as the thickness of subcutaneous adipose tissue at the subscapular location on the trunk continues to increase in most boys during this time. Similar measures on girls show a continuous increase in adipose tissue thickness, with a marked increase after 12 years of age. For girls, adipose tissue grows about as rapidly as do muscle and bone, and this allows an increase to occur in skinfold measures of subcutaneous adipose tissue on the arms and legs.

SKELETAL GROWTH

There are three basic types of bones in the skeleton: long, round or irregular, and flat bones. Long bones are in the arms and legs, and round or irregular bones are the carpals in the wrist, tarsals in the ankle, and the vertebrae. Flat bones

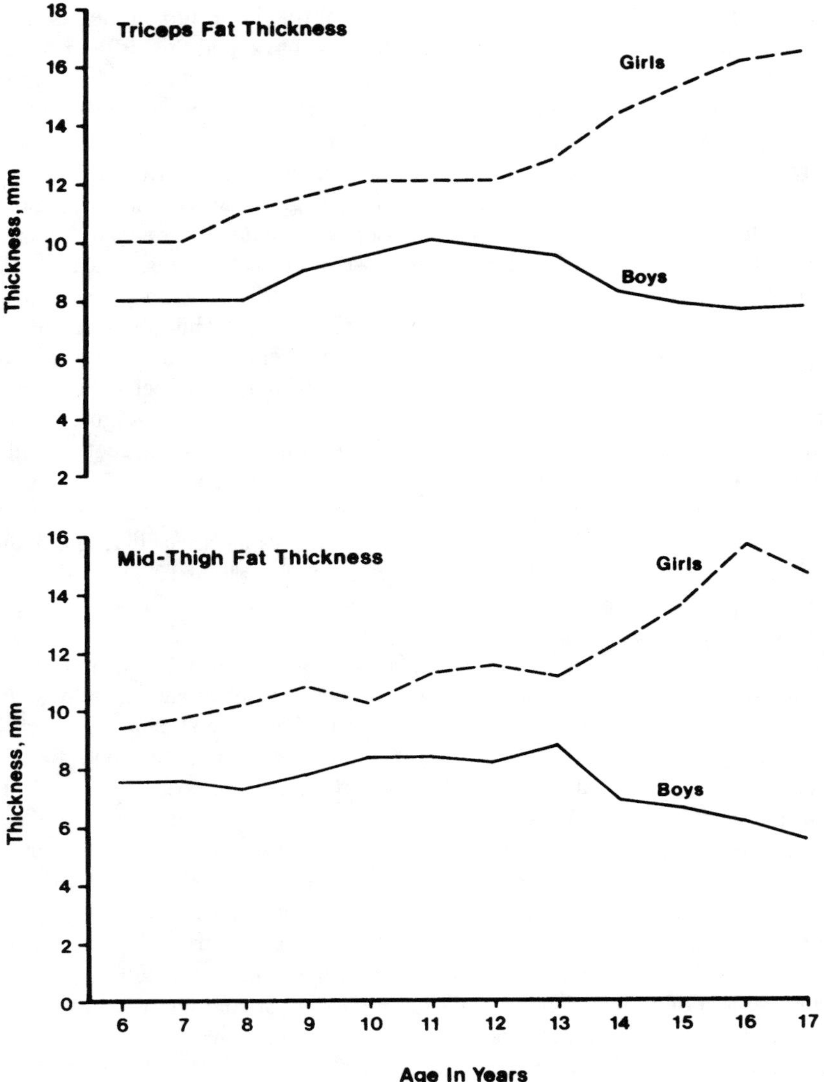

Figure 1-5 Skinfold thickness from the trunk of boys and girls. *Source:* Johnston FE, Hamill PVV and Lemeshow S, *Skinfold Thickness of Children 6–11 Years* and *Skinfold Thickness of Youths 12–17 Years,* USPHS Pub Nos 120 and 132, 1972, 1974.

---

are found mainly in the vault of the skull and the pelvis.

The long bones of the legs and the vertebrae are the major locations of growth in stature. Bone growth is rather steady during the adolescent growth spurt, but late in adolescence, bone growth slows. By about 18 years of age for girls and around 20–22 years of age for boys, the epiphyses or growth plates at the ends of most long bones have fused to the shaft or diaphysis. The

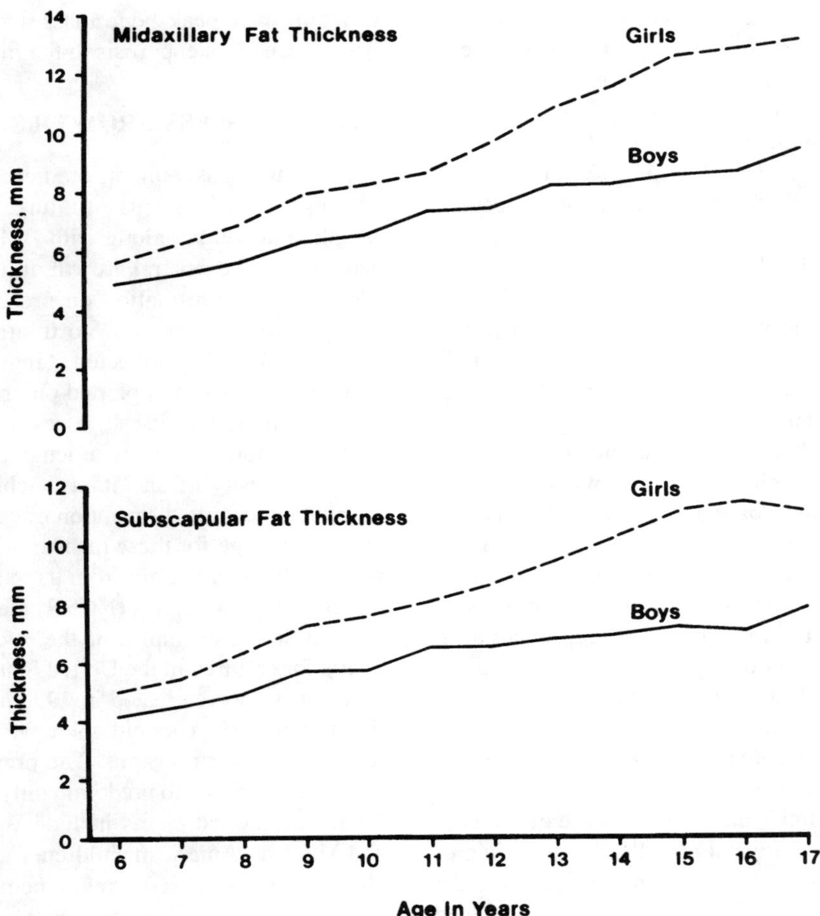

Figure 1-6 Skinfold and fat thicknesses (x-ray) on the arms and legs (respectively) of boys and girls. *Source:* Johnston FE, Hamill PVV and Lemeshow S, *Skinfold Thickness of Youths 12–17 Years,* USPHS Pub No 132, 1974.

cartilage of the growth plates where growth in bone length occurs, has been replaced by bone, which prevents any further elongation.

Skeletal growth is a continuous process, and repeated assessment of the levels of skeletal maturation known as *skeletal age* can help monitor this growth and provide an index of a child's biologic age. Two children of the same chronologic age may have different levels of skeletal maturation, or skeletal ages, just as they may also have different rates of muscle growth, weight gain, and sexual maturation. Skeletal age is highly correlated with aspects of physical and sexual maturation. For example, a child who is more mature sexually than another will generally have a more advanced skeletal age, although both children may have the same chronologic age. Skeletal maturation can be assessed by the degree to which the growth plates or epiphyses have fused. Many parts of the skeleton can be used to estimate skeletal age, but the most commonly used areas are the hand-wrist and knee.

The hand-wrist has a long history in the study of skeletal maturation, even predating the use of radiography. However, the use of the knee in assessing skeletal maturity is important because it is a major site for growth in stature. Several of the techniques for assessing skeletal age are sample-specific and require training for accurate use.

Bones in the skeleton do not grow at the same uniform rate, but their growth is coordinated. Growth of the vault of the skull is, in part, a function of the growth of the nervous system. By about 7 years of age, the skull, like the average brain, has completed approximately 95% of its growth. The bones of the vault of the skull do not experience a rapid period of growth during adolescence, but the base of the skull and the jaw, or lower face, have a growth spurt during adolescence. Differential growth of bones in the skeleton also contributes, in part, to changes in body proportions between the sexes, eg, longer arms and broader shoulders in boys than in girls. Bones start or stop growing at different ages, depending on their location. For example, at a given age, the hand is nearer its adult length than is the upper arm.

The skeleton is the body's reserve of calcium. One aspect of skeletal growth is the building of this calcium reserve. The importance here for children is that those girls and boys who end growth with a low calcium reserve are at an increased risk for developing osteoporosis. Peak bone mass is the maximum mineral mass attained by the skeleton. This peak occurs at some time in the third decade of life, but by maturity, the majority of peak bone mass has been reached. In the past, it was impossible to measure the amount of calcium in the bones of children or the density of their bones. With the widespread availability of DXA, this is now possible, and limited reference data for bone mineral content and density are now available for children at many ages. These data and the use of DXA, along with calcium supplementation, provide mechanisms for monitoring the growth of the skeleton and its calcium content. This information may help children with low calcium intakes to attain their peak bone mass and reduce the prevalence of osteoporosis in the future.

HOW TO ASSESS GROWTH STATUS

Accurate measurements are necessary for assessing growth status. Stature, recumbent length, and weight, along with BMI, are representative of the general growth of the body, and they provide information on present status or any progress or response to treatment. These measures should be collected at regularly scheduled age intervals and plotted on growth charts. Growth charts provide an assessment or comparison of how the stature or length, weight, and level of obesity of an infant or child compare with the percentile distribution of other children at the same age for these measures. The correct growth charts to use are from the National Center for Health Statistics (NCHS) (see Appendix M). These are examples of the revised growth charts for children in the United States. The previous charts were created in 1977 and, in addition to being 20 years old, there were numerous reasons for their revisions. The previous charts had been restricted to predominantly White children. The revised charts include White, Black, and Mexican-American children. In revising the charts, the increased prevalence of obesity among American children was recognized, and recently, obese children were excluded from the construction of the new growth charts. The inclusion of obese children would have inflated the levels of the growth curves and made it difficult to identify obese children. These charts do not reflect the current obese state of American children, so that obese children plotted on the charts still will appear as obese.

There are significant group differences in growth among Black, White, and Mexican-American children. These differences tend to be more obvious at the extremes. There are also some group differences in the growth of Chinese- or Japanese-American children or American children of other racial or ethnic groups, compared with that of White, Black, or Mexican-American children. The available national growth data from NCHS does not allow the construction of race- or ethnic-specific growth charts. The sample sizes of these different groups of children, although several hundred in number, are too small for the construction of adequate percentile growth charts from birth to 20 years of age. It is recommended that the growth of children in the United States be plotted on the revised growth charts. If a child is healthy, he or she should track along the percentile lines on the charts. The child's position on the chart, however, will be displaced as a function of the difference in his or her genetic background and that of the children used to construct the charts.

Most normal children living in an adequate environment will maintain a level of growth from 1 year of age to the next, relative to that of other children at the same chronologic age. For example, a child whose stature is at the 75th percentile at age 6 years will have a stature at approximately the same percentile at age 12 years and again at age 16 years. However, the growth of a child can be irregular and still be considered normal, due to differences in the rate of growth and maturation that can occur among children at the same chronologic age. Significant deviations in a child's growth, however, may be due to sickness or over- or undernutrition. Another growth characteristic in the United States has been that each generation of children was taller as adults than the previous generation. In the United States, this secular trend in height has stopped for the majority of children, but children and adults are continuing to increase in weight. For children of some ethnic groups who are recent immigrants, the trend in height may still appear, as it will for weight.

For premature infants or infants who are small at birth, it is important to account for their gestational age in plotting their growth data. This is done by subtracting the amount of prematurity from the infant's chronologic age. For a child with a gestational age of 28 weeks, this is a difference of 3 months. After about 2.5 years of age, it is generally no longer necessary to make an adjustment for gestational age for most premature children who are healthy. This is because the difference in body measurement values is less than the error for the measurements. Also, there are charts now available for plotting the growth of preterm low-birthweight infants.[9] These charts include measures of weight, recumbent length, and head circumference (see Appendix A).

GROWTH VELOCITY

If growth is measured at repeated visits, the amount of change in a pair of measurements or increments in stature, length, weight, and head circumference from one visit to the next can be quantified. This information provides an additional perspective on the growth of a child. Growth velocity can be used to measure a child's response to nutritional intervention. Plots of increments are records of the velocity or the rate of growth per unit of time. Increment growth charts are available for boys and girls.[10] For children aged 3 years and younger, there are increment charts for weight, recumbent length, and head circumference; for older children there are charts for stature and weight. Use of the increment charts helps to determine whether a child's rate of growth is unusual by comparison with that of other normal American children at the same ages.

The increment charts are distributions of growth increments from a group of healthy children, but there is no proof that children represented at the median (50th percentile) are healthier than other children at other percentiles at the same or other ages. These charts should be used to supplement the revised growth charts in which attained size is plotted relative to chronologic age. The primary purpose of both these types of charts is to help identify children in need of further investigation or treatment and to monitor the results of such treatment (see Appendix B).

Subcutaneous adipose tissue can be measured at a variety of sites as the thickness of a skinfold. One of the most common sites for measuring a skinfold is on the back of the arm over the triceps muscle, and another possible location is just below the scapula. The triceps and subscapular skinfolds are highly correlated with total body fatness. Measuring skinfolds on an infant can be a problem because it is sometimes difficult to get a good separation of subcutaneous adipose tissue from the muscle tissue. Reference data are available for skinfold thickness of White, Black, and Hispanic children older than 2 months of age from NCHS. There are also charts for plotting measures of triceps, subscapular skinfold thicknesses, and midarm circumference.[5] These charts use data from the first National Health and Nutrition Examination Survey (NHANES I). These charts are from 2 to 18 years of age, with separate charts for boys and girls. There are race differences in the thickness of subcutaneous adipose tissue among Whites, Blacks, and Hispanics. These differences are most significant at extreme percentile values, so these charts can be used for White, Black, and Hispanic children (see Appendix H).

SPECIAL CHILDREN

A difficult problem is assessing the growth status of children with "problems," eg, Down syndrome, cerebral palsy, contractures, braces, mental retardation, etc. Because of the heterogeneity of these conditions among children, there is limited recommended standard methodology and limited or no specific reference data.[11] If the child can stand, possibly standard methods can be used. If the child is nonambulatory, one can attempt to use recumbent methods. The reference data from the NCHS needs to be interpolated, depending on the condition of the child in question.

Two major problems to face in making a growth assessment of a handicapped child are how to make maximum use of the information collected and how to keep errors of measurement to a minimum. For example, one measurement is probably not going to be sufficient. It may be necessary to take several measurements, especially the more difficult the measurement or the more uncooperative the child. For children with some specific conditions such as trisomy 21 (Down syndrome), there are available growth charts (see Appendix C).[12] For other groups of children, such as those with cerebral palsy, growth charts are being developed (see Chapter 14).

CONCLUSIONS

Childhood is a period of steady growth for the body, without significant changes. In adolescence, a child copes with his or her body as it grows, enlarges, changes shape, and matures from what he or she had grown accustomed to over the past 12 or so years. This new body is similar but with different and exciting capabilities and functions. Unfortunately, these changes may not be readily accepted as fact for several years. The emotional upheavals of puberty and adolescence for an individual, his or her family, and society might be avoided if growth and its changes were drawn out over a longer period of time. However, the ability to procreate necessitates the ability to carry a fetus to term and then to provide child care afterward. Thus, the adult body must follow shortly on the heels of sexual maturity.

REFERENCES

1. Troiano RP, Flegal KM, Kuczmarski RJ, Campbell SM, Johnson CL. Overweight prevalence and trends for children and adolescents. *Arch Pediatr Adolesc Med.* 1995;149:1085–1091.
2. Guo SS, Chumlea WC, Roche AF, Siervogel RM, Gardner JD. The predictive value of childhood body mass index values for overweight at 35 years. *Am J Clin Nutr.* 1994;59:810–819.
3. Lohman TG, Roche AF, Martorell R, eds. *Anthropometric Standardization Reference Manual.* Champaign, IL: Human Kinetics Publishers; 1988.
4. Wickelgren I. Obesity: How big a problem? *Science.* 1998;280:1364–1367.
5. Moore WM, Roche AF. *Pediatric Anthropometry*, 3rd ed. Columbus, OH: Ross Laboratories; 1987.
6. Whitaker RC, Wright JA, Pepe MS, Seidel KD, Dietz WH. Predicting obesity in young adulthood from childhood and parental obesity. *N Engl J Med.* 1997;337: 869–873.

7. Beunen G. Muscular strength development in children and adolescents. In: Froberg K, Lammert, O, Hansen, H, Blimkie, CJR, eds. *Exercise and Fitness-Benefits and Risks*. Denmark: Odense University Press; 1997:192–207.
8. Guo S, Chumlea WC, Roche AF, Siervogel RM. Age- and maturity-related changes in body composition during adolescence into adulthood: The Fels Longitudinal Study. *Int J Obesity*. 1997;21:1167–1175.
9. Guo SS, Roche AF, Chumlea WC, Casey PH, Moore WM. Growth in weight, recumbent length, and head circumference for preterm low-birthweight infants during the first three years of life using gestation-adjusted ages. *Early Hum Dev*. 1997;47:305–325.
10. Roche AF, Himes JH. Incremental growth charts. *Am J Clin Nutr*. 1980;33:2041–2052.
11. Stevenson RD, Hayes RP, Cater LV, Blackman JA. Clinical correlates of linear growth in children with cerebral palsy. *Dev Med Child Neurol*. 1994; 36:135–142.
12. Cronk C, Crocker AC, Pueschel SM, Shea AM, Zackai E, Pickens G, et al. Growth charts for children with Down Syndrome: 1 month to 18 years of age. *Pediatrics*. 1988;81:102–110.

SUGGESTED READING

Behnke AR, Wilmore JH. *Evaluation and Regulation of Body Build and Composition*. Englewood Cliffs, NJ: Prentice-Hall; 1974.

Falkner F, Tanner JM, eds. *Human Growth*. Vol. 2. New York: Plenum Press; 1986.

Hamill PVV, Johnson CL, Reed RB, Drizd TA, Roche AF. *NCHS Growth Curves for Children Birth-18 Years*. US Public Health Service No. 165. Washington, DC: US Government Printing Office; 1977.

Johnston FE, Hamill PVV, Lemeshow S. *Skinfold Thickness of Children 6–11 Years*. US Public Health Service No. 120. Washington, DC: US Government Printing Office; 1972.

Johnston FE, Hamill PVV, Lemeshow S. *Skinfold Thickness of Youths 12–17 Years*. US Public Health Service No. 132. Washington, DC: US Government Printing Office; 1974.

MacMahon B. *Age at Menarche*. US Public Health Service No. 133. Washington, DC: US Government Printing Office; 1973.

Malina RM, Bouchard C. *Growth, Maturation, and Physical Activity*. Champaign, IL: Human Kinetics Books; 1991.

Malina RM, Hamill PVV, Lemeshow S. *Body Dimensions and Proportions, White and Negro Children 6–11 Years*. US Public Health Service No. 143. Washington, DC: Government Printing Office; 1974.

Reynolds EL. The distribution of subcutaneous fat in childhood and adolescence. *Monogr Soc Res Child Dev*. 1951;15.

Reynolds EL, Wines JF. Physical changes associated with adolescence in boys. *Am J Dis Child*. 1951;82:529.

Roche AF, Chumlea WC, Thissen D. *Assessing Skeletal Maturity of the Hand-Wrist: Fels Method*. Springfield, IL: Charles C Thomas; 1988.

Roche AF. *Growth, Maturation and Body Composition. The Fels Longitudinal Study 1929–1991*. Cambridge, England: Cambridge University Press; 1992.

Sinclair D. *Human Growth after Birth*. London: Oxford University Press; 1978.

Tanner JM. *Growth at Adolescence*. Oxford, England: Blackwell Publishers; 1962.

Chapter 2

Nutritional Assessment

Susan Bessler

Increased awareness of the role of nutrition in health maintenance, recognition of malnutrition among the United States population, and improved nutrition support technology have resulted in major changes in both the availability and the delivery of nutritional care. Today, the assessment of nutritional status has become an integral component of pediatric health care. The accurate collection and interpretation of nutritional assessment data are instrumental in providing quality care. The assessment identifies nutritionally depleted or at-risk infants and children, provides essential information for developing achievable nutritional care plans, and serves as a mechanism for evaluating the effectiveness of nutritional care.

SCREENING

The completion of in-depth nutritional assessments on all children served by a health care system is neither practical nor essential for providing quality nutrition care. Well-designed nutritional screening performed by trained personnel is effective in identifying children who are at an elevated nutritional risk and, therefore, may require a more comprehensive nutritional assessment.[1–5] Nutritional screenings can also function to predict outcome in specific diagnoses.[6] The information gathered for screening includes indices of nutritional status routinely collected during scheduled health care appointments or upon admission to a health care facility.[7,8]

Nutritional screening protocols must be adapted to the needs of the specific population served, staff and facility resources, and imposed credentialing requirements.[9] The participation of administrative, medical staff, nursing staff, and often family members is essential in developing a nutritional screening program. Since the measurement and documentation of many of the parameters involve nonnutrition personnel and equipment, the success of the program depends on the coordinated efforts of the multidisciplinary team in completing assigned responsibilities.[1,10]

Key issues to be resolved when planning a nutritional screening program include designation of team member responsibilities, selection of nutritional parameters to be screened, timing of the screening, and determination of how the data will be analyzed and the intended action once the data has been evaluated. In the hospital setting, a dietetic technician may collect the selected data by interview and from the patient's medical record, whereas a clinic or extended care facility may have nursing complete nutritional screening. Family-administered screening instruments that have the child's primary caretaker report data have been developed for use in the community setting.[11] Most pediatric nutrition screening tools routinely include age, weight, length or height, and head circumference. Information about the child's medical history, as well as diet and feeding ability, are also routinely queried. The routine collection of lab values depends on the needs of the population and the laboratory support available. Once the nutritional data have been obtained, the child is assessed for nutritional risk, and the appropriate referral or action plan is made. Exhibit 2–1 is an example of a hospital screening form that weighs the criteria and dictates the next appropriate step in the care plan. Other systems have all nutritional screening reviewed by registered dietitians for determination of nutritional risk.[2] The nutrition screening process generally takes place at or soon after a clinic visit or hospital admission. Additionally, extended care facilities and hospitals with long-term patients may perform periodic rescreening to monitor changes in nutritional risk status.[12]

NUTRITIONAL ASSESSMENT

The assessment of a child's nutritional status is based on pertinent information collected from the medical history, anthropometric data, laboratory data, physical findings, and dietary interview. The forthcoming indices vary in time, invasiveness, and expense. Based on the patient and clinical setting, the practitioner should weigh the cost of the assessment tool with its potential benefit.

Medical History

Approximately 10–15% of children in the United States have special health care needs, defined as "having, or being at risk for congenital or acquired conditions that affect physical and/or cognitive growth and development."[13] These children may be at risk for associated nutrition sequelae (see Table 2–1). A child's medical history should further include a review of social history, growth, acute or chronic illnesses, history of preexisting nutrient deficiencies, history of surgical or diagnostic procedures, and history of relevant therapies, such as chemotherapy or radiation.[14] Medications should be reviewed for potential drug-nutrient interactions.

Growth Data

Weight, Height, and Head Circumference

Age-appropriate growth is the hallmark of adequate nutrition. Monitoring growth through measurement of weight, length or height, and head circumference (in children 3 years of age or less) is a routine practice in most pediatric health care systems. These data are plotted on growth charts according to age for comparison with growth of a reference population of healthy, normal infants and children (see Chapter 1 and Appendix M).

Upper Arm and Skinfold Measurements

Upper arm measurements and skinfold measurements (which include those on the triceps, biceps, subscapular, and abdomen) are used to predict and monitor body fat and muscle stores, clarify other anthropometric findings, and, in some settings, predict morbidity and mortality.[15]

The upper arm measurements most commonly evaluated include triceps skinfold (TSF), midarm circumference (MAC), and midarm muscle circumference (MAMC). The TSF measurements are taken at the midpoint between the acromion and olecranon in the midline on the posterior aspect of the right upper arm. A double fold of the skin and underlying subcutaneous tissue parallel to the longitudinal axis of the arm is measured. The standard position has the child sitting or standing with the arm extended along the trunk. The MAC measurement is taken at the midpoint between the acromion and olecranon of the right arm and recorded in centimeters to the nearest 0.1 cm. MAMC is calculated using the following equation.

$$\text{MAMC(cm)} = \text{MAC(cm)} - (.314 \times \text{TSF(mm)})$$

MAMC can be more simply determined using the nomogram in Appendix G.

Exhibit 2–1 Nutrition Screening Profile

Children's Hospital Oakland

NUTRITION SCREENING PROFILE

CATEGORY		POINTS
ADMITTING DIAGNOSIS		______
Group 1 (8 points)	Group 2 (4 points)	
Burns ≥ 20%, Eating disorders	Anemia, BPD, Burns < 20%	
DM(new), FTT, Immunodeficiency,	CP, Cranial-Facial Surgery,	
Inborn Errors of Metabolism	CHD, DM(f/u), GE Reflux,	
Inflammatory Bowel Disease, CF	Malabsorption, Liver Disease	
Short Bowel Syndrome,	Pregnancy, Renal Disease	
Malnutrition, Nutritional Rickets	Oncologic Disease	
DIET ORDER		______
TPN, Tube Feeding or *NPO/CL >3 Days	(8 points)	
Modified/ Special Diet	(3 points)	
Food Allergies	(1 point)	
Mechanical Feeding Problems	(1 point)	
ANTHROPOMETRICS wt: kg %, ht:	cm %	______
wt/ht: %, HC:	cm %	
wt, ht, wt : ht ≤ 5% (NCHS Percentiles)	(5 points)	
wt : ht ≥ 95% (NCHS Percentiles)	(0 points)**	
Recent wt loss / gain ≥ 10% BW	(5 points)	
Recent wt loss / gain ≥ 5 % BW	(2 points)	
wt% & ht% disparity > 2 percentile bands	(2 points)	
HC < 5%	(1 point)	
LABORATORY STUDIES Hgb: g/dl (nl=	)	______
Hgb 3 g/dl less than normal	(1 point)	
Albumin ≤ 3 g/dl	(3 points)	
ADDITIONAL INFORMATION		______
Age ≤ 2 years old	(1 point)	
Diarrhea or Emesis > 5 days	(3 points)	
	TOTAL POINTS	______

CONCLUSION

______ PRIORITY #1 (8 or more points) Patient at high nutritional risk.
NUTRITION INTERVENTION RECOMMENDED

______ PRIORITY #2 (5 to 7 points) Patient at some nutritional risk.
Registered Dietitian to monitor nutritional status.

______ PRIORITY #3 (0 to 4 points) Patient at low nutritional risk.
Dietetic Technician to monitor nutritional status.

* ______ Recheck in 2 days.
** ______ Consider outpatient nutrition clinic for weight counselling

______________________, DT; Date: ______

______________________, RD: Date: ______

8345-019 (10/94)

White: Patient's Medical Record Pink: Nutrition Care Record

Source: Courtesy of the Clinical Nutrition Service, Children's Hospital Oakland, Oakland, California.

Table 2–1 Examples of Nutritional Risk Factors associated with Selected Disorders

	Growth			*Diet*			*Medical*	
	Under-weight	*Over-weight*	*Short Stature*	*Low Energy Needs*	*High Energy Needs*	*Feeding Problems*	*Constipation*	*Chronic Medications*
Autism	✓[a]					✓		✓
Bronchopulmonary dysplasia	✓				✓			✓
Cerebral palsy	✓	✓	✓	✓	✓	✓	✓	✓
Cystic fibrosis	✓		✓		✓			
Down syndrome		✓		✓		✓		
Fetal alcohol syndrome	✓		✓					
Heart disease (congenital)	✓				✓			
HIV/AIDS[b]	✓				✓			✓
Prader-Willi syndrome		✓	✓	✓				
Premature birth	✓		✓		✓	✓		
Seizure disorder								✓
Spina bifida	✓	✓	✓	✓			✓	

[a] May be present
[b] HIV = human immunodeficiency virus; AIDS = acquired immunodeficiency syndrome

Source: M.T. Baer and A.B. Harris: Pediatric Nutrition Assessment: Identifying Children at Risk. Copyright The American Dietetic Association. Reprinted by permission from *JOURNAL OF THE AMERICAN DIETETIC ASSOCIATION*, Vol. 97, (suppl 2): S107–S115, 1997.

Midarm area (A), midarm muscle area (M), and midarm fat area (F) are less commonly referenced but are thought to show greater changes with age than do diameter or circumference.[16] They are calculated by the following equations.

$$A=(\Pi/4 \times MAC/\Pi)^2$$

$$M=(MAC-\Pi\ (TSF)^2/4\Pi$$

$$F=A-M$$

The standards most commonly used for ages 1–75 years are those revised by Frisancho et al.,[16] based on data from the National Health and Nutritional Examination Survey (NHANES I) (Appendix H).[17] Standards for children under 1 year of age have been published, based on data from American[18] and British children.[19,20] Oakley et al.'s standards for children at 37–42 weeks gestation are based on both age and weight.[21] Triceps, biceps, subscapular, and abdominal measurements from a population of preterm infants at 24–42 weeks gestation data have been determined.[22]

Along with comparison to reference standards, skinfold measurements can be checked and monitored using a child as his or her own control. This can provide qualitative information regarding individual changes in body composition (eg, during rapid weight loss or weight gain).

Though useful, these measurements are not without their limitations. Caution must be used in comparing a child to the reference data. The data published by Frisancho et al.[16] include measurements for a solely Caucasian population and, therefore, use with other ethnic populations that may have different body compositions [23–26] may be erroneous. Even within the same reference population (ie, ethnicity), mean body composition measurements can change over time.[19] Accurate skinfold measurements require both precise instruments that require checking and calibration frequently and trained anthropometrists. Therefore, even under favorable conditions, varying compressibility of fat may make these measurements challenging to obtain and reproduce,[27] especially in an obese or active child.

Body Mass Index

The body-mass index (BMI), also known as the *Quetelet Index,*[28] is derived from dividing weight in kilograms by height in meters squared (wt/ht^2). For example, the BMI of a 14-year-old female who is 5'1" and 110 lb is $50/(1.54)^2$ or 21. Standardized percentile curves have been developed based on children from the United States[29,30], as well as for children from China,[31] Great Britain,[32] Italy,[33] India,[34] Vietnam,[35] Sweden,[36] and Brazil.[37] Based on the NHANES I data,[17] mean BMI decreases from age 1 year to age 4–6 years, at which point it increases. There is some evidence that children who rebound from this trough at earlier ages are at a higher risk for obesity later in life.[38] In adults, the BMI is considered a reliable and valid measurement of adiposity.[39] An expert committee has suggested that BMI be used as a screening criterion for overweight in adolescents, with overweight defined as BMI equal to or in excess of the 90th percentile or greater than 30kg/m^2, whichever is smaller.[40] As of yet, no such criterion exists for younger children. Though BMI is strongly associated with total body fat (TBF) and, to a lesser extent, percentage body fat (PBF),[41–43] individual children with similar BMI may have very different TBF and PBF.[41] Additionally, BMI may underpredict the prevalence of excess adiposity in children with disease states.[42] Therefore, whereas BMI allows a quick and simple method for obesity screening in the normal population, caution should be used in employing a single BMI to predict a child's adiposity. (See Apendixes E and F.)

Incremental Growth

Incremental growth charts and tables have been developed for comparing short-term rates of growth to those of a reference population at specified age intervals.[44–47] Unlike conventional growth charts, in which attained growth measurements are expected to follow a growth channel, growth increments usually show variability at successive age intervals within an individual. The prolonged maintenance of rates of gain for any growth parameter in excess of or below the 50th percentile may indicate abnormal growth patterns and require further evaluation. In addition to identifying abnormal growth patterns, incremental growth assessments are helpful in evaluating individual response to nutritional intervention or other therapies that may alter growth rates.

When using incremental growth charts or tables, measurements must be mathematically adjusted for the reference time increment. For example, if the time between weight measurements is 200 days, adjustment for a 6-month weight increment is made by dividing the measured change in weight by 200 and multiplying the result by 182 (number of days in 6 months). Appendix B contains 6-month incremental growth charts developed from the Fels longitudinal study of normal white American children from birth through 18 years.[44]

Other Considerations

Obtaining and interpreting anthropometric indices of children with developmental indices may require specialized equipment and standards. This is detailed further in Chapter 14.

The developmental maturity of the child must be considered when interpreting anthropometric data. Correction for gestational age at birth is essential in the assessment of infants born prematurely (refer to Chapter 3). Children evaluated for delayed or precocious growth often have bone age assessments based on radiographic studies, which should be considered. For the older child, data relating to the stage of sexual maturity can alter assessment findings.[47,48] Appendix I presents a summary of Tanner's staging of the progression of sexual development.[49] Acceleration in rates of incremental growth is directly related to the onset of puberty.[49] In boys, a prepubescent increase in fat stores is often reflected in triceps skinfold measurements.[50,51]

Laboratory Measurements

Some laboratory measurements of nutritional status are routinely collected as part of a normal health care evaluation. Others are performed when the diagnosis, medical history, or nutritional history indicates nutritional risk. Appendix J lists laboratory norms based on age categories for selected tests of nutritional status.[52] The interpretation of laboratory findings must take into consideration the present and past medical status of the child. Many biochemical indices of nutritional status for normal individuals are altered by acute or chronic disease.

Serum Proteins

Albumin is the serum protein most commonly measured for assessment of nutritional status because it is inexpensive and readily available. However, due to a relatively long half-life of approximately 2 weeks and reduced degradation during periods of low protein intake, diagnosis of nutritional depletion can be missed or delayed if based solely on serum albumin levels. Likewise, a serum albumin level serves as a relatively late indicator of nutritional repletion. Serum albumin may be decreased during malnutrition, due to inadequate availability of precursors.[53] However, independent of nutritional status, albumin can be depressed during infection, trauma, enteropathy, liver disease, or renal disease and elevated in dehydration, third spacing, and after administration of exogenous albumin.[53,54] Serum proteins with shorter half-lives, including transferrin, retinal-binding protein, and thyroxin-binding pre-albumin, more rapidly assess response to nutritional therapy, though, like serum albumin, they may also be low during stress, sepsis, and acute illnesses secondary to fluid shifts and preferential synthesis of acute phase proteins.[53,55,56] Measurement of the acute phase protein C-reactive protein (CRP) may help determine whether a low serum protein level is caused by stress or nutritional deficiency.[57,58] Fibronectin and somatomedin have half-lives of less than 1 day but may not be ideal indicators of nutritional repletion once adequate protein and caloric intake is attained. They are used more in the research rather than the clinical setting.[58,59] Table 2–2 lists half-life and normal reference values for serum proteins commonly used for nutritional assessment.

Table 2–2 Serum Proteins Used in Assessing Nutritional Status

Protein	*Half-Life*	*Normal Value*	*Factors Known to Alter Concentration**
Albumin	18–20 days	Preterm: 2.5–4.5 g/dL Term: 2.5–5.0 g/dL 1–3 mo.: 3.0–4.2 g/dL 3–12 mo.: 2.7–5.0 g/dL > 1 year: 3.2–5.0 g/dL	↓ inflammation, infection, trauma, liver disease, renal disease, protein-losing enteropathy; altered by fluid status
Transferrin†	8–9 days	180–260 mg/dL	↓ inflammation, liver disease; ↑ iron deficiency; altered by fluid status
Prealbumin	2–3 days	20–50 mg/dL	↓ liver disease, cystic fibrosis, hyperthyroidism, infection, trauma
Retinol binding protein	12 hours	30–40 μg/mL	↓ liver disease, zinc or vitamin A deficiency, infection; ↑ renal disease

* Any condition that can alter a protein's rate of synthesis, degradation, or excretion has potential to alter the serum concentration.
† Transferrin may be calculated from total iron binding capacity (TIBC): (0.8 × TIBC) – 43

Source: Data from references 55, 99, and 100.

Creatinine Height Index

Creatinine height index is an indirect measure of somatic protein status.[60,61] The Index is calculated as (24-hour excretion of creatinine [in mg]/ creatinine excretion of normal individuals of same height and sex) × 100. Values of 80% and 60% of standard indicate moderate and severe depletion. Even in the situation of low somatic protein stores, urine creatinine may be elevated during sepsis, trauma, malignancy, and other conditions that increase protein breakdown. Because of this (and due to the difficulty of obtaining the required 24-hour urine collection), this index is infrequently used. Table 2–3 lists normal values for 24-hour creatinine excretion.[62]

Iron Status

Iron deficiency anemia is the most common pediatric nutritional problem in the United States[62] and is routinely assessed in the inpatient and community setting. Hemoglobin and/or hematocrit measurements are commonly used to assess iron nutrition. These are easily and relatively inexpensively monitored but are decreased only during later stages of iron deficiency and may be decreased for reasons other than iron deficiency. Other reasons for low hemoglobin and hematocrit include acute blood loss, acute or chronic infections, chronic inflammation, other micronutrient deficiencies (such as B_{12} or folate), or hereditary defects in red blood cell production (eg, thalassemia major or sickle cell disease).[65,66] Serum ferritin level is highly correlated with total body stores of iron and is the most sensitive index of iron status among healthy individuals. An elevated free erythrocyte protoporophyrin level and a decreased serum iron/total iron-binding capacity ratio and transferrin saturation occur when iron stores are depleted. These biochemical findings are present before changes in hemoglobin and in red blood cell morphology. With the exception of serum ferritin level, which rises, laboratory indicators for iron deficiency decrease during infection and chronic inflammation.[67–69] Table 2–4 summarizes iron status and hematologic abnormalities in states of negative iron balance.

Table 2–3 Normal Values for 24-Hour Creatinine Excretion

Height (cm)	Creatinine Values (mg/24 hr)		
	*Both Sexes**	*Males†*	*Females†*
55	50.0		
60	65.2		
65	80.5		
70	97.5		
75	118.0		
80	139.6		
85	167.6		
90	199.9		
95	239.8		
100	278.7		
105	305.4		
110	349.8		
115	394.5		
120	456.0		
125	535.1		
130		448.1	525.2
135		480.1	589.2
140		556.3	653.1
145		684.3	717.2
150		812.3	780.9
155		940.3	844.8
160		1,068.3	908.8
165		1,196.3	
170		1,324.3	
175		1,452.3	
180		1,580.3	

* Data from reference 61.
† Data from reference 60.

Source: Reprinted from R Merritt and G Blackburn, Nutritional assessment and metabolic response to illness of the hospitalized child, in *Textbook of Pediatric Nutrition* by R Suskind (ed) with permission of Lippincott Williams & Wilkins, © 1981.

Immunologic Function

Protein-energy malnutrition, as well as subclinical deficiencies of one or more nutrients, can impair immune response and increase risk for infection. The measurement of functional parameters of the immune system can, therefore, be useful to assess nutritional status. Among the immunologic indexes that are associated with nutritional status are levels of T-lymphocytes and leukocyte terminal deoxynucleotidyl transferase, appearance of delayed cutaneous hypersensitivity, opsonic function, salivary immunoglobulin A (IgA), and total lymphocyte count. These tests vary in sensitivity for detecting nutritional depletion.[70] The total lymphocyte count (TLC) is the index of immune function most readily available for hospitalized patients. This value can be calculated from white blood cell (WBC) counts, as follows:

$$\text{WBC/mm}^3 \times \%\ \text{lymphocytes} = \text{TLC/mm}^3$$

Values less than 1,500 are associated with nutritional depletion. In infants less than 3 months of age, values of less than 2,500 may be abnormal.[71] Independent of nutritional status, values of immunologic function may be altered during trauma, chemotherapy, immunosuppressant drug therapy, and lack of previous exposure to antigen (in the case of delayed cutaneous hypersensitivity).[70]

Clinical Evaluation

Examination and evaluation of general appearance and specific systems is an essential part of the nutritional assessment. In most cases, severe nutritional deprivation is easily detectable. Milder, nonspecific signs of malnutrition are more commonly observed but may be harder to detect. The presence of a suspected clinical deficiency is often reflected in the diet history and should be further supported by biochemical evaluation.[70,72] Table 2–5 lists clinical signs associated with nutrient deficiencies and specifies laboratory findings recommended to substantiate the diagnosis.

Dietary Evaluation

Components of a Pediatric Diet Evaluation

The thorough collection of dietary data should include the quantity and quality of foods, psychosocial factors impacting food selection and intake, and clinical or physical factors related to

Table 2–4 Iron Status and Hematologic Abnormalities in States of Negative Iron Balance*

	Normal	*Iron Depletion*	*Iron Deficiency*	*Iron Deficiency Anemia* Early	*Iron Deficiency Anemia* Advanced
Storage iron	NL	DECR	DECR	DECR	DECR
Erythron iron	NL	NL	DECR	DECR	DECR
Hemoglobin, Hematocrit, RBC count	NL	NL	NL	DECR	DECR
RBC indices	NL	NL	NL	NL	DECR

* NL, normal; DECR, decrease; RBC, red blood cell.

Source: Adapted with permission from A.J. Cecalupo and H.J. Cohen, Nutritional anemias, in *Pediatric Nutrition Theory and Practice,* R.J. Grand, J.L. Sutphen and W.H. Dietz, eds, p. 491 © 1987, Butterworth Heinemann, Newton, Massachusetts.

nutritional status (see Exhibit 2–2). Specific factors include:[71–73]

Food related factors
- chronologic feeding history from birth or onset of nutritional problem
- current nutrient intake
- feeding skills
- history of prescribed or self-imposed diets and outcome
- food allergies or intolerances

Psychosocial factors
- family history and dynamics
- socioeconomic status, including use of supplemental food programs
- patient's self-perception of nutritional status and/or caretaker's perception of child's nutritional status
- religious or cultural beliefs impacting food intake

Clinical/physical factors
- vitamin supplements and medication
- stooling habits and characteristics
- activity
- sleep patterns

The diet history can be comprehensive, encompassing most of the aforementioned factors or specific to support a suspected diagnosis. For example, to implicate a dietary basis for iron deficiency anemia in a 9-month-old infant, the interview may focus on age of introduction to cow's milk, volume of cow's milk consumed, and use and quantity of iron-containing solid foods.

Complementary Medicine

During the last decade and a half, the interest in and practice of complementary medicine has increased.[74] Complementary medicine may include, but is not limited to: homeopathic medicine, natural products, macrobiotics, megavitamins, and herbal medicine.[75] Families whose children have an acute or chronic condition may especially be seeking complementary medicine to augment routine medical treatment. Information on a family's past or present use of a complementary medicine is important, though it may not be readily volunteered by the family. Specific questions as are outlined in Exhibit 2–3 may be useful to elicit this information. Any ap-

Table 2–5 Clinical Signs and Laboratory Findings in the Malnourished Child and Adult*

Clinical Sign	*Suspect Nutrient*	*Supportive Objective Findings*
Epithelial		
Skin		
Xerosis, dry scaling	Essential fatty acids	Triene/tetraene ratio >0.4
Hyperkeratosis, plaques around hair follicles	Vitamin A	↓ Plasma retinol
Ecchymoses, petechiae	Vitamin K	Prolonged prothrombin time
	Vitamin C	↓ Serum ascorbic acid
Hair		
Easily plucked, dyspigmented, lackluster	Protein-calorie	↓ Total protein
		↓ Albumin
Nails		↓ Transferrin
Thin, spoon-shaped	Iron	↓ Serum Fe
		↑ TIBC
Mucosal		
Mouth, lips, and tongue	B vitamins	
Angular stomatitis (inflammation at corners of mouth)	B_2 (riboflavin)	↓ RBC glutathione reductase
Cheilosis (reddened lips with fissures at angles)	B_2	See above
	B_6 (pyridoxine)	↓ Plasma pyridoxal phosphate†
Glossitis (inflammation of tongue)	B_6	See above
	B_2	See above
	B_3 (niacin)	↓ Plasma tryptophan
		↓ Urinary N-methyl nicotinamide†
Magenta tongue	B_2	See above
Edema of tongue, tongue fissures	B_3	See above
Gums		
Spongy, bleeding	Vitamin C	↓ Plasma ascorbic acid
Ocular		
Pale conjunctivae secondary to anemia	Iron	↓ Serum Fe, ↑ TIBC, ↓ serum folic acid, or ↓ RBC folic acid
	Folic acid	
	Vitamin B_{12}	↓ Serum B_{12}
	Copper	↓ Serum copper
Bitot's spots (grayish, yellow, or white foamy spots on the whites of the eye)	Vitamin A	↓ Plasma retinol
Conjunctival or corneal xerosis, keratomalacia (softening of part or all of cornea)	Vitamin A	↓ Plasma retinol

continues

Table 2–5 continued

Clinical Sign	*Suspect Nutrient*	*Supportive Objective Findings*
Musculoskeletal		
Craniotabes (thinning of the inner table of the skull); palpable enlargement of costochondral junctions ("rachitic rosary"); thickening of wrists and ankles	Vitamin D	↓ 25-OH-vit D ↑ Alkaline phosphatase ± ↓ Ca, ↓ PO_4 Long bone films
Scurvy (tenderness of extremities, hemorrhages under periosteum of long bones; enlargement of costochondral junction; cessation of osteogenesis of long bones)	Vitamin C	↓ Serum ascorbic acid Long bone films
Skeletal lesions	Copper	↓ Serum copper X-ray film changes similar to scurvy since copper is also essential for normal collagen formation
Muscle wasting, prominence of body skeleton, poor muscle tone	Protein-calorie	↓ Serum proteins ↓ Arm muscle circumference
General		
Edema	Protein	↓ Serum proteins
Pallor 2° to anemia	Vitamin E (in premature infants)	↓ Serum vitamin E ↑ Peroxide hemolysis Evidence of hemolysis on blood smear
	Iron	↓ Serum Fe, ↑ TIBC
	Folic acid	↓ Serum folic acid Macrocytosis on RBC smear
	Vitamin B_{12}	↓ Serum B_{12} Macrocytosis on RBC smear
	Copper	↓ Serum copper
Internal systems		
Nervous		
Mental confusion	Protein	↓ Total protein, ↓ albumin, ↓ transferrin
	Vitamin B_1 (thiamine)	↓ RBC transketolase
Cardiovascular Beriberi (enlarged heart, congestive heart failure, tachycardia)	Vitamin B_1	Same as above

continues

Table 2–5 continued

Clinical Sign	*Suspect Nutrient*	*Supportive Objective Findings*
Tachycardia 2° to anemia	Iron Folic acid B_{12} Copper Vitamin E (in premature infants)	See above
Gastrointestinal		
Hepatomegaly	Protein-calorie	↓ Total protein, ↓ albumin, ↓ transferrin
Glandular		
Thyroid enlargement	Iodine	↓ Total serum iodine: inorganic, PBI†

* Fe, iron; PBI, protein-bound iodine; RBC, red blood cells; TIBC, total iron-binding capacity.
† Bio Science Laboratories, 7600 Tyrone Avenue, Van Nuys, CA 91405.

Source: Reprinted with permission from A. Kerner, *Manual of Pediatric Parenteral Nutrition,* pp. 22–23 © 1983, W.B. Saunders Company.

pearance of being judgmental may inhibit disclosure and discussion.[76]

Collection of Current Intake Data

Several approaches to quantitate nutrient intake data are available. A diet history is designed to determine pattern of usual food intake. This type of history requires a detailed interview by a trained nutritionist.[77,78] From the collected data, an estimate of nutrient intake is calculated. Studies indicate that this method yields higher estimated values than does the 24-hour recall and diet record.

A 24-hour recall provides an estimate of nutrient intake based on the individual's recollection of food consumed over the previous day. This method has been used successfully for groups of individuals. However, it is less valid in evaluating diet adequacy for an individual as the 24-hour period assessed may not be representative of the usual diet. Nutrient intakes calculated from 24-hour recalls are lower than those based on dietary histories or food records.[79–83]

Three-day to 7-day food records provide prospective food intake data. These are recorded by the parent, child, or other caregiver and are returned to the nutritionist for analysis. Food records encompassing 7 days may provide more accurate information than one of shorter duration, due to the inclusion of both weekend and weekday meal patterns; however, accuracy of diet record keeping often deteriorates over time. When a 7-day food record is not possible, use of shorter time periods, including selected days of the week, is an adequate alternative.[84]

In inpatient facilities, nutrient intake analyses (calorie counts) are frequently ordered to assess a child's food intake. These are used to determine the ability of a child to consume a sufficient amount of food for growth or to verify the achievement and adequacy of a prescribed feeding regimen. These records, however, do not provide data representative of intake within the home environment.

Food frequencies estimate the frequency and amount of specific foods eaten. These often consist of questionnaires that can be self-adminis-

Exhibit 2–2 Dietary Interview Summary Portion of a Nutrition Clinic Evaluation

NUTRITION CLINIC EVALUATION

Date of Visit: ______ Age: ______
Diagnosis: ______ Onset: ______
Concomitant Conditions: ______
______ Ref. Phys. ______
Problem: ______

Concerns of Parents or Patient: ______

Nutrition History: ______

Recent Nutrition History: ______

Formula: Kind ______ Amount ______ Cal. Density ______
Food Intake: ______

Food Summary (no. of servings/day):
Meat ______ Milk ______ Fr/Veg ______ Grains ______

Fever/Vomiting: ______ Elimination: ______
Appetite: ______
Feeding Ability/Concerns: ______

Vitamin Mineral Supp: ______
Activity level 1–8, 8 high ______

Social Setting in regard to meal prep: ______

Social History: ______

Pertinent family medical/weight history: ______

Source: Courtesy of the Clinical Nutrition Services, Children's Hospital Medical Center, Cincinnati, OH.

Exhibit 2–3 Sample Questions to Elicit Information on Use of Complementary Medicine

1. Is your child receiving any herbal preparations? If yes:
2. What is the name (if known)?
3. For what purpose?
4. How are they administered (tea, tincture, fluid extract, tablet, or capsule)?
5. How much? How often?
6. How prescribed/recommended? Where is it purchased?
7. How well tolerated? Any side effects noted?
8. Is your child receiving any additional vitamins or minerals? (if yes, questions 2–7 apply)
9. Are there any foods or vitamins you specifically avoid for your child?
10. Who are the people involved in your child's health care (caretakers and health providers)?
11. Do you have any questions regarding complementary or alternative health care?

tered and, therefore, reduce professional interview time. The questionnaire generally cannot retrieve unique details of an individual's diet unless designed to do so.[85] Overreporting of food intake is common with this method.[79,80,86,87]

New methods of capturing dietary intake are being explored using such technology as portable computers, videotapes, and tape recorders.[87–90]

Dietary Intake Evaluation

Estimated intakes of specific nutrients are calculated using values derived from food composition tables or computerized nutrient analysis programs. The calculated intake is evaluated for adequacy by comparing it with a reference intake. The 1989 Recommended Dietary Allowances (RDAs) are the most commonly used reference allowances in the United States[91] but are currently being revised. The revised Dietary Reference Intakes (DRIs) actually refer to at least four types of reference values: RDAs, Adequate Intake (AI), Estimated Average Requirement (EAR), and Tolerable Upper Intake Level (UL). The DRIs are based on contemporary studies, which address not only preventing classic nutritional deficiencies but reducing the risk of chronic diseases, promoting optimal health, and preventing nutrient toxicities.[92] The RDA is the dietary intake level that is sufficient to meet the nutrient requirements of nearly all healthy persons and is designed to include a wide margin of safety above amounts required to prevent deficiency.[93] Therefore, a healthy child whose estimated intake for a nutrient falls below the RDA may not have a nutritional deficiency or even a nutritional risk unless this intake is substantially below the RDA for a sufficient length of time.[91] When assessing the adequacy of diets for infants and children with acute or chronic disease, potential alterations in nutrient requirements should be considered. In cases where sufficient scientific evidence is not available to estimate an average requirement, AIs have been set and should be used as a goal for intake where no RDAs exist. The EAR is the intake value that is estimated to meet the requirement defined by a specified indicator of adequacy in 50% of an age- and gender-specified group. The UL is the maximum level of daily nutrient intake that is unlikely to pose risks of adverse health effects to almost all of the individuals. The DRIs are being evaluated and released as seven nutrient groups. These groups are:

- Calcium, vitamin D, phosphorus, magnesium, fluoride
- Folate and other B vitamins
- Antioxidants
- Macronutrients
- Trace elements
- Electrolytes and water
- Other food components (eg, fiber, phytoestrogens)

The 1989 RDAs and the current DRIs are summarized in Appendix K.

Calculation of Energy Requirements

Overview

Accurate prediction of energy requirements is important for the healthy child, and its importance is magnified in such clinical situations as treating the obese or failure-to-thrive (FTT) child and implementing enteral or parenteral nutrition support in the acutely or chronically ill child.[94] Energy needs can be estimated using the RDAs, though, notably, RDAs are based on populations of normal, healthy subjects and may not be applicable to the child with altered activity or with potential alterations in needs related to clinical status.[91]

Many equations have been generated to predict energy needs and to which the clinician can add factors accounting for activity and stress. In a subgroup of children with illnesses and concomitant malnutrition, energy expenditure may be most accurately predicted by the use of indirect calorimetry.[95]

Definition of Terms

Total energy expenditure (TEE) consists of the energy required to meet the basal metabolic rate (BMR), diet induced thermogenesis, activity, and growth.[96] BMR assumes the following basal conditions.[97]

1. fasting (at least 10–12 hours after the last meal)
2. awake and resting in a lying position (measurements are taken shortly after awakening)
3. normal body and ambient temperature
4. absence of psychologic or physical stress

Diet-induced thermogenesis, also referred to as the *specific dynamic action of food*, is the energy necessary for digestion, transport, and storage of nutrients. It accounts for 5–10 % of daily energy expenditure.[101]

Resting energy expenditure (REE) is the energy expenditure of an individual at rest and in conditions of thermal neutrality. REE may include the thermal effect of a previous meal. BMR and REE usually differ by less than 10%.[91,97]

Standardized Equations

Equations have been developed to predict the BMR and REE of infants and children. The most commonly used are summarized in Table 2–6.[102–107] BMR and REE estimates using standard calculations are based on the assumption that the individual is free of pathology and fever that affect energy expenditure and, therefore, applying these equations to the ill pediatric patient requires an additional stress factor. Table 2–7[106–117] highlights a sampling of current findings in potential alterations in energy expenditure with different disease states. This body of knowledge is dynamic, and it behooves the clinician to stay abreast. Regular reevaluation of energy needs should be completed as clinical status changes. Caution must be taken not to overfeed a critically ill child as excess nutritional delivery can potentially increase pulmonary and hepatic pathophysiology.[118]

The final factor in determining energy needs is activity. This can be accomplished by determining the amounts of time spent performing various types of activities and calculating an activity factor based on a 24-hour time period. Activity factors of 1.3 are associated with sedentary lifestyles, whereas activity factors equal to or greater than 2.0 represent lifestyles high in physical activity. Children under normal unconstrained conditions are considered to be active with activity factors ranging from 1.7 to 2.0 × REE. Table 2–8 lists the approximate energy expenditure for various activities in relation to REE. Table 2–9 demonstrates the method of calculating an activity factor and the TEE.

In using BMR and REE equations, it is important to note that individual variation exists. The majority of variation in REE/BMR of individuals of the same age, weight, and sex is related to lean body mass. The person with the higher lean body mass will have the higher energy expenditure.[91] In numerous studies, researchers have concluded that these standardized formulas may

Table 2–6 Equations for Predicting Energy Requirements of Children

Origin	*Energy Determination*	*Gender*	*Age*	*Equation*
Harris, Benedict[102]	BMR	Male	unspecified	66.47 + 13.75 W + 5.0 H – 6.76 A
		Female		655.1 + 9.65 W + 1.85 H – 4.68 A
World Health Organization (WHO)[103]	REE	Male	0–3 yr	60.9W – 54
			3–10 yr	22.7W + 495
		Female	0–3 yr	61 W – 51
			3–10 yr	22.5 W + 499
Schofield[104]	REE	Male	<3 yr	0.167 W + 1.517 H – 617.6
			3–10 yr	19.59 W + .1303 H + 414.9
			10–18 yr	16.25 W + .1372 H + 515.5
		Female	<3 yr	16.252 W + 1.0232 H – 413.5
			3–10 yr	16.969 W + 161.8 H + 371.2
			10–18 yr	8.365 W + 4.65 H + 200.0
Altman and Dittmer[105]	REE	Male	3–16 yr	19.56 W + 506.16
		Female		18.67 W + 578.64
Maffeis et al.[106]	REE	Male	6–10 yr	1287 + 28.6 W + 23.6 H – 69.1 A
		Female		1552 + 35.8 W + 15.6 H – 36.3 A
Pierro et al. (for surgical infants)[107]	REE	unspecified	Infants	Cal/min = –74.436 + 34.661 W + 4.96 × HR + (0.78 × age in days)

Weight = weight in kilograms; A = age in years; H = Height in centimeters; HR = heart rate in beats per minute

Source: Data from references 102 to 107.

not be accurate in predicting individual energy needs for children with FTT, obesity, and some acute or chronic illnesses.[95,98,119,120]

Indirect Calorimetry

Many health care facilities are using indirect calorimetry to predict the energy needs for the subset of patients whose energy needs are elusive. This subset includes but is not limited to patients who are failing to thrive despite meeting predicted needs, obese patients, critically ill patients on nutrition support, and patients unable to be weaned from the ventilator. Indirect calorimetry measures oxygen consumption (VO_2) and carbon dioxide production (VCO_2.) Most indirect calorimeters are open-circuit systems in which the patient breathes room air or air supplied from a mechanical ventilator and expires into a gas sampling system that eventually vents the expired air back into the room.[121] Indirect calorimetry provides two pieces of information: REE and a measure of substrate utilization, as reflected in the respiratory quotient (RQ).

The following abbreviated Weir equation calculates REE:[122]

$$\text{REE (kcal/min)} = 3.94 \times VO_2 + 1.11 \times VCO_2$$

Table 2–7 Potential Changes in Energy Expenditure associated with Different Diagnoses

Diagnosis	*Research*	*Population*	*Potential Stress Factor*
Closed Head Injury. Postinjury day 1–14	Phillips et al. (1987)[106]	2–17 yr	Measured energy expenditure averaged 1.3 times value predicted by Harris and Benedict
Inflammatory Bowel Disease	Kushner et al. (1991)[107]	19–40 yr	No significant increase in energy needs
Cystic Fibrosis	Ramsey et al. (1992)[108]	Not specified	Normal lung function—energy expenditure increased about 50% Moderate lung disease 70% Severe lung lung disease 80% (Includes activity and assumes sedentary activity)
Extrahepatic Biliary Atresia	Pierro et al. (1989)[109]	2–73 mo	Energy expenditure was 29% higher than normal
Spastic Quadriplegic Cerebral Palsy	Stallings et al. (1996)[110]	2–18 yr	Nonbasal energy expenditure was minimal
Burns	Mayes et al. (1996)[111]	0.5–10 yr (mean 30% BSA burns)	Supports application of an additional 30% REE
Postsurgery	Powis et al. (1998)[112]	0–3 yr (major abdominal surgery)	No increase in metabolic rate after major abdominal operations
	Jones et al. (1993)[113]	0–4 mo (various surgeries)	Mean increase of 15% REE following surgery.
Congenital Heart Defects	Barton et al. (1994)[114]	<6 mo (severe congenital heart disease)	Needs 40% greater than RDA for age
HIV	Various	Mostly adult	Results of adult literature inconclusive, with some studies showing increased REE[115] and others decreased.[116] No evidence that pediatric HIV disease in and of itself increases REE (see Chapter 21)
Fevers	Dubois EF (1954)[117]	—	REE increases 13% for each degree Centigrade of fever (7.2% for each degree Fahrenheit)

Source: Data from references 106 to 117.

Table 2–8 Approximate Energy Expenditure for Various Activities in Relation to Resting Needs for Males and Females of Average Size*

Activity Category†	*Representative Value for Activity Factor per Unit Time of Activity*
Resting	REE × 1.0
Sleeping, reclining	
Very light	REE × 1.5
Seated and standing activities, painting trades, driving, laboratory work, typing, sewing, ironing, cooking, playing cards, playing a musical instrument	
Light	REE × 2.5
Walking on a level surface at 2.5 to 3 mph, garage work, electrical trades, carpentry, restaurant trades, house-cleaning, child care, golf, sailing, table tennis	
Moderate	REE × 5.0
Walking 3.5–4 mph, weeding and hoeing, carrying a load, cycling, skiing, tennis, dancing	
Heavy	REE × 7.0
Walking with load uphill, tree felling, heavy manual digging, basketball, climbing, football, soccer	

* Data from references 26 and 33.
† When reported as multiples of basal needs, the expenditures of males and females are similar.

Source: Reprinted with permission from *Recommended Dietary Allowances,* 10th edition, © 1989 by the National Academy of Sciences. Published by National Academy Press.

Measured REE in children accounts for their current clinical status (ie, level of stress) and may require reevaluation as this changes. Additional energy should be added if the measurement was taken while the child was intubated and is subsequently extubated. Work of breathing normally accounts for 2–3% of REE and may be as high as 25% in respiratory failure.[123] Activity will also alter REE. Being awake and alert increases energy expended by 10%.[124] Routine nursing procedures, such as baths, positioning, and dressing changes can increase energy expenditure by 20–30%, although these activities tend to be short in duration.[125,126] Ambulatory hospitalized individuals require an increase in energy of 25–30% to allow for activity.[127] Measured REE does not account for anabolism or growth. In the adult or older child, this represents a fraction of total energy needs. In the very young infant, this potential energy has been measured to be 2.73 kcal/g tissue synthesized,[128] though in the very sick or traumatized child, growth may be inhibited, and applying growth factors may result in overfeeding.[118] Indirect calorimetry can also evaluate how the body is using fuel, as reflected by the RQ, which is the ratio of carbon dioxide produced to oxygen consumed.

$$RQ = (VCO_2/VO_2)$$

Glucose oxidation is associated with an RQ of 1.0, fat oxidation with an RQ of 0.7, and protein metabolism with an RQ of 0.8. Alcohol or ketone metabolism may reduce the RQ to 0.67, whereas overfeeding with lipogenesis may increase the RQ to 1.3. Knowledge of inefficient

Table 2–9 Example of Calculation for Total Energy Expenditure in an 11-Year-Old Boy*

Activity Type	*REE Multiple*	*Duration (h)*	*Weighted REE Factor*
Resting	1.0	9	9
Very light	1.5	8	12
Light	2.5	4	10
Moderate	5.0	2	10
Heavy	7.0	1	7
TOTALS		24	48

Activity factor = weighted REE ÷ hours
= 48 ÷ 24
= 2.0

Total energy expenditure:

Gender	*Age (yr)*	*Wt (kg)*	*REE† (kcal/d)*	×	*Activity Factor*	=	*TEE (kcal/d)*
Male	11	35	1263.5	×	2.0	=	2527

* Hypothetical activity pattern.
† Calculated from equations in Table 2-6.

Source: Reprinted from S. Krug-Wispé, Nutritional Assessment, in *Handbook of Pediatric Nutrition,* P. Queen and C.E. Lang, eds., p. 45, © 1993, Aspen Publishers, Inc.

substrate utilization and subsequent reduction of RQ through alteration of energy substrates can be medically advantageous.[127–129]

DATA EVALUATION AND PLAN

The assessment of nutritional status is based on the careful evaluation of all gathered information. Interrelationships between the health status of the child, feeding abilities, eating habits, anthropometric data, and laboratory findings should be considered.[130–132] Exhibit 2–4 is an example of a nutrition assessment summary sheet.

Protein-Energy Malnutrition

The identification of the presence and severity of protein-energy malnutrition (PEM) among children in hospitals and clinics is a valuable function of nutritional assessment. Table 2–10 outlines anthropometric indices that have been developed to quantitate the severity of chronic and acute PEM. Children may present with one or both forms of PEM. Acute but not chronic PEM may increase morbidity and increase length of hospital stay.[133] Children may present with increased morbidity and increased length of hospital stay. For more information on "standard" reference values, refer to Chapter 18.

Marasmus and Kwashiorkor

Marasmus and kwashiorkor are two classifications of severe acute PEM. Marasmus develops over a period of weeks or months and is characterized by a wasted appearance, due to diminished subcutaneous fat. Infants and children with marasmus have normal or low levels of se-

Exhibit 2–4 Nutritional Assessment Summary for Hospitalized Infant or Young Child

NUTRITIONAL ASSESSMENT
(Birth to 36 months)

Date of Birth ____________ Admitting Diagnosis ________________________
Significant Medical Problems __________________ % Weight change in _________
Growth History: Previous Weights Previous Lengths

date	kg	%ile	date	cm	%ile
___	___	___	___	___	___
___	___	___	___	___	___
___	___	___	___	___	___

Previous Growth Velocity: ______________________________

Date					NUTRITIONAL RISK CRITERIA
Age					
Length (cm)					<5th %ile suggests growth retardation
%ile					
Weight (kg)					<5th %ile
%ile					
Weight/Lenth Index (actual weight + ideal weight for length)					80% to 90%; Mild PEM* 70% to 80%l Moderate PEM* <70%; Severe PEM*
Ideal Weight for Length					
Head Circumference (cm)					<5th %ile
%ile					
Arm Circumference/ Head Circumference Ratio					.28 to .31; Mild PEM* .25 to .28; Moderate PEM* <.25%; Severe PEM*
Arm Circumference (cm)					<5th %ile
%ile					
Arm Muscle Circumference (mm)					<5th %ile
%ile					
Arm Muscle Area (mm^2)					<5th %ile
%ile					
Tricep Skinfold (mm)					<5th %ile
%ile					
Subscapular Skinfold (mm)					<5th %ile
%ile					

Date					NUTRITION RISK CRITERIA
Albumin					0–6 MO <2.9 gm/dl; 6 mo–3yr <3.5 gm/dl
Transferrin					<200 mg/dl
Pre Albumin					
Retinol Binding Protein					
Total Lynphocyte Count					
					<1500 mm^3
Intake					
Dates ______					
Kcal/kg ______					
gm pro/kg ______					

Oxygen consumption: Date: ________ REE = ________
NUTRITIONAL NEEDS* ______ Kcal/kg ______ gm pro kg
Based on ______________________
(*energy needs increase 7% per degree F.)
Expected rate of weight gain for size: ______________

Comments:

*PEM: Protein Energy Malnutrition

Source: Courtesy of the Clinical Nutrition Services, Children's Hospital Medical Center, Cincinnati, OH.

Table 2–10 Anthropometric Indexes Associated with Protein-Energy Malnutrition

Type PEM	Anthropometric Index	Degree of PEM: Normal	Mild	Moderate	Severe
Chronic (stunting)					
	Height for age as % standard*	95	90–94	85–89	<85
Acute (wasting)					
	Weight for age as % standard*	90	75–89	60–74	<60
	Weight for height as % standard*	90	80–89	70–79	<70
	Arm circumference/ head circumference ratio†	>0.31	0.28–0.31	0.25–0.28	<.25

* Original data for determining degree of PEM used the 50th percentile of Boston growth data as standard. The 50th percentile on NCHS growth charts is now commonly used as the standard with these assessments.
† Ratio has been found to correlate with weight for age in children 3 months to 4 years of age.

Source: Adapted with permission from Gomez F, Galvan R, Frenks, Munoz JC, Chavez R, Vasquez J. Mortality in second and third degree malnutrition. *J Trop Pediatr.* 1956;2:77 and Waterlow J. Classification and definition of protein calorie malnutrition. In Beaton G, Bengoa X, eds. *Nutrition in Preventive Medicine.* WHO monograph series No. 62. Geneva: WHO; 1976.

rum albumin and other transport proteins and no evidence of edema. Liver size is normal.[130–133]

Conversely, kwashiorkor develops acutely, often in conjunction with an infection. Levels of serum albumin, other transport proteins, and lymphocytes are reduced. Edema is present over the trunk, extremities, and face. These infants and children often have subcutaneous fat stores that mask muscle wasting. Dermatitis and hair changes (flag sign) are usually present. In severe cases, fatty infiltration of the liver occurs.[130–133]

Marasmic kwashiorkor is the classification used to describe the presence of symptoms of kwashiorkor in a child with a weight for height less than 70% of standard or a weight for age less than 60% of standard. This condition often develops following acute stress and is associated with high mortality.[133]

Other Nutritional Diagnoses

Other nutritional diagnoses, such as obesity and failure to thrive, as well as other diagnoses requiring therapeutic diet intervention, will be further discussed in the forthcoming chapters.

Care Plan

The nutritional care plan is developed to correct nutritional problems or reduce nutritional risks identified through the assessment. Basic information included in the medical and dietary histories provides a foundation for designing a plan that is reasonable and achievable within a given setting. The effectiveness of the nutritional intervention is determined through periodic nutritional reassessment. The care plan is modified as needed for changes in nutritional status/risk.

CONCLUSIONS

The provision of quality nutritional services to children is dependent on identifying those who are nutritionally depleted or at nutritional risk. In-depth nutritional assessments include a medical history, a clinical evaluation, evaluation of anthropometric indices, and a dietary evaluation. Biochemical indices may be evaluated as part of a routine nutritional screen or to confirm a suspected nutritional aberration. Assessment data are used to identify specific nutritional problems and to develop workable care plans targeted to improve nutritional status.

REFERENCES

1. Shapiro LR. Streamlining and implementing nutritional assessment. The dietary approach. *J Am Diet Assoc.* 1979;75:230–237.
2. Hunt DR, Maslovitz A, Rowlands BJ, Brooks B. A simple nutrition screening procedure for hospital patients. *J Am Diet Assoc.* 1985;85:332–335.
3. Christensen KS, Gstundtner KM. Hospital-wide screening improves basis for nutrition intervention. *J Am Diet Assoc.* 1985;85:704–706.
4. DeHoog S. Identifying patients at nutritional risk and determining clinical productivity; essentials for an effective nutrition care program. *J Am Diet Assoc.* 1985; 85:1620–1622.
5. Hedberg AM, Garcia N, Trejus IJ, Weinmann-Winkler S, Gabriel ML, Lutz AL. Nutrition risk screening: development of a standardized protocol using dietetic technicians. *J Am Diet Assoc.* 1988;88:1553–1556.
6. Mezoff A, Gamm L, Konek S, Beal KG, Hitch D. Validation of a nutritional screen in children with respiratory syncytial virus admitted to an intensive care complex. *Pediatr.* 1996;97:543–546.
7. Fomon SJ. *Nutritional Disorders of Children.* Rockville, MD: Public Health Services No. (HAS)75-5612. US Department of Health and Human Services, Education and Welfare; 1976:1–610.
8. Christakis G. Nutritional assessment in health programs. *Am J Public Health.* 1973;63(suppl):1–56.
9. Joint Commission. *Comprehensive Accreditation Manual of Hospitals*, May Update. Oakbrook Terrace, IL: *JCAHO*; 1998;PE7,PE8.
10. Kamath SK, Lawler M, Smith AE, Kalat T, Olson R. Hospital malnutrition: a 33 hospital screening study. *J Am Diet Assoc.* 1986;86:203–206.
11. Campbell MC, Kelsey KS. The PEACH Survey: a nutrition screening tool for use in early intervention programs. *J Am Diet Assoc.* 1994:1156–1158.
12. Noel MB, Wojnarosk SM. Nutrition screening for long-term care patients. *J Am Diet Assoc.* 1987;87: 1557–1558.
13. Baer MT, Farnan S, Mauer AM. Children with special health care needs. In: Shorbaugh Co., ed. *Call to Action: Better Nutrition for Mothers, Children and Families.* Washington, DC: National Center for Education in Maternal and Child Health; 1991:191–208.
14. Klawittler BM. Nutrition assessment of infants and children. In: Williams CD, ed., *Pediatric Manual of Clinical Dietetics.* Library of Congress; 1998: 19–34.
15. Alam N, Wojtyniak B, Rahaman MM. Anthropometric indicators and risk of death. *Am J Clin Nutr.* 1989;49: 884–888.
16. Frisancho AR. New norms of upper limb fat and muscle areas for assessment of nutritional status. *Am J Clin Nutr.* 1981;34:2540–2545.
17. National Center for Health Statistics. Plan and operation of the Health and Nutrition Examination Survey, United States, 1971–73. *Vital Health Statistics.* 1973; 10a,10b.
18. Ryan AS, Martinez GA. Physical growth of infants 7–12 mos of age: results from a national survey. *Am J Phys Anthropol.* 1987;73:449–457.
19. Paul AA, Cole TJ, Ahmed EA, Whithead RG. The need for revised standards for skinfold thickness in infancy. *Arch Dis Child.* 1998;78:354–358.
20. Tanner JM, Whitehouse RH. Revised standards for triceps and subscapular skinfolds in British children. *Arch Dis Child.* 1975;50:142–145.
21. Oakley RR, Parsons RJ, Whitelaw AOC. Standards for skinfold thickness in British newborn infants. *Arch Dis Child.* 1977;52:287–290.
22. Vaucher YE, Grigsby Harrison G, Udall JN, Morrow G. Skinfold thickness in North American infants 24–41 weeks gestation. *Hum Biol.* 1984;56:713–731.
23. Cronk CE, Roche AF. Race- and sex-specific reference data for triceps and subscapular skinfolds and weight/stature. *Am J Clin Nutr.* 1982;35:347–354.
24. Owen GM, Lubin AH. Anthropometric differences between black and white preschool children. *Am J Dis Child.* 1973;162:168–169.
25. Ryan AS, Martinez GA, Baumgartner RN, Roche AF, Guo S, Chumlea WC, Kuczumarski RJ. Median skinfold thickness distributions and fat-wave patterns in Mexican-American children from the Hispanic

Health and Nutrition Examination Survey (HHANES 1982–1984). *Am J Clin Nutr.* 1990;51:925s–935s.

26. Ryan AS, Martinez GA, Roche AF. An evaluation of the associations between socioeconomic status and the growth of Mexican-American children data from the Hispanic Health and Nutrition Examination Survey (HHANES 1982–1984). *Am J Clin Nutr.* 1990;51: 944s–952s.
27. Bray GA, Greenway FL, Molitech ME. Use of anthropometric measures to assess weight loss. *Am J Clin Nutr.* 1978;31:769–773.
28. Quatelet LAJ. Physique Sociale. Vol 2. Brussels: C Muquardt; 1869.
29. Hammer LD, Kraemer HC, Wilson DM, Ritter PL, Dornbusch SM. Standardized percentile curves of Body-Mass Index for children and adolescents. *Am J Clin Nutr.* 1997;145:259–263.
30. Rosner B, Prineas R, Loggie J, Daniels SR. Percentiles for body mass index in US children 5 to 17 years of age. *J Pediatr.* 1998;132:211–222.
31. Leung SS, Cole TJ, Tse LY, Lau JT. Body mass index reference curves for Chinese children. *Ann Hum Biol.* 1998;25:169–174.
32. Cole TJ, Freeman JV, Preece MA. Body mass index reference curves for the UK 1990. *Arch Dis Child.* 1995;73:25–29.
33. Luciano A, Bressan F, Zoppi G. Body mass index reference curves for children ages 3–19 years from Verona, Italy. *Eur J Clin Nutr.* 1997;51:6–10.
34. Bhalla AK, Walia BN. Percentile curves for body-mass index of Punjabi infants. *Indian Pediatr.* 1996;33:471–476.
35. Aurelius G, Khan NC, Truc DB, Ha TT, Lindren G. Height, weight, and body mass index (BMI) of Vietnamese (Hanoi) schoolchildren aged 7–11 years related to parents occupation and education. *J Trop Pediatr.* 1996;42:21–26.
36. Lindgren G, Strandell A, Cole T, Healy M, Tanner J. Swedish population reference standards for height, weight and body mass index attained at 6–16 years (girls) or 19 years (boys). *Acta Paediatrica.* 1995;84: 1019–1028.
37. Sichieri R, Recine E, Everhart JE. Growth and body mass index of Brazilians ages 9 through 17 years. *Obes Res.* 1995;3:117s–121s.
38. Rolland-Cachera MF, Deheeger M, Bellisle F, Semp M, Guilloud-Bataillem M, Patois E. Obesity rebound in children: a simple indicator for predicting obesity. *Am J Clin Nutr.* 1984;39:129–135.
39. Garrow JS, Webster J. Quetelets index (W/H2) as a measure of fatness. *Int J Obes Relat Metab Disord.* 1985;9:147–153.
40. Himes JH, Dietz WH. Guidelines for overweight in adolescent preventive services. Recommendations from an expert committee. *Am J Clin Nutr.* 1994;59: 307–316.
41. Pietrobelli A, Faith MS, Allison DB, Gallagher D, Chiumello G, Heymsfield SB. Body mass index as a measure of adiposity among children and adolescents: a validation study. *J Pediatr.* 1998;132:204–210.
42. Warner JT, Cowan FJ, Dunstan FD, Gregory JW. The validity of body mass index for the assessment of adiposity in children with disease states. *Ann Hum Biol.* 1997;24:209–215.
43. Hannan WJ, Wrate RM, Cowen SJ, Freman CPL. Body mass index as an estimate of body fat. *Int J Eating Disord.* 1995;18:91–97.
44. Roche AF, Guo S, Moore WM. Weight and recumbent length from 1 to 12 mos of age: reference data for 1 mo increments. *Am J Clin Nutr.* 1989;49:599–607.
45. Baumgartner RN, Roche AF, Himes JH. Incremental growth tables. *Am J Clin Nutr.* 1986;43:711–722.
46. Roche AF, Guo S, Moore WM. Weight and recumbent length from 1–12 mos of age: reference data for 1 mo increments. *Am J Clin Nutr.* 1989;49:599–607.
47. Tanner JM, Davis PSW. Clinical longitudinal standards for North American children. *J Pediatr.* 1985; 107:317–329.
48. Tanner JM. Issues and advances in adolescent growth and development. *J Adolesc Health Care.* 1987;8:470–478.
49. Gong EJ, Spear BA. Adolescent growth and development: implication for nutritional needs. *J Nutr Educ.* 1988;20:273–278.
50. Jensen TG, Dudrick SJ, Johnston DA. A comparison of triceps skinfold and upper arm circumference measurements taken in standard and supine positions. *J Parenter Enter Nutr.* 1981;5:519–521.
51. Roche AF, Guo S, Baumgartner RN, Chumlea WC, Ryan AS, Kuczmarski RJ. Reference data for weight/stature^2 in Mexican-Americans from the Hispanic Health and Nutrition Examination Survey (HHANES 1982–1984). *Am J Clin Nutr.* 1990;51:917s–924s.
52. Behrman RE, Vaughan, eds. *Nelsons Textbook of Medicine.* 13th ed. Philadelphia, PA: WB Saunders Company, 1987.
53. Russell MS. Serum proteins and nitrogen balance: evaluating response to nutrition support. *Diet Nutr Support Newsletter* (practice group for the American Dietetic Association). 1995;17:3–7.
54. Dowliko J, Nomplegsi DJ. The role of albumin in human physiology and pathophysiology. III. Albumin and disease states. *J Parenter Enter Nutr.* 1991: 15:477–487.
55. Golden MHN. Transport proteins as indices of protein status. *Am J Clin Nutr.* 1982;35:1159–1165.

56. Yoder MC, Anderson DC, Gopalakrishna GS, Douglas SD, Polin RA. Comparison of serum fibronectin, prealbumin and albumin concentrations during nutritional repletion in protein-calorie malnourished infants. *J Pediatr Gastroenterol Nutr.* 1987;6:84–88.

57. Joyce DL, Waites KB. Clinical applications of c-reactive protein in pediatrics. *Pediatr Infect Dis J.* 1997; 16:735–747.

58. Collier SB, Hendricks KM. Nutrition Assessment. In: Baker RD, Baker SS, Daris AY, eds. *Pediatric Parenteral Nutrition.* New York: Chapman & Hall; 1997:42–63.

59. Buopane EA, Brown RO, Boucher BA, Fabian TC, Luther RW. Use of fibronectin and somatomedin C as nutritional markers in the enteral support of traumatized patients. *Crit Care Med.* 1989;17:126–132.

60. Graystone JE. Creatinine excretion during growth. In: Cheek DB, ed. *Human Growth.* Philadelphia: Lea & Febiger; 1968:182–197.

61. Viteri FE, Alvarado J. The creatinine height index: its use and the estimation of the degree of preterm depletion and repletion in protein calorie malnutrition. *Pediatrics.* 1970;46:696–706.

62. Merritt RJ, Blackburn GL. Nutritional assessment and metabolic response to illness of the hospitalized child. In: Suskind R, ed. *Textbook of Pediatric Nutrition.* New York: Raven Press; 1981:296.

63. Cecalupo AJ, Cohen HJ. Nutritional anemias. In: Grand RJ, Sutphen JL, Dietz WH. *Pediatric Nutrition.* Stonehaven, MA: Butterworth Heinemann; 1987:489–499.

64. Expert Scientific Working Group. Summary of a report on assessment of the iron nutritional status of the United States population. *Am J Clin Nutr.* 1985;42:1318–1330.

65. Recommendations to prevent and control iron deficiency in the United States. *CDC MMWR Morb Mortal Wkly Rep.* 1983;47(RR-3):1–25.

66. Dallman RR, Yip R, Johnson C. Prevalence and causes of anemia in the United States, 1976–1980. *Am J Clin Nutr.* 1984;39:437–445.

67. Yip R, Johnson C, Dallman PR. Age-related changes in laboratory values used in the diagnosis of anemia and iron deficiency. *Am J Clin Nutr.* 1984;39:427–436.

68. Yip R, Dallman PR. The roles of inflammation and iron deficiency as causes of anemia. *Am J Clin Nutr.* 1988;48:1295–1300.

69. Cecalupo AJ, Cohen HJ. Nutritional anemias. In: Grand RJ, Sutphen JL, Dietz WH Jr, eds. *Pediatric Nutrition: Theory and Practice.* Boston: Butterworth Publishing; 1987:491.

70. Puri S, Chandra RK. Nutritional regulation of host resistance and predictive value of immunologic tests in assessment of outcome. *Pediatr Clin North Am.* 1985; 32:499–515.

71. Hattner JT, Kerner JA Jr. Nutritional assessment of the pediatric patient. In: Kerner JA Jr, ed. *Manual of Pediatric Parenteral Nutrition.* New York: John Wiley & Sons; 1983:19–60.

72. Christakis G. Nutritional assessment in health programs. *Am J Public Health.* 1973;63(suppl):1–56.

73. Pipes PL, Bumbalo J, Glass RP. Collecting and assessing food intake information. In: Pipes P, ed. *Nutrition in Infancy and Childhood.* St. Louis, MO: Mosby; 1989:58–85.

74. Barrocas A. Complementary and alternative medicine: friend, foe, or OWA. *J Am Diet Assoc.* 1997;98:1373–1376.

75. *Alternative Medicine: Expanding Medical Horizons. Workshop on Alternative Medicine.* GPO No. 017-040-00537-7. Pittsburgh, PA: US Government Printing Office; 1994.

76. Eisenberg DM. Advising patients who seek alternative medical therapies. *Ann Int Med.* 1997;127:61–67.

77. Burke BS. The dietary history as a tool in research. *J Am Diet Assoc.* 1947;23:1041.

78. Frank GC, Hollatz AT, Webber LS, Berenson GS. Effect of interviewer recording practices on nutrient intake—Bogalusa Heart Study. *J Am Diet Assoc.* 1984;84:1432–1439.

79. Medlin C, Skinner JD. Individual dietary intake methodology; a 50-year review of progress. *J Am Diet Assoc.* 1988;88:1250–1257.

80. Block G. A review of validations of dietary assessment methods. *Am J Epidemiol.* 1982;114:492–504.

81. Persson LA, Carlgren G. Measuring children's diets: evaluation of dietary assessment techniques in infancy and childhood. *Int J Epidemiol.* 1984;113:506–517.

82. Carter RL, Sharbaugh CO, Stapell CA. Reliability and validity of the 24-hour recall. *J Am Diet Assoc.* 1981; 79:542–547.

83. Emmons L, Hayes M. Accuracy of 24-hr recalls of young children. *J Am Diet Assoc.* 1973;62:409–415.

84. St Jeor SR, Guthrie HA, Jones MB. Variability in nutrient intake in a 28-day period. *J Am Diet Assoc.* 1983:83;155–162.

85. Rockett HRH, Colditz GA. Assessing diets of children and adolescents. *Am J Clin Nutr.* 1997;65:1116–1122.

86. Willett WC, Sampson L, Stampfer MJ, et al. Reproducibility and validity of a semiquantitative food frequency questionnaire. *Am J Epidemiol.* 1985;122: 51–65.

87. Larkin FA, Metzner HL, Thompson FE, Flegal KM, Guire KE. Comparison of estimated nutrient intakes by food frequency and dietary records in adults. *J Am Diet Assoc.* 1989;89:215–223.

88. Fong AK, Kretsch MJ. Nutrition evaluation scale system reduces time and labor in recording quantitative dietary intake. *J Am Diet Assoc.* 1990;90:664–670.

89. Brown JE, Tharp TM, Dahlber-Luby EM, et al. Videotape dietary assessment: validity, reliability and comparison of results with 24-hour dietary recalls from elderly women in a retirement home. *J Am Diet Assoc.* 1990;90:1675–1679.

90. Ammerman AS, Kirkley BG, Dennis B, et al. A dietary assessment for individuals with low literacy skills using interactive touch-scan computer technology. *Am J Clin Nutr.* 1994;59:289S.

91. Subcommittee on the Tenth Edition of the RDAs, Food and Nutrition Board, National Research Council. *Recommended Dietary Allowances.* 10th ed. Washington, DC: National Academy Press; 1989.

92. Yates AA, Schlicker SA, Suitor CW. Dietary reference intakes: the new basis for recommendations for calcium and related nutrients, B vitamins, and chorine. *J Am Diet Assoc.* 1998;98:699–706.

93. Guthrie HA, The 1985 Dietary Allowance Committee; an overview. *J Am Diet Assoc.* 1985;85:1646–1648.

94. Garrel DR, Jobin N, De Jorge LHM. Should we still use the Harris and Benedict equations? *Nutr Clin Prac.* 1996;11:99–103.

95. Kaplan AS, Zemal BS, Neiswender KM, Stallings VA. Resting energy expenditure in clinical pediatrics; measured versus prediction equations. *J Pediatr.* 1995;127: 200–205.

96. World Health Organization. *Energy and Protein Requirements. Report of a Joint FAO/WHO/ UNU Expert Consultation.* WHO Technical Report Series No. 724. Geneva: World Health Organization; 1985.

97. Bursztein S, Elwyn DH, Askanazi J, Kinney JM. The theoretical framework of indirect calorimetry and energy balance. *Energy Metabolism, Indirect Calorimetry and Nutrition.* Baltimore: Williams & Wilkins; 1989:27–83.

98. Pencharz PB, Azcue MP. Measuring resting energy expenditure in clinical practice. *J Pediatr.* 1995;127: 269–271.

99. Cole CH, ed. *The Harriet Lane Handbook: A Manual for Pediatric House Officers.* 10th ed. Chicago: Year Book Medical Publishers; 1984:354.

100. Williams CS. Laboratory values and their interpretation. In: Krey SH, Murray RL, eds. *Dynamics of Nutrition Support: Assessment, Implementation, Evaluation.* Norwalk, CT: Appleton-Century-Crofts; 1986: 83–97.

101. Pencharz MB, Azcue MP. Measuring resting energy expenditure in clinical practice. *J Pediatr.* 1995;127: 269–271.

102. Harris JA, Benedict FG. *A Biometric Study of Basal Metabolism in Men.* No. 279. Carnegie Institute of Washington; 1919.

103. World Health Organization. *Energy and Protein Requirements.* WHO Technical Report Series No. 724. Geneva: World Health Organization; 1985.

104. Schofield WN. Predicting basal metabolic rate, new standards and review of previous work. *Hum Nutr Clin Nutr.* 1985;39c(1s):5–42.

105. Pierro MO, Hammond JP, Donnell SC, Lloyd DA. A new equation to predict the resting energy expenditure of surgical infants. *J Pediatr Surg.* 1994;29:1103–1105.

106. Phillips R, Ott K, Young B. Nutritional support and measured energy expenditure of the child and adolescent with head injury. *J Neurol Surg.* 1987;67: 846–851.

107. Kushner RF, Schoeller DA. Resting and total energy expenditure in patients with inflammatory bowel disease. *Am J Clin Nutr.* 1991;53:161–165.

108. Ramsey BW, Farrell PM, Pencharz P. Nutritional assessment and management in cystic fibrosis; a consensus report. *Am J Clin Nutr.* 1992;55:108–116.

109. Pierro A, Koletzko B, Carnielli V, Superine RA, Roberts EA, Filler RM, et al. Resting energy expenditure is increased in infants and children with extrahepatic biliary atresia. *J Pediatr Surg.* 1989;24:534–538.

110. Stallings VA, Zemol BS, Davies JC, Cronk CE, Charney EB. Energy expenditure of children and adolescents with severe disabilities; a cerebral palsy model. *Am J Clin Nutr.* 1996;64:627–634.

111. Mayes, TM, Gottschlich MM, Khoury J, Warren GD. Evaluation of predicted and measured energy requirements in burned children. *J Am Diet Assoc.* 1996;96: 24–29.

112. Powis MR, Smith K, Rennie M, Halliday D, Pierro A. Effect of major abdominal operations on energy and protein metabolism in infants and children. *J Pediatr Surg.* 1998;33:49–53.

113. Jones MO, Pierro P, Hammond P, Lloyd DA. The metabolic response to operative stress in infants. *J Pediatr Surg.* 1993;28:1258–1262.

114. Barton JS, Hindmarsh PC, Scrimseour CM, Rennie MJ, Preece MH. Energy expenditure in congenital heart disease. *Arch Dis Child.* 1994;70:5–9.

115. Grunfeld C, Feingold RR. Metabolic disturbances and wasting in the acquired immunodeficiency syndrome. *N Engl J Med.* 1992;327:329–337.

116. Kotler DP, Tierney AR, Brenner SK, Couture S, Wang J, Pierson RM. Of short-term energy balance in clinically stable patients with AIDS. *Am J Clin Nutr.* 1990; 51:7–13.

117. Dubois EF. Energy metabolism. *Ann Rev Physiol.* 1954;16:125–134.

118. Chwals, WJ. Overfeeding the critically ill child: fact or fantasy? *New Horizons.* 1994;2:147–155.

119. Coss-Bu JA, Jefferson LS, Walding D, Yadin D, Smith EO, Klish W. Resting energy expenditure in children in a pediatric intensive care unit: comparison of Harris-Benedict and Talbot predictions with indirect calorimetry values. *Am J Clin Nutr.* 1998; 67:74–80.

120. Bandini LG, Morelli JA, Must A, Dietz WH. Accuracy of standardized equations for predicting metabolic rate in premenarchal girls. *Am J Clin Nutr.* 1995;62: 711–714.

121. Matarese LE, Indirect calorimetry: technical aspects. *J Am Diet Assoc.* 1997;97:S154–160.

122. Weir JB. New methods for calculating metabolic rate with special reference to protein metabolism. *J Physiol.* 1949;109:1–9.

123. McClure SA, Snider TL. Use of indirect calorimetry in clinical nutrition. *NCP.* 1992;7:207–221.

124. Weissman C, Kemper M, Elwyn DH. The energy expenditure of the mechanically ventilated critically ill patient—an analysis. *Chest.* 1986;89:254–259.

125. Weisman C, Kemper M, Damask MC, et al. Effect of routine intensive care interactions on metabolic rate. *Chest.* 1984;86:815–818.

126. Swinamer DL, Phang PT, Jones RL, et al. Twenty-four hour energy expenditure in critically ill patients. *Crit Care Med.* 1987;15:637–643.

127. Bursztein S, Elwyn DH, Askanazi J, Kinney JM. The theoretical framework of indirect calorimetry and energy balance. *Energy Metabolism, Indirect Calorimetry and Nutrition.* Baltimore: Williams & Wilkins; 1989:27–83.

128. Porter C, Cohen NH. Indirect calorimetry in critically ill patients. Role of the clinical dietitian in interpreting results. *Am J Diet Assoc.* 1996;96:49–57.

129. Ireton-Jones CS, Turner WW Jr. The use of respiratory quotient to determine the efficacy of nutrition support systems. *J Am Diet Assoc.* 1987;87:180–183.

130. Waterlow JC. Classification and definition of protein-calorie malnutrition. *Br Med J.* 1972;3:566–569.

131. Mclaren DS, Read WWC. Classification of nutritional status in early childhood. *Lancet.* 1972;2:146–148.

132. Waterlow JC. Note on the assessment and classification of protein-energy malnutrition in children. *Lancet.* 1973;2:87–89.

133. Pollack MM, Ruttimann UE, Wiley JS. Nutritional depletions in critically ill children; associations with physiologic instability and increased quantity of care. *J Parenter Enter Nutr.* 1985;9:309–313.

Chapter 3

Nutrition for Premature Infants

Diane M. Anderson

Premature infants are defined as infants born before 37 weeks of gestation, as compared with full-term infants born from 38–42 weeks.[1] The physiologic immaturity of premature infants renders them susceptible to a number of problems (see Table 3–1), many of which imperil their nutrition and growth (see Table 3–2). Low birth weight (LBW) refers to infants with a birth weight of less than 2,500 g; very-low-birth-weight (VLBW) infants weigh less than 1,500 g, and extremely low-birth-weight (ELBW) infants weigh less than 1,000 g.[1,2] Infants can be LBW but yet be full term, due to poor intrauterine growth.

Assessment of intrauterine growth is determined by plotting the infant's birth weight by gestational age on various charts (see Appendix A). On the Lubchenco chart, infants who are small-for-gestational-age (SGA) have a birth weight less than the 10th percentile.[3] Large-for-gestational-age (LGA) infants have a birth weight greater than the 90th percentile.[3] Infants who are appropriate for gestational age are between the 10th and 90th percentiles. On the Babson Growth Chart, SGA and LGA are defined as two standard deviations from the mean birth weight.[4] Table 3–3 lists etiologies for SGA and Table 3–4 lists factors associated with LGA infants. The Babson chart can be used to follow the premature infant's growth through the first year of life. These assessments are used to anticipate medical and

Table 3–1 Potential Problems of the Premature Infant

Undernutrition	Asphyxia
Anemia	Respiratory distress syndrome
Retinopathy of prematurity	Uncoordinated suck and swallow
Poor temperature control	Hyperbilirubinemia
Apnea	Hypocalcemia
Glucose instability	Periventricular leukomalacia
Necrotizing enterocolitis	Infection
Intraventricular hemorrhage	Fat malabsorption
Decreased gastric motility	Limited renal function
Osteopenia	Hypotension
Patent ductus arteriosus	Bronchopulmonary dysplasia

Source: Data taken from references 2 and 61.

Table 3–2 Premature Infants' Risk Factors for Nutritional Deficiencies

1. Decreased nutrient stores
   - Premature infants are born before anticipated quantities of nutrients are deposited.
   - Low stores include glycogen, fat, protein, fat soluble vitamins, calcium, phosphorus, magnesium, and trace minerals.
2. Increased growth rate
   - Full-term infants often triple their birthweight by 1 year of age; for the preterm infant a tenfold increase may be needed to achieve optimal catch-up growth.
   - With rapid growth, energy and nutrient needs will be increased.
3. Immature physiological systems
   - Digestion and absorption capabilities are decreased due to low concentrations of lactase, pancreatic lipase, and bile salts.
   - Gastrointestinal motility and stomach capacity are decreased, which limits gastric emptying and feeding volume.
   - A coordinated suck and swallow is not developed until 32–34 weeks' gestation.
   - Hepatic enzymes are decreased, which may make specific amino acids conditionally essential (cysteine) or toxic (phenylalanine), due to the inability to synthesize or degrade.
   - Renal concentrating ability is limited.
4. Illnesses
   - Respiratory distress syndrome delays the introduction of enteral feedings because of the increased risk of aspiration. Gastrointestinal motility will also be decreased, and feedings may not be tolerated.
   - Patent ductus arteriosus often requires fluid restriction, which limits caloric intake. Infants are usually made NPO when a ductus is treated with indomethacin because the clinically significant ductus alters mesenteric blood flow. The infant is at risk for necrotizing enterocolitis.
   - Necrotizing enterocolitis forces nutrition management to parenteral nutrition for bowel rest. With refeeding, an elemental infant formula is often indicated. Some infants may develop short-gut syndrome as a complication and require extensive nutritional management for malabsorption.
   - Bronchopulmonary dysplasia leads to an increased energy demand with fluid restriction. Calorically dense formulas are often utilized. Chronic diuretic use will create electrolyte and calcium depletion.
   - Hyperbilirubinemia may be treated by phototherapy, which increases the infant's insensible water loss and fluid requirement. If exchange transfusion is needed, introduction of enteral feedings will be delayed. Necrotizing enterocolitis has been reported as a complication of exchange transfusion therapy.
   - Sepsis and suspected sepsis will result in withholding all enteral fluids until it is established that the infant is stable. The affected infant may have an altered mesenteric blood flow, which can result in necrotizing enterocolitis, or may have apnea, which may cause aspiration of feedings.

Source: Klaus MH and Fanaroff AA, *Care of the High-Risk Neonate,* ed 3, 1986, WB Saunders.

---

nutritional problems and management needs of the infant (see Table 3–5). For example, consider an infant born at 34 weeks' gestation whose birth weight is 1,200 g. This infant is premature as the gestational age is less than 37 weeks. On both the Lubchenco and Babson growth grids, the infant is SGA because birth weight is less than the 10th percentile or less than two standard deviations from the mean birth weight.

SGA infants are further classified by their body length and head circumference as symmetrically or asymmetrically growth retarded.[5] The symmetrically SGA infant's birth weight, head circumference, and body length are all classified as small, whereas the asymmetrically SGA infant has a small body weight but an appropriate head circumference and body length. The asymmetrically SGA infant is more likely to have catch up growth because poor intrauterine

Table 3–3 Etiologic Factors for SGA Births

Normal variation	High altitude
Pregnancy-induced hypertension	Elevated maternal hematocrit
Chronic hypertension	Multiple gestation
Chronic renal disease	Congenital malformations
Diabetes with vascular complications	Chromosomal abnormalities
Intrauterine infection	Placental insufficiency
Maternal malnutrition	Twin-to-twin transfusion
Cigarette smoking	Placental and cord defects
Drug or alcohol abuse	Short interpregnancy interval

Source: Data from reference 50.

Table 3–4 Factors Associated with LGA Births

Infant of diabetic mother	Genetic predisposition
Beckwith's syndrome	Rh isoimmunization
Transposition of the great vessels	High prepregnancy weight with large pregnancy weight gain
Miscalculation of expected day of confinement	

Source: Data from references 65 and 66.

growth has been of shorter duration.[5] This period of poor growth represents the last trimester of pregnancy and often results from placental insufficiency. The symmetrically SGA infant has frequently sustained an early insult to growth and development, such as infection, genetic abnormality, severe placental insufficiency, or maternal drug abuse.[6] Infants who experience these types of growth retardation usually do not obtain their full potential for physical growth and are at greater risk for poor neurologic development.[5]

Early studies suggested that catch-up growth for premature infants is limited to the first few years of life, but one recent report demonstrated that catch-up weight and length growth can continue through adolescence.[7,8] In another report, premature infants at 8 years of age were at approximately 50% for weight and height on the National Center for Health Statistics' growth charts, but they remained smaller than a comparison group of term infants who were matched for age and social economic status.[9] A suboptimal head circumference measurement at 8 months of age has been independently associated with decreased intellectual quotients, cognitive functioning skills, and behavior problems at school age.[10] Additional factors associated with poor developmental outcome include lower socioeconomic status, lower maternal education, and neurologic impairment of the infant.[5,11]

Premature infants represent a heterogeneous population for nutrition management. Intrauterine growth establishes nutritional status at birth, and gestational age determines physiologic nutrient need and feeding modality employed. Postnatally, as the infant matures, nutrient need and feeding modality will vary. Finally, the infant's clinical condition can change acutely and alter nutrition care. Due to these factors, their nutrition management is a day-to-day decision-making process regarding what to feed, what volume and nutrient density to provide, and how to administer nourishment. The goal is to provide nutrition for optimal growth and development to take place. The intrauterine growth rate and weight gain composition without meta-

Table 3–5 Anticipated Problems for SGA and LGA Infants

Problems	*Issues*
Small for gestational age	
Perinatal asphyxia	Enteral feedings may be delayed because of the risk of necrotizing enterocolitis.
Hypoglycemia	Caused by: Low glycogen stores Decreased gluconeogenesis Increased metabolic rate Decreased glycogenolysis Decreased counter-regulatory hormones Hyperinsulinemia
Increased energy demand	Caused by: Increased metabolic rate Increased growth rate Increased energy cost of growth
Heat loss	Caused by: Relatively large surface area Decreased subcutaneous fat
Large for gestational age	
Birth trauma	Shoulder dystocia, fractured clavicle, depressed skull fracture, brachial plexus palsy, facial paralysis
Hypoglycemia	Caused by hyperinsulinism

Source: Data from references 26, 28, 63, 65, and 67.

bolic complications has been advocated as the goal for premature infant nutrition.[12]

PARENTERAL NUTRITION

Parenteral nutrition is often indicated and initiated in the first few days of life to allow the premature infant to adapt to the extrauterine environment before enteral feedings are begun. It may also supplement enteral feedings, for premature infants have decreased enteral feeding tolerance and small gastric capacities, which limit volume intakes and advancements. Premature infants are at risk for necrotizing enterocolitis (NEC), and enteral feedings will be cautiously advanced.[12] Parenteral nutrition should be initiated within the first 24 hours of life to promote energy intake and glucose homeostasis, to establish nitrogen balance, and to prevent essential fatty acid deficiency.[13,14] The provision of amino acids as part of parenteral nutrition within the first 24 hours of life has been associated with nitrogen balance, improved glucose tolerance, increased protein synthesis, and normal plasma amino acid levels.[13,15] Tables 3–6 and 3–7 give suggested guidelines for parenteral administration of specific nutrients. Table 3–8 briefly describes a protocol for parenteral nutrition management.

For the premature infant who is not fluid restricted, adequate nutrition can be provided via a peripheral intravenous line. A central venous

Table 3–6 Parenteral Nutrition Guidelines: Energy, Energy Nutrients, and Minerals per Day

Nutrient	*Unit/kg*
Energy (kcal)	80–90
Glucose (mg/kg/min)	6-12
Fat (g)	0.5–3.0
Protein (g)	2.7–3.8
Sodium (mEq)	2–4
Potassium (mEq)	2–3
Chloride (mEq)	2–3
Calcium (mg)	60–100
Phosphorus (mg)	43–70
Magnesium (mg)	3.0–7.2
Zinc (μg)	400
Copper (μg)	20
Chromium (μg)	0.05–0.2
Manganese (μg)	1
Selenium (μg)	1.5–2.0
Molybdenum (μg)	0.25
Iodide (μg)	1

Source: Data taken from references 12 and 68.

Table 3–7 Parenteral Vitamin Guidelines per Day

Vitamin	*Dose/kg*	*Maximum Dose per Day**
Vitamin A (μg)	280	700
Vitamin E (mg)	2.8	7
Vitamin K (μg)	80	200
Vitamin D (μg)	4	10
Vitamin C (mg)	32	80
Thiamin (mg)	0.48	1.2
Riboflavin (mg)	0.56	1.4
Niacin (mg)	6.8	17
Vitamin B_6 (mg)	0.4	1
Folate (μg)	56	140
Vitamin B_{12} (μg)	0.4	1
Biotin (μg)	8	20
Pantothenic Acid (μg)	2	5

* Preterm infants receive 40% of the daily dose (2 mL/kg/d) MVI Pediatric (Armour Pharmaceuticals) per kg until the maximum daily dose (5 mL) is achieved at 2.5 kg.

Source: Data taken from references 12 and 69.

catheter is required for the infant who requires prolonged parenteral nutrition, has limited venous access, is fluid restricted, or has an increased nutrient demand that cannot be met by peripheral nutrition. The peripherally inserted central catheters (PICC) are frequently used with premature infants for the PICC line can be placed at an infant's bedside. A PICC line can reduce the stress to the infant of repeated insertion of peripheral lines and facilitate the delivery of concentrated parenteral nutrients.[16] A tunneled, central venous catheter must be placed surgically under anesthesia and is used when a PICC line cannot be inserted or a prolonged course of parenteral nutrition is planned.

Management Concerns and Medical Problems

Fluid management is very individualized for the preterm infant. Insensible water losses will be high, and the infant's renal function and neuroendocrine control will be immature.[17] Fluid overload should be avoided to prevent the development of NEC, bronchopulmonary dysplasia, patent ductus arteriosus, and intraventricular hemorrhage.[17] Table 3–9 gives laboratory parameters that should be observed in guiding parenteral nutrition therapy.

Insensible fluid losses are high for many reasons.[18] First, the premature infant's skin offers little protection from evaporative losses. The skin of a premature infant has a high water content, and the epidermis is thin and highly permeable. Second, environmental factors in the newborn intensive care unit increase insensible fluid losses, eg, the use of radiant warmers, phototherapy, and high or low ambient temperature.[18] These losses can be decreased by the use of humidified incubators, plastic shields, and plastic wraps or clothing.

Preterm infants have a limited ability to hydrolyze triglycerides. Elevated serum triglycer-

Table 3–8 Parenteral Nutrition Progression

	DOL to Begin	*Beginning Quantity*	*Increase*	*Maximum or Goal*	*Considerations*
Fluid (mL/kg/d)	1	80–100	10–20	140–160	
Glucose (mg/kg/min)	1	4–6	1–2	11–12	• Begin on DOL 1 to prevent hypoglycemia. • Decrease glucose load for hyperglycemia. Glucose homeostasis will usually improve in 1–2 days. • Insulin infusions should be used with caution. The dose is 0.05–0.1 U/kg/hr.
Sodium Chloride (mEq/kg)	2–5	1–3	—	2–5	• Allow diuresis to occur the first few days of life to decrease extracellular blood volume. • Start sodium to prevent hyponatremia.
Potassium (mEq/kg)	2	1–3	—	2–3	• Excretion of potassium is not obligatory on DOL 1. • Add potassium after urine flow is established and serum potassium level is normal. • Check for hyperkalemia as the ELBW infant has a decreased glomerular filtration rate, acidosis, and the release of nitrogen and potassium secondary to negative nitrogen balance.
Amino Acids (g/kg/d)	1	1.5	1.0	3.5–3.8	
Lipids (g/kg/d)	1	0.5	0.5	3.0	• Provide at rate no greater than 0.12–0.15 g/kg/d. • Provide over an 18–24 hr period. • With hyperbilirubinemia, limit to 0.5 g/kg/d.
Vitamins and Minerals	1				

DOL, day of life; ELBW, extremely low birth weight.

Parenteral nutrition progression may be slowed with fluid and electrolyte imbalance, renal failure, the anticipation of enteral feedings, or the initiation and tolerance of enteral feedings.

Source: Data from references 12, 13, 28, 43, 68, and 70.

Table 3–9 Fluid and Electrolyte Monitoring Parameters

Fluid intake	80–150 mL/kg†
Urine output	1–4 mL/kg/h, up to 6–9 mL/kg/h for ELBW‡
Daily body weights	Allow 1–3% daily weight loss or 10–20 % maximum total weight loss
Serum sodium	135–145 mEq/L
Serum potassium	3.5–5.0 mEq/L
Serum chloride	98–108 mEq/L
Serum creatinine	0.3–1.0 mg/dL
Blood urea nitrogen	3–25 mg/dL
Urine specific gravity	1.005–1.015
Urine osmolality	100–500 mOsm

† The critically ill premature infant has highly variable fluid needs. This range represents the usual volume of fluid administered. To prevent over- or underhydration, fluids should be provided to keep the other monitoring parameters within normal levels.

‡ ELBW = extremely low birth weight

Source: Data from references 18, 43, 63, 71, and 72.

ide levels are more frequently found with decreasing gestational age, infection, surgical stress, malnutrition, and with the SGA infant.[16] In addition, intravenous lipid administration should be limited for the premature infant suffering from hyperbilirubinemia.[12] It is believed that the free fatty acids released from the lipids will compete with the indirect bilirubin for binding onto the albumin molecule. Without binding to albumin, bilirubin can cross the blood–brain barrier and cause kernicterus. A dosage of 0.5 g/kg/day has been suggested, and this level will prevent essential fatty acid deficiency.[16]

Several amino acid solutions are formulated for the pediatric patient.[19] These solutions contain a larger percentage of total nitrogen as essential amino acids and branched-chain amino acids, and a balanced pattern of nonessential amino acids instead of a single amino acid concentration. Improved weight gain and nitrogen balance have been associated with its use.[20] The addition of cystine to Trophamine (Kendall McGraw Laboratories), one of the pediatric amino acid solutions, has suggested improved nitrogen balance[13] which may reflect the reformulation of Trophamine with N-acetyl-L-tyrosine.[16] The addition of cysteine hydrochloride has not consistently improved nitrogen balance.[21]

Transition to Enteral Feedings

Weaning to enteral feedings is a slow process that is necessary to facilitate feeding tolerance and to prevent the development of necrotizing enterocolitis.[22] Enteral feedings are gradually increased in volume and strength as parenteral fluids are decreased at a similar volume. The two fluid types are coordinated to keep stable the total fluids provided until enteral feedings provide adequate nutrition for growth. Parenteral fluids are discontinued at approximately 100–120 mL/kg/day of enteral feedings. The infant should receive full enteral feedings within 3 days.

ENTERAL NUTRITION

Enteral feeding is initiated when the infant has become clinically stable. Table 3–10 outlines factors in deciding to initiate enteral feeding, and Table 3–11 describes some of the risks and benefits of enteral feedings. Minimal or trophic feedings have been advocated with the premature infant.[12,22–24] These feedings are small volumes of feedings given to nourish the gut but which do not serve as a major source of nutrition. The concerns listed in Table 3–10 are often ignored with the introduction of trophic feedings. When the infant's condition stabilizes, feedings are advanced. On the other hand, feedings can be safely initiated and advanced during the first week of life for many infants. Feeding advancement for the VLBW infant is often limited to 20 mL/kg/day or less as rapid feeding advancement has been associated with NEC.[12,25–28] Trophic feedings have not been associated with the development of NEC.[12]

Table 3–10 Traditional Considerations in Initiating Enteral Feedings

1. Vital signs stable
2. Bowel sounds present
3. Abdomen not distended
4. Medical risk factors
   - Absence of asphyxiation or low Apgar scores
   - Respiratory distress syndrome
   - Apnea and bradycardia
   - Acute sepsis
   - Hypotension
5. Equipment barriers or procedures
   - Ventilators (inhibit feeding by mouth)
   - Oxygen therapy
   - Intubation/extubation
   - Exchange transfusion
   - Umbilical arterial catheter
6. Experience of staff
   - Dictates when feeds will be started
   - Dictates which feeding methods can be employed
7. Physical development
   - Dictates method of feeding
   - Coordinated suck and swallow present at 32–34 weeks of gestation
   - Small gastric size and slow emptying, which limit feed volume and rate

Source: Data from references 12, 26, 47, 62, and 73.

Table 3–11 Risks and Benefits of Introducing Enteral Feedings

Risks	*Benefits*
Necrotizing enterocolitis	Shortens physiologic jaundice
Aspiration	Prevents cholestatic jaundice
Feeding intolerance	Stimulates gastrointestinal tract development
Intestinal perforation with transpyloric feedings	Allows full-volume feeds earlier
	Increases weight gain
	Lowers alkaline phosphatase activity levels

Source: Data from references 12 and 22–24.

The type of formula selected depends on individual factors and can sometimes involve complex decisions. Table 3–12 lists factors that must be considered. Whatever formula is chosen, it should provide appropriate amounts of energy, protein, minerals, and vitamins (see Table 3–13). The goal is to promote growth and to prepare the infant for discharge. In Table 3–14 selected nutrients are compared (at 150 mL of milk or formula). This value represents the average volume of intake for a premature infant on full enteral feedings. Fortified human milk or premature infant formulas will meet the needs of most premature infants.

The premature infant's vitamin need will be met by the use of fortified human milk or premature infant formula without additional supplementation.[12] Iron needs will be met by the consumption of 120 kcal/kg of an iron-fortified premature infant formula; this will provide 2 mg/kg of iron, which is within the 2–4 mg/kg/day goal.[12] For the infant receiving human milk, iron supplementation can be initiated at 2–4 mg/kg/day, once full-volume feedings have been achieved. The human milk fortifiers do not contain iron. The infant receiving a combination of human milk and formula can be given 2 mg/kg/day of iron. Depending on formula intake, the infant will receive a total of 2–4 mg/kg/day from all sources.

Pharmacologic dosage of vitamin E (50–100 mg/kg/day) for premature infants to prevent retinopathy of prematurity, bronchopulmonary dysplasia (BPD), or intraventricular hemorrhage is not recommended.[12,29] Although vitamin E is an antioxidant, it has not consistently prevented these illnesses, and complications associated with its pharmacologic dosing include NEC, sepsis, intraventricular hemorrhage, and death.[29] With the use of erythropoietin therapy, iron has been provided at 6 mg/kg/day to facilitate red cell production and a vitamin E supplement of 15 IU/day has been given to prevent hemolytic anemia.[30]

A daily intake of 1,500–2,800 IU/kg/day of vitamin A has been suggested to prevent bronchopulmonary dysplasia by this vitamin's me-

Table 3–12 Milk and Formula Selection Indications and Concerns

	Indications	*Concerns*
Human milk	• Nutrients are readily absorbed. • Anti-infective factors are present. • The incidence of necrotizing enterocolitis is decreased. • Hormones, enzymes and growth factors are present. • Nutrient composition is unique. • Maternal–infant attachment may be enhanced. • Maternal emotional support by the family and health care team is indicated to facilitate lactation.	• Milk from mothers who deliver prematurely will often contain a higher protein concentration than that found in the milk from mothers who deliver at term. This elevated protein concentration decreases by 28 days of lactation and may not meet the protein needs of the rapidly growing premature infant. • The concentration of protein, calcium, phosphorus, and sodium is too low to meet the needs of many premature infants. To increase nutrient density, human milk fortifiers should be added to the milk. • Milk volume production may be inadequate to nourish the infant.
Formulas for premature infants	• Glucose polymers comprise 50–60% of the carbohydrate calories, which decreases the lactose load presented to the premature infant for digestion. Glucose polymers also decrease the osmolality of the formula. • Lactose comprises 40–50% of the carbohydrate calories, which facilitates calcium absorption. • Medium chain triglycerides (MCTs) are 40–50% of the fat calories. MCTs do not require pancreatic lipase or bile salts for digestion and absorption. • Protein is at a higher concentration than that incorporated into standard infant formulas to meet the increased protein needs of the preterm infant. • The protein is a 60/40 whey/casein ratio, as compared with the 18/82 whey/casein ratio found in bovine milk. This whey predominance prevents the elevation of plasma phenylalanine and tyrosine levels.	• Feeding volumes and strengths should be advanced slowly with the very LBW infant. • The bottle of formula must be shaken prior to use to suspend the minerals. • With any signs of feeding intolerance, feedings should be discontinued, diluted, decreased, or not advanced.

continues

Table 3–12 continued

	Indications	*Concerns*
	• Calcium and phosphorus are 2–3 times the concentration found in standard infant formulas. These levels will maintain normal serum calcium and phosphorus levels, prevent osteopenia, and promote calcium and phosphorus accretion at the fetal rate. • Sodium, potassium, and chloride concentrations are greater than in standard infant formulas to meet the increased electrolyte needs of the premature infant. • Vitamins, trace minerals, and additional minerals are incorporated into these formulas at a high concentration to meet the infant's increased nutrient need while facilitating a limited volume intake. • Iron-fortified formulas are available, which decreases the number of high-osmolar supplements that must be provided to the premature infant. • Formula osmolarity is within the physiologic range at 210–270 mOsm/L, which facilitates formula tolerances and decreases the risk of necrotizing enterocolitis. • Infants with osteopenia may be discharged home on these formulas. • Premature formulas can be used until the infant reaches 2.5–3.6 kg, depending on the formula vitamin concentration and volume intake.	
Transition formulas	• Designed for the premature infant at discharge. The infant should weigh at least 1.8 kg when this formula is provided.	• It is unclear how long infants should remain on the transition formula.

continues

Table 3–12 continued

	Indications	*Concerns*
	• Formula should be initiated at least 2 days prior to discharge to document formula tolerance and weight gain. • Formulas have the nutrient composition that is between the concentrated premature formulas and the standard infant formulas. • Glucose polymers comprise 50–60% of the carbohydrate calories, and lactose comprises 40–50%. • MCTs are 20–25% of the fat calories. • The protein is either a 60/40 or a 50/50 whey/casein ratio. • Improved bone mineral concentration and greater weight and length gains were documented with premature infants fed a transition formula for the first 9 months of life.	
Standard infant formulas	• They were fed to premature infants after discharge from the hospital, but the transition formulas are often used.	• Nutrient content is inadequate for the small premature infant during the neonatal period. • During the early neonatal period, these formulas may not be tolerated well. Lactose is the sole carbohydrate source, and only long chain fatty acids are incorporated into these formulas.
Elemental infant formulas	• Premature infants who do not tolerate premature formulas will often benefit from a formula containing glucose polymers, protein hydrolysate, and MCT oil. • Infants who are recovering or suffering from gastrointestinal disorders can benefit from elemental infant formulas.	• Nutrient content is inadequate for the premature infant, with special reference to calcium and phosphorus levels. • The time to switch to a premature formula must always be considered to improve nutrient intake. Depending on the infant's feeding history, the formulas can be switched or a stepwise approach of mixing the two formulas with altering parts per solution can be used.

continues

Table 3–12 continued

	Indications	*Concerns*
Soy formulas		• These formulas are not indicated for premature infants who weigh <1.8 kg. • The premature infant is at risk for osteopenia. The phytates in the formula bind phosphorus and make it unavailable for absorption. • The amino acid profile may be inappropriate for the premature infant. • Decreased weight gain and length growth have been reported when soy formulas were fed to premature infants.

Source: Data from references 12, 27, 47, and 74–84.

Table 3–13 Enteral Nutrient Guidelines per kg/day

Nutrient	*Amount*	*Nutrient*	*Amount*
Energy (kcal)	105–130	Molybdenum (μg)	0.3
Protein (g)	3–4	Iodine (μg)	6–60
Carbohydrate (g)	10.8–16.8	Vitamin A (IU)	90–1500
Fat (g)	5.4–7.2	Vitamin D (IU)	150–400
Sodium (mEq)	2.0–3.5	Vitamin E (IU)	1.3–12
Potassium (mEq)	2–3	Vitamin K (μg)	4.8–10
Chloride (mEq)	2–3	Vitamin C (mg)	18–42
Calcium (mg)	120–230	Thiamin (μg)	48–240
Phosphorus (mg)	60–140	Riboflavin (μg)	72–360
Magnesium (mg)	7.9–15	Niacin (mg)	0.3–4.8
Iron (mg)	2–4	Vitamin B_6 (μg)	42–210
Zinc (μg)	600–1000	Folate (μg)	25–50
Copper (μg)	108–125	Vitamin B_{12} (μg)	0.18–0.3
Chromium (μg)	0.1–0.5	Biotin (μg)	1.8–6.0
Manganese (μg)	6.0–7.5	Pantothenic acid (mg)	0.36–1.8
Selenium (μg)	1.3–3.0		

Source: Data taken from references 12 and 68.

Table 3–14 Selected Nutrient Comparison per 150 mL of Milk or Formula

Guidelines (per kg)	*Human*	*Standard*	*Transition*	*Premature*
120 kcal	101	101	111–112	121
3.5–4.0 g protein	1.6–2.1	2.1	2.9–3.2	3.3–3.6
2.5–3.5 mEq sodium	1.2–1.7	1.0–1.2	1.6–1.7	2.0–2.3
210 mg calcium	38–42	79	118–134	200–218
110 mg phosphorus	20–21	43–54	69–74	100–109
270 IU vitamin D	3.0	61	78–89	181–327

Source: Data from references 74 and 85.

diation of cell differentiation, but benefits have not been consistently reported.[31,32] These studies of relatively small sample sizes do not reflect today's practices of giving prenatal steroids, surfactants, and/or corticosteroids to premature infants.[33] These variables may affect the incidence of BPD, and the use of corticosteroids will increase the release of retinol and retinol-binding protein from tissue. The American Academy of Pediatrics states that additional vitamin A may be helpful, but further investigation is necessary.[12] A randomized control trial with a large sample size that reflects today's care in the newborn intensive care unit is needed to determine whether larger doses of vitamin A would be helpful and safe.[33]

Osteopenia or poor bone mineralization is commonly reported for premature infants when the intake of calcium and phosphorus is inadequate or when mineral losses are excessive, adding to their poor nutrient stores at birth.[34] Risk factors include prolonged parenteral nutrition, diets of unfortified human milk, and/or chronic diuretic therapy. A diet of fortified human milk or premature infant formula will meet the infant's needs.[12,34] Vitamin D intake at 200–400 IU per day with the calcium- and phosphorus-enriched premature formula is adequate.[35] With osteopenia, vitamin D at 800 IU per day can be safely provided but does not appear necessary.[34]

Premature infants are at risk for trace mineral deficiency, due to their poor nutrient stores at birth, rapid growth, and dependence on adequate intake. With use of today's parenteral guidelines and premature infant formula or fortified human milk, deficiencies should be uncommon. Infants who have excessive losses via an ileostomy drainage or high urine output related to renal failure could need 2–3 times the recommended guidelines for zinc.[36] Additional cases of zinc deficiency have been reported when the mother's milk had an extremely low zinc content or when the infant had been provided with oral copper and/or iron supplements, which will compete with zinc for absorption.[37]

The feeding method employed will depend on the nursery staff experience and on the infant's gestational age and clinical condition.[12] Table 3–15 describes methods in use, and Table 3–16 gives guidelines for amounts and rates of feedings. Due to the infant's constantly changing clinical condition and development, several feeding methods may be used. Both continuous and bolus infusions are used with gavage feedings.[38] The use of transpyloric feedings dictates the use of continuous infusion to prevent the presenting of an osmotic load to the intestine,

Table 3–15 Methods of Feeding a Premature Infant

Type	*Considerations*
Breast/bottle	Most physiological methods Infant at least 32–34 weeks' gestation Infant medically stable Infant's respiratory rate less than 60 breaths per minute
Gavage	Supplement to breast/bottle feedings Suggested for infants less than 32 weeks gestation Use when respiratory rate less than 80 breaths per minute Use for intubated infant Use for neurologically impaired neonate
Transpyloric	Employ when gavage feedings not tolerated Use when the infant is at risk for aspiration Infant intubated Use for the infant with decreased gut motility Must wait for passage of tube to begin feedings Requires radiographic assessment to check placement Complications include dumping syndrome, altered intestinal microflora, nutrient malabsorption, perforation of intestine
Gastrostomy	Use for gastrointestinal malformation Use for neurologically impaired infant

Source: Data from references 12, 27, 42, and 49.

Table 3–16 Suggested Feeding Guidelines*

Weight (g)	*Feeding Interval*	*Beginning Volume (cc/kg/d)*	*Feeding Increments (cc/kg/d)*	*Days to Full Feedings*†
<1,000	q 2 h	10	10	16
1,000–1,500	q 2–3 h	10–20	15–20	10–7
1,501–1,800 sick‡	q 3 h	10–20	20–30	7–5
1,501–1,800 healthy‡	q 3 h	20–40	30–50	5–3
>1,800 sick‡	q 3 h	20–40	30–75	5–2

* Data obtained from guidelines used at The Children's Hospital Medical University of South Carolina. Advancement of feedings should occur only as the infant demonstrates tolerance of enteral feedings. Clinical signs of feeding intolerance or illness dictate discontinuing feedings or holding the advancement of feedings. Clinical signs are discussed in the nutritional assessment section of this chapter. Infants are started on either full-strength human milk or 20 kcal/oz premature formula. At 120–150 mL/kg, fortifier is added to human milk, and the premature infant formula is changed to the 24 kcal/oz formula. Iron supplements are added at 2–4 mg/kg for the human milk fed infant.[12]

† *Full feedings* are defined as 120 kcal/kg of a 24 kcal milk.

‡ *Sick* refers to infants who have had symptoms of any medical or surgical condition, other than uncomplicated prematurity. *Healthy* refers to term or preterm infants who have had no symptomatic medical or surgical conditions.

Source: Data from The Children's Hospital, Medical University of South Carolina.

with subsequent dumping.[12] The delivery of nutrients to the infant is decreased with continuous infusion.[12] Specifically, human milk fat, fat additives, and minerals in the human milk fortifier adhere to or precipitate in the delivery system.[12,27,39] The use of a syringe pump with the syringe in an upright position will increase fat delivery.[27,40] Numerous studies have been completed on feeding methodologies, but there is no consensus on which method is best or whether there are different results from continuous infusion and bolus feedings.[12,38] Each method has its benefits, but neither is superior in promoting feeding tolerance for all premature infants.

Breastfeeding

Mothers who want to breastfeed their premature infant must usually express their milk. During the infant's prolonged hospitalization, it will be difficult for the mother to be available for 24-hour breastfeeding. Many premature infants are too weak or too small to breastfeed. Family members, friends, and nursery staff must provide support for these women to enable them to be successful in providing milk during this stressful period (see Table 3–17). Kangaroo care (skin-to-skin contact between the parent and the infant) will facilitate parent-infant bonding and has been linked to a longer period of lactation by the mother who delivers prematurely.[41] A lactation consultant can be called upon to offer guidance and ongoing support.

NUTRITIONAL ASSESSMENT

Dietary Considerations

Assessments must be made daily to determine need for changing feeding volume, solution strength, or feeding method. Intake is evaluated against nutrient guidelines. Finally, feeding technique should be advanced to the most physiologic method possible for the infant. Breast or

Table 3–17 Steps To Support Lactating Women

1. Instruction
   - Methods of milk expression
   - Sterilization of expression equipment
   - Storage and transport of milk
   - Diet for lactation
   - Tips for relaxation
2. Tips to help with let down prior to expression
   - Showering
   - Hand massaging of the breasts
   - Applying warm washcloths to the breasts
   - Consuming warm beverages
   - Visiting the infant
   - Talking to the infant's nurse by phone
   - Placing the infant's picture on the pump
3. Nursery staff and nursery support
   - Electric pump and breastfeeding room conveniently available to the nursery
   - Hand pumps available for purchase
   - Education of nursery staff on milk expression
   - Mother's milk used to feed the infant whenever it is available
   - Help mother with the initiation of nursing
   - Promote kangaroo care
4. Initiation of breastfeeding
   - Wake baby up
   - Express a little milk prior to nursing so nipple is easier to grasp by the small infant
   - Position infant so mother and infant are stomach to stomach
   - Allow mother to room in with baby prior to discharge to establish breastfeeding pattern

Source: Data from reference 41, 86, and 87.

bottle feedings are introduced as the infant's coordination of sucking, swallowing, and breathing is developed at 32–34 weeks of gestation.[12] The number of oral feedings should be increased per day as the infant demonstrates the ability to feed effectively. Feedings are usually limited to 20 minutes per feeding period to prevent fatigue and excessive energy expenditure.[42] Feedings may be limited to once a day until the infant demonstrates successful feeding.

Anthropometric Measurements

Anthropometric measurements are difficult to perform on a premature infant, principally due to the infant's small size and clinical condition. Medical equipment can interfere with the measurement or can add to the recorded weight. Also, the infant is at risk for cold stress during these procedures, which diverts energy from growth to heat production.

Daily weights should be recorded on a premature infant growth grid (see Appendix A). Weights will be influenced by the medical equipment attached to the infant, the use of different scales, the infant's hydration status, and the infant's total nutrient intake. Weights taken at the same time each day will avoid recording diurnal variations. Initial weight loss, which reflects the loss of extracellular fluid, ranges from 10% to 20% of birth weight during the first week of life.[43] After regaining birth weight, the weight gain goal is 10–20 g/kg/day or 15–30 g/day.[44] When the infant weighs 2.5 kg, a weight gain of 20–30 g/day is appropriate.[27]

Head circumference should be measured weekly. Alterations in measurement will occur from birth to week 1 of life, due to head molding or edema. Additional errors are introduced when scalp intravenous lines are employed or the head has been shaved. The measurement should be recorded on a premature growth grid (see Appendix A). The goal is 0.5–0.8 cm/wk.[44] Length measurements are difficult to obtain accurately. Length should increase by 1 cm/wk.[27]

Skinfolds and midarm circumference measurements do not change rapidly enough to be more helpful than weight measurements for diet changes. These measurements are generally not employed for routine clinical care but are indicated for growth studies. There are limited standards for these measurements.[45,46]

Assessing Inadequate Weight Gain

When a series of daily measurements indicates inadequate weight gain, a search must be made for the cause. Table 3–18 outlines areas to check.

Table 3–18 Possible Etiologies of Inadequate Weight Gain

1. Nutrient calculations are incorrect.
2. Infant is not receiving ordered diet.
   - Intravenous fluid administration has been interrupted to give blood or drugs, or the intravenous line has become infiltrated.
   - Infant is unable to consume what is ordered by bottle, and no gavage supplements were provided.
   - Feedings were held because the infant's respiratory rate increased or body temperature instability developed.
3. Infant does not tolerate given formula.
4. Calculated nutrient guidelines are inadequate for the infant due to growth retardation, illness, or high physical activity.
5. Infant is cold stressed.
6. Infant has outgrown previous diet order.
7. Nutrition solution was not prepared correctly.
8. Incorrect formula was provided to infant.

Assessment of Feeding Tolerance

Feeding intolerance and clinical compromise are common for the premature infant, so constant surveillance is required to detect early signs of feeding intolerance, sepsis, or NEC.[47] Depending on the findings, feedings may be held, decreased, diluted, or discontinued; or their frequency may be changed. Feedings will often be held upon signs of illness, including persistent apnea and bradycardia or temperature instability. Clinical parameters are discussed below.

Gastric residuals are often present; however, exactly what constitutes an unacceptable volume is difficult to define. Some infants have small aspirates, no matter what the feeding volume and yet are tolerating feedings.[48] With bolus feedings, a residual of up to 50% of the feeding volume or the hourly rate for continuous feeding is often accepted. Mucus residuals are not a concern and are present in the infant recovering from lung disease. Undigested formula may indicate that the feeding volume is too large, that the infant does not tolerate this formula, that the infant has poor gastrointestinal motility, or that the infant has NEC or intestinal obstruction. Residuals containing bile are not uncommon when the infant is fed transpylorically.[47,49]

Abdominal girth circumference increases will occur with growth, air swallowing, feeding intolerance, infrequent stooling, or NEC. An increase of 1.5 to 2 cm is considered significant, and feedings should be held.[50,51] A workup for sepsis and NEC may be considered when other signs of feeding intolerance or increase in abdominal tone are noted. Visible loops of bowel may indicate illness.

Blood in the stool is a concern and should be evaluated. Blood may be a sign of illness, feeding tube irritation of the intestine, anal fissure, or blood swallowed during delivery.

Assessment of Nutrient Adequacy and Tolerance

Both the specific clinical signs of nutrient deficiency/toxicity and the associated laboratory values should be regularly assessed. Vitamin assays should be performed when pharmacologic dosing of vitamins is underway to permit detection of vitamin toxicity or when a deficiency is suspected.[52] There are several reviews on clinical signs.[29,53–55] Acceptable standards for laboratory values are difficult to establish because premature infants differ by their physical maturity, clinical condition, and nutrient stores. For example, serum proteins will vary by the infant's hepatic maturity, energy and protein intake, vitamin and mineral nutritional status, and clinical condition.

During the first week of life, serum electrolytes, glucose, creatinine, and urea nitrogen, are monitored daily, and serum Ca, P, Mg levels may be examined twice per week. Blood levels will be checked more frequently when values are abnormal. As these blood parameters stabilize, they can be examined twice weekly or with changes in parenteral nutrition formulation and as needed for infants on enteral feedings.[56] Serum electrolytes are assessed for those infants receiving diuretics. Additional parameters monitored when parenteral nutrition is being administered include serum triglycerides to check lipid tolerance, direct bilirubin to detect cholestatic jaundice, and serum alanine aminotransferase (ALT, serum glutamic-pyruvic transaminase) to evaluate hepatic function.[52] Serum calcium, phosphorus, and alkaline phosphatase levels are monitored in infants at risk for osteopenia. Infants at risk are those fed unfortified human milk or nonpremature infant formulas, those receiving long-term parenteral nutrition, or those being treated with chronic diuretic therapy. Hematocrit and hemoglobin levels are checked as needed.

DISCHARGE CONCERNS

The premature infant is ready for discharge from the hospital when body temperature can be maintained, breastfeeding or bottle feeding supports growth, and cardiorespiratory function is mature and stable.[57] Additionally, the caretaker must be ready to care for this high-risk infant. Twenty-four-hour visitation allows the parents to become active in caring for their infants. Rooming in with the infant will help to facilitate care and give confidence to the parent.[58]

The infant should be evaluated for participation in the Special Supplemental Nutrition Program for Women, Infants, and Children (WIC) and for enrollment in a developmental follow-up program for premature infants. The follow-up program should monitor the infant's growth and development, offer aid with chronic illness management, provide early detection of problems, make referrals to specialized services as indicated, and give the parents support and guidance in caring for their prematurely born infant.[59] A primary care physician must be identified to provide well-baby and sick care, and an appointment should be established prior to discharge to home.[57] Most infants will be discharged home on human milk, standard infant formula, or transition formula. The breastfed infant should receive a multiple vitamin with iron supplement, and the infant who is fed formula with iron will not require additional supplementation. Infants who have osteopenia should be discharged home on premature infant formula until the osteopenia resolves. Infants suffering from bronchopulmonary dysplasia may need a nutrient-dense formula. The transitional formulas can be concentrated easily to 24 or 27 kcal per ounce.

CONCLUSIONS

Although premature infants begin life in a compromised nutritional state, nutrition and medical therapies that enhance the infant's potential for optimal growth and development continue to evolve.[60] Daily nutrition evaluation of the premature infant is necessary to ensure that appropriate nutrition therapy can be provided.

REFERENCES

1. American Academy of Pediatrics and American College of Obstetricians and Gynecologists. *Guidelines for Perinatal Care.* 4th ed. Elk Grove, IL: American Academy of Pediatrics; 1997.
2. Fanaroff AA, Martin RJ, eds. Neonatal-Perinatal Medicine. *Diseases of the Fetus and Infant.* Vol. 1, 6th ed. St. Louis, MO: Mosby; 1997.
3. Battaglia FC, Lubchenco LO. A practical classification of newborn infants by weight and gestational age. *J Pediatr.* 1967;71:159–163.
4. Babson SG, Benda GI. Growth graphs for the clinical assessment of infants of varying gestational age. *J Pediatr.* 1976;89:814–820.
5. Bernstien S, Heimler R, Sasidharan P. Approaching the management of the neonatal intensive care unit graduate through history and physical assessment. *Pediatr Clin North Am.* 1998;45:79–105.
6. Frieman AA, Bernbaum JC. Growth outcome of critically ill neonates. In: Polin RA, Fox WW, eds. *Fetal and Neonatal Physiology.* Vol. 1, 2nd ed. Philadelphia: W.B. Saunders Company; 1998:394–400.
7. Hack M, Merkatz IR, McGrath SK, Jones PK, et al. Catch-up growth in very-low-birth-weight infants. *Am J Dis Child.* 1984;138:370–375.
8. Hirata T, Bosque E. When they grow up: The growth of extremely low birth weight (≤1,000 gm) infants at adolescence. *J Pediatr.* 1989;132:1033–1035.
9. Hack M, Weissman B, Borawski-Clark E. Catch-up growth during childhood among very low-birth-weight

children. *Arch Pediatr Adolesc Med.* 1996;150:1122–1129.

10. Hack M, Breslau N, Weissman B, Aram D, et al. Effect of very low birth weight and subnormal head size on cognitive abilities at school age. *N Engl J Med.* 1991;325:231–237.
11. Kitchen WH, Doyle LW, Ford GW, Callanan C, et al. Very low birth weight and growth to age 8 years. II: Head dimensions and intelligence. *Am J Dis Child.* 1992;146:46–50.
12. American Academy of Pediatrics Committee on Nutrition. Nutritional needs of preterm infants. In: Kleinman RE, ed. *Pediatric Nutrition Handbook.* 4th ed. Elk Grove Village, IL: American Academy of Pediatrics. 1998:55–88.
13. Rivera A, Bell EF, Bier DM. Effect of intravenous amino acids on protein metabolism of preterm infants during the first three days of life. *Pediatr Res.* 1993;33:106–111.
14. Murdock N, Crighton A, Nelson LM, Forsyth JS. Low birthweight infants and total parenteral nutrition immediately after birth. II. Randomised study of biochemical tolerance of intravenous glucose, amino acids, and lipid. *Arch Dis Child.* 1995;73:F8–F12.
15. Rivera A, Bell EF, Stegink LD, Ziegler EE. Plasma amino acid profiles during the first three days of life in infants with respiratory distress syndrome: Effect of parenteral amino acid supplementation. *J Pediatr.* 1989;115:464–468.
16. Heird WC, Gomez MR. Parenteral nutrition in low-birth-weight infants. *Annu Rev Nutr.* 1996;16:471–499.
17. ASPEN Board of Directors. Guidelines for the use of parenteral and enteral nutrition in adult and pediatric patients. Section VII. Nutrition support for low-birth-weight infants. *J Parenter Enteral Nutr.* 1993; 17(Suppl):1SA–52SA.
18. Bell EF, Oh W. Fluid and electrolyte management In: Avery GB, Fletcher MA, MacDonald MG, eds. *Neonatology: Pathophysiology and Management of the Newborn,* 4th ed. Philadelphia: JB Lippincott; 1994:312–329.
19. Heird WC. Amino acid and energy needs of pediatric patients receiving parenteral nutrition. *Pediatr Clin North Am.* 1995;42:765–789.
20. Helms RA, Christensen ML, Mauer EC, Storm MC. Comparison of a pediatric versus standard amino acid formulation in preterm neonates requiring parenteral nutrition. *J Pediatr.* 1987;110:466–472.
21. Zlotkin SH, Bryan MH, Anderson GH. Cysteine supplementation to cysteine-free intravenous feeding regimens in newborn infants. *Am J Clin Nutr.* 1981;34: 914–923.
22. Berseth CL. Minimal enteral feedings. *Clin Perinatol.* 1995;22:195–206.
23. Dunn L, Hulman S, Weiner J, Kliegman R. Beneficial effects of early hypocaloric enteral feeding on neonatal gastrointestinal function: preliminary report of a randomized trial. *J Pediatr.* 1988;112:622–629.
24. Meetze WH, Valentine C, McGuigan JE, Conlon M, et al. Gastrointestinal priming prior to full enteral nutrition in very low birth weight infants. *J Pediatr Gastrointest Nutr.* 1992;15:163–170.
25. Anderson DM, Kliegman RM. The relationship of neonatal alimentation practices to the occurrence of endemic necrotizing enterocolitis. *Am J Perinatol.* 1991; 8:62–67.
26. Pereira GR. Nutritional care of the extremely premature infant. *Clin Perinatol.* 1995;22:61–76.
27. Schanler RJ. The low-birth-weight infant. In: Walker WA, Watkins JB, eds. *Nutrition in Pediatrics.* 6th edition. Malden, MA: B.C. Decker, Inc.; 1997:392–412.
28. Denne SC, Clark SE, Poindexter BB, Leitch CA, et al. Nutrition and Metabolism in the High-Risk Neonate. In: Fanaroff AA, Martin RJ, eds. *Neonatal-Perinatal Medicine Diseases of the Fetus and Infant.* Vol. 1, 6th ed. St. Louis, MO: Mosby; 1997:562–619.
29. Greer FR. Special needs and dangers of fat soluble vitamins A, E and K. In: Tsang RC, Zlotkin SH, Nichols BL, Hansen JW, eds. *Nutrition During Infancy: Principles and Practice.* 2nd ed. Cincinnati, OH: Digital Educational Publishing; 1997:285–312.
30. Shannon KM, Keith JF, Mentzer WC. Recombinant human erythropoietin stimulates erythropoiesis and reduces erythrocyte transfusions in very low birth weight preterm infants. *Pediatrics.* 1995;95:1–8.
31. Shenai JP, Kennedy KA, Chytil F, Stalman MR, et al. Clinical trial of vitamin A supplementation in infants susceptible to bronchopulmonary dysplasia. *J Pediatr.* 1987;111:269–277.
32. Pearson E. Trial of vitamin A supplementation in very low birth weight infants at risk for bronchopulmonary dysplasia. *J Pediatr.* 1992;121:420–427.
33. Kennedy KA, Stoll BJ, Ehrendranz RA, Oh W, et al. Vitamin A to prevent bronchopulmonary dysplasia in very-low-birth-weight infants: has the dose been too low? *Early Hum Dev.* 1997;49:19–31.
34. Koo WWK, Steichen JJ. Osteopenia and rickets of prematurity. In: Poland RA, Fox WW, eds. *Fetal and Neonatal Physiology.* Vol. 2, 2nd ed. Philadelphia: W.B. Saunders Company; 1998:2335–2349.
35. Koo WWK, Krug-Wispe S, Neylan M, Succop P, et al. Effect of three levels of vitamin D intake in preterm infants receiving high mineral-containing milk. *J Pediatr Gastroenterol Nutr.* 1995;21:182–189.
36. Zlotkin SH, Atkinson S, Lockitch G. Trace elements in nutrition for premature infants. *Clin Perinatol.* 1995;22: 223–240.

37. Atkinson SA, Zlotkin S. Recognizing deficiencies and excesses of zinc, copper, and other trace elements. In.: Tsang RC, Zlotkin SH, Nichols BL, Hansen JW, eds. *Nutrition During Infancy: Principles and Practice.* 2nd ed. Cincinnati, OH: Digital Educational Publishing; 1997:209–232.

38. Asuncion M, Silvestre A, Morbach CA, Brans YW, et al. A prospective randomized trial comparing continuous versus intermittent feeding methods in very low birth weight neonates. *J Pediatr.* 1996;128:748–752.

39. Bhatia J, Rassin DK. Human milk supplementation: delivery of energy, calcium, phosphorus, magnesium, copper, and zinc. *Am J Dis Child.* 1988;142:445–447.

40. Schanler RJ. Suitability of human milk for the low-birthweight infant. *Clin Perinatol.* 1995;22:207–222.

41. Hurst NM, Valentine CJ, Renfro L, Burns P, et al. Skin-to-skin holding in the neonatal intensive care unit influences maternal milk volume. *J Perinatol.* 1997;17:213–217.

42. Price PT, Kalhan SC. Nutrition and selected disorders of the gastrointestinal tract. In: Klaus MH, Fanaroff AA, eds. *Care of the High-Risk Neonate.* 4th edition. Philadelphia: W.B. Saunders Company; 1993:130–175.

43. Costarino AT, Baumgart S. Water as nutrition. In: Tsang RC, Lucas A, Uauy R, Zlotkin S, eds. *Nutritional Needs of the Preterm Infant.* Baltimore: Williams & Wilkins; 1993:1–14.

44. Crouch JB. Anthropometric assessment. In: Groh-Wargo S, Thompson M, Cox JH, eds. *Nutritional Care for High-Risk Newborns.* Revised ed. Chicago: Precept Press; 1994:9–14.

45. Vaucher YE, Harrison GG, Udall JN, Morrow G. Skinfold thickness in North American infants 24–41 weeks gestation. *Hum Biol.* 1984;56:713–731.

46. Sasanow SR, Georgieff MK, Pereira GR. Midarm circumference and midarm/head circumference ratios: Standard curves for anthropometric assessment of the neonatal nutritional status. *J Pediatr.* 1986;109:311–315.

47. Anderson DM. Nutrition support for neonates. In: Matarese LE, Gottschlich MM, eds. *Contemporary Nutrition Support Practice.* Philadelphia: W.B. Saunders Company; 1998:333–346.

48. Rickard K, Gresham E. Nutritional considerations for the newborn requiring intensive care. *J Am Diet Assoc.* 1975;66:592–600.

49. Ernest JA, Gross SJ. Types and methods of feeding for infants: In: Polin RA, Fox WW, eds. *Fetal and Neonatal Physiology.* Vol 1, 2nd ed. Philadelphia: W.B. Saunders Company; 1998:363–383.

50. Currao WJ, Cox C, Shapiro DL. Diluted formula for beginning the feeding of premature infants. *Am J Dis Child.* 1988;142:730–731.

51. Robertson AF, Bhatia J. Feeding premature infants. *Clin Pediatr.* 1993;32:36–44.

52. Kerner JA, Poole RL. Metabolic monitoring and nutritional assessment. In: Yu VYH, MacMahon RA, eds. *Intravenous Feeding of the Neonate.* London: Edward Arnold; 1992:207–233.

53. Ernst JA, Neal PR. Minerals and trace elements. In: Poland RA, Fox WW, eds. *Fetal and Neonatal Physiology.* 2nd ed. Philadelphia: W.B. Saunders Company; 1998:332–343.

54. Schanler RJ. Who needs water-soluble vitamins? In: Tsang RC, Zlotkin SH, Nichols BL, Hansen JW, eds. *Nutrition During Infancy: Principles and Practice.* 2nd ed. Cincinnati, OH: Digital Educational Publishing; 1997:255–284.

55. Koo WWK, Tsang RC. Building better bones: Calcium, magnesium, phosphorus, and vitamin D. In: Tsang RC, Zlotkin SH, Nichols BL, Hansen JW, eds. *Nutrition During Infancy: Principles and Practice.* 2nd ed. Cincinnati, OH: Digital Educational Publishing; 1997:175–208.

56. Heird WC, Gomez MR. Parenteral nutrition. In: Tsang RC, Lucas A, Uauy R, Zlotkin S, eds. *Nutritional Needs of the Preterm Infant.* Baltimore: Williams & Wilkins; 1993:225–242.

57. American Academy of Pediatrics Committee on Fetus and Newborn. Hospital discharge of the high-risk neonate-proposed guidelines. *Pediatrics.* 1998;102:411–417.

58. Klaus MH, Kennell JH. Care of the mother, father, and infant. In: Fanaroff AA, Martin RJ, eds. *Neonatal-Perinatal Medicine. Diseases of the Fetus and Infant.* Vol. 1, 6th ed. St. Louis, MO: Mosby; 1997:548–561.

59. Hack M. Follow-up for high-risk neonates. In: Fanaroff AA, Martin RJ, eds. *Neonatal-Perinatal Medicine. Diseases of the Fetus and Infant.* Vol. 2, 6th ed. St. Louis, MO: Mosby; 1997:952–957.

60. Berry MA, Abrahamowicz M, Usher R. Factors associated with growth of extremely premature infants during initial hospitalization. *Pediatrics.* 1997;100:640–646.

61. Fanaroff AA, Martin RJ, eds. *Neonatal-Perinatal Medicine. Diseases of the Fetus and Infant.* Vol. 2, 6th ed. St. Louis, MO: Mosby; 1997.

62. Pereira GR, Balmer D. Feeding the critically ill neonate. In: Spitzer AR, ed. *Intensive Care of the Fetus and Neonate.* St. Louis, MO: Mosby; 1996:823–833.

63. Thureen PJ, Hay WW. Conditions requiring special nutritional management. In: Tsang RC, Lucas A, Uauy R, Zlotkin S, eds. *Nutritional Needs of the Preterm Infant.* Baltimore: Williams & Wilkins; 1993:243–266.

64. Davis AM. Pediatrics. In: Matarese LE, Gottschlich MM, eds. *Contemporary Nutrition Support Practice.* Philadelphia: W.B. Saunders Company; 1998:347–364.

65. Pittard WP. Classification of the low-birth-weight infant. In: Klaus MH, Fanaroff AA, eds. *Care of the High-Risk Neonate.* 4th ed. Philadelphia: W.B. Saunders Co; 1993:86–113.

66. Subcommittee on Nutritional Status and Weight Gain During Pregnancy, Subcommittee on Dietary Intake and Nutrient Supplements During Pregnancy, Committee on Nutritional Status During Pregnancy and Lactation. Food and Nutrition Board. Institute of Medicine, National Academy of Sciences. *Nutrition During Pregnancy. I. Weight Gain. II. Nutrient Supplements.* Washington, DC: National Academy Press; 1990.

67. Kliegman RM. Intrauterine growth retardation. In: Fanaroff AA, Martin RJ, eds. *Neonatal-Perinatal Medicine. Diseases of the Fetus and Infant.* Vol. 1, 6th ed. St. Louis, MO: Mosby; 1997:203–240.

68. Hansen JW. Consensus recommendations. In: Tsang RC, Lucas A, Uauy R, Zlotkin S, eds. *Nutritional Needs of the Preterm Infant.* Baltimore: Williams & Wilkins; 1993:288–289.

69. Greene HL, Hambidge KM, Schanler R, Tsang RC. Guidelines for the use of vitamins, trace elements, calcium, magnesium, and phosphorus in infants and children receiving total parenteral nutrition: Report of the Subcommittee on Pediatric Parenteral Nutrient Requirements from the Committee on Clinical Practice Issues of The American Society for Clinical Nutrition. *Am J Clin Nutr.* 1988;48:1324–1342.

70. Brans YW, Andrew DS, Carrillo DW, Dutton EP, et al. Tolerance of fat emulsions in very-low-birth-weight neonates. *Am J Dis Child.* 1988;142:145–152.

71. Nicholson JF, Pesce MA. Laboratory testing and reference values in infants and children. In: Behrman RE, Kliegman RM, Arvin AM, eds. *Nelson Textbook of Pediatrics.* 15th ed. Philadelphia: W.B. Saunders Company; 1996:2031–2084.

72. Oh W. Fluid, electrolytes, and acid-base homeostasis. In: Fanaroff AA, Martin RJ, eds. *Neonatal-Perinatal Medicine. Diseases of the Fetus and Infant.* Vol. 1, 6th ed. St. Louis, MO: Mosby; 1997:622–638.

73. Anderson DM, Pittard WP. Update on neonatal nutrition therapy. *Topics in Clinical Nutrition.* 1997;13:8–20.

74. *NEONOVA Nutrition Optimizer.* Version 4.1. Columbus, OH: Ross Laboratories; 1997.

75. *Pediatric Products Handbook.* Evansville, IN: Mead Johnson Nutritionals; 1996.

76. *Ross Products Handbook.* Columbus, OH: Ross Products Division, Abbot Laboratories; January 1994.

77. Lucas A, Bishop NJ, King FJ, Cole TJ. Randomized trial of nutrition for preterm infants after discharge. *Arch Dis Child.* 1992;67:324–327.

78. Bishop NJ, King FJ, Lucas A. Increased bone mineral content of preterm infants fed with a nutrient enriched formula after discharge from hospital. *Arch Dis Child.* 1993;68:573–578.

79. American Academy of Pediatrics Committee on Nutrition. Soy protein-based formulas: Recommendations for use in infant feeding. *Pediatr.* 1998;101:148–153.

80. Lucas A, Cole TJ. Breast milk and neonatal necrotising enterocolitis. *Lancet.* 1990;336:1519–1523.

81. Churella H, Blenneman B. *Meeting the Special Needs of Premature Infants after Discharge.* Columbus, OH: Ross Product Division, Abbott Laboratories; 1994.

82. Sheni JP, Jhaveri BM, Reynolds JW, Huston RK, et al. Nutritional balance studies in very-low-birth-weight infants: role of soy formula. *Pediatr.* 1981;67:631–637.

83. Jew RK, Owen D, Kaufman D, Balmer D. Osmolality of commonly used medications and formulas in the neonatal intensive care unit. *Nutr Clin Pract.* 1997;12:158–163.

84. Wirth FH, Numerof B, Pleban P, Neylan MJ. Effect of lactose on mineral absorption in preterm infants. *J Pediatr.* 1990;117:283–287.

85. *Nutrient Levels of Mead Johnson Formulas.* Evansville, IN: Mead Johnson Nutritionals; 1998.

86. Anderson DM. Nutrition care for the premature infant. *Top Clin Nutr.* 1987;2:1–9.

87. Kubit JG. Lactation issues. In: Groh-Wargo S, Thompson M, Cox JH, eds. *Nutritional Care For High-Risk Newborns.* Revised ed. Chicago: Precept Press; 1994:194–205.

CHAPTER 4

Normal Nutrition During Infancy

Susan M. Akers and Sharon L. Groh-Wargo

New discoveries in infant nutrition challenge feeding traditions and invite updated guidelines. At no other time in the life cycle is nutrition delivery more important for future health, growth, and development than during infancy. Most issues revolving around nutrient needs and delivery are consistent for all healthy infants. However, not all infants will develop or adapt to change at the same rate. The most positive feeding experiences are those that meet the nutritional demands of the infant while focusing on the individual developmental readiness of the infant. The objectives of this chapter are to cover current recommended feeding practices for healthy, full-term infants and to discuss common feeding problems encountered during the first year.

BREASTFEEDING

Breastfeeding is the recommended method of feeding for virtually all infants. Both the American Academy of Pediatrics (AAP)[1] and the American Dietetic Association[2] continue to support breastfeeding as the best source of infant nutrition. Recent studies indicate that the number of women choosing to breastfeed their infants is once again rising. The number of women breastfeeding their newborns increased through the 1970s and 1980s. With a slight decline in the early 1990s, the percentage of women breastfeeding has rebounded, with an all-time high of 62.4% in 1997.[3]

As positive as these initiation rates appear, there is still a significant decrease in the numbers of women breastfeeding through 6 months of age. The rate of infants being breastfed at 6 months increased through the 1970s, reaching a high of 27.1% in 1982. These numbers decreased for 8 consecutive years to a low in 1990 of 17.6%. Since that time, the rate of women breastfeeding until 6 months steadily increased once again to 26.0% in 1997. Although these statistics have shown improvement in the last 7 years, they still indicate an overall decrease of breastfeeding from birth to 6 months of 42%.[3]

The distribution of women breastfeeding continues to vary among different cultures, ethnic backgrounds, education levels, and ages. In-hospital breastfeeding rates are highest among households with mothers who are: over the age of 30, college educated, not Women, Infants and Children (WIC) participants, and living in the Mountain or Pacific census regions.[3] African-Americans, the poor, the less educated, and those younger than 20 years of age choose to breastfeed less often.[3] Education and support can help these groups make informed choices. Health professionals must often fill this role and, therefore, need to be knowledgeable about both the science and the art of breastfeeding.

Informed Choice

To make an informed decision, each mother, ideally with the baby's father or other significant family member, needs to weigh the implications of feeding choices. This process is ideally completed early in the pregnancy. Studies have shown that women's attitudes and decisions regarding breastfeeding are influenced more by familial and social opinions than by sociodemographic factors.[4] Advantages commonly listed for human milk and breastfeeding are:

- superior nutritional composition[2,5]
- provision of immunologic and enzymatic components[2,5,6,7]
- health benefits for mothers[2,8]
- lower cost and increased convenience[2]
- enhanced maternal-infant bonding[2,5,7]
- decreased incidence of respiratory and gastrointestinal infections[5,6,9]
- leaner body composition for infants at 1 year of age[10]
- improved cognitive development[5]

Evidence also exists that breastfed infants develop fewer allergies,[5,11] although this is controversial.[12]

Human Milk Composition

Human milk is not a uniform body fluid but a secretion of the mammary gland of changing composition.[5] Not only does the composition of human milk vary from individual to individual, but also with stage of lactation, time of day, time into feeding, and maternal diet. Laboratory techniques continue to improve, allowing the over 200 constituents of maternal milk to be analyzed and identified.[8] The four stages of human milk expression include colostrum, transitional milk, mature milk, and extended lactation, each containing its own significant biochemical components and properties.

- Colostrum is the milk produced during the first several days following delivery. It is lower in fat and energy than mature milk, but higher in protein, fat-soluble vitamins, minerals, and electrolytes.[7,13] This early stage of lactation also provides a rich source of antibodies.[7,13]
- Transition milk begins from approximately 7 to 14 days postpartum, when the composition of human milk changes with a decrease in the concentration of immunoglobins and total proteins and an increase in the amount of lactose, fat, and total calories. [5,8]
- The third phase, beginning at about 2 weeks postpartum, referred to as *mature milk*, continues throughout lactation until about 7–8 months.[8]
- Extended lactation (7 months to 2 years) results in milk different from colostrum, transitional, and mature human milk. Its carbohydrate, protein, and fat content remain relatively stable, but concentrations of several vitamins and minerals decrease.[7,14,15]

Milk production has been found to be higher during the day,[16] and fat content increases toward the end of each feeding.[17]

Table 4–1 summarizes the content of major nutrients in mature human milk. There is wide variation in the composition data reported in the literature, and older data may be inaccurate, due to inferior analysis techniques that were commonly used.

Maternal Diet During Breastfeeding

Throughout pregnancy, the maternal body is preparing for lactation by increasing the development of the breast tissue and storing additional nutrients and energy. The Subcommittee on the 10th Edition of the Recommended Dietary Allowances (RDAs) of the Food and Nutrition Board (National Research Council, National Academy of Sciences) offered the most widely recognized nutrition standards for the lactating woman (see Appendix K). In 1997, the Standing Committee on the Scientific Evaluation of Dietary Reference Intakes (DRI Committee) of the Food and Nutrition Board (Institute of Medicine, National Academy of Sciences) published preliminary data on revised nutrient requirements for North Americans and Canadians,

Table 4–1 Composition of Mature Human Milk and Cow Milk

Nutrient	*Human Milk (100 mL)*	*Cow Milk (100 mL)*
Macronutrients		
Energy (kcal)	62–70	61
Protein (g)	0.9	3.3
Carbohydrate (g)	7.3	4.7
Fat (g)	3–5	3.3
Vitamins		
Vitamin A (IU)	133–177	126
ß-Carotene (μg)	16–21	N/A
Vitamin D (IU)	2.5–5.0	41*
Vitamin E (IU)	0.48	0.06
Vitamin K (μg)	0.1–0.23	6.0
Vitamin C (mg)	5.0–6.0	0.94
Thiamine (μg)	18.3–20	38
Riboflavin (μg)	31.0–50	162
Vitamin B_6 (μg)	10.7–20	42
Vitamin B_{12} (μg)	0.02–0.06	0.36
Nicotinic acid (μg)	0.18	0.08
Folic acid (μg)	4.2–5.0	5.0
Pantothenic acid (μg)	261	314
Biotin (μg)	0.53	N/A
Minerals		
Calcium (mg)	29.4	119
Phosphorus (mg)	13.9	93
Magnesium (mg)	3.0	13
Iron (mg)	0.02–0.04	0.05
Zinc (mg)	0.15–0.25	0.38
Manganese (μg)	0.41	2–4
Copper (μg)	31	30
Chromium (μg)	0.03	0.8–1.3
Selenium (μg)	1.6	0.5–5.0
Fluoride (μg)	0.5–1.0	N/A
Sodium (mg)	11.2–14	49
Potassium (mg)	44.3	152
Chloride (mg)	37.3	N/A
Other composition data		
Protein source	80% whey; 20% casein	18% whey; 82% casein
% Calories protein	6	21
Carbohydrate source	Lactose	Lactose
% Calories carbohydrate	39	31
Fat source	Human	Butterfat
% Calories fat	55	48
Osmolality (mOsm/kg H_2O)	300	288

*Vitamin D added.
NA, not available

Source: Data from references 7, 39, 67, and 108 to 122.

including lactating women. The intent of the DRIs is to replace the RDAs, which have been published since 1941 by the National Academy of Sciences. The DRI are to be issued in seven separate nutrient groups. The first group of nutrients consists of calcium, phosphorus, magnesium, vitamin D, and fluoride. Publication of these nutrient recommendations is expected by the year 2000. Requirements are being established to meet the additional demands of lactation without compromising the nutrient stores of the mother. Revisions have not been developed for all nutrients. Therefore, the 1989 RDAs are still being used as a guide for assessing the adequacy of pregnant and lactating women. Overall, recommendations for maternal diet during lactation include a well-balanced diet comparable to that of a nonlactating woman, with an additional need for about 500 calories and vitamin/mineral supplementation for those not consuming a variety of foods. Lactation will not produce a net drain on the mother if the amount of energy available and the requirement of any given nutrient are replaced in the diet.[5]

The additional calories indicated in the RDAs assumes an average daily milk production of 750–800 mL and a store of 2–3 kg of body fat from weight gain during pregnancy.[5,19] Energy requirements are greater if weight gain during the pregnancy was low, weight during lactation falls below standards for height and age, and/or more than one infant is being nursed. There is some evidence that successful lactation can be maintained at energy intakes somewhat lower than the RDAs without adversely affecting lactation performance or infant growth.[5,8,20]

Increases in protein, vitamin, and mineral requirements can be met by consuming the appropriate number of servings from the Food Guide Pyramid (see Table 4–2) and choosing nutritious foods for the additional calories needed to support lactation. For those mothers not motivated to eat a well-balanced diet or for those avoiding primary food groups, continuation of prenatal vitamin and/or calcium supplementation, is recommended. It is suggested that iron supplementation be continued postpartum, whether breastfeeding or not, to replenish iron stores depleted by pregnancy.[8]

Most breastfeeding women experience increased thirst. This should naturally result in additional intake of fluids. There are no data to support the idea that forcing fluids will increase or restricting fluids will decrease milk production.[5,19] Regular exercise and weight loss up to 2 kg per month should not affect milk production,[19] but both should be kept within moderate levels to help conserve the mother's energy to care for the infant.

Although the quality of human milk is remarkably preserved, even when the mother is poorly nourished, maternal diet can affect composition in the following ways:

Table 4–2 Maternal Diet During Breastfeeding

Food Group	*Number of Servings*
Milk (and milk substitutes)	4 cups (6 cups teens) or equivalent
Meat (and meat substitutes)	Two 2- to 3-oz servings or equivalent
Fruits	2–3 1/2-cup servings (vitamin C source daily)
Vegetables	2–3 1/2-cup servings (vitamin A source 3–4 times/week)
Breads and cereals	6–11 servings (serving equal to one slice of bread or 1/2–3/4 cup of cereal)
Fats	In moderation

Source: Based on United States Department of Agriculture Food Guide Pyramid, 1992

- decreased milk volume from a diet low in energy, carbohydrate, and/or protein[13,21,22]
- altered fatty acid composition that mirrors maternal intake[19,23]
- varied content of some vitamins and minerals (see Table 4–3)[19]
- appearance of colic symptoms in babies whose mothers drink a lot of cow's milk, due to transmission of allergens into the milk[24]
- passage of caffeine, nicotine, and alcohol into milk, possibly causing adverse affects in the baby when maternal consumption is high[25–27]
- passage of medications, drugs, and environmental contaminants[5,8,22,28,29]

Table 4–3 Effect of Changes in Maternal Diet on Vitamin and Mineral Composition of Human Milk

Yes Maternal Diet Can Change Composition	*No Maternal Diet Cannot Change Composition*
Vitamins	
Vitamin A	
Vitamin D	
Vitamin C	
Thiamine	
Vitamin K	
Folate	
Riboflavin	
Niacin	
Vitamin E	
Pyridoxine	
Biotin	
Pantothenic Acid	
Cyanocobalamin	
Minerals	
Manganese	Sodium
Iodine	Calcium
Fluoride	Phosphorus
Selenium	Magnesium
	Iron
	Zinc
	Copper

Source: Data from references 7, 19, 21, 123, and 124.

Management of Breastfeeding

Successful lactation is greatly influenced by the motivation and confidence of the mother, and by support from those around her, including the father, other family members, and medical professionals. The ability to lactate is a natural characteristic of all mammals, and infants have the capability to suckle even in utero. Infant suckling stimulates release of the hormones from the pituitary: prolactin, responsible for milk production, and oxytocin, responsible for milk release. To establish and sustain lactation, therefore, it is necessary to allow the baby access to the breast on demand. The more a mother nurses, the more milk she will produce. The following list offers some tips for ensuring breastfeeding success:

1. *Initial breastfeeding.* Ideally, this should take place as soon after delivery as possible.
2. *Positioning.* Have the mother find a comfortable position, either lying down or sitting up. Use pillows to support the baby's body and the mother's back and arms. Change the position of the baby with every feeding during the first few weeks so that pressure and friction on the mother's nipples are rotated. The mother should use one hand to support and guide her breast and put the other around the baby and on the baby's bottom to support and move the baby.
3. *Latching on.* The mother can stimulate the rooting reflex by touching the baby's closest cheek. When the mouth is open wide, pull the baby close. Be sure the baby's mouth latches on to suckle the mother's entire nipple, with the lips well behind the nipple. The baby's lower lip should be turned out. Rapid sucking, followed by slower, rhythmic sucking and swallowing will stimulate the let-down reflex, or the actual release of milk. Signs that let-down has occurred include tingling in the breast, tightening in the

uterus, milk around the baby's mouth, or milk dripping from the other breast. Don't pull the baby off the breast; first have the mother use her little finger to break the suction before moving the baby.

4. *Timing.* In the first few weeks, nurse the baby 8–12 times a day, or about every 2–3 hours. The feedings will become less frequent after breastfeeding is established. Build up to at least 10–15 minutes per breast per feeding and offer both breasts at each feeding, rotating sides where feeding is initiated. It takes several minutes to elicit the let-down reflex. The majority of the milk volume is emptied after 5–7 minutes of sucking.
5. *Assessing adequacy* (or "How do I know if my baby is getting enough?"). The following are signs that a baby is receiving adequate fluid and calories.[30–32] The baby will:
   a.) have at least 6–8 thoroughly wet diapers a day
   b.) have regular bowel movements
   c.) nurse 8–12 times a day
   d.) seem satisfied after nursing
   e.) grow at a relatively predictable rate

A number of situations arise during the early weeks of breastfeeding that, if unanticipated and poorly managed, can jeopardize a successful nursing experience. Table 4–4 points out the most frequent complaints from breastfeeding mothers.

Many new mothers return to work or school after their babies are born. They can continue to breastfeed by these methods:

- arranging to go to the baby or having the baby brought to them
- pumping and saving the milk
- discontinuing the feeding(s) when they are away but continuing to nurse at other times

Ruth Lawrence's book, *Breastfeeding, A Guide for the Medical Profession,* and a book by Margit Hamosh et al., *Breastfeeding and the Working Mother: Effect of Time and Temperature of Short-Term Storage on Proteolysis, Lipolysis, and Bacterial Growth in Milk,* are interesting resources that discuss alternatives to discontinuing breastfeeding, as well as issues related to milk storage.[5,35]

BOTTLE FEEDING

When breastfeeding is not chosen, is unsuccessful, or is stopped before 1 year of age, bottle feeding with a commercially prepared, iron-fortified infant formula is the recommended alternative. A wide variety of products is available.

Infant Formula Composition

Both the AAP[37] and the United States Food and Drug Administration (FDA)[38] have identified nutrient requirements for infants. Tables 4–5—4–9 list the nutrient requirements for infant formulas and the composition of the most common ones. Formulas are grouped by the following categories: standard, soy, protein hydrolysate, and follow-up formulas.

Standard Formulas

The most common human milk substitutes are standard formulas. They are made from cow's milk that is altered by removing the butterfat, adding vegetable oils and carbohydrate, and decreasing protein. Some standard formulas contain demineralized whey. This produces a whey/casein ratio of 60:40. Human milk has a ratio of about 80:20 in colostrum[40] and decreases to about 55:45 in mature human milk.[41] Standard formulas without the demineralized whey have a ratio of 20:80. Although the addition of the demineralized whey appears to make those formulas closer to human milk, there are no clear scientific data to support superior performance when they are fed to babies.[40–42]

The current requirements for protein in infant formulas range from 1.8 to 4.5 g per 100 calo-

Table 4–4 Most Frequent Complaints from Breastfeeding Mothers

Problem	*Description*	*Treatment*
Sore Nipples	These are most often the result of improper positioning.	Involves nursing on the least sore nipple first and changing the position of the baby's mouth on the mother's nipple.
Engorgement	This painful swelling of the breast can occur as mature milk production begins and is accompanied by an increase in blood flow and fluid accumulation.	Frequent nursing may help to minimize the discomfort until the breast adjusts. Expressing more milk than is necessary to relieve the pressure will only result in increased milk production and should be discouraged.
Jaundice	In the newborn, this is associated with an elevated bilirubin level and is often the result of inadequate feeding. [5,33]	Early and frequent feedings will facilitate a good milk supply and stimulate increased gut motility, thus decreasing the absorption of bilirubin. Supplemental water has not been shown to be an effective treatment and may interfere with establishing breastfeeding skills in the baby and, therefore, a good milk supply in mother. [33,34]
Poor Milk Supply	This is probably more a theoretical concern than an actual problem because many mothers are insecure with their ability to successfully provide adequate nutrition without tangible evidence of consumption.	Information about assessing adequacy should be presented in a positive and supportive manner. Frequent feedings and adequate rest will do more to promote milk production than forcing fluids or increasing calories in the mother, unless the diet is severely restricted. Overuse of pacifiers, swings, and other calming devices may deter the mother from offering the breast as comfort. If there is still concern regarding actual milk consumption, the infant can be weighed before and after a feeding to determine intake.

Source: Adapted from S. L. Groh and K. Antonelli, Normal Nutrition During Infancy, in *Handbook of Pediatric Nutrition,* P.M. Queen and C.E. Lang, eds., © 1993, Aspen Publishers, Inc.

ries.[43] There is some evidence that the amount of protein found in standard formulas is excessive and that, unless the quantity is lowered, the ideal protein quality will be difficult to determine precisely.[43,44] Taurine, a free amino acid derived from cysteine, present in human milk, is often added to standard formulas.[7] Standard formulas are marketed as iron fortified (12 mg/quart) and low iron (1 mg/quart). Only the iron-fortified variety meets the iron requirements of infancy. Although only about 4% of the iron in iron-fortified formula is absorbed,[45] its generous content makes it an adequate source of iron for the entire first year of life.

Table 4–5 Composition of Selected Standard Formulas

	Enfamil with Iron		*Improved Similac with Iron*		*Store Brand Infant Formula*	
	per 100 kcal	*per 100 mL*	*per 100 kcal*	*per 100 mL*	*per 100 kcal*	*per 100 mL*
Macronutrients						
Energy(kcal)	100	67	100	67	100	67
Protein (g)	2.2	1.5	2.2	1.5	2.2	1.5
Carbohydrate (g)	10.3	7.0	10.7	7.2	10.6	7.2
Fat (g)	5.6	3.8	5.4	3.6	5.3	3.6
Linoleic acid (g)	1.1	0.7	1.3	0.9	0.5	0.3
Vitamins						
Vitamin A (IU)	310	209	300	202	300	202
Vitamin D (IU)	62	42	60	40	60	40
Vitamin E (IU)	3.1	2.1	3.0	2.0	1.4	0.9
Vitamin K (μg)	8.6	5.8	8.0	5.4	8.0	5.4
Vitamin C (mg)	8.1	5.5	9.0	6.1	8.5	5.7
Thiamine (μg)	78	53	100	67	100	67
Riboflavin (μg)	156	105	150	101	150	101
Vitamin B_6 (μg)	62	42	60	40	63	43
Vitamin B_{12} (μg)	0.2	0.2	0.2	0.2	0.2	0.1
Niacin (μg)	1250	844	1050	709	750	506
Folic acid (μg)	16	10	15	10	7.5	5.1
Pantothenic acid (μg)	470	317	450	304	315	213
Biotin (μg)	2.3	1.6	4.4	3.0	2.2	1.5
Choline (mg)	16	10	16	11	15	10.1
Inositol (mg)	4.7	3.2	4.7	3.2	4.7	3.2
Minerals						
Calcium (mg)	69	47	78	51	63	43
Phosphorus (mg)	47	32	42	39	42	28
Magnesium (mg)	7.8	5.3	6.0	4.0	7	4.7
Iron (mg)	1.9	1.3	1.8	1.2	1.8	1.2
Zinc (mg)	0.8	0.5	0.8	0.5	0.8	0.5
Manganese (μg)	16	10	5.0	3.4	22	15
Copper (μg)	94	63	90	61	70	47
Iodine (μg)	10	7	15	10	9	6
Sodium (mg)	27	18	24	19	22	15
Potassium (mg)	108	73	105	73	83	56
Chloride (mg)	62	42	65	44	55	38
Other composition data						
Protein source	Cow milk; 60% whey		Cow milk; 82% casein		Cow milk; 60% whey	
% Calories protein	9		9		9	
Carbohydrate source	Lactose		Lactose		Lactose	
% Calories carbohydrate	41		43		43	

continues

Table 4–5 continued

	Enfamil with Iron		*Improved Similac with Iron*		*Store Brand Infant Formula*	
	per 100 kcal	*per 100 mL*	*per 100 kcal*	*per 100 mL*	*per 100 kcal*	*per 100 mL*
Fat source	Palm olein, soy, coconut, & high oleic sunflower oils		Soy, coconut oils, & safflower		Coconut, safflower, soybean oils, & oleo	
% Calories fat	50		48		48	
Osmolality (mOsm/kg H_2O)	300		300		300	
Manufacturer/Distributor	Mead Johnson		Ross		Wyeth-Ayerst	

Source: Adapted from S. L. Groh-Wargo and K. Antonelli, Normal Nutrition During Infancy, in *Handbook of Pediatric Nutrition,* P.M. Queen and C.E. Lang, eds., © 1993, Aspen Publishers, Inc.

Soy Formulas

Indications for using soy-based infant formulas are limited; nevertheless, the number of infants being fed soy formulas in the United States has nearly doubled in the last decade, and soy formulas currently represent 25% of the infant formula market.[46] The three major indications for its use include: intolerance to cow's milk protein, galactosemia, and lactose intolerance. Soy formulas have been used for milk protein allergies; however, current studies suggest that at least 50–60% of infants with milk protein intolerance will also have a soy intolerance.[46,47] Lactose intolerance can be due to either primary congenital lactase deficiency (rarely) or secondary lactase deficiency as a result of an acute gastritis. In the latter case, the use of soy formula may be indicated for the short term until the small intestine regenerates lactase. This practice is controversial (see Chapter 8, Food Hypersensitivities).

Soy formulas contain methionine, carnitine, and taurine-fortified soy protein isolate, vegetable oils, and a carbohydrate source other than lactose. All are iron-fortified and meet the requirements for vitamins and minerals established by the AAP and the FDA. The protein content of soy formulas is higher than standard formulas because the biologic value of soy protein is lower than cow's milk protein.

Though all soy formulas are lactose-free, some are also sucrose-free or corn-free. Soy phytates and fiber oligosaccharides contained in soy formulas have been found to interfere with the absorption of calcium, phosphorus, zinc, and iron. For this reason, calcium and phosphorus levels in soy formulas have been increased by 20% over those of cow's-milk-based formulas and are fortified with zinc and iron.[46] Overall, studies have confirmed that soy formulas are adequate for promoting normal growth and development when fed to full-term, healthy infants.[46] However, some serious concerns have been raised regarding the use of soy formulas with preterm infants secondary to aluminum content, risk of osteopenia, and negative influences on growth.[46]

Table 4–6 Composition of Selected Soy Formulas

	Isomil		*Prosobee*		*Store Brand Soy*	
	per 100 kcal	*per 100 mL*	*per 100 kcal*	*per 100 mL*	*per 100 kcal*	*per 100 mL*
Macronutrients						
Energy (kcal)	100	67	100	67	100	67
Protein (g)	2.7	1.8	3.0	2.0	3.1	2.1
Carbohydrate (g)	10.1	6.8	10.0	6.7	10.2	6.9
Fat (g)	5.5	3.7	5.3	3.6	5.3	3.6
Linoleic acid (g)	1.3	0.9	1.0	0.7	0.5	0.3
Vitamins						
Vitamin A (IU)	300	202	310	209	300	202
Vitamin D (IU)	60	40	62	42	60	40
Vitamin E (IU)	3.0	2.0	3.1	2.1	1.4	0.9
Vitamin K (μg)	15	10	16	10	15	10
Vitamin C (mg)	9.0	6.1	8.1	5.5	8.5	5.7
Thiamine (μg)	60	40	78	53	100	67
Riboflavin (μg)	90	61	94	63	150	101
Vitamin B_6 (μg)	60	40	62	42	63	43
Vitamin B_{12} (μg)	0.4	0.3	0.3	0.2	0.3	0.2
Niacin (μg)	1350	911	1250	844	750	506
Folic acid (μg)	15	10	16	10	7.5	5.1
Pantothenic acid (μg)	750	506	470	317	450	304
Biotin (μg)	4.5	3.0	7.8	5.3	5.5	3.7
Choline (mg)	8.0	5.4	7.8	5.3	13	8.8
Inositol (mg)	5.0	3.4	4.7	3.2	4.1	2.8
Minerals						
Calcium (mg)	105	71	94	63	90	61
Phosphorus (mg)	75	51	74	50	63	43
Magnesium (mg)	7.5	5.1	11	7.4	10	6.7
Iron (mg)	1.8	1.2	1.9	1.3	1.7	1.2
Zinc (mg)	0.8	0.5	0.8	0.5	0.8	0.5
Manganese (μg)	30	20	25	17	30	20
Copper (μg)	75	51	94	63	70	47
Iodine (μg)	15	10	10	6.9	9.0	6.1
Sodium (mg)	44	30	36	24	30	20
Potassium (mg)	108	73	122	82	105	71
Chloride (mg)	62	42	83	56	56	38
Other composition data						
Protein source	Soy isolate & L-methionine		Soy isolate & L-methionine		Soy isolate & L-methionine	
% Calories protein	11		12		12	
Carbohydrate source	Corn syrup & sucrose		Corn syrup solids		Sucrose	

continues

Table 4–6 continued

	Isomil		*Prosobee*		*Store Brand Soy*	
	per 100 kcal	*per 100 mL*	*per 100 kcal*	*per 100 mL*	*per 100 kcal*	*per 100 mL*
% Calories carbohydrate	40		40		41	
Fat source	Soy & coconut oils		Palm olein, soy, coconut, & high oleic sunflower oils		Oleo, coconut, safflower, & soy oils	
% Calories fat	49		48		47	
Osmolality (mOsm/kg H_2O)	240		200		296	
Manufacturer	Ross		Mead Johnson		Wyeth-Ayerst	

Source: Adapted from S. L. Groh-Wargo and K. Antonelli, Normal Nutrition During Infancy, in *Handbook of Pediatric Nutrition,* P.M. Queen and C.E. Lang, eds., © 1993, Aspen Publishers, Inc.

Protein Hydrolysates

When an infant is allergic to the intact protein of cow's milk and/or soy protein, a casein hydrolysate may be appropriate. Casein hydrolysates contain nonantigenic peptides of <1,200 molecular weight[48] and have a successful history of use for over 40 years. Enzymatic hydrolysates of whey contain peptides of >2,000 molecular weight, have limited clinical use, and may be an acceptable alternative for only those infants who are sensitive but not truly allergic to cow's milk or soy protein.[48]

Sources of carbohydrate and fat vary among the protein hydrolysates and should be considered when they are fed for indications other than protein allergy or sensitivity. The AAP does not support the use of hypoallergenic formulas for the treatment of colic, sleeplessness, or irritability because of insufficient data connecting these common symptoms and immune-mediated reaction to cow's milk protein.[48]

Follow-Up Formulas

The original "follow-up formulas" were designed for infants older than 6 months who were taking solid foods but not enough to meet all essential nutrients needed for optimal growth and development. Currently, the only follow-up formula on the market for infants 6 months and older in the United States is Carnation Follow-up Formula. It has a higher percentage of calories from protein (3 g/100 kcal) and carbohydrates, and a lower percentage of calories from fat (3.9 g/100 kcal). This seems inappropriate as protein requirements go down during the second half of the first year, and typical solid foods fed to infants, eg, cereals, fruits, and vegetables, are low in fat and high in carbohydrates. It does offer a good source of vitamins and iron, if those are lacking in the solid foods that the infant likes. The AAP has stated that, though nutritionally adequate, this type of follow-up formula offers no clearly established superiority over currently used feedings for infants at this age.[49] This opinion has been restated by Zeigler.[50] In the last 4 years, infant formula manufacturers have developed follow-up formulas for premature infants. These formulas are more caloric and nutrient dense. For more information on prematurity and special formulas, see Chapter 3, Nutrition for Premature Infants.

Table 4–7 Composition of Selected Protein Hydrolysate Formulas

	Nutramigen		*Pregestimil*		*Alimentum*		*Good Start*	
	per 100 kcal	*per 100 mL*	*per 100 kcal*	*per 100 mL*	*per 100 kcal*	*per 100 mL*	*per 100 kcal*	*per 100 mL*
Macronutrients								
Energy (kcal)	100	67	100	67	100	67	100	67
Protein (g)	2.8	1.9	2.8	1.9	2.8	1.9	2.4	1.6
Carbohydrate (g)	13.4	9.0	10.3	7.0	10.2	6.9	11.0	7.4
Fat (g)	3.9	2.6	5.6	3.8	5.5	3.7	5.1	3.4
Linoleic acid (g)	2.0	1.4	0.8	0.5	1.6	1.1	0.4	0.3
Vitamins								
Vitamin A (IU)	310	209	375	253	300	202	300	202
Vitamin D (IU)	62	42	75	51	60	40	60	40
Vitamin E (IU)	3.1	2.1	3.8	2.5	3.0	2.0	1.2	0.8
Vitamin K (μg)	16	10	19	13	15	10	8.2	5.5
Vitamin C (mg)	8.1	5.5	12	7.9	9.0	6.1	8.0	5.4
Thiamine (μg)	78	53	78	53	60	40	60	40
Riboflavin (μg)	94	63	94	63	90	61	135	91
Vitamin B_6 (μg)	62	42	62	42	60	40	75	51
Vitamin B_{12} (μg)	0.3	0.2	0.3	0.2	0.4	0.3	0.2	0.2
Niacin (μg)	1250	844	1250	844	1350	911	750	506
Folic acid (μg)	16	10	16	10	15	10	9.0	6.1
Pantothenic acid (μg)	470	317	470	317	750	506	450	304
Biotin (μg)	7.8	5.3	7.8	5.3	4.5	3.0	2.2	1.5
Choline (mg)	13	9.0	13	9.0	8.0	5.4	12	8.1
Inositol (mg)	4.7	3.2	4.7	3.2	5.0	3.4	6.1	4.1
Minerals								
Calcium (mg)	94	63	94	63	105	71	64	43
Phosphorus (mg)	62	42	62	42	75	51	36	24
Magnesium (mg)	11	7.4	11	7.4	7.5	5.1	6.7	4.5
Iron (mg)	1.9	1.3	1.9	1.3	1.8	1.2	1.5	1.0
Zinc (mg)	0.8	0.5	0.9	0.6	0.8	0.5	0.8	0.5
Manganese (μg)	31	21	31	21	30	20	7.0	4.7
Copper (μg)	94	63	94	63	75	51	80	54
Iodine (μg)	7.0	4.7	7.0	4.7	15	10	8.0	5.4
Sodium (mg)	47	32	47	32	44	30	24	16
Potassium (mg)	109	74	109	74	118	80	98	66
Chloride (mg)	86	58	86	58	80	54	59	40
Other composition data								
Protein source	Casein hydrolysate		Casein hydrolysate		Casein hydrolysate		Whey hydrolysate	
% Calories protein	11		11		11		10	

continues

Table 4–7 continued

	Nutramigen		*Pregestimil*		*Alimentum*		*Good Start*	
	per 100 kcal	*per 100 mL*	*per 100 kcal*	*per 100 mL*	*per 100 kcal*	*per 100 mL*	*per 100 kcal*	*per 100 mL*
Carbohydrate source	Corn syrup solids & corn starch		Corn syrup solids, glucose & starch		Sucrose & tapioca starch		Maltodextrin & lactose	
% Calories carbohydrate	54		40		40		44	
Fat source	Corn oil		MCT; corn & high oleic safflower oils		MCT; safflower & soy oils		Palm, high oleic safflower & coconut oils	
% Calories fat	35		49		49		46	
Osmolality (mOsm/kg H_2O)	320		320		370		265	
Manufacturer	Mead Johnson		Mead Johnson		Ross		Carnation	

Note: MCT, medium-chain triglycerides.

Source: Adapted from S. L. Groh-Wargo and K. Antonelli, Normal Nutrition During Infancy, in *Handbook of Pediatric Nutrition,* P.M. Queen and C.E. Lang, eds., © 1993, Aspen Publishers, Inc.

Evaporated Milk Formulas

The AAP does not currently support the use of evaporated milk preparations for infants because of their inadequate nutrient composition.[51] Although not recommended, a home-prepared formula of evaporated milk is probably better than unmodified cow's milk when a commercial formula or breast milk is unavailable. The usual recipe is one can of evaporated whole milk (13 oz), 19½ oz of water, and 3 tablespoons of sugar or corn syrup.[52] The evaporation process denatures the protein, rendering a softer and more digestible curd. Adding the sugar or corn syrup improves the ratio of protein/fat/carbohydrate.

Evaporated milk formula has the same disadvantages for infants as unmodified cow's milk: poorly digested fat, low concentration of iron and vitamin C, and excessive amounts of sodium and phosphorus. A vitamin A and D supplement is needed unless the evaporated milk is fortified; additional vitamin C and iron are needed unless the infant takes sufficient quantities of the appropriate solid foods; and supplemental fluoride is needed after 6 months if the water used is not fluoridated.[52,53,63] A vitamin A+D+C supplement drop with iron and/or fluoride is appropriate. Table 4–10 lists the products not recommended for infant feeding.

Management of Bottle Feeding

Pediatric professionals should not assume that parents are familiar with how to purchase or prepare infant formulas. Bottle-feeding parents need information about how infant formulas are packaged in relation to cost and how formulas are prepared and stored. They may also need advice on bottles and nipples and on appropriate feeding techniques.

Preparation of Infant Formulas

Infant formulas usually come packaged in three ways:

1. ready-to-feed (32-oz. cans) and single-use 8-oz. cans for select formulas

Table 4–8 Composition of Selected Follow-Up Formulas

	Follow-Up Formula	
	per 100 kcal	*per 100 mL*
Macronutrients		
Energy (kcal)	100	67
Protein (g)	3.0	2.0
Carbohydrate (g)	13.2	8.9
Fat (g)	3.9	2.6
Linoleic acid (g)	0.7	0.5
Vitamins		
Vitamin A (IU)	250	169
Vitamin D (IU)	65	44
Vitamin E (IU)	0.8	0.5
Vitamin K (μg)	8.1	5.5
Vitamin C (mg)	8.0	5.4
Thiamine (μg)	80	54
Riboflavin (μg)	96	65
Vitamin B_6 (μg)	66	45
Vitamin B_{12} (μg)	0.3	0.2
Niacin (μg)	1280	864
Folic acid (μg)	16	11
Pantothenic acid (μg)	480	324
Biotin (μg)	1.5	1.0
Choline (mg)	—	—
Inositol (mg)	—	—
Minerals		
Calcium (mg)	135	91
Phosphorus (mg)	90	61
Magnesium (mg)	8.4	5.7
Iron (mg)	1.9	1.3
Zinc (mg)	0.6	0.4
Manganese (μg)	7.0	4.7
Copper (μg)	76	51
Iodine (μg)	5.7	3.8
Sodium (mg)	39	26
Potassium (mg)	135	91
Chloride (mg)	90	61
Other composition data		
Protein source	Cow milk; 82% casein	
% Calories protein	12	
Carbohydrate source	Lactose & corn syrup solids	
% Calories carbohydrate	53	

continued

Table 4–8 continued

	Follow-Up Formula	
	per 100 kcal	*per 100 mL*
Fat source	Palm, corn, & high oleic safflower oils	
% Calories fat	35	
Osmolality (mOsm/kg H_2O)	N/A	
Manufacturer	Carnation	

Note: N/A, not available.

Source: Adapted from S. L. Groh-Wargo and K. Antonelli, Normal Nutrition During Infancy, in *Handbook of Pediatric Nutrition,* P.M. Queen and C.E. Lang, eds., © 1993, Aspen Publishers, Inc.

2. concentrated liquid (13-oz. cans)
3. powder (12- to 16-oz. cans)

Ready-to-feed formulas provide the convenience of offering sterile, accurately mixed formulas for those who do not have the capability of preparing formulas at the time of a feeding (eg, while traveling). Concentrated liquid formulas are cheaper than ready-to-feed formulas, are readily available, mix easily, and can be the vehicle for fluoridated water. Powder is convenient if only a small amount of formula is desired and may be the cheapest form of formula. Powdered formula is popular among breastfeeding mothers who may have to miss a feeding. Manufacturers recommend boiling the water for 1–5 minutes and cooling it before mixing. In practice, some clinicians do not feel boiling water for formula preparation is necessary for healthy babies. The prepared formulas can be kept in the refrigerator for 24–48 hours after opening; however, it is safest to consume formula within 24 hours. Powders have a 30-day shelf life after opening. Although often recommended at the time of discharge from the hospital, sterilization of equipment is probably not carried out and is unnecessary if:

1. The formula source is a sterile, commercially prepared formula.
2. The water source is from a supervised city filtration plant.
3. Hands are washed during preparation and before feeding.
4. Equipment is washed well in warm, soapy water and rinsed thoroughly or washed in a dishwasher.
5. Formula is promptly refrigerated after preparation.[54,55]

There is currently no evidence that babies prefer warmed milk; however, most caregivers do not feed cold bottles from the refrigerator. Warming is best done quickly under a stream of hot water or in a pan of hot water. Microwave heating is not recommended because it is difficult to monitor the actual temperature of formula in the center of the bottle. In addition, steam building within the bottle can result in

Table 4–9 Nutrient Requirements for Infant Formulas

	Per 100 kcal	
	Minimum	*Maximum*
Macronutrients		
Protein (g)	1.8	4.5
Carbohydrate (g)	—	—
Fat (g)	3.3	6.0
Linoleic acid (g)	0.3	—
Vitamins		
Vitamin A (IU)	250	750
Vitamin D (IU)	40	100
Vitamin E (IU)	0.7	—
Vitamin K (μg)	4	—
Vitamin C (mg)	8	—
Thiamine (μg)	40	—
Riboflavin (μg)	60	—
Vitamin B_6 (μg)	35	—
Vitamin B_{12} (μg)	0.15	—
Niacin (μg)	250*	—
Folic acid (μg)	4	—
Pantothenic acid (μg)	300	—
Biotin (μg)	1.5†	—
Choline (mg)	7†	—
Inositol (mg)	4†	—
Minerals		
Calcium (mg)	60	—
Phosphorus (mg)	30	—
Magnesium (mg)	6	—
Iron (mg)	0.15	3
Zinc (mg)	0.5	—
Manganese (μg)	5	—
Copper (μg)	60	—
Iodine (μg)	5	75
Sodium (mg)	20	60
Potassium (mg)	80	200
Chloride (mg)	55	150

* Includes nicotinic acid and niacinamide.
† Required only for nonmilk-based formulas.

Source: Data from reference 38.

an explosion and spraying of hot liquid. Reports have associated facial and palatal burns of babies with the heating of bottles of formula in a microwave, and the practice should be discouraged.[56,57]

Feeding Techniques and Schedules

Good bottle-feeding technique includes holding the infant so that face-to-face contact is maximized and tilting the bottle so that the

Table 4–10 Products *Not* Recommended for Infant Feeding

Nutrient Distribution	*Ideal**	*Goat's Milk†*	*Evaporated Milk‡*	*Whole Cow's Milk†*	*Skim Milk*	*Low-Fat Milk†*
Kcal/100 mL	67	67	66	62	35	43
% Pro	7–16	20	16	21	38	31
% CHO	35–65	26	42	30	57	45
% Fat	30–55	54	45	49	5	24
Nutrient excesses		Protein	Butterfat	Protein	Protein	Protein
Nutrient deficiencies		Folic acid Iron	Vitamin C Iron	Vitamin C Iron	Vitamin C Iron Fat	Vitamin C Iron Fat
Daily supplementation required						
Vitamin C‖		+	+	+	+	+
Folic acid¶		+	–	–	–	–
Iron¶		+	+	+	+	+
Comments		High renal solute load with mineral composition similar to cow's milk*#	Cost is similar to powdered commercial infant formulas*#	High renal solute load. Guaiac-positive stools may develop, precipitating iron deficiency anemia#	Unacceptable feeding alternative during infancy#	Unacceptable feeding alternative during infancy#

* Data from reference 131.
† Data from reference 119.
‡ One can (13 oz) evaporated milk with 3 tbsp corn syrup and 19½ oz water.
‖ May be given as fruit juice (3.5 oz/d infant juice or 2 oz/d regular orange juice).
¶ See RDA for age.
# See text.

Source: Adapted with permission from R.J. Grand, J.L. Sutphen, and W.H. Dietz, *Pediatric Nutrition Theory and Practice,* p. 334, © 1987, Butterworth-Heinnemann, Newton, Massachusetts.

nipple is filled with milk. Interaction between caregiver and infant can be just as intimate during bottle feeding as with breastfeeding.

The bottle should never be propped. This practice removes the socialization aspect of feeding and can lead to dental caries[58] and increased risks of ear infection.[59] There is also an increased risk of ear infections with feedings in the supine position with either breast or bottle feedings.[59] Infants should be fed in a semi-upright position.

The addition of sugar to the formula or sucrose-containing fluids to the bottle also increases the risk of dental disease.[7] Adding solids, such as cereal, also is not recommended. Many view this practice as a form of force-feeding and also an indication that the infant may not be ready for spoon feeding yet.[60]

Most infants can finish a bottle in 15–20 minutes. If most feedings exceed this time frame, it is recommended that a pediatric feeding specialist evaluate the infant to rule out any severe oral or motor delay or dysfunction. Other possible reasons for slow feeding include a nipple with a hole that is too small or clogged, or a collapsed nipple. Burping is usually done midway through the feeding and at the end of the feeding. Partially used bottles should be discarded after the feeding, not saved for the next feeding time. Table 4–11 gives a suggested bottle-feeding schedule for infants.

SUPPLEMENTATION OF VITAMINS AND MINERALS FOR ALL INFANTS

Because the human race has evolved over the centuries on an infant diet of human milk, the argument can be made that no routine supplementation should be necessary. There are several nutrients, however, for which this may not be entirely true of the breastfed infant. In addition, there are some vitamin and mineral supplemental issues for the formula-fed infant. Table 4–12 summarizes the most up-to-date vitamin and mineral supplementation recommendations. They include vitamin K, vitamin D, iron, and fluoride. Table 4–13 lists the composition of selected infant vitamin and mineral drops.

A one-time intramuscular dose of vitamin K at birth (0.5–1.0 mg) is effective protection against hemorrhagic disease of the newborn.[61] This is recommended for both breastfed and bottle-fed infants.

The need for supplemental vitamin D in exclusively breastfed infants is controversial. Though some do not believe it is necessary,[62] most support the practice.[7,63] Infants particularly at risk are those who:

1. live in northern urban areas, especially during the winter
2. are dark skinned
3. are kept covered due to cultural practices or beliefs

Table 4–11 Suggested Number and Volume of Bottle Feedings for a Normal Infant

Age	*Number*	*Volume*
Birth–1 week	6–10	30– 90 mL
1 week–1 month	7–8	60–120 mL
1 month–3 months	5-7	120–180 mL
3 months–6 months	4–5	180–210 mL
6 months–9 months	3–4	210–240 mL
10 months–12 months	3	210–240 mL

Source: Reprinted from *Manual of Pediatric Nutrition* (p 38) by DG Kelts and EG Jones, 1984, Little, Brown, and Company, with permission from Lippincott Williams & Wilkins.

Table 4–12 Suggested Vitamin and Mineral Supplementation for Full-Term Infants (0–12 Months)

	Infants Fed Human Milk	*Infants Fed Commercial Formula*
Vitamin K	Single dose at birth: IM 0.5–1.0 mg PO 1.0–2.0 mg	Single dose at birth: IM 0.5–1.0 mg PO 1.0–2.0 mg
Vitamin D	400 IU/d Especially at-risk infants*	
Iron	1 mg/kg/d to maximum 15 mg/d by 4–6 months; iron drops are best source	1 mg/kg/d to maximum 15 mg/d by 4 months; iron-fortified formula is best source†
Fluoride	0.25 mg/d after 6 months if local H_2O has < 0.3 ppm Fl	0.25 mg/d after 6 months if local H_2O has <0.3 ppm Fl or ready-to-feed formula is used

* See text for definition of at-risk infants.
† An iron-fortified formula (20 kcal/oz and 12 mg iron per quart) supplies approximately 2 mg/kg iron when fed at 120 kcal/kg.

Source: Data from references 36, 38, 53, 61-66, and 123.

Table 4–13 Composition of Selected Infant Vitamin and Mineral Drops

Product and Suggested Dose	*Vitamin D (IU)*	*Vitamin C (mg)*	*Vitamin A (IU)*	*Fe (mg)*	*Fl (mg)*
ADC drops 1.0 mL eg: Tri-Vi-Sol (Mead Johnson); Vi-Daylin ADC (Ross)	400	35	1500	—	—
ADC drops with iron 1.0 mL eg: Tri-Vi-Sol with iron (Mead Johnson); Vi-Daylin ADC plus iron (Ross)	400	35	1500	10	—
ADC drops with fluoride 1.0 mL* eg: Tri-Vi-Flor 0.25 mg (Mead Johnson); Vi-Daylin/F ADC (Ross)	400	35	1500	—	0.25
ADC drops with fluoride and iron* 1.0 mL eg: Tri-Vi-Flor 0.25 mg with iron (Mead Johnson); Vi-Daylin/F ADC plus iron (Ross)	400	35	1500	10	0.25
Iron drops: Fer-In-Sol (Mead Johnson) 0.6 mL	—	—	—	15	—
Fluoride drops Pediaflor (Ross)* eg, 0.5 mL	—	—	—	—	0.25

*Prescription required.

Source: Data from product handbooks by Mead Johnson Nutritional Division and Ross Laboratories, 1990.

4. have little exposure to sunlight[7,63]
5. have mothers with inadequate intakes of vitamin D or little exposure to sunlight.

Although the amount of iron in human milk is minimal, its bioavailability is quite high. About 50% of the iron is absorbed.[5,64,65] Some studies suggest that exclusively breastfed term infants remain iron sufficient for up to 9–12 months.[62,63] Most authorities, however, recommend another source of iron by 4–6 months of age to prevent the possibility of deficiency.[63–65] Iron deficiency anemia is associated with cognitive and motor impairments that may be irreversible.[7,64,66] It seems prudent to supply generous iron during the first year before the vigorous infant 'connoisseur' becomes the 'picky' toddler. Infants exclusively breastfed should receive additional iron supplementation after the age of 6 months. The AAP now supports the use of iron-fortified formulas as an acceptable alternative to feeding infants if breastfeeding is not chosen.[37] There are currently no data to support the opinion that iron-fortified formulas are not as well tolerated as low-iron formulas.

At 4–6 months, with the introduction of solids, infant cereal is probably the most convenient source of iron. However, iron drops are a more reliably absorbed source.[65] Iron-fortified infant cereals should be encouraged during of the first year of life until infants' diets include foods with good sources of heme-iron.

The Committee on Nutrition of the AAP no longer recommends fluoride supplementation for any infants, breastfed or formula fed, from birth until 6 months of age. Commercial formulas do not contain fluoride, and if after 6 months they are mixed with fluoridated water, no supplement is needed. The AAP recommends daily supplements for those infants over 6 months of age living in areas where water supplies contain less than 0.3 ppm of fluoride or those exclusively fed ready-to-feed formulas.[53] The current recommendation for infants over 6 months of age consuming nonfluoridated water (eg, well water, bottled water) is a daily supplement of 0.25 mg fluoride.[53]

Diets of breastfeeding mothers should be assessed for adequacy of vitamin B_{12} if the mother is following a meat-restricted diet, especially those who comply with vegan diets. When the mother takes a limited diet in any nutrient, supplementation is indicated for both the mother and infant (see Chapter 7, Vegetarianism in Children).

WEANING AND FEEDING PROGRESSION

The introduction of solids into an infant's diet should balance nutrient needs with a variety of foods and textures while encouraging feeding skills development. The goal of weaning is the transition from a liquid diet to a well-balanced table food diet. Readiness generally occurs during the first 4–6 months of life, but observations of physical and psychologic development are better determinants of readiness than age alone.

Nutrient Needs

In the absence of physical or developmental hindrance, a neonate can usually obtain the necessary calorie requirement from human milk or infant formula alone. As the infant reaches 4–6 months, nutrient needs become greater than human milk or formula can provide. Supplemental foods become necessary for adequate satiety.

During infancy, distribution of calories is generally recommended to be 40–50% fat[67] and 7–11% protein, with the remainder from carbohydrate. The recommended water/energy ratio is 1.5 mL/kcal. Both human milk and infant formulas resemble these distributions, as seen in Table 4–1 and Tables 4–5 to 4–8. Adding supplemental foods to the diet may alter the distribution of nutrients. This is a significant factor when deciding on the type and amount of solids to add to the diet.

Vitamin and mineral intake is also affected by the introduction of solid foods, especially as the solids begin to replace the volume of milk taken daily by the infant. At this point in the changing infant's diet, the solids are relied upon to provide adequate vitamins and minerals. For this reason, any solids fed should be nutrient-dense items. It has been estimated that infants about 6 months old who are consuming age-appropriate solids still rely on about 80% of their energy intake from formula and 20% from beikost, or food other than breast milk and formula. By 10 months of age, it is assumed that this infant will be able to take about 50% of energy intake from formula and 50% from other foods.[68]

Physical Readiness for Solids

Before 4 or 5 months of age, infants possess an extrusion reflex that enables them to swallow only liquid foods.[69] Around 4–6 months of age, an infant learns oral and gross motor skills that aid in accepting solid foods. Oral motor skills have evolved from the reflexive suck to the ability to swallow nonliquid foods and to transfer food from the front of the tongue to the back. Gross motor advancement includes sitting independently and maintaining balance while using hands to reach and grasp objects.[70] At this stage, the infant is ready to sit in a high chair and grasp pieces of food; however, the infant still lacks the hand-to-mouth coordination necessary to feed himself or herself.[71]

Psychologic Readiness for Solids

Independent eating behaviors are encouraged as the infant advances from reflexive and imitative behaviors to more independent and exploratory behaviors. This transitional milestone occurs sometime during the fourth month of life.[70] By 6 months, an infant is able to indicate a desire for food by opening his or her mouth, leaning forward to indicate hunger, and leaning back and turning away to show disinterest or satiety. Until an infant can express these feelings, feeding of solids will probably represent a type of forced feeding,[64] potentially leading to overfeeding and obesity.

In addition to determining the quantity of feedings, the infant should be encouraged to develop more independence with feeding in the following ways:

- self-feeding of soft finger foods
- sipping from a cup by 6–8 months of age[72]
- holding the bottle or cup independently
- controlling the timing of feeds in an effort to promote self-regulation of hunger and satiety[73]

Later in infancy, a variety of foods is introduced into the diet. These introductions of unfamiliar foods are noteworthy as they allow the infant to gain experience with various tastes and textures, promoting successful weaning to the family diet. The importance of diversifying the diet at specific intervals during the infant's psychologic development can be observed in deprived environments in which the eating pattern is unvaried and monotonous, or where weaning is delayed. Both of these situations fail to stimulate interest in solid foods[73,74] or self-feeding.

First Foods

Around 4–6 months of age, infants are generally ready for the introduction of solids. Two indicators that an infant is ready for solids include the ability to hold the head up without support and disappearance of extrusion reflex. Commercial infant rice cereal thinned to a semiliquid consistency with breast milk or infant formula is generally recommended as an infant's first food, as it is an unlikely allergen.[7] The cereal is traditionally introduced on a small spoon. Resistance to the initial spoon-feeding is common as the infant is unaccustomed to the spoon as a dispenser of food. Holding the infant in one's arms, rather than sitting him or her in a high chair, may relieve some of the initial apprehension the infant may experience. A gag reflex of varying degrees is apparent until about the age of 7–9 months. At this time, most infants are beginning to chew and tolerate smooth to chunky foods, and normal gag is developing. Choking, however, indicates that, despite the infant's chronologic age, he or she is not ready for the transition to solid foods.

When initiating rice cereal as the first solid food in the infant's diet, it should be fed for 2–3 days while examining the infant for symptoms of intolerance, such as skin rashes, vomiting, diarrhea, or wheezing. In the absence of such symptoms, the quantity, frequency, and consistency of cereal feedings are increased, and a second food, such as oatmeal or barley cereal, is presented. Refer to Table 4–14 for further recommendations regarding the progression of solid foods.

Market Choices

Many commercial baby food products are available in markets today. Virtually all are prepared without added sodium and many without added sugar. Juices are generally enriched with vitamin C, and cereals are enriched with iron, thiamine, riboflavin, niacin, calcium, and phosphorus. Those advertised as "first foods" are single-ingredient foods, in contrast to "dinners," baked goods, desserts, "junior foods," and some cereals, which contain a combination of ingredients. Textures from strained to chunky are available, along with foods designed for teething.

Commercial baby foods are a time-efficient means of providing an infant with solids and, if chosen wisely, can supply a nutrient-dense diet. Certain items will provide more nutrients than seemingly comparable choices. For example, plain meats contain from 220% to 250% of the protein and up to 200% of the iron of "meat dinners." The nutrient contents of selected commercial baby foods are listed in Table 4–15.

Home Preparation of Baby Foods

Home-prepared baby foods are an alternative to commercially prepared foods. They are more economic and allow greater flexibility in altering food consistency, but preparation can be time-consuming. Families should not be encouraged to prepare baby foods from their own meals if they lack variety in their diet, lack refrigeration and freezing, or have poor sanitation in their homes.[76] Home-grown foods should not be prepared for infants if the lead concentration of soil in residential areas is excessive.[77] These precautions are to ensure a varied diet and to prevent nutrient deficiencies, food-borne illness, and lead toxicity. Table 4–16 provides detailed instructions for the home preparation of baby foods.

DENTAL CARIES IN INFANCY

Baby bottle tooth decay (BBTD) is an oral health disorder characterized by rampant dental caries associated with inappropriate infant feeding practices (see Figure 4–1). The disorder affects the primary teeth of infants and young children, particularly those who are permitted to fall asleep with a bottle filled with juice or other fermentable liquid.[75,78] Nursing caries, similar to tooth decay caused by BBTD from formulas, can also occur with prolonged or inappropriate breastfeeding at naptime. Certain feeding practices can be altered to prevent BBTD.

Providing liquids concentrated in mono- and disaccharides, such as juice and sweetened beverages, is a leading cause of BBTD.[7] While sleeping with a bottle in his or her mouth, an infant's swallowing and salivary flow decrease. This creates a pooling of liquid around the teeth.

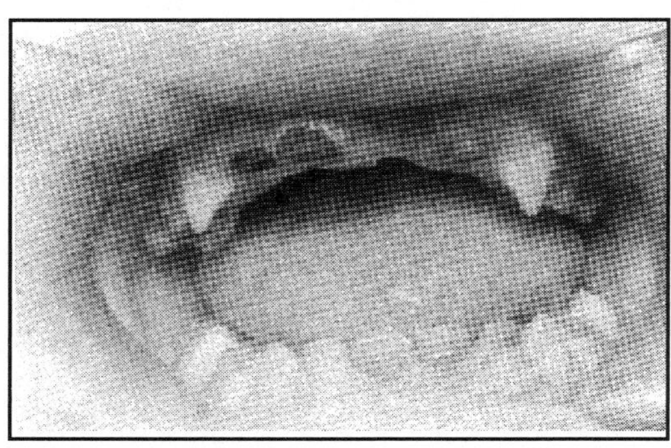

Figure 4–1 Baby bottle tooth decay.

Source: S. L. Groh and K. Antonelli, Normal Nutrition During Infancy, in *Handbook of Pediatric Nutrition,* P.M. Queen and C.E. Lang, eds., ©1993, Aspen Publishers, Inc.

Table 4–14 Guidelines for Progression of Solid Foods

Years in Months	*Feeding Skills*	*Oral Motor Skills*	*Types of Food*	*Suggested Activities*
B–4		Rooting reflex Sucking reflex Swallowing reflex Extrusion reflex	Breast milk Infant formula	Breastfeeding or bottle feeding
5	Able to grasp objects voluntarily Learning to reach mouth with hands	Disappearance of extrusion reflex		Possible introduction of thinned cereal
6	Sits with balance while using hands Ready for high chair	Transfers food from front of tongue to back Closes lips around spoon	Infant cereal Strained fruit Strained vegetables	Prepare cereal with formula or breast milk to a semiliquid texture Use spoon Feed from a dish Advance to 1/3–1/2 cup cereal before adding fruits or vegetables
7	Improved grasp Drinks from cup with help	Mashes food with lateral movements of jaw	Infant cereal	Thicken cereal to lumpier texture
		Learns side-to-side or “rotary” chewing	Strained to junior texture of fruits, vegetables, and meats	Sit child in high chair with feet supported Introduce cup
8–10	Holds bottle without help Drinks from cup without spilling Decreases fluid intake and increases solids Coordinates hand-to-mouth movement	Swallows with closed mouth	Juices Soft, mashed, or minced table foods	Begin finger foods Do not add salt, sugar, or fats to food Present soft foods in chunks ready for finger feeding
10–12	Feeds self with fingers and spoon Holds cup without help	Tooth eruption Improved ability to bite and chew	Soft, chopped table foods	Provide meals in pattern similar to rest of family Use cup at meals

Source: Data from references 7, 70, and 125.

Table 4–15 Nutrient Content of Selected Commercial Baby Food Products

Food	*Amount (g)*	*Calories*	*Protein (g)*	*Carbohydrate (g)*	*Fat (g)*	*Iron (mg)*	*Sodium (mg)*
Infant cereal	100 (7 Tbsp.)	55	1.7	9.9	0.9	5.3	8
Strained juices	100 (3.2 oz.)	46	0	11.2	*	*	*
Strained fruits "first foods"	100	56	*	13.3	*	*	*
Strained vegetables "first foods"	100	35	0.9	6.9	0.3	0.2	37
Strained meat	100	103	11.7	4.4	4.3	1.3	44
Strained meat dinner	100	68	3.0	9.9	1.8	0.7	22
Strained dinner	100	62	2.4	10.4	1.4	0.4	13

*insignificant content

Note: Mean values derived from data provided by Gerber Products Company, 1998 Nutrient Values, Fremont, MI 49413.

Table 4–16 Steps in the Home Preparation of Baby Foods

1. Choosing appropriate foods
   - Use fresh or unsalted frozen foods. Do not use canned foods as they may contribute excessive sodium to the infant diet.
   - Spinach, carrots, broccoli, and beets should not be pureed at home because they may contain sufficient nitrite to cause methemoglobinemia in young infants.
2. Preparing fruits and vegetables
   - Thaw frozen vegetables/wash fresh produce.
   - Remove peels, cores, and seeds.
   - Steam or boil.
   - Puree in blender to desired consistency. Use liquid from cooking to preserve nutrients otherwise lost in cooking. Do not overblend as this may cause excessive oxidation of nutrients.
3. Preparing meats
   - Bake, broil, or stew.
   - Remove all skins.
   - Chop into small pieces.
   - Puree in blender to desired consistency.
4. Storing prepared foods
   - Keep refrigerated in a covered container. Use refrigerated foods within 48 hours.
   - Freeze in 2 tbsp portions by pouring pureed food into an ice cube tray. Thaw desired portions in refrigerator before using.

Source: Data from references 125, and 127 to 129.

Sweet fluid contacting the teeth for a prolonged period of time provides plaque-forming bacteria, particularly *Streptococcus mutans*, with energy.[78,79] The outcome is otherwise known as *dental plaque*.

Infants who refuse cold foods or grimace when chewing should be examined for BBTD. Those afflicted will have tooth discoloration varying from yellow to black. Preventive measures include the following:

- feeding only infant formula or water from a bottle
- cleaning the infant's teeth and gums with a damp washcloth or gauze pad after each feeding
- giving juices with a cup rather than a bottle
- filling bedtime bottles with water

WHOLE COW'S MILK

The most recent recommendations by the AAP Committee on Nutrition suggest that, to maintain optimal nutrition status, infants should be provided breast milk for the first 6–12 months, with the only alternative being iron-fortified formulas.[50,51] Early introduction of whole cow's milk is associated with increased risks of milk protein allergy, gastrointestinal blood loss, poor iron delivery, and overall poor nutritional status of the infant.[7,79]

When the infant's diet is changed to cow's milk after the first year, it should be whole cow's milk, as opposed to 2% or skim (see Table 4–10) to provide essential fat and calories. Incidence of cow's milk protein allergy is 1–2% during the first 2 years of life.[79,80] Very early exposure to cow's milk increases the risk of developing the allergy to milk protein and possibly to other foods as well. Resistance to allergy increases with gastrointestinal maturity,[7,81] so that at 6 months of age, cow's milk can be introduced into the infant's diet with somewhat less risk of allergy. However, risks of iron deficiency anemia[7,81] and inadequate nutrient delivery are increased when cow's milk replaces breast milk or formula before 12 months of age.

Occult loss of blood from the gastrointestinal tract is associated with the introduction of cow's milk in both early and later infancy. Blood loss, along with the lower concentration and bioavailability of iron in cow's milk, predisposes the infant to iron deficiency anemia.[7,82] Neonatal iron stores become depleted by about 4–6 months in a term infant.[51] Iron-fortified infant cereal is traditionally introduced into the diet at this time or shortly thereafter and is an excellent source of iron. However, the bioavailability of the electrolytic iron powders presently fortifying the cereal is currently being scrutinized.[7,83,84,85] Heme-iron in meat is a reliable source of iron.[85] Until meat can be incorporated into the diet, infants fed cow's milk or unfortified formula should be provided with an iron supplement. Cow's milk is also a poor source of vitamin C, vitamin E, and essential fatty acids (EFAs). When an infant is changed to cow's milk, high-vitamin-C foods such as fruits, fruit juices, and vegetables should be a regular part of the diet, or a supplement with vitamin C should be prescribed. The AAP recommends 2.7% of calories as EFAs in infancy.[37] Meeting this requirement and the RDAs for vitamin E may be difficult for the infant on cow's milk until a fairly wide variety of table foods is introduced into the diet.[7]

Lastly, the additional protein and electrolytes in cow's milk increases the renal solute load and places the infant at risk for dehydration during periods of vomiting, diarrhea, or exposure to dry heat in winter or to the sun in the summer. For all of the above reasons, it is best to delay the introduction of cow's milk until the infant is 1 year old.

JUICE CONSUMPTION DURING INFANCY

There is considerable controversy regarding the consumption of fruit juices during infancy. The debate revolves around the influence of fruit juice on failure to thrive and malabsorption versus its role relieving constipation.

The carbohydrate source in fruit juice is primarily from a combination of fructose, glucose, and sorbitol. See Table 4–17 for the carbohydrate sources in various fruit juices.[7] Studies summarized by Fomon suggest that infants have greater absorption and tolerance to juices containing fructose when found in combination with sucrose and glucose.[7,86] Fruit juices containing these sugars appear to have beneficial effects similar to those of fiber for infants suffering from constipation. Juices containing the greatest amounts of fructose and sorbitol include apple and pear juice.[87,88]

Table 4–17 Carbohydrate Sources in Select Juices (g/100g of food) (mOsm/kg H_2O)

	Fructose	*Glucose*	*Sucrose*	*Sorbitol*	*Osmolality*
Apple Juice	6.0	2.4	2.5	0.5	638
Pear Juice	6.6	2.0	3.7	2.2	764
White Grape	7.5	7.1	0.6		1030

Values may vary depending on the dilution of the juice and type of fruit used.

Sources: From references 7, 87, and 130.

Consumption of fruit juices may displace the intake of nutrient-dense formulas essential for delivering the majority of an infant's nutritional needs. It is not uncommon to obtain a diet history from a caregiver of an infant with poor weight gain and to discover an excessive intake of fruit juice in the diet. Excessive fruit juice consumption for infants and toddlers is defined as an amount greater than 12 oz per day.[89] Some risks involved with overconsumption of juices include dental caries, failure to thrive, short stature, and obesity later in the preschool years.[89]

FEEDING PROBLEMS

Formula intolerance, constipation, acute diarrhea, and food refusal are common feeding problems encountered during infancy. These problems can usually be resolved through simple measures. If ignored, the problems may become exacerbated and cause detrimental effects to an infant's nutritional status.

Milk Allergy

Intolerance to lactose must not be confused with milk protein allergy. Lactose intolerance has an enzymatic etiology, whereas milk allergy is based on immunologic mechanisms. Gastrointestinal disturbance is common to both disorders. Diarrhea is frequently observed in both, but vomiting is exclusive to milk allergy. In addition to gastrointestinal symptoms, dermatologic, respiratory, and possibly systemic reactions, such as anaphylactic shock (although this is rare), may occur in milk allergy.[90]

The usual onset of milk allergy occurs in the first 4 months of infancy. This onset is due to the immaturity of both the gastrointestinal tract and the immune system. In early infancy, the gastrointestinal tract adapts to the extrauterine environment, protecting against the penetration of harmful substances such as bacteria, toxins, and antigens within the intestinal lumen.[91] Mechanisms act to control and maintain the epithelium as an impermeable barrier to the uptake of such antigens as β-lactoglobulin and α-lactalbumin found in cow's milk.

Treatment of milk allergy involves the elimination of suspected foods from the diet until 1 or 2 years of age, at which time a challenge with cow's milk is done to determine whether the allergy persists. Goat's milk has been used in the past for the treatment of cow's milk allergy. If the reaction to cow's milk is truly allergic, however, the infant will most likely react to goat's milk in the same way.[7] Unpasteurized, unfortified goat's milk also is not recommended because it contains inadequate folic acid, is excessive in protein and electrolytes, and is not reliably hypoallergenic (see Table 4–10). Canned goat's milk may be fortified but is still high in protein and not reliably hypoallergenic. Casein hydrolysate formulas are the feeding of choice in true cow's milk allergy.

Food Allergy

Presence of milk protein allergy may correlate with allergies to other foods. Withholding the more allergenic foods from the diet for the first 6–12 months of life can be a prophylactic measure. Restricting these allergenic foods until the milk allergy has resolved may be indicated for more severe cases. The most common allergenic foods include the following: eggs, soy, nuts, peas, fish, chocolate, citrus fruit, corn products, wheat, chicken, and fish (see Chapter 8 for further information on food sensitivities).

Constipation

There are many reasons an infant may experience constipation. The most common influencing factors include inappropriate fluid intake, excessive fluid losses, allergic etiology,[92] and medications. It is recommended that constipation be considered a symptom and not a diagnosis.[90] In simplest terms, it is defined as infrequent stooling as compared with usual number of bowel movements for that infant or as extremely dry, hard, or small stools. Normal stooling patterns vary from infant to infant and with differences in dietary intake. Constipation is rare in the breastfed infant but more common in the bottle-fed infant.[69] Refer to Tables 4–18 and 4–19 for normal stooling patterns and colors in relation to type of infant formula or milk being consumed.

Treating nonanatomic constipation requires dietary intervention. Five measures can be taken, in the following sequence:

1. Verify constipation through family interview.
2. Ensure the proper diet, including free fluid intake versus fluid losses.

Table 4–18 Stool Characteristics

Protein Source	*Stool Characteristic*
Breast Milk	Pasty, yellow, soft
Modified skim milk	Formed, greenish brown, very little free water
Whey, casein	Small volume, pasty yellow, some free water (similar to breast milk stool)
Whey, casein (with iron)	Soft, formed, yellowish green
Soy protein isolate	Soft, yellowish green
Casein hydrolysate	Green, some mucus, small volume
Sodium caseinate	Formed, greenish brown, little free water

Source: Reproduced with permission from *Pediatrics,* Vol. 95, pages 50–54, 1995.

Table 4–19 Stool Frequency and Weight in Normal Infants

	1 Week	*8–28 Days*	*1–12 Months*	*13–24 Months*
No. stools/24 hr.	4	2.2	1.8	1.7
Weight (g)	4.3	11	17	35
Water content (%)	72	73	75	73.5

Source: Reprinted from *Gastrointestinal Problems in the Infant* by J Grybowski and WA Walker with permission of WB Saunders, © 1983.

3. Ensure accurate preparation of formula if infant is bottle fed.
4. Feed two additional ounces of water after each feeding.
5. Provide two oz of pear or apple juice (refer to discussion on fruit juice during infancy).

If there is no relief from the above recommendations and the infant appears to be in pain or cramping, a physician should be notified.

Acute Diarrhea

Acute infantile diarrhea is defined as the sudden onset of increased stool frequency, volume, and water content.[93] The cause can be bacterial, viral, parasitic, or a result of large-dose antibiotics.[94,95] Diarrhea lasting more than 4 days, or resulting in greater than 10% dehydration may still require intravenous fluid therapy. However, bottle-fed infants suffering from mild to moderate diarrhea can be rehydrated with an oral rehydration solution for 4–6 hours. Refer to Table 4–20 for the nutrient comparison of clear liquids and rehydration solutions.

The AAP recommends the reintroduction of age-appropriate foods and liquids after a brief rehydration period.[96] Studies revealed that this approach did not worsen stool output and helped with maintaining nutritional status.[97] Beverages such as juice, broth, carbonated beverages, or Gatorade should not be fed as their high osmolalities may induce osmotic diarrhea, exacerbating the initial problem.[98] Continued breastfeeding is beneficial, despite controversial concerns related to secondary lactose intolerance during acute diarrhea. Infants on formula should resume with their previous full-strength formulas.[97]

Stool Characteristics in Relation to Infant Formulas

It is not uncommon to obtain an infant's diet history and have a caregiver report various formula changes secondary to "formula intolerance." The frustration around this situation is that the perceived intolerance is usually nonspecific. A common complaint involves alterations in stool characteristics. Caregivers may fail to understand that different types of infant feedings are expected to produce variations in stool patterns. Infants being breastfed or receiving hydrolyzed protein formulas typically experience between 1 and 12 bowel movements a day.[98] This can be at least twice as many stools as infants consuming cow's-milk-based or soy-based formulas.[99] The frequency of stools usually decreases considerably as infants reach their first

Table 4–20 Nutrient Comparison of Clear Liquids and Rehydration Solutions

Product	*Na (mEq/L)*	*K (mEq/L)*	*Cl (mEq/L)*	*Sugar (g/L)*	*Starch (g/L)*	*Osmolality (mOsm/L)*
Cola	1.7	0.1–0.6	—	53–58.5	—	750
Apple juice	4.6	26	1.1	39.5	—	747
Gatorade	20–23	2.5–3	23	25–28	—	330–365
Chicken broth	250	8	—	—	—	500
Rehydralyte	75	20	65	25	—	305
Pedialyte	45	20	35	25	—	250
Ricelyte	50	25	45	—	30	200

Source: Data from references 94 and 126 and from product information provided by Ross Laboratories and Mead Johnson Nutritionals.

birthdays. (See Table 4–19.) Studies also suggest a variation in stool consistency in relation to type of formula. Infants fed soy-based formulas tend to have more stools, which are hard and firm.[99] Whether the perceived intolerance is valid or not, parents should be discouraged from "formula jumping." This only causes confusion for the infant and professional attempting to distinguish between a "fussy" infant and a true allergic finding. Refer to Table 4–18 for common stool characteristics.

Gastroesophageal Reflux

Gastroesophageal reflux (GER), or chalasia, affects many infants. GER is otherwise referred to as *regurgitation* or *spitting up*. A clinical definition is the presence of gastric contents in the esophagus proximal to the stomach.[100] All infants experience some degree of GER. Most infants have no significant complications associated with it, whereas others may develop failure to thrive, anemia, or pulmonary aspiration with pneumonia. GER can potentially cause asthma or apnea.[100] Mild GER may be treated with modifications in feeding positions and dietary regimens. More severe GER may require pharmaceutical or surgical interventions.

An upright position during feeding may prevent GER. In this position, gravity may aid in gastric emptying. When an infant is placed in the semi-upright position of an infant seat, however, reduced truncal tone, common in early infancy, may result in slumping.[100] Slumping submerges the infant's posterior gastroesophageal junction into the stomach, increasing abdominal pressure and GER. A truly upright position is most reliable in preventing GER.[101] Studies indicate that infants maintained in an upright position for at least 15 minutes after a feeding have a lower incidence of earaches.[59] If this is not possible, a prone position with the head elevated to a 30° angle may also be effective.[102]

Thickening formula with cereal has been routine practice in preventing GER. There has been documentation of anecdotal responses to this treatment, including decreased emesis and crying time, and increased sleeping time in the postprandial period. However, there has been no proof of its efficacy in clinical studies, and it may even increase the frequency of asymptomatic reflux.[103–105] The clinician must also be aware that cereal increases the caloric concentration of formula, interferes with breastfeeding, and may delay gastric emptying.

Food Refusal

Two important milestones during infancy are self-feeding and developing a positive relationship with food and eating. If these do not occur, a spiral effect of food refusal and poor nutrient intake can ensue. It is currently estimated that feeding problems may occur in up to 25–35% of infants and children.[106] Food refusal can occur in infancy because of physical or emotional stress and is more typically classified as organic, indicating a medical etiology, or functional, referring to environmental influences. Illness and unfavorable atmospheres for feeding are typical contributors to food refusal. The consequence of this problem is failure to thrive (see Chapter 18).

During illness, infants become irritable due to fever, congestion, or lack of sleep. At these times, food refusal is inevitable. The encouragement of fluids and possibly administration of parenteral fluids are necessary to prevent/treat dehydration. Although food refusal of this nature can still cause significant weight loss and deplete nutrient stores, if identified early, it is usually self-limited.

Food refusal originating from excessive or deficient stimulation is more difficult to discern. Commotion and overly aggressive or restrictive caregivers can cause development of negative associations with feeding. Routine negative interactions at mealtime can keep an infant from wanting to explore and advance with the normal self-feeding progression. As the stages of eating advance from complete liquid and dependence as a newborn to table foods as a toddler, the "balance of power" also shifts in the feeding relationship.[107] Similarly, a caregiver may restrict the infant's exploration of food and/or rush through a meal, disrupting the feeding pace. Under these circumstances, it is not uncommon for an infant to begin to refuse food entirely. Concerned that the infant is feeding poorly or losing weight, caregivers become tense. This tension only exacerbates the reluctance to feed.

The most effective means of treating feeding disorders after identification is to increase appropriate behavior and decrease maladaptive behavior between infant and caregiver, and infant and feeding.[108] Most literature related to feeding disorders promotes a calm, interactive, and supportive environment and one that encourages the most positive relationship with infant feeding.

CONCLUSIONS

Issues related to breastfeeding, bottle feeding, vitamin and mineral supplementation, the introduction and progression of solids, and common feeding problems have all been discussed in this chapter. Translating this scientific information into practical suggestions for parents is a necessity to ensure good nutrition for adequate growth and development.

REFERENCES

1. American Academy of Pediatrics. The promotion of breastfeeding. *Pediatrics.* 1982;69:654.
2. Position of the American Dietetic Association. Promotion of breastfeeding. *J Am Diet Assoc.* 1997;97:662.
3. *Mother's Survey,* Ross Products Division, Abbott Laboratories; 1998.
4. Scott JA, Binns CW, Aroni RA. The influence of reported paternal attitudes on the decision to breast-feed. *J Paediatr Child Health.* 1997;33:305–307.
5. Lawrence RA. *Breastfeeding, A Guide for the Medical Profession.* 4th ed. St Louis, MO: Mosby; 1994.
6. McVeagh P, Miller B. Review Article: Human milk oligosaccharides: Only the breast. *J Paediatr Child Health.* 1997;33:281–286.
7. Fomon SJ. *Nutrition of Normal Infants.* St Louis, MO: Mosby; 1993.
8. Institute of Medicine. *Nutrition During Lactation.* Washington, D.C.: National Academy of Sciences; 1991.
9. Scariati PD, Grummer-Strawn LM, Fein SB. A longitudinal analysis of infant morbidity and the extent of breastfeeding in the United States (Abstract) *Pediatrics.* 1997;99(6):862.
10. Dewey KG, Heinig MJ, Nommsen LA, et al. Breast-fed infants are leaner than formula-fed infants at 1 year of age: the DARLING Study. *Am J Clin Nutr.* 1993;57:140–145.
11. Gruskay FL. Comparison of breast, cow and soy feedings in the prevention of onset of allergic disease. *Clin Pediatr.* 1982;21:486.
12. Kramer MS. Does breast feeding help protect against atopic disease? Biology, methodology, and a golden jubilee of controversy. *J Pediatr.* 1988;112:181.
13. Lawrence RA. *Breastfeeding: A Guide for the Medical Profession.* 3rd ed. St Louis, MO: Mosby; 1989.
14. Dewey KG, Finley DA, Lonnerdal B. Breast milk volume and composition during late lactation (7–20 months). *J Pediatr Gastroenterol Nutr.* 1984;3:713–720.
15. Karra MV, Udipi SA, Kirksey A, Roepke JLB. Changes in specific nutrients in breast milk during extended lactation. *Am J Clin Nutr.* 1986;43:495–503.
16. Brown KH. Clinical and field studies of human lactation: methodological considerations. *Am J Clin Nutr.* 1982;35:745.
17. Hall B. Changing composition of human milk and early development of appetite control. *Lancet.* 1975;1:779.
18. Standing Committee on the Scientific Evaluation of Dietary Reference Intakes. *Dietary Reference Intakes (for Various Nutrients).* Food and Nutrition Board, Institute of Medicine. Washington, DC: National Academy Press; 1998.
19. Jensen RG. *Handbook of Milk Composition.* San Diego: Academic Press; 1995.
20. Lourdes B, Butte NF, Villalpando S, et al. Maternal energy balance and lactation performance of Mesoamerindians as a function of body mass index. *Am J Clin Nutr.* 1997;66:575–583.
21. American Academy of Pediatrics, Committee on Nutrition. Nutrition and lactation. *Pediatrics.* 1981;68:435–443.
22. Worthington-Roberts BS. Lactation and Human Milk: nutritional considerations. In: Worthington-Roberts BS, Williams SR, eds. *Nutrition in Pregnancy and Lactation.* 4th ed. St Louis, MO: Mosby; 1989:244–322.
23. Mellies MJ, Ishikawa TT, Gartside PS, et al. Effects of varying maternal dietary fatty acids in lactating women and their infants. *Am J Clin Nutr.* 1979;32:299.
24. Jakobsson I, Lindberg T. Cow's milk proteins cause infantile colic in breast-fed infants: a double-blind crossover study. *Pediatrics.* 1983;71:268.

25. Berlin CM, Denson HM, Daniel CH, Ward RM. Deposition of dietary caffeine in milk, saliva, and plasma of lactating women. *Pediatrics.* 1984;73:59.

26. Luck W, Nau H. Nicotine and cotinine concentrations in serum and urine of infants exposed via passive smoking or milk from smoking mothers. *J Pediatr.* 1985;107:816.

27. Binkiewicz A, Robinson MJ, Senior B. Pseudo-Cushing syndrome caused by alcohol in breast milk. *J Pediatr.* 1978;93:965.

28. Nehlig A, Debry G. Consequences on the newborn of chronic maternal consumption of coffee during gestation and lactation: A Review. *J Am Coll Nutr.* 1994;13(1):6–21.

29. LeGuennec JC, Billon B. Delay in caffeine elimination in breast-fed infants. *Pediatrics.* 1987;79(2):264–268.

30. Ahn CH, MacLean WC. Growth of the exclusively breast-fed infant. *Am J Clin Nutr.* 1980;33:183.

31. Matheny R, Picciano MF. Feeding and growth characteristics of human milk-fed infants. *J Am Diet Assoc.* 1986;86:327.

32. Dewey KG, Peerson JM, Brown KH, et al. Growth of breast-fed infants deviates from current reference data: A pooled analysis of US, Canadian, and European data sets. *Pediatrics.* 1995;96(3):495–503.

33. Freed GL, Landers S, Schanler RJ. A practical guide to successful breastfeeding. *Am J Dis Child.* 1991;145:917–921.

34. Kuhr M, Paneth N. Feeding practices and early neonatal jaundice. *J Pediatr Gastroenterol Nutr.* 1982;1:485.

35. Hamosh M. Breast feeding and the working mother. *Pediatrics.* 1996;97:492–498.

36. Fomon SJ. Reflections on infant feeding in the 1970s and 1980s. *Am J Clin Nutr.* 1987;46:171.

37. Forbes GB, Woodruff CW, eds. *Pediatric Nutrition Handbook.* 2nd ed. Elk Grove Village, IL: American Academy of Pediatrics; 1985.

38. Food and Drug Administration. Rules and regulations. Nutrient requirements for infant formulas. *Fed Register.* 45106-8. 21 CFR Sec 107. 1985;50:100.

39. Lonnerdal B, Forsum E. The casein:whey ratio of human milk. *Fed Proc.* 1984;43:468.

40. Jarvenpaa A-L, Rassin DK, Raiha NCR. Milk protein quantity and quality in the term infant, II. Effects on acidic and neutral amino acids. *Pediatrics.* 1982;70:221.

41. Voltz VR, Book LS, Churella HR. Growth and plasma amino acid concentrations in term infants fed either whey predominant formula or human milk. *J Pediatr.* 1983;102:27.

42. Jarvenpaa A-L, Raiha NCR, Rassin DK, et al. Milk protein quantity and quality in the term infant, I: Metabolic response and effects on growth. *Pediatrics.* 1982;70:214.

43. Raiha N, Axelsson I. Protein nutrition during infancy. *Pediatr Clin North Am.* 1995;42(4):745–763.

44. Janas LM, Picciano MF, Hatch TF. Indices of protein metabolism in term infants fed human milk, whey predominant formula, or cow's milk formula. *Pediatrics.* 1985;75:775.

45. Dallman PR, Siimes MA, Stekel A. Iron deficiency in infancy and childhood. *Am J Clin Nutr.* 1980;33:86.

46. American Academy of Pediatrics, Committee on Nutrition. Soy protein-based formulas: Recommendations for use in infant feeding. *Pediatrics.* 1998;101(1):148–153.

47. Burks AW, Casteel HB, Fiedorek SC, et al. A prospective food challenge study of two different types of soy protein isolates in patients with possible milk or soy protein intolerance. (Abstract) *J Allergy Clin Immunol.* 1996;87:175.

48. American Academy of Pediatrics, Committee on Nutrition. Hypoallergenic infant formulas. *Pediatrics.* 1989;83:1068.

49. American Academy of Pediatrics, Committee on Nutrition. Follow-up or weaning formulas. *Pediatrics.* 1989;83:1067.

50. Ziegler EE. Milk and formulas for older infants. *J Pediatr.* 1990;117:S76.

51. American Academy of Pediatrics. The use of cow's milk in infancy. *Pediatrics.* 1992;89:6.

52. Fomon SJ, Filer LJ, Anderson TA, Ziegler EE. Recommendations for feeding normal infants. *Pediatrics.* 1979;63:52.

53. American Academy of Pediatrics, Committee on Nutrition. Fluoride supplementation for children: interim policy recommendations. *Pediatrics.* 1995;95:777–778.

54. *Preparation of Infant Formulas: Guidelines for Health Care Facilities.* Chicago: The American Dietetic Association; 1991.

55. Gerber MA, Berliner BC, Karolus JJ. Sterilization of infant formulas. *Clin Pediatr.* 1983;22:344.

56. Hibbard RA, Blevins R. Palatal burn due to bottle warming in a microwave oven. *Pediatrics.* 1988;82:382.

57. Puczynski M, Rademaker D, Gatson RL. Burn injury related to the improper use of a microwave oven. *Pediatrics.* 1983;72:714.

58. Shelton PG, Berkowitz RJ, Forrester DJ. Nursing bottle caries. *Pediatrics.* 1977;59:777.

59. Tully SB, Bar-Halm Y, Bradley RL. Abnormal tympanography after supine bottle feeding. *J Pediatr.* 1995;126:S105–S111.

60. Satter E. *Child of Mine: Feeding with Love and Good Sense.* Palo Alto, CA: Bull Publishing; 1986.
61. Greer FR. Improving the Vitamin K status of breastfeeding infants with maternal Vit K supplements. *Pediatrics.* 1997;99:88–92.
62. Park MJ. Bone mineral content is not reduced despite low vitamin D status in breast milk-fed infants versus cow's milk based formula-fed infants. *J Pediatr.* 1998;132:641–645.
63. American Academy of Pediatrics, Committee on Nutrition. Vitamin and mineral supplement needs in normal children in the United States. *Pediatrics.* 1980;66:1015.
64. Tsang R, Zlotkin SH, Nichols BL, et al. *Nutrition during Infancy, Principles and Practice.* 2nd ed. Cincinnati, OH: Digital Education Publishing; 1997.
65. Newman V. *Iron Needs of the Breastfed Infant. Building Blocks for Life.* Pediatric Nutrition Practice Group, Chicago: American Dietetic Association. 1993;17:3.
66. Walter T, DeAndraca I, Chadud P, et al. Iron deficiency anemia: adverse effects on infant psychomotor development. *Pediatrics.* 1989;84:7.
67. Fomon SJ. *Infant Nutrition.* 2nd ed. Philadelphia, PA: WB Saunders Company; 1974.
68. Fomon SJ, Sanders KD, Ziegler EE. Formulas for older infants. *J Pediatr.* 1990;116:690–696.
69. Lipsitt L, Crook C, Booth C. The transitional infant: behavioral development and feeding. *Am J Clin Nutr.* 1985;41:485.
70. Marlow D. *Textbook of Pediatric Nursing.* 6th ed. Philadelphia, PA: WB Saunders Company; 1988.
71. Cloud H. Feeding problems of the child with special health care needs. In: Ekvall SW. *Pediatric Nutrition in Chronic Diseases and Developmental Disorders: Prevention, Assessment, and Treatment.* New York: Oxford University Press; 1993:203–218.
72. Chatoor I, Hirsch R, Persinger M. Facilitating internal regulation of eating: A treatment model of infantile anorexia. *Infants Young Child.* 1997;9(4):12–22.
73. Underwood B. Weaning practices in deprived environments: the weaning dilemma. *Pediatrics.* 1985;75 (suppl):194.
74. Pipes P, Trahms CM. *Nutrition in Infancy and Childhood.* 5th ed. St. Louis, MO: Mosby; 1993.
75. Alvarez JO, Naviaj JM. Nutritional status, tooth eruption, and dental caries: a review. *Am J Clin Nutr.* 1989; 49:417–426.
76. Oskarsson A. *Exposure of Infants and Children to Lead.* Rome, Italy: Food and Agriculture Organization of the United Nations; 1989.
77. Shils ME, Olson JA, Shike M. *Modern Nutrition in Health and Disease.* 8th ed. Philadelphia, PA: Lea & Febiger; 1994.
78. Nowak A. What pediatricians can do to promote oral health. *Contemp Pediatr.* 1993;10:90–106.
79. Foucard T. Development of food allergies with special reference to cow's milk allergy. *Pediatrics.* 1985; 75(suppl):177.
80. Committee on Nutrition, American Academy of Pediatrics. The use of whole cow's milk in infancy. *Pediatrics.* 1983;72:253.
81. Tunnessen WW, Oski FA. Consequences of starting whole cow milk at 6 months of age. *J Pediatr.* 1987; 111:813–816.
82. Ziegler EE, Fomon SJ, Nelson SE, et al. Cow milk feeding in infancy: further observations on blood loss from the gastrointestinal tract. *J Pediatr.* 1990;116:11.
83. Fomon S. Bioavailability of supplemental iron in commercially prepared dry infant cereals. *J Pediatr.* 1987; 110:660.
84. Rios E, Hunter R, Cook J, et al. The absorption of iron as supplements in infant cereal and infant formulas. *Pediatrics.* 1975;55:686.
85. Monsen E. Iron nutrition and absorption: dietary factors which impact iron bioavailability. *J Am Diet Assoc.* 1988;88:786.
86. Hoeksttra JH, van Kempen AAMW, Kneepkens CMF. Apple juice malabsorption: fructose or sorbitol? *J Pediatr Gastroenterol Nutr.* 1993;16:39–42.
87. Smith MM, Davis M, Chasalow FI, et al. Carbohydrate absorption from fruit juice in young children. *Pediatrics.* 1995;95:340–344.
88. Lifschitz CH. Fruit juice. (Letter to the editor) *Pediatrics.* 1995;96:376.
89. Levine AA. Excessive fruit juice consumption: How can something that causes failure to thrive be associated with obesity? (Selected summary) *J Pediatr Gastroenterol Nutr.* 1997;25:554–555.
90. Wyllie R, Hyams JS. *Pediatric Gastrointestinal Diseases.* Philadelphia, PA: WB Saunders Company; 1993.
91. Walker A. Absorption of protein and protein fragments in the developing intestine: role in immunologic/allergic reactions. *Pediatrics.* 1985;75(suppl):167.
92. Iacono G, Carroccio A, Cavataio F, et al. Chronic constipation as a symptom of cow milk allergy. *J Pediatr.* 1995;126:34–39.
93. Moffet H, Shulenburger BH, Burkholder BE. Epidemiology and etiology of severe infantile diarrhea. *J Pediatr.* 1968;72:1–14.
94. Snyder J. Oral rehydration therapy for acute diarrhea. *Semin Pediatr Gastroenterol Nutr.* 1990;1:8.
95. Provisional Committee on Quality Improvement, Subcommittee on Acute Gastroenteritis. Practice parameter: the management of acute gastroenteritis in young children. *Pediatrics.* 1996;97:424–436.
96. Duggan C, Nurleo S. "Feeding the gut:" The scientific basis for continued enteral nutrition during acute diarrhea. *J Pediatr.* 1997;131:801–808.

97. Moutos D. *Diarrhea. Building Blocks for Life.* Pediatric Nutrition Practice Group. Chicago: American Dietetic Association; 1996;20,3.
98. Hyams J, Treem WR, Etienne NL, et al. Effects of infant formula on stool characteristics of young infants. *Pediatrics.* 1995;95:50–54.
99. Hillemier C. Gastroesophageal reflux. *Pediatr Clin North Am.* 1996;43:1.
100. Herbst J. Gastroesophageal reflux. *J Pediatr.* 1981; 98:859.
101. Orenstein S, Whitington P. Positioning for prevention of infant gastroesophageal reflux. *J Pediatr.* 1983;103:534.
102. Bailey D, Andres J, Danek G, Pineiro-Carrero V. Lack of efficacy of thickened feeding as treatment for gastroesophageal reflux. *J Pediatr.* 1987;110:187.
103. Orenstein S, Magill H, Brooks P. Thickening of infant feedings for therapy of gastroesophageal reflux. *J Pediatr.* 1987;110:181.
104. Ulshen M. Treatment of gastroesophageal reflux: is nothing sacred? *J Pediatr.* 1987;110:254.
105. Benoit D. Phenomenology and treatment of failure to thrive. *Child Adolesc Psychiatr Clin North Am.* 1993; 2:61–73.
106. Burklow KA, Phelps AN, Schultz JR, et al. Classifying complex pediatric feeding disorders. *J Pediatr Gastroenterol Nutr.* 1998;27:143–147.
107. Babbitt RL, Hoch TA, Coe DA, et al. Behavioral assessment and treatment of pediatric feeding disorders. *J Dev Behav Pediatr.* 1994;15:278–291.
108. Hollis BW, Ross BA, Draper HH, Lambert PW. Occurrence of vitamin D sulfate in human milk whey. *J Nutr.* 1981;111:384.
109. Jansson L, Akesson B, Holmberg L. Vitamin E and fatty acid composition of human milk. *Am J Clin Nutr.* 1981;34:8.
110. Haroon Y, Shearer MJ, Rahim S, Gunn WG, McEnergy G, Barkhan P. The content of phylloquinone (vitamin K1) in human milk, cow's milk and infant formula food determined by high-performance liquid chromatography. *J Nutr.* 1982;112:1102.
111. Moran JR, Vaughan R, Stroop S, et al. Concentrations and total daily output of micronutrients in breast milk of mothers delivering preterm: a longitudinal study. *J Pediatr Gastroenterol Nutr.* 1983;2:629.
112. Ford JE, Zechalko A, Murphy J, Brooke OG. Comparison of the B vitamin composition of milk from mothers of preterm and term babies. *Arch Dis Child.* 1983; 58:367.
113. Butte NF, Garza C, Smith EO, et al. Macro- and trace-mineral intakes of exclusively breast-fed infants. *Am J Clin Nutr.* 1987;45:42.
114. Lemons JA, Moye L, Hall D, Simmons M. Differences in the composition of preterm and term human milk during early lactation. *Pediatr Res.* 1982;16:113.
115. Casey CE, Hambidge KM, Neville MC. Studies in human lactation: zinc, copper, manganese and chromium in human milk in the first month of lactation. *Am J Clin Nutr.* 1985;41:1193.
116. Smith AM, Picciano MF, Milner JA. Selenium intakes and status of human milk and formula fed infants. *Am J Clin Nutr.* 1982;35:521.
117. Ericsson Y, Hellstrom I, Hofvander Y. Pilot studies on the fluoride metabolism in infants on different feedings. *Acta Paediatr Scand.* 1972;61:459.
118. Tomarelli RM. Osmolality, osmolarity, and renal solute load of infant formulas. *J Pediatr.* 1976;88:454.
119. United States Department of Agriculture. *Composition of Foods: Dairy and Egg Products, Raw, Processed, Prepared.* Washington, DC: Agricultural Research Service; 1976. Handbook 8-1, Item No. 01-078.
120. Casey CE, Hambidge KM. Nutritional aspects of human lactation. In: *Lactation: Physiology, Nutrition and Breastfeeding.* New York: Plenum Press; 1983.
121. Lammi-Keefe CJ, Jensen RG. Lipids in human milk: a review, II: Composition and fat-soluble vitamins. *J Pediatr Gastroenterol Nutr.* 1984;3:172.
122. Gebre-Medhin M, Vahlquist A, Hofvander Y, et al. Breast milk composition in Ethiopian and Swedish mothers, I: vitamin A and B-carotene. *Am J Clin Nutr.* 1976;29:441.
123. Specker BL, Tsang RC, Hollis BW. Effect of race and diet on human-milk vitamin D and 25-hydroxyvitamin D. *Am J Dis Child.* 1985;139:1134.
124. Greer FR, Tsang RC, Levin RS, et al. Increasing serum calcium and magnesium concentrations in breast-fed infants: longitudinal studies of minerals in human milk and in sera of nursing mothers and their infants. *J Pediatr.* 1982;100:59.
125. Hinton S, Kerwin D. *Maternal and Child Nutrition.* Chapel Hill, NC: Health Sciences Consortium Corporation; 1981.
126. Swedberg J, Steiner J. Oral rehydration therapy in diarrhea: not just for Third World children. *Postgrad Med.* 1983;74:336.
127. American Academy of Pediatrics. *Pediatric Nutrition Handbook.* 4th ed. Evanston, IL: American Academy of Pediatrics; 1998;47.
128. American Academy of Pediatrics, Committee on Nutrition. Infant methemoglobinemia: the role of dietary nitrate. *Pediatrics.* 1970;46:475.
129. Kerr C, Reisinger K, Plankey F. Sodium concentration of homemade baby foods. *Pediatrics.* 1978;62:331.
130. Hyams JS, Etienne NL, Leichtner AM, et al. Carbohydrate malabsorption following fruit juice ingestion in young children. *Pediatrics.* 1988;82:64–68.
131. American Academy of Pediatrics, Committee on Nutrition. Iron supplementation for infants. *Pediatrics.* 1976;58:765.

CHAPTER 5

Normal Nutrition from Infancy through Adolescence

Betty Lucas

The ages 1 through adolescence incorporate most of the growing years. This includes physical, cognitive, and social-emotional growth. The 1-year-old toddler is taking his or her first steps into the bigger world, becoming more independent in self-help skills, and rapidly learning to communicate. At the other end of the spectrum, the 18-year-old is also taking steps into the wide world, becoming more independent and self-sufficient in many areas, and planning for the future. This chapter will focus on the nutritional needs and issues of normal, healthy children during these growing years.

PROGRESS IN GROWTH AND DEVELOPMENT

After the rapid growth of infancy, there is a considerable slowing in physical growth during the preschool and school years. The elementary school years are often referred to as the *latent period* prior to the pubertal growth spurt of adolescence. Children will have individual growth patterns, which may be erratic at times, with spurts in height and weight followed by periods of little or no growth. These patterns usually correspond to similar changes in appetite and food intake in healthy children and teenagers. Parents and other caregivers need to realize that these changes are normal so that they can avoid struggles over food and eating.

Developmental progress during the growing years influences many aspects of food and eating. The very young child prefers food that can be picked up or doesn't have to be chased across the plate. Food jags may be more an expression of independence than of actual likes and dislikes. In older children, the influence of peers and of the media will affect snack choices. Teenagers want foods that fit into their lifestyles, are quick and easy to fix, and are inexpensive. Understanding the developmental characteristics and milestones at any particular age will help parents and professionals to set realistic expectations, support eating behavior and food decisions that are developmentally appropriate, and avoid unnecessary conflicts. Satter[1] has described well the feeding relationship between parents and children of all ages, which incorporates these developmental aspects.

Nutrient Needs

A child's rate and stage of growth usually parallel nutrient needs and are primary factors in determining needs. Other factors include physical activity, body size, basal energy expenditure, and state of illness. There is a wide range of actual needs based on individual characteristics. The Dietary Reference Intakes (DRIs), which include the Recommended Dietary Allowances (RDAs) and Adequate Intake (AI), serve as a guide to prevent deficiency and/or to provide positive health benefits.[2,3] Many of the data for children and adolescents, however, are extrapolated values. Because these guidelines provide a margin of safety greater than the physiologic requirements for most children in the United States, they are not meant to be marker goals for individual children. Intakes less than these guidelines do not presume inadequacies or adverse effects (see Appendix K).

Energy

Energy needs are the most variable, due to individual differences in basal metabolism, growth, physical activity, onset of puberty, and body size. The RDAs provide an average energy allowance, based on a reference weight for each age group.[2] However, recent studies using doubly labeled water to assess energy expenditure show evidence that the RDA for children may be overestimated by as much as 25%.[4] Up to age 10 years, there is no distinction between sexes, but at age 11 and above, allowances for energy are based on sex and puberty.

Age alone is not a good criterion for determining energy needs, especially in the pubertal years, when the growth spurt occurs at varying times. Weight is also a limited standard because of over- or underweight status. Height, however, is a useful reference in determining appropriate energy intakes for individual children. Use of kilocalories per centimeter of height (kcal/cm), as shown in Table 5–1, is a good clinical tool for both assessing and estimating energy needs. This is applicable in situations of failure-to-thrive and catch-up growth, as well as in planning for weight loss or weight maintenance.

Protein

Adequate protein intake is needed to provide for optimal growth in children and adolescents. National surveys have reported actual protein intakes to be in the range of 10-16% of energy for these ages.[5,6] This level assumes that enough energy is provided so that protein is spared for growth. Protein needs decrease as the growth rate slows after infancy, then increase again at puberty. Total protein intake increases steadily until about 12 years of age in girls and 16 years of age in boys.

In the United States, protein intakes usually exceed recommended allowances. Some children and adolescents, however, may be at risk for protein malnutrition, ie, those receiving inadequate calories, (extreme use of low-fat diets, limited access to food, dieting to lose weight, athletes in training who limit food), those who

Table 5–1 Energy Intake per Centimeter of Height*

	Males (Percentiles)			*Females (Percentiles)*		
Age	*10th*	*50th*	*90th*	*10th*	*50th*	*90th*
1	10.3	14.1	18.8	10.6	13.6	17.6
2–3	11.6	15.0	20.2	10.5	13.5	17.9
4–6	12.3	15.2	20.4	10.7	13.8	18.6
7–10	12.8	16.7	22.3	10.4	14.1	18.4
11–14	12.4	16.8	22.2	9.0	13.0	18.2
15–16	11.4	15.9	21.1	7.4	11.8	17.3

* These energy intakes (kcal) are means of the age groups listed. The data were collected on normal, healthy children involved in a prospective study.

Source: Adapted from VA Beal, Nutritional intake, in *Human Growth and Development* (p 63) by RW McCammon (ed) with permission of Charles C Thomas Publishers, © 1970.

are strict vegetarians, and some with food allergies] so that protein is used for energy. Dietary evaluation of protein intake should include the growth rate, energy intake, and quality of the protein sources.

Minerals and Vitamins

Although clinical signs of vitamin or mineral deficiency are rare in the United States, dietary intake studies have reported that the nutrients most likely to be low or deficient in the diets of children and adolescents are calcium, iron, vitamin A, folic acid, zinc, and vitamin B_6.[6,7] Certain populations of children, such as low-income, Native American, and other groups with limited food and health resources (eg, the homeless), are more at risk for poor diet and nutrient deficiencies.

Calcium

Primarily needed for bone mineralization, calcium needs are determined by growth velocity, rates of absorption, and other nutrients, such as phosphorus, vitamin D, and protein. Because of individual variability, a child receiving less than the recommended allowance of calcium is not necessarily at risk. Approximately 100 mg of calcium per day is retained as bone in the preschool years. This doubles or triples for adolescents during peak growth periods.[8] Adolescence is a critical period for optimal calcium retention to achieve peak bone mass, especially for females who are at risk for osteoporosis in later years. Calcium intake, however, often decreases during the teen years. Balance studies indicate that young adolescent girls (less than 16 years of age) may need to consume as much as 1600 mg per day to achieve maximum calcium intake and calcium balance.[8] Even pre-pubertal children have demonstrated increased bone mineral density when their diets have been supplemented with calcium.[9] The Food and Nutrition Board recommends an AI of 1,300 mg of calcium per day for ages 9–18 years to support optimal bone mineralization.[3]

Because dairy products are the major sources of calcium, those who consume no or limited amounts of these foods are at risk for calcium deficiency. Some adolescents may also receive less calcium than needed because of rapid growth, dieting practices, and substituting carbonated beverages for milk. In assessing calcium status, vitamin D intake should be considered because of its major role in calcium metabolism. For children with limited sunshine exposure, dietary intake is critical. Vitamin D-fortified milk is the primary food source of this nutrient; other dairy products are not usually made with fortified milk. A child may be receiving adequate calcium from cheese and yogurt but taking very little fluid milk and, thus, receiving minimal dietary vitamin D. Table 5–2 contains a list of calcium food sources.

Iron

Requirements for iron are determined by the rate of growth, iron stores, increasing blood volumes, and rate of absorption from food sources. Menstrual losses, as well as rapid growth, increase the need in adolescent females. To reach adulthood with adequate storage of iron, recommended daily intakes are 10 mg for children, 12 mg for pubertal males, and 15 mg for pubertal females.[2,10] (See Iron Deficiency Anemia discussion in this chapter.)

Vitamins

Vitamins function in numerous metabolic processes. Vitamin needs are often dependent on energy intake or other nutrient levels. Most of the recommended allowances for children and adolescents have been extrapolated from studies on infants and adults.

Vitamin-Mineral Supplements

After infancy, the use of supplements decreases but is still a common practice in the United States. About 54% of preschool children take supplements, typically a multivitamin-

Table 5–2 Calcium Equivalents

1 cup whole milk =	1 cup skim milk* 1 cup 1% or 2% milk 1 cup buttermilk 1 cup (8 oz) yogurt	= 300 mg calcium (approximately)
3/4 cup milk =	1 oz cheddar, jack, or Swiss cheese	
2/3 cup milk =	1 oz mozzarella or American cheese 2 oz canned sardines (with bones)	
1/2 cup milk =	2 oz canned salmon (with bones) 1/2 cup custard or milk pudding 1/2 cup cooked greens (mustard, collards, kale)	
1/4 cup milk =	1/2 cup cottage cheese 1/2 cup ice cream 3/4 cup dried beans, cooked or canned	

* Some low-fat or skim milks and some low-fat yogurts have additional nonfat dry milk (NFDM) solids added. Some labels will read "fortified." Such products will contain more calcium than indicated here.

mineral preparation with iron.[11] The use of supplements is generally less in older children and adolescents. Children taking supplements do not necessarily represent those who need them most. Higher rates of use are found in families with more education and income. The supplements may not be providing the marginal or deficient nutrients either; ie, a child may be taking a children's vitamin but may actually need extra calcium, not always provided in a supplement.

Except for fluoride supplementation in nonfluoridated areas, the American Academy of Pediatrics does not support routine supplementation for normal, healthy children.[12] It does, however, identify four groups at nutritional risk who might benefit from supplementation. These include: (1) children and adolescents from deprived families, especially those abused or neglected; (2) children and adolescents with anorexia, poor appetites, or who consume fad diets; (3) children with chronic disease, ie, cystic fibrosis, inflammatory bowel disease; (4) children using diets to manage obesity; and (5) pregnant teenagers. Both the American Medical Association and the American Dietetic Association have also recommended that nutrients for healthy children should come from food, not supplements.[13,14]

Dietary evaluation will determine the need for supplements. Children with food allergies, those who omit entire food groups, and those with limited food acceptances will be likely candidates for supplementation. No risk is involved if parents wish to give their children a standard pediatric multivitamin. Megadose levels of nutrients should be discouraged and parents counseled regarding the dangers of toxicity, especially of fat-soluble vitamins. Because many children's vitamins look and taste like candy, parents should be educated to keep them out of reach of children.

FOOD INTAKE PATTERNS AND GUIDELINES

Because appetite usually follows the rate of growth, food intake is not always smooth and consistent. After a good appetite in infancy, parents frequently describe their preschool children as having fair to poor appetites, a response to a slower growth rate. There is a wide variability in nutrient intake in healthy children. Daily energy intake of preschool children is surprisingly constant, despite a high variability from meal to meal. One longitudinal study found that the maximum intake of energy, carbohydrate, fat, and protein was two to three times the minimum intake. For ascorbic acid and carotene, the maximum/minimum ratios were 10:1 and 20:1, all in healthy children.[15] With such variability (especially in micronutrient intake) being the norm for children, nutrition professionals need to use dietary assessment tools that include intake over time.

Just as there are changing trends of dietary patterns in the general public, similar patterns are seen in children. National dietary studies have shown decreased intake of whole milk and eggs, greater use of low-fat and nonfat milk, more snacking, and more eating away from home among children and adolescents.[6] These shifts in intake, however, still do not meet national recommendations such as the United States Dietary Guidelines, or the Food Guide Pyramid (see Appendix L). Using national data, one study reported an average of 35% of energy intake from fat, and only about one-third of the group met recommendations for fruit, vegetable, grain, and meat intake.[16]

Factors Influencing Food Intake

Food intake and habits are determined by numerous factors. Major influences for children include the family, peers, media, and body image.

Family

Eating habits and food likes and dislikes are formed in the early years and often continue into adulthood. Parents and siblings are primary models for young children to imitate behavior. Mealtime atmosphere, both positive and negative, can influence how a child approaches and handles family meals. As children move into adolescence, they eat fewer meals at home.

With more women employed outside the home, there may be less time available for food preparation and more use of fast food, eating out, and prepared foods. Mothers' employment, however, is not associated with poorer dietary intakes for their children.[17] There is also a larger percentage of single-parent families, usually headed by women. This usually translates into lower income, with less money available for food.

Media

Television is the primary media influence on children of all ages. It has been estimated that by the time the average American child graduates from high school, he or she will have watched about 15,000 hours of television, compared with spending 11,000 hours in the classroom. One-half of all commercials are for food, with an even higher percentage found in children's programs.[18] The food items generally advertised to young audiences are sweetened cereals, fast food, snack foods, and candy—foods high in sugar, fat, and salt.

The commercial messages are not based on nutrition but on an emotional/psychologic appeal, ie, fun, gives you energy, yummy taste. Younger children generally cannot discriminate between the regular program and commercial messages, frequently giving more attention to the latter because of their fast, attention-getting pace. Television viewing has been suggested as a factor in the rising rate of obesity among American children and teenagers.[19] In addition to encouraging inactivity, there is the steady presentation of food and eating cues.

Peers

As children move into the world, their food choices are influenced by others. In preschool, the group snack time may encourage a child to try a new food. During school years, participation in the school lunch program may be decided by friends rather than the menu. Peer influence is particularly strong in adolescence as teenagers strive for more independence and eating becomes a more social activity outside the home. A chronic illness or disorder that requires diet modification, such as diabetes, phenylketonuria, or food allergies, can be a problem for children and teenagers when they want to be part of the group. These individuals need education regarding diet rationale appropriate to their developmental level, as well as problem-solving methods to explain it to their peers.

Body Image

Puberty is the period of greatest awareness of body image. It is normal for teens to be uncomfortable and dissatisfied with their changing bodies. The media and popular idols offer a standard that adolescents compare themselves with, no matter how unrealistic it may be (eg, magazine models and store mannequins are usually size 8 or 10). Even pre-pubertal school-age girls have been increasingly preoccupied with body image and "dieting." To change their body image, they may try restrictive diets, purchase weight loss products, or in the case of males, try supplements or diets in the hope of increasing their muscles. Some of these dietary measures may put them at risk for poor nutritional status.

Feeding the Toddler and Preschool Child

Parents often become concerned when their toddler refuses some favorite foods and appears to be disinterested in eating. These periods (food jags) vary in intensity from child to child and may last a few days or years. At the same time, the child is practicing self-feeding skills, with frequent spills, and is often resorting to the use of fingers. These changes and behaviors during the preschool years are a normal part of the development and maturation of young children. When parents understand this, they are more likely to avoid struggles, issues of control, and negative feedback around food and eating.

Portion sizes for young children are small by adult standards. Table 5–3 provides a guide for foods and portion sizes. A long-standing rule of thumb is to initially offer 1 tablespoon of each food for every year of age for preschool children, with more provided according to appetite.

Because of smaller capacities and fluctuating appetites, most children eat four to six times a day. Snacks contribute significantly to the total day's nutrient intake and should be planned accordingly. Foods that make nutritious snacks are listed in Table 5–4. Foods chosen for snacks should be those least likely to promote dental caries.

Parents of young children frequently become concerned about the adequacy of their child's intake—plain meats are often refused because they are more difficult to chew, very little or too much milk may be consumed, cooked vegetables are pushed away. Table 5–5 offers nutrition solutions to these common, normal variations in eating behaviors.

Just as important as providing adequate nutrients to young children is supporting a positive feeding environment, both physically and emotionally, so that, as they grow, they acquire skills, develop positive attitudes, and have control over food decisions as appropriate for their developmental level. General guidance in this area is listed in Table 5–6.

Children under age 4 are at greatest risk for choking on food. In some cases, this can lead to death from asphyxiation.[20] Foods most likely to cause choking are those that are round, hard, and do not readily dissolve in saliva, such as hot dogs, grapes, raw vegetables, popcorn, peanut butter, nuts, and hard candy. Other foods can also cause choking problems if too much is stuffed into the mouth, if the child is running while eating, or if the child is unsupervised. Choking episodes can be prevented by common-sense management of foods and eating environment. Table 5–7 outlines the preventive approaches.

Fruit juice, especially apple, has become a common beverage for young children, usually replacing water and frequently replacing milk. Excessive fruit juice consumption has been linked to chronic diarrhea and failure to thrive.[21,22] Both conditions improved when juice

Table 5–3 Feeding Guide for Children

The following is a guide to a basic diet. Fats, sauces, desserts, and snack foods will provide additional energy to meet the growing child's needs. Foods can be selected from this pattern for both meals and snacks.

Food	*2- to 3-Year Olds*		*4- to 6-Year Olds*		*7- to 12-Year Olds*		*Comments*
	Portion Size/Servings		*Portion Size/Servings*		*Portion Size/Servings*		
Milk and dairy products	1/2 cup (4 oz.)	4–5	1/2–3/4 cup (4–6 oz.)	3–4	1/2–1 cup (4–8 oz.)	3–4	The following may be substituted for 1/2 cup liquid milk: 1/2-3/4 oz. cheese, 1/2 cup yogurt, 2½ Tbsp. nonfat dry milk.
Meat, fish, poultry, or equivalent	1–2 oz.	2	1–2 oz.	2	2 oz.	3–4	The following may be substituted for 1 oz. meat, fish or poultry: 1 egg, 2 Tbsp. peanut butter, 4–5 Tbsp. cooked legumes.
Fruits and vegetables		4–5		4–5		4–5	Include one green leafy or yellow vegetable for vitamin A, such as carrots, spinach, broccoli, winter squash. Include one vitamin-C-rich fruit, vegetable, or juice, such as citrus juices, orange, grapefruit, strawberries, melon, tomato, broccoli.
Vegetables							
Cooked	2–3 Tbsp.		3–4 Tbsp.		1/4–1/2 cup		
Raw*	Few pieces		Few pieces		Several pieces		
Fruit							
Raw	1/2–1 small		1/2–1 small		1 medium		
Canned	2–4 Tbsp.		4–6 Tbsp.		1/4–1/2 cup		
Juice	3–4 oz.		4 oz.		4 oz.		
Bread and grain products		3–4		3–4		4–5	The following may be substituted for 1 slice of bread: 1/2 cup spaghetti, macaroni, noodles, or rice; 5 saltines; 1/2 English muffin or bagel; 1 tortilla.
Whole-grain or enriched bread	1/2–1 slice		1 slice		1 slice		
Cooked cereal	1/4–1/2 cup		1/2 cup		1/2–1 cup		
Dry cereal	1/2–1 cup		1 cup		1 cup		

* Do not give to young children until they can chew well.

Source: Adapted from Lowenberg ME, Development of food patterns in young children, in *Nutrition Infancy and Childhood*, ed 4 (pp 146–147) by PL Pipes (ed) with permission of Times Mirror/Mosby College Publishing, © 1989 with permission of W.B. Saunders Company.

Table 5–4 Foods that Make Nutritious Snacks

Protein Foods	Fruits†
Natural cheese	Apple wedges*
Milk	Bananas
Plain yogurt	Pears
Cooked turkey or beef	Berries
Unsalted nuts and seeds*	Melon
Peanut butter*	Oranges and other citrus fruits
Hard-cooked eggs	Grapes*
Cottage cheese	Unsweetened canned fruit
Tuna	Unsweetened fruit juices
Breads and Cereals†	**Vegetables**
Whole-grain breads	Carrot sticks*
Whole-grain, low-fat crackers	Celery*
Rice crackers	Green pepper strips*
English muffins	Cucumber slices*
Bagels	Cabbage wedges*
Tortillas	Tomatoes
Pita bread	Jicama*
Popcorn*	Vegetable juices
	Cooked green beans
	Broccoli and cauliflower flowerettes*

* Foods that are hard, round, and do not easily dissolve can cause choking. Do not give to children under 3 years of age. (Peanut butter is more dangerous when eaten in chunks or spread thickly rather than thinly spread on crackers or bread.)

† Fruits, juices, and most cereal/bread products contain fermentable carbohydrate, which is a factor in the development of dental caries. Try to limit these foods to one serving in a snack.

intake was limited. A recent report of preschool children found an association between short stature or obesity and the consumption of more than 12 ounces of juice daily.[23] It is understandable that frequent juice intake could dull the appetite enough to result in less food consumed at regular meals, or, for some children, the energy from juice (instead of water) in addition to other foods could cause excess weight gain. Parents should be given general guidelines to limit juice to no more than 12 ounces per day.

Feeding the School-Age Child

The years from 6–12 are a period of slow but steady growth, with increases in food intake as a result of appetite (see Table 5–3). Most food behavior problems from early childhood have been resolved except for extreme cases, but food dislikes may persist, especially if attention is given to them.

Because children are in school, they may eat fewer times in the day, but after-school snacks usually are a routine. Breakfast-skipping may begin in these years, with contributing factors such as time constraints, children left to get themselves off to school, and school starting early. With participation in organized sports, music lessons, and other activities, having a family meal may be less frequent.

An emerging trend in the United States is the increased responsibility of children not yet in their teens to do family shopping and cooking. Some children are frequently responsible for their own breakfasts, lunches, snacks, and even the dinner meal. They also do food shopping on a regular basis and influence the family food purchases. Several factors contribute to this trend, including working parents,

Table 5–5 Common Feeding Concerns in Young Children

Common Concerns	*Possible Solutions*
Refuses meats	• Offer small, bite-size pieces of moist, tender meat or poultry • Incorporate into meat loaf, spaghetti sauce, stews, casseroles, burritos, pizza • Include legumes, eggs, cheese • Offer boneless fish (including canned tuna and salmon)
Drinks too little milk	• Offer cheeses and yogurt, including cheese in cooking, eg, macaroni and cheese, cheese sauce, pizza • Use milk to cook hot cereals; offer cream soups, milk-based puddings and custards • Allow child to pour milk from a pitcher and use a straw • Include powdered milk in cooking and baking, eg, biscuits, muffins, pancakes, meat loaf, casseroles
Drinks too much milk	• Offer water if thirsty between meals • Limit milk to one serving with meals or offer at end of meal; offer water for seconds • If bottle is still used, wean to cup
Refuses vegetables and fruits	• If child refuses vegetables, offer more fruits, and vice-versa • Prepare vegetables that are tender but not overcooked • Steam vegetable strips (or offer raw if appropriate) and allow child to eat with fingers • Offer sauces and dips, eg, cheese sauce for cooked vegetables, dip for raw vegetables, yogurt to dip fruit • Include vegetables in soups and casseroles • Add fresh or dried fruit to cereals • Prepare fruit in a variety of ways, eg, fresh, cooked, juice, in gelatin, as a salad • Continue to offer a variety of fruits and vegetables
Eats too many sweets	• Limit purchase and preparation of sweet foods in the home • Avoid using as a bribe or reward • Incorporate into meals instead of snacks for better dental health • Reduce sugar by half in recipes for cookies, muffins, quick breads, etc. • Work with staff of day care, preschools, etc, to reduce use of sweets

increased use of microwave ovens, more money available to spend on convenience and prepared foods, and less emphasis on family meals. Along with this trend, increasingly sophisticated advertising is being aimed at these children.

Children usually participate in the school lunch program or bring a packed lunch from home. The National School Lunch Program is administered by the United States Department of Agriculture (USDA) and supported by means of reimbursements and supplemental commodity

Table 5–6 Tips for a Happy Mealtime

Physical Setting

- Schedule meals at regular times.
- Avoid having a child get too hungry or too tired before mealtime.
- Snacks should be at least 1½ to 2 hours before meals.
- Child should be able to sit up to the table comfortably without reaching.
- Provide support for the legs and feet, such as a booster seat, stool, etc.
- Use nonbreakable, sturdy dishes with sides to push food against.
- Spoons and forks should be blunt with broad, short handles.
- Use cups that are nonbreakable, broad based, and small.

Social-Emotional

- Serve a new food with familiar ones—don't be surprised by an initial rejection.
- Offer at least one food at a meal that you know your child will eat, but do not cater to his or her likes and dislikes.
- Avoid coaxing, nagging, bribing, or any other pressure to get your child to eat.
- Serve dessert (if any) with the meal—it becomes less important and cannot be used as a reward.
- Let children determine when they are full; amounts eaten will vary from child to child and day to day.
- Use the child's developmental stage to determine expectations for neatness and manners, but set limits on inappropriate behaviors, eg, throwing food, playing.
- Attempt to have family meals be as pleasant as possible; avoid arguments and criticism.
- Allow children to help set the table or do part of the meal preparation.

Table 5–7 Guidelines for Feeding Safety—Preschool Children

1. Insist that children eat sitting down. It lets them concentrate on chewing and swallowing.
2. An adult should supervise children while they eat.
3. Food on which preschoolers often choke, such as hot dogs, peanut butter, hard pieces of fruit and vegetables, should be avoided for children under 3 years of age.
4. Well-cooked foods, modified so that the child can chew and swallow without difficulty, should be offered.
5. Eating in the car should be avoided. If the child starts choking, it is hard to get to the side of the road safely.
6. Rub-on teething medications can cause problems with chewing and swallowing because the muscles in the throat may also become numb. Children who receive such medications should be carefully observed during feeding.

Source: Reprinted from *Nutrition in Infancy and Childhood*, ed 4 (p 126) by PL Pipes (ed) with permission of Times Mirror/Mosby College Publishing, © 1989 with permission from W.B. Saunders Company.

foods. Federal guidelines are established for food groups and portion sizes so that the lunch provides approximately one-third of the RDAs for students. About 70% of schools also participate in the School Breakfast Program. Free and reduced-price meals are available for low-income children. Problems with the school lunch program have included plate waste, poor menu acceptance by students, competition from vending machines, and concerns regarding the amount of fat, sugar, and salt in the food. These problems have been addressed by including students in menu planning, offering popular items more frequently (ie, pizza, tacos, hamburgers, salad bars), and allowing students to refuse one or two items from the menu. Incorporating the U.S. Dietary Guidelines into child nutrition programs has also encouraged menus with a lower fat content, more fresh fruits, vegetables, and whole grain products.[24] A sack lunch prepared at home will likely provide fewer nutrients than will the school lunch meal.[25] The same favorite foods tend to be packed with less variety, and foods are limited to those that don't require heating or refrigeration.

Feeding the Adolescent

Adolescents in their rapid-growth period seem to eat all the time. Their appetite usually guides their intake. As teenagers achieve more independence and spend more time away from home, they have more variable intakes and irregular eating patterns. Meal-skipping is greatest in this age group, particularly for breakfast and lunch. On the other hand, snacking tends to be a common characteristic. Whether they are called snacks or meals, adolescents who eat less than three times a day have poorer diets than do those eating more often.

Although fast foods are popular with all segments of the population, they appeal most to teenagers. The food is inexpensive, well accepted, and can be eaten informally without utensils or plates. Fast food restaurants are also socially acceptable and a common employer of adolescents. Generally, the menu items tend to be energy-dense, high in fat (some items have more than 50% of their calories as fat), high in sodium, and low in fiber, vitamin A, ascorbic acid, calcium, and folate. Although these establishments now offer more salads and lower-fat sandwiches, these foods are not necessarily chosen by teens. Any negative impact of fast foods on the diets of adolescents will depend on how frequently they are eaten and the choices made.

NUTRITION ISSUES

As children grow and develop, various nutrition-related issues or problems arise. These are not uncommon in otherwise healthy children, and they can be prevented or managed with minimal intervention. Other specific problems, eg, obesity, allergies, and chronic diseases, are discussed in other chapters.

DIET AND DENTAL HEALTH

Despite successful efforts in the past few decades, dental caries remain a common oral health disease in the pediatric population. National Health and Nutrition Examination Survey III (NHANES III) data reveal that 45% of children and adolescents have caries.[26] The rate changes with age; 62% of children ages 2–9 were caries-free, while only 33% of adolescents ages 12–17 were caries-free.

Dental caries develop in the presence of carbohydrate, bacteria, and a susceptible tooth. The process of decay begins with the interaction of bacteria (*Streptococcus mutans*) and fermentable carbohydrate on the tooth surface. When the bacteria within the dental plaque (the gelatinous substance on the tooth surface) metabolizes the carbohydrate, organic acids are produced. When the acid reduces the pH to 5.5 or less, demineralization of the tooth enamel occurs.[27] Some individuals seem to be more susceptible to caries than others, suggesting a hereditary influence. About 80% of the caries in 5–17 year olds is found in only 25% of the children and adolescents.[26] Individual salivary counts of *S. mutans* that are high appear to be a risk for caries.[28]

Sucrose is the most common carbohydrate recognized in the caries process. Although starch is considered less cariogenic than sucrose, it can easily be broken down into fermentable carbohydrate by salivary amylase. Also, many foods high in starch often contain sucrose or other sugars, which may make the food more cariogenic than sugar alone because starch is retained longer in the mouth. Honey is just as cariogenic as sucrose.

The cariogenicity of specific foods depends not only on the type and amount of fermentable carbohydrate but also on the retentiveness of foods to the tooth surface and the frequency of eating. Dental researchers believe that all of these factors influence the length of time the teeth are exposed to an acidic environment, which leads to tooth decay.[27]

Some protein foods, eg, nuts, hard cheeses, eggs, and meats, do not decrease plaque pH and are thought to have a protective effect against caries.[29] Eating these foods at the same time as high-sugar foods prevents a reduction in plaque pH. Why these foods are protective is not known, but theories include the presence of protein and lipids in these foods, the presence of calcium and phosphorus, and the stimulation of alkaline saliva. Chewing gum sweetened with xylitol or sorbitol after a sugar-containing snack may also counteract the decrease in pH and reduce caries.[30]

Prevention of Caries

Because children of all ages eat frequently, snacks should emphasize foods that are low in sucrose, are not sticky, and stimulate saliva flow, thereby limiting acid production in the mouth (Table 5-4). Including protein foods such as cheese and nuts may provide nutritional as well as dental benefits. Desserts, when consumed, should be eaten with meals. School-age children and adolescents may benefit from chewing sugarless gum after snacks containing fermentable carbohydrate.

Good oral hygiene complements the efforts of dietary control. In infancy, parents can clean the gums and teeth with a clean cloth. The toothbrush should be introduced in the toddler period. The key is to incorporate brushing and flossing as a regular, consistent routine, with parental supervision in the early years. If the water supply is not fluoridated, a fluoride supplement is recommended into the teen years. See Table 5–8 for recommended fluoride dosages.

Baby Bottle Tooth Decay

Children under 3 years of age are most likely to have baby bottle tooth decay (BBTD). In some nonfluoridated communities, the prevalence is about 20%; in Native American and Native Alaskan preschool children, the rate is more than 50%.[31] Rampant caries develop on the primary upper front teeth (incisors) and often on the cheek surface of primary upper first molars. Children from poor families are at highest risk for BBTD. A history of BBTD seems to increase the risk for future caries.

The primary cause of BBTD is prolonged exposure of the teeth to a sweetened liquid (formula, milk, juice, soda pop, sweetened drinks). This occurs most often when the child is rou-

Table 5–8 Fluoride Supplementation Schedule*

	Fluoride Concentration in Local Water Supply (ppm)		
Age	*less than 0.3*	*0.3–0.6*	*greater than 0.6*
6 mo to 3 yr	0.25†	0.00	0.00
3–6 yr	0.50	0.25	0.00
6 yr to at least 16 yr	1.00	0.50	0.00

*Must know fluoride concentration in patient's drinking water before prescribing fluoride supplements.
†All values are milligrams of fluoride supplement per day.

Source: Used with permission of the American Academy of Pediatrics, *Pediatric Nutrition Handbook, 4th ed.,* © 1998, American Academy of Pediatrics.

tinely given a nursing bottle at bedtime or during naps. During sleep, the liquid pools around the teeth, saliva flow decreases, and the child may continue to suck liquid over an extended period of time. Although BBTD has been documented in ad libitum breastfeeding, the occurrence is believed to be less than with bottle feeding.[31] Toddlers who hold their own bottle and have access to it anytime throughout the day are also at high risk. Dental treatment of BBTD is expensive, often requires a general anesthetic, and may be traumatic for the child and family.

Education is the primary strategy to prevent BBTD. Parents should be counseled about the disorder early in infancy and encouraged to avoid putting a baby to sleep with a bottle, as previously addressed in Chapter 4. Juices and liquids other than milk or formula should be offered in a cup. In typically developing infants, weaning from the bottle should begin at about 1 year of age. Day care providers and other caregivers should also be informed of the threat to oral health posed by use of the nursing bottle as a pacifier. For this educational approach to be successful, families often need help with positive parenting strategies and behavioral counseling.

Iron Deficiency Anemia

Iron deficiency anemia is most common in children between 1 and 3 years of age, with a prevalence of about 9%.[32] Other high-risk groups are young adolescent males and females of childbearing age. Reported trends have shown an overall decrease in the prevalence of iron deficiency anemia, both in low-income and middle-class pediatric populations.[33] Factors influencing this positive trend include increased and prolonged use of iron-fortified infant formulas, more breastfeeding, increased iron intake from other food sources, and the Women, Infants, and Children (WIC) food program.

Despite the encouraging trends, some young children, especially those in low-income households, are at high risk for iron deficiency. Although the relationship between iron deficiency and cognitive/behavioral function has been debated for a long time, poorer cognitive performance and delayed psychomotor development have been reported in infants and preschool children with iron deficiency, compared with children without iron deficiency.[34,35] Iron deficiency in infancy may have long-term consequences, as demonstrated by poorer performance on a developmental test at the age of 5 years.[36] Children who are iron deficient are also at risk for increased lead absorption when exposed to sources of lead.

Dietary factors, as well as growth and physiologic needs, play a role in development of anemia. Some toddlers consume a large volume of milk, to the exclusion of solids; plain meats are often not well accepted by preschool children because they require more chewing. For many of these children, most dietary iron comes from nonheme sources such as vegetables, grains, and cereals. Because the typical American mixed diet contains approximately 6 mg iron per 1,000 calories, adolescents dieting to lose weight will have minimal iron intake, especially if animal protein is limited.

Absorption of iron from food depends on several factors. One is the iron status of the individual; those with low iron stores will have a higher absorption rate. There is a higher rate of absorption from heme-iron (in meat, fish, and poultry) than from nonheme-iron (in vegetables, grains, and animal tissue). Absorption of nonheme-iron can be increased by two enhancing factors: (1) ascorbic acid and (2) meat, fish, or poultry (MFP).[37] The presence of an ascorbic-acid-rich food and/or MFP in a meal will increase the rate of nonheme iron absorption. Other food or compounds inhibit iron absorption. Table 5–9 identifies good iron sources as well as absorption enhancers and inhibitors. Simple but conscientious menu planning can help improve iron availability to children and teenagers.

Hemoglobin or hematocrit are the main biochemical screening tests for iron deficiency anemia. The American Academy of Pediatrics recommends either universal or selective screening

Table 5–9 Food Sources of Iron

	Iron (mg)
Meat, Fish and Poultry* (1 oz)	
Chicken liver	2.8
Beef liver	2.2
Turkey, roasted	1.7
Beef pot roast	1.3
Hamburger	1.1
Fresh pork, roasted	1.1
Ham	0.7
Chicken	0.6
Tuna, canned	0.5
Hot dog	0.3
Salmon	0.3
Fish stick	0.1
Cereals, Grains, Vegetables, Fruits†	
Cooked cereals (1/2 cup)	0.7–1.3
Ready-to-eat cereals (3/4 cup)	0.3–9.0
Whole-wheat bread, enriched bread (1 slice)	0.6–0.8
Legumes, cooked (1/2 cup)	1.3–3.0
Greens (spinach, mustard, beet), cooked (1/2 cup)	1.5–2.0
Green peas, cooked (1/2 cup)	1.3
Dried fruit (1/4 cup)	1.0–1.5
Nuts, most kinds (2 tbsp)	1.0
Wheat germ (1 tbsp)	0.5
Molasses, light (1 tbsp)	0.9

Dietary Enhancers of Nonheme Iron Absorption

- Meat, fish, poultry
- Ascorbic acid

Dietary Inhibitors of Nonheme Iron Absorption

- Tea (tannic acid)
- Antacids
- Sequestering additives (such as EDTA used in fats and soft drinks to clarify and prevent rancidity)

* Heme iron sources (approximately 40% of the iron in these foods); well-absorbed.

† Nonheme sources; lower level of absorption; enhancers eaten at the same time will increase absorption.

for infants between 9 and 12 months of age, with a second screening 6 months later.[38] Universal screening for children up to two years of age is recommended for communities and populations with significant levels of iron deficiency anemia or for infants whose diets put them at risk. Selective screening would be based on individual risk factors such as prematurity, low-birth-weight infants, and dietary intake. Routine screening is not recommended after age two except for risk factors, ie, poor diet, poverty/limited access to food, special health care needs. Guidelines for treatment and follow-up of iron deficiency anemia have been developed.[38]

EFFECT OF DIET ON LEARNING AND BEHAVIOR

What impact does a child's diet have on his or her school performance and behavior? For decades people have debated whether skipping breakfast affects classroom learning. Food additives, sugar, and allergies have been suggested as causes of hyperactivity in children. Although these are controversial issues, some scientific studies have examined them.

Diet and Learning Behavior

Although severe malnutrition early in life is known to negatively affect intellectual development, the impact of marginal malnutrition, skipping meals, or hunger has been more difficult to document. Experimental studies have used standardized tests to measure cognitive functions (eg, problem solving, attention, and memory) in healthy school-age children who were given either breakfast or no breakfast. The "fasted" children had slower memory recall, increased errors, and slower stimulus discrimination.[39] Similar studies comparing healthy children to those stunted, those who suffered severe malnutrition early in life, and those currently wasted (low weight for height) showed even poorer results for the malnourished/undernourished children when they missed breakfast.[39,40]

In a community study, standardized achievement test scores were compared before and after implementation of the School Breakfast Program in six schools in a predominantly low-income community.[41] Children participating in the breakfast program demonstrated improved academic performance compared with those qualified but not participating. The findings also noted decreased tardiness and absenteeism among the children in the breakfast program. These results indicate that efforts of nutrition education and feeding programs should be targeted to children at risk so that they might be better able to achieve in school.

The impact of diet and nutrition on a child's behavior has been a controversial topic for some time. Although malnourished children and those experiencing iron deficiency anemia often demonstrate decreased attention and responsiveness, less interest in their environment, and reduced problem solving ability, the effects of periodic hunger or "food insecurity" is less clear. A recent report of families from a large Community Childhood Hunger Identification Project (CCHIP) found that the "hungry" children were three times more likely than "at-risk for hunger" children, and seven times more likely than "not hungry" children, to have scores indicating irritability, anxiety, aggression, and oppositional behavior.[42] Although other unstudied factors could also be related to these negative behaviors, they could be tied to the family's food insecurity. With federal welfare reform legislation, more low income families are likely to be at risk for limited food resources, and without broad policies to ensure children their basic needs, these children may suffer worsening behavioral and academic functioning.

Attention Deficit Hyperactivity Disorder

Commonly known as hyperactivity, attention deficit hyperactivity disorder (ADHD) is a clinical diagnosis with specific criteria, ie, inattention, impulsivity, hyperactivity, onset before 7 years of age, and duration of at least 6 months. The etiology of ADHD is not clear, and some dietary factors have been proposed as causes, such as food additives, sugar, and food allergies. Although treatment usually includes behavioral management, medication, and/or special education, various dietary treatments have been proposed.

The Feingold diet, popularized in the 1970s, theorized that artificial colorings and flavorings in the food supply caused hyperactivity. Treatment was to remove from the child's diet those substances, natural salicylates (found mostly in fruits), and some preservatives (BHA, BHT). Although initial anecdotal reports were popular, controlled double-blind challenge studies have not supported the Feingold hypothesis.[43] It is generally accepted that a small percentage (no more than 5–10%) of hyperactive children (usually preschoolers) may benefit from the diet. One report, using a total diet replacement design with crossover between experimental and control diets, suggested a greater diet impact.[44] The experimental diet was the Feingold diet plus elimination of foods that the family thought were bothersome to their child, eg, chocolate, sugar, or caffeine. Almost 50% of the preschool hyperactive boys showed some improvement in behavior using accepted rating scales. The modified Feingold diet, including fruits, has been evaluated favorably according to nutrient content and thus poses little risk for the child.[45] Families using the diet should receive nutritional counseling and should not disregard other helpful treatment for their child's ADHD.

Sugar (sucrose) is popularly believed to cause hyperactivity in children or behavior problems and delinquency in adolescents. Controlled challenge studies, however, have failed to show any negative behavioral effects from sucrose.[46] In one study, children receiving the sugar were less active and quieter afterward than were those receiving the placebo.[47] A double-blind challenge study with juvenile delinquents did not show impaired behavioral performance after a sucrose load.[48] There are many good reasons for reducing sugar consumption, including improved dental health and diets that are more nutrient dense. This can be reinforced with families, while helping them remain objective about a sugar-behavior relationship. There is always the rare possibility that a child may have an individual intolerance to sugar.

Stimulant medications, such as methylphenidate (Ritalin) or dextroamphetamine (Dexedrine) are commonly used to treat ADHD. They usually result in improvement of motor restlessness, short attention span, and irritability. Anorexia is a side effect that has been shown to cause suppression of physical growth.[49] Over time, there seems to be more tolerance for a medication's negative effect on growth, but the response is individual. Data suggest that there is a direct relationship between dosage of the medication and the degree of reduced growth.[50] Although the mechanisms involved are not clear, decreased energy intake is a factor. Children receiving these medications should have regular monitoring of growth, and the efficacy of the drug effect should be reassessed routinely. Because the effect of the medication will be noted about half an hour after being ingested and is usually absent after 4–6 hours, food should be offered to take advantage of the child's optimal appetite; ie, the medication should be given with or after meals.

Megavitamin therapy has been promoted for many disorders, including ADHD and behavior problems. Of the controlled studies done, none have supported the use of megavitamins, and there is the potential for vitamin toxicity or other negative effects.[51]

Food allergies as a factor in ADHD or behavioral difficulties in children are unclear. Many reports are subjective, and the validity and interpretation of allergy tests can be controversial. It is certainly possible that children suffering from allergies may manifest behaviors (irritability, poor attention) seen in children with ADHD, but whether elimination diets alleviate these symptoms is not clear. Children suspected of having food allergies should be seen by an allergist for diagnosis. Periodic nutrition evaluations are warranted for any child using an atypical dietary regimen.

ADOLESCENT PREGNANCY

Although pregnancy is a normal physiologic state, there are more risks and complications for pregnant teens compared to any other age group. They have higher rates of low-birth-weight infants, especially among those younger than 15 years old. Birth rates among adolescents have been declining during the 1990s; there were 34 births per 1000 in 1996.[52] The biggest decline was in adolescent Black females ages 15–17. The nutritional status of the pregnant adolescent is influenced by both physiologic and environmental/social factors. There is evidence that young pregnant teenage girls are still growing, creating a maternal-fetal competition for nutrients, and thus indicating increased nutrient needs in addition to pregnancy.[53] Other risk factors include a low prepregnancy weight and minimal nutrient stores at the time of conception. Many social factors can also affect the health and nutritional status of the teen, including late or no prenatal care, little financial support, limited food resources, poor eating habits, family difficulties, and various other emotional stresses.

For a positive outcome of pregnancy, weight gain for the pregnant adolescent needs to be more than the usual 25–35 pounds. The Committee on Nutritional Status during Pregnancy and Lactation of the Food and Nutrition Board recommends that pregnant teens should gain at the upper end of the recommended range for their prepregnancy weight[54] (see Appendix D). The pattern of weight gain is important, with weight gain in the first and early second trimesters being related to improved birth weights.[55] Recent studies, however, document that weight gain in adolescent pregnancy results in a reduced birth weight infant and greater maternal stores than would be expected in the pregnant adult.[56]

Dietary guides for pregnant teens have usually added the pregnancy RDAs to the RDAs for 15–18-year-old females (see Appendix K). Energy needs can vary greatly, depending on pubertal maturation and physical activity. An adequate weight gain is the best indicator of an appropriate energy intake. The pregnancy RDA for protein is 60 g, which is 14–16 g more than the RDA for teenage females.[2] Higher protein intakes may be needed, depending on body build and growth needs. A sufficient energy intake will protect the protein to be used for growth. Individualized nutrition assessments will help identify the nutrition and diet concerns to be prioritized for ongoing nutrition counseling and education. An iron supplement is routinely recommended for the second and third trimesters, and vitamins B_6, C, folate, and calcium may be indicated in the presence of dietary and social-environmental risk factors.[57]

Education and counseling are needed for the teen to accept the needed weight gain, plus the likelihood of a higher postpartum weight as part of a healthy pregnancy. Pregnant teenagers are best served by an interdisciplinary health care team to deal with their multiple health, psychosocial, and economic issues. This is most effective when provided as accessible prenatal care targeted to the teenage population in their own communities.[58] Because most of them keep their babies, education and resource referrals are needed regarding infant care and feeding, continued schooling of the mother, parenting, and financial services.

SUBSTANCE ABUSE

Alcohol, tobacco, and marijuana are the most widely used substances among teenagers. During the 1990s there was an increase in the percentages of 8th, 10th, and 12th graders who smoked daily, drank heavily, or used illegal drugs.[52] Alcoholism in adolescence is a significant public health problem. More than 90% of teenagers have had some experience with alcohol by the 12th grade, with many having their first exposure as early as 12 years of age.[59] Any negative effect on nutritional status will depend on the frequency and amount of drinking as well as usual food habits. A survey of teenage males who were alcohol and marijuana abusers did not show significant differences in biochemical measures, but decreased intakes of milk, fruits, and vegetables were reported, as well as more snack food consumption and more symptoms of poor nutrition (tiredness, bleeding gums, muscle weakness).[60] For the female who consumes alcohol and becomes pregnant, there is risk of fetal alcohol syndrome in her infant.

Despite a decrease in cigarette smoking among adults in recent years, smoking remains relatively popular among teenagers. There may be increased need for some nutrients such as ascorbic acid, and smoking during pregnancy can reduce infant birth weight. Smokeless (chewing) tobacco has become popular with both school-age children and adolescents. Not a benign substance, regular use is related to periodontal disease, oral cancer, dependence, and hypertension.[61]

The negative nutritional consequences of a substance user's habit will depend on factors such as lifestyle, available food, and money to buy food. During a nutrition evaluation, the areas of alcohol consumption, tobacco use, and illegal drug use should be considered. Information will most likely be shared if a matter-of-fact, nonthreatening approach is used. Depending on the individual's situation, nutrition education and counseling can focus on improving health and nutrition. Other teenagers will need comprehensive treatment programs, which include a nutrition component.

HEALTH PROMOTION

Americans have been gradually altering their eating habits as a result of increased interest in their health and their concern about preventing heart disease, cancer, obesity, and hypertension. The federal government and nonprofit organizations have provided recommendations, such as the Dietary Guidelines, to promote healthy eating. To what degree, if any, should this advice be applied to growing children and adolescents?

The federally sponsored National Cholesterol Education Program (NCEP) recommends that everyone over 2 years of age follow a diet that includes no more than 30% of calories as fat (10% or less from saturated fat, up to 10% from unsaturated fat, 10%–15% from monounsaturated fat) and no more than 300 mg cholesterol per day.[62] The panel also recommends cholesterol screening for children at risk: those with parents or grandparents diagnosed with coronary heart disease or a cardiac event before age 55, and those with one or both parents having a serum cholesterol of 240 mg or more. Although controversy exists regarding universal versus selective cholesterol screening,[63] screening in childhood appears to be a sensitive predictor of adult lipid levels.[64]

For children identified by screening, the NCEP intervention is dependent on low-density lipoprotein (LDL) cholesterol categories.[62] For those with an acceptable level (less than 110 mg/dL), the recommended dietary pattern (step-one diet) is suggested, with a repeat lipoprotein analysis in 5 years. Children with a borderline level of LDL cholesterol (110–129 mg/dL) would be provided with a step-one diet prescribed and individualized for them and a reevaluation in 1 year. Those with high LDL cholesterol levels (greater than 130 mg/dL) would initially be given the step-one diet, and if necessary the step-two diet (further reduction to less than 7% saturated fat and less than 200 mg cholesterol per day).

Some experts believe that these recommendations are not appropriate, especially for the young child.[65] Failure to thrive has been seen in some infants and toddlers whose parents, well intentioned but misguided, restricted their children's diet to prevent atherosclerosis, obesity, and poor eating habits.[66] (See Chapter 13.) Although there is little evidence that dietary intervention in the growing years will decrease serum cholesterol levels or modify other risk factors later in life,[67] young children appear to be able to consume low-fat diets (less than 30% of calories as fat) without negatively influencing the level of energy or micro-nutrients consumed.[68] It seems appropriate to recommend a gradual transition to a diet meeting the NCEP guidelines for children over 2 years of age.

Prevention of osteoporosis begins with optimal calcium intake and maximal bone density in the growing years. However, many young people, especially adolescents, do not receive the recommended AI of 1,300 mg calcium. Since dairy products are the major sources of calcium, those who consume no or limited amounts of these foods are at risk for calcium deficiency. Some adolescents may also receive less calcium than needed because of rapid growth, dieting practices, and substituting carbonated beverages for milk. Nutrition education public media campaigns are being used to improve these diet trends.

National diet intake data have shown that children and adolescents consume less than desirable intake of fiber, similar to the adult population. A current recommendation is "age plus five"—children over two years of age should take in minimum dietary fiber of age plus five grams per day, up to a maximum safe intake of age plus 10 grams per day.[69] Increasing dietary fiber can also help prevent constipation, and often results in greater intake of fruits and vegetables.

For overall health promotion, moderation and common sense continue to be the best policy. Although prevention of obesity and other chronic conditions is a worthy goal, there are no conclusive data to support a massive change in the diets of growing children. For healthy, growing children, the use of low-fat dairy products and fewer high-fat foods is appropriate for those over 2 years of age. Limiting the intake of fermentable carbohydrate will enhance dental health. Increasing the intake of fruits, vegetables, whole-grain products, and legumes above the usual reported levels can have several benefits: reducing the percentage of fat in the diet, increasing the fiber content, increasing the amount of beta-carotene and other dietary factors that may help prevent cancer, and making the total diet more nutrient dense. The more varied the diet, the more likely that the child's nutrient needs will be met.

NUTRITION EDUCATION

Children first learn about food and nutrition from their families in their own homes. This begins in an informal manner, with parental attitudes, foods commonly served (eg, potatoes or tortillas may be served daily; okra or bok choy may never be served), and family opinions about what foods are good for us. Later, more formal nutrition education occurs in preschools, Head Start programs, day care, schools, and clubs such as 4-H. Information is also assimilated from the media, advertising, written materials, and peers.

A child's developmental level should be taken into account when teaching nutrition concepts. For example, Piaget's learning theory can be used to correlate developmental periods and cognitive characteristics with progress in feeding and nutrition.[70] Younger children definitely do best with hands-on personal experience with food, not abstract nutrition concepts. A personal approach works well with children and adolescents, such as the use of computer software to examine their own dietary profiles. Using theoretical concepts to design nutrition education programs and evaluating the effectiveness of these programs is necessary to have an impact on the target population.[71] Lastly, nutrition education efforts for children should not overlook parents and the family as a whole. (See Chapter 6.)

REFERENCES

1. Satter E. *How to Get Your Kid to Eat...But Not Too Much.* Palo Alto, CA: Bull Publishing Co; 1987.
2. *Food and Nutrition Board. Recommended Dietary Allowances.* 10th ed. Washington, DC: National Academy of Sciences, National Research Council; 1989.
3. Food and Nutrition Board, Institute of Medicine, National Academy of Sciences. *Dietary Reference Intakes: Calcium, phosphorus, magnesium, vitamin D and fluoride.* Washington, DC: National Academy Press; 1997.
4. Cryan J, Johnson RK. Should the current recommendations for energy intake in infants and young children be lowered? *Nutr Today.* 1997;32:69–74.
5. Albertson AM, Tobelmann RC, Engstrom A, et al. Nutrient intakes of 2- to 10-year-old American children: 10-year trends. *J Am Diet Assoc.* 1992;92:1492–1496.
6. U.S. Department of Agriculture, Agricultural Research Service. *Data tables. results from USDA's 1994-96 continuing survey of food intakes by individuals and 1994-96 diet and health knowledge survey*, (Online). ARS Food Surveys Research Group. (Available at http://www.barc.usda.gov/bhnrc/foodsurvey/home.htm)
7. Alaimo K, McDowell MA, Briefel RR, et al. *Dietary intake of vitamins, minerals, and fiber of persons ages 2 months and over in the United States: Third National Health and Nutrition Examination Survey, phase I,*

1988-1991, Advance Data from Vital Statistics; No. 258(PHS) 95-1250 Hyattsville, MD: National Center for Health Statistics; 1994.

8. Matkovic V, Fontana D, Tominac C. Factors that influence peak bone mass formation: A study of calcium balance and the inheritance of bone mass in adolescent females. *Am J Clin Nutr*. 1990;52:878–888.
9. Johnston CC, Miller JZ, Slemenda CW, et al. Calcium supplementation and increases in bone mineral density in children. *N Engl J Med*. 1992;327:82–87.
10. Herbert V. Recommended dietary intakes (RDI) of iron in humans. *Am J Clin Nutr*. 1987;45:679–686.
11. Yu SM, Kogan MD, Gergen P. Vitamin-mineral supplement use among preschool children in the United States. *Pediatrics*. 1997;100(5):e4.
12. Vitamins. In: American Academy of Pediatrics. Committee on Nutrition. *Pediatric Nutrition Handbook*. 4th ed. Elk Grove Village, IL: The American Academy of Pediatrics; 1998:267–281.
13. American Dietetic Association. Position of the American Dietetic Association: Vitamin and mineral supplementation. *J Am Diet Assoc*. 1996;96:73.
14. American Medical Association, Council on Scientific Affairs. Vitamin preparations as dietary supplements and as therapeutic agents. *JAMA*. 1987;257:1929.
15. Beal VA. Dietary intake of individuals followed through infancy and childhood. *Am J Public Health*. 1961;51:1107–1117.
16. Munoz KA, Krebs-Smith SM, Ballard-Barbash R, et al. Food intakes of U.S. children and adolescents compared with recommendations. *Pediatrics*. 1997;100:323–329.
17. Johnson RK, Crouter AC, Smiciklas-Wright H. Effects of maternal employment on family food consumption patterns and children's diets. *J Nutr Educ*. 1993;25:130–133.
18. Kotz K, Story M. Food advertisements during children's Saturday morning television programming: Are they consistent with dietary recommendations? *J Am Diet Assoc*. 1994;94:1296–1300.
19. Kohl HW, Hobbs, KE. Development of physical activity behaviors among children and adolescents. In Hill JO, Trowbridge FL. The causes and health consequences of obesity in children and adolescents. *Pediatrics*. 1998;101(suppl):549–554.
20. Harris CS, Baker SP, Smith GA. Childhood asphyxiation by food: A national analysis and overlook. *JAMA*. 1984;251:2231–2235.
21. Smith MM, Davis M, Chasalow FI, et al. Carbohydrate absorption from fruit juice in young children. *Pediatrics*. 1995;95:340–344.
22. Smith MM, Lifshitz F. Excess fruit juice consumption as a contributing factor in nonorganic failure to thrive. *Pediatrics*. 1994;93:438–443.
23. Dennison BA, Rockwell HL, Baker SL. Fruit juice consumption by preschool-aged children is associated with short stature and obesity. *Pediatrics*. 1997;99:15–22.
24. United States Department of Agriculture. Child Nutrition Programs: School meal initiatives for healthy children. *Federal Register,* 7CFR, Part 220, Food and Consumer Service, USDA, 1995.
25. Ho CS, Gould RA, Jensen LN, et al. Evaluation of the nutrient content of school, sack and vending lunch of junior high students. *Sch Food Serv Res Rev*. 1991;15:85–90.
26. Kaste LM, Selwitz RH, Oldakowski RJ, et al. Coronal caries in the primary and permanent dentition of children and adolescents 1-17 years of age: United States, 1988-1991. *J Dent Res*. 1996;75:631–641.
27. White-Graves MV, Schiller MR. History of foods in the caries process. *J Am Diet Assoc*. 1986;86:241–245.
28. Garcia-Closas R, Garcia-Closas M, Sera-Majem L. A cross-sectional study of dental caries, intake of confectionery and foods rich in starch and sugars, and salivary counts of *Steptococcus mutans* in children in Spain. *Am J Clin Nutr*. 1997;66:1257–1263.
29. Navia JM. Carbohydrates and dental health. *Am J Clin Nutr*. 1994;59(suppl):719S–727S.
30. Makinen KK, Hujoel PP, Bennett CA, et al. A descriptive report of the effects of a 16-month xylitol chewing-gum programme subsequent to a 40-month sucrose gum programme. *Caries Res*. 1998;32:107–112.
31. Johnsen D, Nowjack-Raymer R. Baby bottle tooth decay (BBTD): Issues, assessment, and an opportunity for the nutritionist. *J Am Diet Assoc*. 1989;89:112–116.
32. Looker AC, Dallman PR, Carroll MD, et al. Prevalence of iron deficiency in the United States. *JAMA*. 1997;277:973–976.
33. Yip R, Walsh KM, Goldfarb MG, et al. Declining prevalence of anemia in childhood in a middle-class setting: a pediatric success story? *Pediatrics*. 1987;80:330–334.
34. Pollitt E, Saco-Pollitt C, Leibel R, et al. Iron deficiency and behavioral development in infants and preschool children. *Am J Clin Nutr*. 1986;43:555–565.
35. Walter T, De Andraca I, Chadud P, et al. Iron deficiency anemia: Adverse effects on infant psychomotor development. *Pediatrics*. 1989;84:7–17.
36. Lozoff B, Jimenez E, Wolf AU. Long-term development outcome of infants with iron deficiency. *N Engl J Med*. 1991;325:687–694.
37. Monsen ER, Hallberg L, Layrisse M, et al. Estimation of available dietary iron. *Am J Clin Nutr*. 1978;31:134–141.
38. Iron deficiency. In: American Academy of Pediatrics. Committee on Nutrition. *Pediatric Nutrition Handbook*. 4th ed. Elk Grove Village, IL: The American Academy of Pediatrics; 1998.

39. Pollit E, Cueto S, Jacoby ER. Fasting and cognition in well- and undernourished school children: a review of three experimental studies. *Am J Clin Nutr.* 1998; 67(suppl):779S–784S.
40. Simeon DT, Grantham-McGregor S. Effects of missing breakfast on the cognitive functions of school children of differing nutritional status. *Am J Clin Nutr.* 1989;49:646–653.
41. Meyers AF, Sampson A, Weitzman M, et al. School breakfast program and school performance. *Am J Dis Child.* 1989;143:1234–1239.
42. Kleinman RE, Murphy J, Little M, et al. Hunger in children in the United States: Potential behavioral and emotional correlates. *Pediatrics.* 1998;101:e3.
43. Lipton MA, Mayo JP. Diet and hyperkinesis: An update. *J Am Diet Assoc.* 1983;83:132–134.
44. Kaplan BJ, McNicol J, Conte RA, et al. Dietary replacement in preschool-aged hyperactive boys. *Pediatrics.* 1989;83:7–17.
45. Harper PH, Goyette CH, Conners CK. Nutrient intakes of children on the hyperkinesis diet. *J Am Diet Assoc.* 1978;73:515–519.
46. Wolraich ML, Wilson DB, White JW. The effect of sugar on behavior or cognition in children: a meta-analysis. *JAMA.* 1995;274:1617–1621.
47. Behar D, Rapoport JL, Adams AJ, et al. Sugar challenge testing with children considered behaviorally sugar reactive. *Nutr Behav.* 1984;1:277–288.
48. Bachorowski J, Newman JP, Nichols SL, et al. Sucrose and delinquency: behavioral assessment. *Pediatrics.* 1990;86:244–253.
49. Mattes JA, Gittelman R. Growth of hyperactive children on maintenance regimen of methylphenidate. *Arch Gen Psychiatry.* 1983;40:317–321.
50. Lucas B, Sells CJ. Nutrient intake and stimulant drugs in hyperactive children. *J Am Diet Assoc.* 1977;70:373–377.
51. Haslam RHA, Dalby JT, Rademaker AW. Effects of megavitamin therapy on children with attention deficit disorders. *Pediatrics.* 1984;74:103–111.
52. Federal Interagency Forum on Child and Family Statistics: *America's Children: Key National Indicators of Well-Being.* U.S. Government Printing Office, Washington, DC. Pub no. 065-000-01162-0; 1998.
53. Hediger ML, Scholl TO, Schall JI. Implications of the Camden study of adolescent pregnancy: Interactions among maternal growth, nutritional status, and body composition. *Ann NY Acad Sci.* 1997;817:281–291.
54. National Academy of Sciences. *Nutrition during Pregnancy.* Washington, DC: National Academy Press; 1990.
55. Hediger ML, Scholl TO, Belsky DH, Ances IG, Salmon RW. Patterns of weight gain in adolescent pregnancy: Effect on birth weight and preterm delivery. *Obstet Gynecol.* 1989;74:6–12.
56. Scholl TO, Hediger ML, Schall JI. Maternal growth and fetal growth: Pregnancy course and outcome in the Camden study. *Ann NY Acad Sci.* 1997;817:292–301.
57. American Dietetic Association. Nutrition care for pregnant adolescents. *J Am Diet Assoc.* 1994;94:449–450.
58. Story M. Promoting healthy eating and ensuring adequate weight gain in pregnant adolescents: Issues and strategies. *Ann NY Acad Sci.* 1997;817:321–333.
59. Johnston LD, O'Malley PM, Bachman JG. *National survey results on drug use from the monitoring the future study, 1975-1995.* Rockville, MD: U.S. Department of Health and Human Services, Public Health Services; 1996.
60. Farrow JA, Rees JM, Worthington-Roberts B. Health, developmental and nutritional status of adolescent alcohol and marijuana abusers. *Pediatrics.* 1987;79:218–223.
61. Connolly GN, Winn DM, Hecht SS, et al. The reemergence of smokeless tobacco. *N Engl J Med.* 1986;314: 1020–1027.
62. National Heart, Lung, and Blood Institute, National Cholesterol Education Program. *Report of the Expert Panel on Blood Cholesterol Levels in Children and Adolescents.* Bethesda, MD: National Heart, Lung, and Blood Institute; 1991.
63. Steiner NJ, Neinstein LS, Pennbridge J. Hypercholesterolemia in adolescents: Effectiveness of screening strategies based on selected risk factors. *Pediatrics.* 1991;88: 269–275.
64. Stuhldreher WL, Orchard TJ, Donahue RP, et al. Cholesterol screening in childhood: Sixteen-year Beaver County Lipid Study experience. *J Pediatr.* 1991;119: 551–556.
65. Olson RE. The folly of restricting fat in the diet of children. *Nutr Today.* 1995;30(6):234–245.
66. Pugliese MT, Weyman-Daum M, Moses N, et al. Parental health beliefs as a cause of nonorganic failure to thrive. *Pediatrics.* 1987;80:175–182.
67. Luepker RV, Perry CL, McKinlay SM, et al. Outcomes of a field trial to improve children's dietary patterns and physical activity. The Child and Adolescent Trial for Cardiovascular Health (CATCH). *JAMA.* 1996;275: 768–776.
68. Dixon LB, McKenzie J, Shannon BM, et al. The effect of changes in dietary fat on the food group and nutrient intake of 4- to 10-year-old children. *Pediatrics.* 1997;100:863–872.
69. Williams CL, Bollella M, Wynder EL. A new recommendation for dietary fiber in childhood. *Pediatrics.* 1995;96(suppl):985–988.

70. Lucas B. Nutrition in childhood. In: Mahan LK, Escott-Stump S, eds. *Krause's Food, Nutrition, & Diet Therapy*. 9th ed. Philadelphia: W.B. Saunders Company; 1996:257.

71. Contento I, Balch GI, Bronner YL, et al. The effectiveness of nutrition education and implications for nutrition education and policy, programs, and research: a review of research. *J Nutr Educ*. 1995;27:298–311.

CHAPTER 6

Nutrition Counseling

Bridget M. Klawitter

COUNSELING CHILDREN VERSUS ADULTS—WHAT IS THE DIFFERENCE?

Historically, the dietetic practitioner received little training to differentiate between nutrition counseling and nutrition education. Often, even less was learned about the distinction between children and adults. Children learn naturally through experience and play. Adults often will be able to identify their concerns and express them to the nutrition counselor, whereas children are more likely to express their concerns and feelings either indirectly, through play, or directly, through behavior. This chapter attempts to distinguish for the reader some of the differences the nutrition counselor may encounter with various age and developmental levels in the pediatric population.[1]

HOW CHILDREN LEARN

Information is processed through attention, perception, memory, thinking, and problem solving.[2] Gullo[3] has provided a discussion of how young children process information using these stages. An expansion of this to the field of nutrition counseling is warranted.

Attention

Before children can respond to something, they must recognize it. For the infant, recognition of a parent and the smile and giggling it elicits is an early example. Pellegrini and Smith[4] suggest that forms of physical activity and play serve a developmental function and have labeled this dimension of activity in infants as *rhythmic stereotypes* that serve to improve control of specific motor patterns.

Perception

As the child grows older, attention to objects and events in the environment elicit more specific responses. Once an element in the environment has the child's attention, the child must be able to make sense of it. For example, the infant and toddler soon learn to associate elements of their environment to foods. The sight of the breast or bottle for the infant or the bright colors on the cereal box for the toddler usually attract attention and elicit a response based on the meaning associated with the item. Counseling strategies aimed at the toddler should focus on attracting attention. For example, brightly colored food models or brightly colored pictures can gain the attention of the toddler who is being asked to identify foods.

Memory

The retention of information over time is one of the primary goals of nutrition counseling. Jackson[5] has outlined four ways to facilitate memory in young children:

1. Make it familiar, meaningful, and containing similar characteristics (such as pictures of fruits).
2. Have the child actively involved with the information (such as playing with food models).
3. Give the child repeated exposure to the information (parents reinforce food groups at home).
4. Make sure the information is of interest, fun, and holds their attention (fruits are cut in different shapes and/or the child is involved in food preparation).

Thinking

This aspect appears to become more evident in the older preschool and school-aged group, and is often illustrated by the decision-making process that children demonstrate. One strategy that uses this skill is having children plan a meal using the Food Guide Pyramid (see Appendix L) or food models. Challenging them to include a food from each group can facilitate the thinking and decision-making processes.

Problem Solving

Through experience, children learn the consequences of their actions and decisions. Skills in problem solving increase with exposure to various situations in the environment. For the older child and adolescent, the nutrition counselor may be able to present scenarios and ask them what actions they would take.

DEVELOPMENTAL STAGES

Children perceive, discern, and react to elements in their environment based on their experiences and level of development. Understandably, their reactions change over time as their base of experience and developmental stage changes. A brief discussion of each age group and the typical developmental stages the counselor may encounter can assist in developing counseling strategies appropriate for the age and developmental stage of the children seen.

Infant and Toddler

Biologic, cognitive, and psychosocial development begins and advances quite rapidly during the infant and toddler years. For infants, the parent or caretaker should become the focus of the nutrition counseling session. Two primary reasons that the nutrition counselor should ask parents to bring the infant or toddler to the counseling session are:[6]

- to assess the child's developmental level
- to evaluate the parent-child or caretaker-child interaction.

Observation and appropriate interview probes can provide the nutrition counselor with valuable information about the infant or toddler. The nutrition counselor should be familiar with the normal course of child development and should be able to determine any deviations from the norm that may influence feeding ability. An evaluation of parenting skills and interactions is invaluable, due to the infant or toddler's total dependence on the parent for nutritional well-being.

For many new parents, learning the normal developmental stages of the infant and the range of individual differences can be quite overwhelming. The infant's growth and development pattern is the most suitable guide to introducing semi-solid foods. The feeding of semi-solid foods should be delayed until the consumption of food is no longer a reflexive process and the infant has the fine, gross, and oral motor skills to appropriately consume non-liquid foods safely. Infants need appropriate stimulation to thrive; thus, they usually love colors, talking, music, and being physically held. The attention span of infants is short, but they enjoy sharing pictures, songs, or nursery rhymes, which can encourage cognitive development. The nutrition counselor has a prime opportunity to assist parents during this stage in learning the importance of stimulation for their infant as well as the importance of consistency in meeting the infant's needs. The skilled nutrition counselor adapts the parent learning experience to include issues that cause stress related to the care of the infant and food.

The toddler stage is a time of rapid development and increasing autonomy. Temper tantrums and negative behaviors are common but usually become tempered as the toddler starts to learn socialization skills. As language skills develop, toddlers gradually start to recall past events and to anticipate the consequences of their actions. By 2 or 3 years of age, the toddler can problem-solve through physical and mental experimentation, differentiate space and colors, and identify symbols. Although the attention span of the toddler is limited, play that involves the toddler can be beneficial. Although the parent will be the primary recipient of nutrition and feeding information, children in the toddler stage are capable of understanding some basic nutrition concepts, especially if they are fun. During the toddler phase, parents must continue to be supported, and the nutrition counselor should provide reinforcement for positive changes. The use of small utensils and dishes that are easily manipulated until motor skills are better developed should be encouraged. The importance of continued parental stimulation and a good parent-child relationship should be emphasized by the nutrition counselor during this period.

Play therapy is a technique that may be useful to help young children express their feelings and to understand basic nutrition facts. Play is one of the most powerful ways young children learn and provides an important base for cognitive, language, and social development. Play is a natural medium for self-expression, and open-ended play encourages children to think and to reflect about their environment. As challenges naturally arise in the course of play, the child seeks meaningful solutions. Play is a voluntary activity, and the child is in control.

Through play, children feel control over situations because they can decide what to play and how long to play. Pretend play allows children to create an imaginary world that they can master. In the early years, children think primarily in concrete terms and have no concept of the abstract. The toddler is unable to reason, and, instead, takes words literally. As vocabulary increases, so does the child's ability to express thoughts, needs, and desires. Play therapy is one method that permits children to express their needs and to discover solutions in a safe, therapeutic environment.

Preschool Children

As the toddler matures, the need for social experiences increases. The preschooler can understand his or her physical needs, such as hunger and tiredness, but usually has a poor perception of time. Preschoolers may be able to express their fears and frustrations but may often use play to express these feelings. As the child enters the preschool years, gross motor skills improve dramatically; fine motor skills remain limited.[7] Social interaction increases as the child more actively participates in play, both real and imaginary. Children begin to interact with one another, as well as to communicate with imaginary playmates. Preschool children continue to develop their own identities and to expand their world through outside social contacts. Social skills start to develop as the child attempts to model observed behaviors. The preschooler's maturing cognitive skills produce endless curiosity, as evidenced by the now-constant question "Why?" Explanations must be kept simple and to the point. The counselor should take this opportunity to involve the child, using language and tools appropriate to the child's developmental level. Opportunities to observe the child at play can provide insight into neuromuscular and cognitive development. At this stage, it is also important for the nutrition counselor to develop a rapport with the child to promote behavior change.

Parents should be provided guidance and encouragement in making appropriate nutrition changes. The nutrition counselor should assess parental nutrition knowledge and attitudes toward food during this period, as the influence of the parent on the child's behavior is tremendous. It is during this time that "food jags" and the parent's response may become a challenge of control. The nutrition counselor becomes a support for parents in understanding usual developmental behavior and effective parental responses.

School-Aged Children

School-aged children rapidly build on motor and social skills as they spend more time away from home and enter the formal education environment. Although the attention span of the school-aged child is longer, the nutrition counselor must be attuned to the length of time the child remains attentive during a counseling session. The school-aged child will begin to establish self-concept and values through interaction with others in their environment. At this stage, children start to realize cause and effect relationships, and, gradually, logical reasoning develops. The school-aged child enjoys learning new words and science principles in simple terms. Children in this age group enjoy play that involves winning; stickers, stars, or "points" may provide an incentive for learning and compliance. By age 10–12 years, the child begins to choose friends more selectively, and the influence of peers becomes more predominant. The nutrition counselor should strive to promote more one-on-one interaction with the child during the counseling session and to have parents reinforce the concepts at home. Parents should be encouraged to foster the child's sense of independence and to praise accomplishments within the nutrition care plan.

It is also during this period that the environment becomes more structured and routine; consequently, physical activity levels may decline, and the incidence of obesity increases. Much research has been done on the growing problem of childhood obesity.[8–10] The nutrition counselor can play a major role in assisting parents to understand the important relationship between diet and physical activity, and the potential negative long-term effects of severe dieting to promote weight loss. It is also a period during which the nutrition counselor can aid the child in learning self-management skills with parental support.

Adolescents

The nutrition counselor may use group therapy or one-to-one interaction with adolescents. Children at this stage are usually able to give facts accurately and are becoming more autonomous in their actions and decisions. Adolescents are usually able to understand abstract ideas and concepts and will sometimes verbalize disagreement with nutrition concepts. The adolescent may readily absorb medical terminology but often needs clarification of definitions. Improving self-esteem may make adolescents more compliant because peer relationships are important as the adolescent strives to "fit in." Adolescents also have difficulty imagining themselves vulnerable to illness or disease, and this may impact compliance with the nutrition plan of care. Thus, it is important to emphasize the importance of nutrition and physical activity in relationship to the adolescent's current lifestyle—not the prevention of disease.

The limits of confidentiality should be established early.[6] Two types of information that nutrition counselors may need to pass on to caregivers include their opinion on the nutritional status of the adolescent and what information the adolescent has revealed either verbally or nonverbally that impacts the nutrition plan of care. Being honest and frank up front with the adolescent aids in establishing trust and can facilitate the interview process. Studies noted by Hayes[11] have found caregivers usually to be receptive to the issue of confidentiality and to recognize its importance in building relationships with a child. In many instances, adolescents will give permission to the counselor to share the details of the session with their parents, and this makes the counseling experience more open. Respecting the individuality of the adolescent can go a long way in establishing the trust needed for a productive nutrition counseling experience.

A strong preoccupation with body image may also accompany this group and interfere with comprehension of healthy lifestyle practices. Growing evidence[12] suggests that body image is just as important to young boys as it is to girls. The primary difference is that boys worry more about not having enough size. Society views being big and powerful as being manly, evidenced by messages sent in films, on television, by rock groups, and in video games. Men in athletics or involved in physical activity are also valued by society in general. Approximately 90% of individuals treated for eating disorders are female; however, the number of males appears to be increasing.[13] The same factors—decreased self-esteem, feeling the need to be "perfect," and the desire to feel in control of the environment—accompany eating disorders in both males and females.

Adolescents are capable of abstract thinking and logical reasoning, and these should become the major focus of the counseling session. Adolescents may rebel against authority as they struggle to establish their own identities. Establishing rapport with the adolescent and facilitating the relationship between the child and the family in following recommendations is perhaps the most challenging aspect of counseling this age group. Parents should be encouraged to set realistic limits for adolescents while fostering independence.

CREATING A LEARNING ENVIRONMENT

Interviewing Techniques

Some general techniques for interviewing children using the five-stage model[14] are provided in Exhibit 6–1.

Interviewing the child or adolescent can present many unique challenges to the nutrition counselor.[6] Interviewing is quite different from counseling the adult, and the younger the client, the greater will be the difference. The nutrition counselor will find that children and adolescents will vary in their cognitive and language skills, at times independent of chronologic age. Children and adolescents (either willing or unwilling) are often brought by others to the counseling experience. Occasionally, an older adolescent will come on his or her own initiative. Children and adolescents may often perceive the nutrition counseling experience as a reflection of misdeeds; that is, "eating wrong" or having an "imperfect body." This perception can lead to barriers that the nutrition counselor must recognize and overcome for the counseling to be effective. Finally, nutrition counseling sessions may involve children or adolescents who have difficulty with communication, either voluntary or involuntary. The skilled nutrition counselor will possess a variety of counseling methodologies to assist the child to participate actively in the learning experience as much as possible.

Establishing rapport is key to the success of the counseling experience. The counselor must be warm, empathetic, and genuine, and should develop a warm and friendly relationship with the child. At the first visit, the primary focus should be the establishment of rapport, rather than simply determining facts about the child. With very young children, it is especially important to explore their world with them before introducing change. Nutrition counselors should take the time to show interest in the child and should genuinely care about who the child is.

It is important for the nutrition counselor to have a flexible approach to counseling children. This includes being aware of feedback that the child may provide, either verbal or nonverbal. The nutrition counselor should be alert to the feelings of the child and should be able to reflect those feelings back to the child in a manner that the child understands.

It is usually possible, through skillful probing, to determine whether a child is ready to learn a particular nutrition concept. The nutrition counselor should respect the child's ability to solve problems when given the opportunity to

Exhibit 6–1 Interviewing children using the five-stage model

Stage 1 Establish rapport
Establish rapport in your own way: Use facial expressions (ie, smile, laugh), play activities, or drawing.

Stage 2 Gather data emphasizing strengths
Paraphrase, reflect child's feelings, summarize frequently. Keep questions and concepts concrete, avoid abstract talk. Identify positive aspects.

Stage 3 Determine goals
Ask what the child wants to happen. Accept a child's goals but focus on concrete, short-term goals. Allow a child to explore the ideal world and discover fantasies and desires.

Stage 4 Generate alternative solutions and actions
Utilize creative brainstorming techniques. Try small groups with children having similar problems. Imagine the future and explore various alternatives.

Stage 5 Generalize
Maintain concrete goals day to day. Homework assignments are useful. Observe behavior and interactions with others.

Source: Adapted with permission from A.E. Ivey, M.B. Ivey, and L. Simek-Morgan. *Counseling and Psychotherapy: A Multicultural Perspective,* 4th ed. Copyright © 1997 by Allyn and Bacon.

do so. As with adults, the responsibility to make choices and to make change rests with the child.

THE COUNSELING EXPERIENCE

Role of the Child

The role of the child is to be him/herself. It is important for the nutrition counselor to realize that the ultimate decision to change rests with the child and that the counseling approach, as well as strategies used, must take this into consideration to be successful.

Role of the Parent

The role of the parent in the counseling experience changes as the child matures. For the infant, the parent's primary role is to engage in social interaction with the child and counselor, and to attend to the needs of the infant on cue. As the child enters the toddler stage, the parental role is to provide opportunities for the child to explore and experiment with his or her environment. Children love mastering a new skill, and the preschooler relishes completing tasks for the parent. The preschooler also enjoys reenacting experiences through imaginary play, and the parental role is to provide props and to acknowledge the child's progress and accomplishments. As the child enters school and takes charge of more activities, the parent becomes a mentor, offering information and assistance. Adolescence is the child's final push for independence as youth "practice" adulthood; the parental role gradually decreases to offering objective, succinct information for the adolescent's decision-making process.

Parents appear to respond best to information that focuses on their specific needs and problems.[15] Verbal suggestions can be effective for conveying brief, concrete nutrition concepts but clearly written information should be provided for both reinforcement and more complex, detailed information. Modeling or role playing may be a useful technique for parents who need visual examples or when the issue involves problematic parent or child behavior. The counselor may ask, "What could you do differently in that circumstance?" These various techniques, if applied wisely and appropriately, can facilitate nutrition and activity behavior changes.

Exercising together as a family should be promoted as an excuse to have fun. Families should find an activity that can be accomplished at varying skill levels and enjoyed on a regular basis. The benefits of an active lifestyle to children include improved motor skills, increased self-confidence, and maximizing time together as a family unit. Inactivity is often accompanied by poor eating habits during childhood and can contribute to a lifetime of health problems. The American Heart Association has issued general guidelines for healthy physical activity that can aid families in increasing physical activity in their children.[16] Some key points to suggest to parents include:

- Encourage regular walking, bicycling, and outdoor play; use of playgrounds and gyms; and interaction with other children.
- Limit watching television or video tapes and video games to less than 2 hours per day.
- Encourage weekly participation in age-appropriate organized sports, lessons, or team activities.
- Seek out daily school or daycare physical activity that includes at least 20 minutes of coordinated large muscle exercise.
- Plan regular family outings that involve walking, cycling, swimming, or other recreational activities.
- Be a positive role model for a physically active lifestyle, and look for other caregivers and school personnel who do the same.

Role of the Counselor

A counselor can help guide the child through an age- and developmentally appropriate play experience to learn basic health concepts and can assist parents or caregivers to discover the correct balance of independence for a child. Certain limits required by family structure and therapeutic diet modifications may also need to be communicated.

Counseling Environment

The nutrition counselor must provide a physical environment that will facilitate the counseling experience for both the parent and the child. Using concepts outlined by Barker,[6] the nutrition interview should be conducted in counseling rooms or playrooms designed for younger children. Key elements include:

- comfortable chairs and tables of sizes suitable for the age of the child being seen
- book shelves with a selection of age-appropriate books, especially those illustrating nutrition and physical fitness concepts
- paper and drawing materials
- child-centered and age-appropriate surroundings
- culturally sensitive toys
- well-designed cupboards and other readily accessible storage space
- cleaning solution to sanitize items between sessions, especially toys and food models

Arrangement of the room, perhaps by age category or developmental level, can assist in directing a child's attention to items that are likely of interest and age-appropriate. Older adolescents are usually comfortable in an adult environment. Elements key to an environment conducive to counseling adults may include such factors as:[1,17]

- adults want to be treated as adults and as individuals
- most adults prefer objectivity and a business-like approach

- adults want counseling to address their perceived needs
- adults need positive reinforcement and feedback
- adults want to be active participants in the counseling experience
- adults prefer a counseling location that is clean, safe, private, and furnished with the adult client in mind

PROVIDING DEVELOPMENTALLY APPROPRIATE EXPERIENCES

Biologic Experiences

As the infant grows and develops, important biologic experiences occur that can influence food habits later on. The process of introducing solid foods is a primary learning ground for food tastes and textures. Caregivers should be prepared for initial refusal of new textures and flavors and counseled on how to encourage an infant without force-feeding. Negative food experiences during this time can often develop into food aversions. Trying foods too early or in a certain order may influence a child's food preferences and acceptance. The role of the nutrition counselor involved during this early period is to assist parents in identifying when their infant is developmentally ready to advance food types and textures, and to assist parents in recognizing cues their infant gives in regard to acceptance of the food.

Physical Experiences

Infants prefer exploring objects with all their senses. Many parents comment that "everything goes in the mouth!" Mobiles, musical toys, and bright colors and shapes all stimulate the infant's senses. As mobility increases, the child's ability to explore increases, and toys should have a variety of colors, shapes, and sizes to stimulate interest. Safety is an important feature during this stage as children explore their environment.

Role playing is evident as the maturing child "pretends" during play. The preschooler often will be found modeling the behavior of the waitress at the restaurant and taking orders for food from stuffed animals. Pretending allows children to recall events in their environment and to translate those into play experiences. The nutrition counselor may want to consider role-playing activities to teach and evaluate basic nutrition concepts.

Pictures, puzzles, and games can challenge children as they develop cognitive and motor skills. For very young children, coloring a picture of the Food Pyramid (Appendix L) or drawing a picture of a favorite food in each group can foster both motor and cognitive skill building. Use of the food pyramid and food models to plan a special meal or to go on a trip to the grocery store can be an exciting activity. School-aged children can often incorporate math and reading skills into food activities by planning the number of servings per day of a food or measuring the ingredients for baking. Cutting out magazine pictures of food and arranging them in a collage or mobile by food group can spur interest in food variety.

Children learn important nutrition concepts through daily food experiences. Cooking can be an enjoyable activity for many children; however, many parents may be reluctant to use this activity, anticipating chaos and inedible results. The nutrition counselor should encourage parents to use this activity and to plan ahead, taking time to help children prepare simple recipes. Cooking helps develop important skills in a number of areas, including language, science, nutrition, art, sensori-motor development, socio-emotional development, social studies, and mathematics.[18] Exhibit 6–2 illustrates some of the concepts that may be reinforced in these developmental areas by involving children in cooking experiences.

Social Experiences

Family meal time can provide high-quality, positive social interactions that facilitate a

Exhibit 6–2 Cooking and Learning Together

Socioemotional Development
- taking turns, sharing
- feeling of competence
- sense of independence
- respect for others' work
- trying new experiences

Sensori-Motor Development
- taste and smell differentiation
- touch and food texture, size
- sight and food appearance
- small muscle coordination (chopping, stirring)
- large muscle coordination (kneading, mixing)

Art
- balance
- aesthetic development
- awareness of color, form, texture, shape

Language
- reading recipes
- asking questions
- learning new vocabulary
- writing and recording
- following written and verbal instructions

Science
- investigating the origins of food
- physical properties of food
- food and temperature changes
- how food changes from one state or form to another
- predicting and testing predictions

Social Studies
- ethnic foods
- regional food
- geography
- meaning of food in different cultures

Nutrition
- trying new and unusual foods
- learning about Canada's Food Guide
- developing positive attitudes about nutrition
- planning a healthy meal or snack

Mathematics
- numbers, fractions
- ordering
- classifying
- measuring
- developing spatial concepts

Source: Reprinted from Resource Sheet #22, "Cooking and Learning Together" published by the Canadian Child care Federation, Winter 1993. This material was adapted by Susan Vaughn from *Cooking With Children,* published by New Brunswick Health and Community Services; and "Creative Food Experiences for Children," in *Health, Safety and Nutrition for the Young Child,* by Lynn R. Marotz, Jeanettia M. Rush and Marie Z. Cross.

child's cognitive abilities, enhance the nurturing process, promote family values, and affirm a sense of identity and security. Unfortunately, many families find it difficult to eat together regularly. The role of the nutrition counselor is to encourage parents to provide at least one family meal time daily, where the child can experience the companionship of family members and a positive feeding environment. To assist families to "reconnect," meals can be planned outside in the yard, at a park, or at a restaurant with as many family members present as possible.

ROLE OF THE PARENT

Developmental Stage of the Parent

The nutrition counselor must assess not only the developmental level of the child, but also that of the parent. Providing complex information that the parent is unable to understand or apply will serve only to stress the family environment and to decrease compliance. In general, the nutrition counselor may want to consider having all initial materials provided to parents to be written at a sixth-grade reading level to facilitate learning and to provide quick access for review at a later time. More complex information can always be provided as the situation demands.

Cultural Influences

In today's multicultural society, sensitivity to the ethnic and religious facets of a child's environment is critical to long-term compliance with the nutrition plan of care. Incorporating ethnic foods into the meal plan can facilitate the entire family unit supporting the diet interventions versus expectations that the child must eat "differently."

Knowledge of cultural and religious traditions and how these can be integrated into day-to-day meals and activity is also an important asset for the nutrition counselor to possess.

Feeding Relationship

The ability to observe the feeding relationship between child and parent can provide tremendous insight into potential barriers to adequate nutrition. For children with feeding difficulties enrolled in rehabilitation programs, observation of a feeding session with a speech therapist can provide valuable information on the parent-child relationship. Asking parents to record a food diary for 2–3 days, including the time of feedings and where the feedings took place, provides information on the structure of the family lifestyle. For older children, input from caregivers or school personnel, where available, can be helpful, as well. In addition, in-depth probing on the parent's feelings toward food and the child's particular feeding issues can assist in developing a successful nutrition care plan.

Psychosocial Relationship with Child

Parents will sometimes comment on the difficulty they have in getting a child to eat or to comply with a modified diet. Careful attention to the feelings of the parent in regard to the child's actions can aid the nutrition counselor in assessing the parent-child psychosocial relationship when it comes to food. Food can become a power struggle—one that usually neither side wins without outside intervention. It is also important to assess the relationship between parents. One parent sabotaging the other's efforts will often be picked up on quickly by the child, making compliance with the nutrition plan difficult and challenging.

Model Behavior

Children look to their parents as role models. The nutrition counselor must help parents to understand that the family must help the child adapt to any needed diet modifications, but, in many cases, the nutrition plan of care can be used by all members of the family to promote health. For the child who is battling a weight problem, having the entire family become more active and follow a low-fat, balanced diet will facilitate compliance and improve the health status of the entire family. In some cases, the nutrition counselor may, in fact, become a role model for the child if the family situation lacks the support and follow-through.

COUNSELING THE CHILD WITH SPECIAL NEEDS

The nutrition counselor who sees children with special needs must be attuned to the developmental stages and cues previously discussed. Chronologic age often does not correlate with the abilities of the child, and the level of parental involvement can vary significantly. The etiology of the disability and its physiologic and psychosocial implications on nutrition status must be determined. The medical nutrition therapy protocols (such as for failure to thrive[19,20]) can provide the nutrition counselor with clinical and functional outcomes to be monitored, as well as with potential interventions that may be considered.

The first step that the nutrition counselor should consider is accommodations required by the population served to make services as accessible as possible. Laurel Hayes[21] outlines many of the general considerations that the counselor should take into account. Specific to the field of nutrition counseling, scales and other equipment should be calibrated to accommodate the nonambulatory client. Reference materials specific to special populations (such as growth grids and activity conversion factors) should be readily available. The nutrition counselor should also have a good working knowledge of the disabilities most frequently encountered and the impact on the family unit as a whole. Play therapy allows many children with special needs to discover what strengths they have in relation to their disabilities. The involvement of parents and/or caregivers becomes key in this population and may also entail coordination of efforts with other health care professionals.

SUMMARY

Developmental considerations are important in determining the interview approach to be used. Flexibility and the establishment of rapport are key to a successful nutrition interview. Key tips for parents to facilitate nutrition learning experiences include:

- establish routines for the feeding experience
- talk to children about how they feel about foods and any necessary diet modifications prescribed by the health care provider
- help children tie their self-worth to actions regarding food selections instead of body looks
- model appropriate behavior, including diet selections and physical activity behavior
- redirect a child's attention or activity by using neutral or positive language (such as, "Potato chips are fine for an occasional snack, but here is some fresh fruit that would be a better snack.")
- acknowledge positive behavior (such as, "You helped me plan a very healthy meal for dinner tonight.")
- do not make food and diet selections a power struggle
- do not use food as a reward or a punishment
- recognize that each child is an individual and is unique

Evers[22] summarizes the most successful approach to pediatric nutrition counseling with what she calls the *FIB* (fun, integrated, behavior change) approach to nutrition education. First, the nutrition counseling experience should be fun for the parent, child, and nutrition counselor. Creating engaging methods to illustrate basic nutrition concepts can be a challenge but an enjoyable one. Secondly, nutrition should be integrated wherever possible. The effective nutrition counselor finds ways for parents and children to integrate the basic nutrition concepts into their daily lifestyle. Change may be gradual but gradual change may be more permanent. Last, but not least, behavior change is key. Possessing the knowledge is one thing; making the necessary lifestyle changes is another. The nutrition counselor must assist the parents in making healthy choices as a family unit, not expecting the change to affect just the child. Changes isolated only to the child foster noncompliance and can potentially influence the child's self-image negatively in the long-term. Involving the family as a whole in making wise food and activity choices can promote a more permanently healthy lifestyle for all involved.

REFERENCES

1. Klawitter B. Counseling and learning: child, adolescent, adult, elderly and family. In: Helm KK, Klawitter B, eds. *Nutrition Therapy: Advanced Counseling Skills.* Lake Dallas, TX: Helm Seminars; 1995:21–47.
2. Yusson SR, Santrock JW. *Child Development: An Introduction.* Dubuque, IA: WC Brown Co; 1982.
3. Gullo DF. *Developmentally Appropriate Teaching in Early Childhood.* Washington, DC: National Education Association; 1992.
4. Pellegrini AD, Smith PK. Physical activity play: the nature and function of a neglected aspect of play. *Child Dev.* 1998;69:577–598.

5. Jackson NE, Robinson HB, Dale PS. *Cognitive Development in Young Children.* Washington, DC: National Institute of Education; 1976.
6. Barker P. *Clinical Interviews with Children and Adolescents.* New York: WW Norton and Company; 1990.
7. Anderson JR. *Cognitive Psychology and Its Implications.* 3rd ed. New York: WH Freeman; 1990.
8. Hill JO, Trowbridge FL. Childhood obesity: future directions and research priorities. *Pediatrics.* 1998;101:570–574.
9. Mei Z, Scanlon KS, Grummer-Strawn LM, Freedman DS, Yip R, Trowbridge, FL. Increasing prevalence of overweight among US low-income preschool children: the Centers for Disease Control and Prevention pediatric nutrition surveillance, 1983 to 1995. *Pediatrics.* 1998;101:E12.
10. Ogden CL, Troiano RP, Briefel RR, Kuczmarski RJ, Flegal KM, Johnson CL. Prevalence of overweight among preschool children in the United States, 1971 through 1994. *Pediatrics.* 1994;99:E1.
11. Hayes LL. Counseling resistant teens. *CTOnline.* 1997;40:1–3.
12. Andersen AE. Eating disorders in males. In: Brownell K, Fairburn CG, eds. *Eating Disorders and Obesity. A Comprehensive Handbook.* New York: Guilford Press; 1995:177–182.
13. Holbrook TL, Weltzin TE. Eating disorders in males: a neglected problem revisited. *Treatment Today.* 1998;10.
14. Ivey AE, Ivey MB, Simek-Morgan L. *Counseling and Psychotherapy: A Multicultural Perspective.* 3rd ed. Boston, MA: Allyn & Bacon; 1993.
15. Glascoe FP, Oberklaid F, Dworkin PH, Trimm F. Brief approaches to educating patients and parents in primary care. *Pediatrics.* 1998;101:E10.
16. American Heart Association. Exercise (physical activity) and children. *AHA Scientific Position.* Chicago, IL: 1998.
17. Helm KK. Business skills that improve your communication and success. In: Helm KK, Klawitter B, eds. *Nutrition Therapy: Advanced Counseling Skills.* Lake Dallas, TX: Helm Seminars; 1995:81–88.
18. Vaughn S. *Cooking and Learning Together.* Resource Sheet #22. Ontario, Canada: Canadian Child Care Federation; 1996.
19. American Dietetic Association and Morrison Healthcare, Inc. *Medical Nutrition Therapy Across the Continuum of Care: Supplement 1.* Chicago, IL: American Dietetic Association; 1997.
20. Dietitians Independent Practice Association. *The Handbook of Medical Nutrition Therapy: Practice Guidelines, Protocols, Codes, and Outcomes.* Lake Dallas, TX: Helm Publishing; 1996.
21. Hayes LL. Counseling individuals with disabilities. *CTOnline.* 1997;40:2–5.
22. Evers CL. *How to Teach Nutrition to Kids.* Tigard, OR: Carrot Press; 1995.

Chapter 7

Vegetarianism in Children

Carol M. Coughlin

Increasingly, nutrition professionals are called upon to counsel vegetarian children. A recent poll indicated that 37% of vegetarians have children under the age of 18.[1] These vegetarian parents may wish to raise their children as vegetarians. Children as young as early elementary age may choose a vegetarian diet for themselves. This chapter will assist nutrition professionals in counseling the vegetarian client. As with any diet for a child, vegetarian diets should be planned appropriately to be nutritionally adequate.

The term *vegetarian* is commonly defined as a person who excludes meat, seafood, and poultry from his or her diet. The most common type of vegetarian is the lacto-ovo vegetarian, who includes dairy products and eggs. Vegans (pronounced "vee-guns") exclude all animal products and by-products, including honey and gelatin. It is common for people to describe themselves as vegetarian when their actual diet ranges anywhere from the typical American diet to one that excludes red meat but includes fish and chicken. Therefore, a dietary assessment of foods included and excluded, typical portions, and frequency of consumption is critical to ascertain dietary adequacy.[2] Nutrition professionals should familiarize themselves with foods typically found in vegetarian and vegan diets (see Table 7–1 for a description of vegetarian foods), as well as cooking techniques, local availability, and nutrient content. This knowledge will greatly assist nutritional counseling.

REASONS FOR CHOOSING A VEGETARIAN DIET

In the general population, the most frequently cited reasons for adopting a vegetarian diet are health benefits and disease prevention.[3] For pregnant women and parents of vegetarian children, moral and religious considerations are more commonly given as the reason.[4] The Seventh Day Adventist religion strongly encourages a lacto-ovo vegetarian diet. Other religions, such as Jain, Hindu, Moslem, and Hare Krishna, have prohibitions against eating some or all forms of meat. Many people adopt a vegan diet because they view the use of animals for food and clothing to be against their ethical beliefs. Alternative medical beliefs, such as Macrobiotics and Ayurveda, recommend a vegetarian or near-vegetarian diet. Health professionals must take these views into consideration when counseling children and parents.

COUNSELING THE VEGETARIAN CLIENT

The first step in counseling clients in general, and vegetarian clients in particular, is to establish rapport.[5] This is impeded if spiritual and health beliefs are not explored and respected. It is important to reinforce positive practices, such as adequate fiber, moderate fat, or the inclusion of adequate amounts of fruits and vegetables, before beginning the discussion of any dietary adjustments that should be made.

Table 7–1 Vegetarian and Vegan Foods

Meat analogs	Made from soy or gluten (wheat protein). Most have less fat and far less saturated fat than the animal product that they resemble. Many have vitamins such as B_{12} added.
Miso	Fermented soybean paste. This high-sodium food is used in small amounts to flavor dishes and as a soup base.
Nutritional yeast	A yellow, flaky powder with a salty/cheesy taste. Do not confuse this with brewer's yeast, which is bitter, brown granules. Some brands (Red Star Vegetarian Support Formula, for example) are fortified with vitamin B_{12}. Others are not. Sprinkle on vegetables, pasta, or salad as Parmesan cheese would be used. Also can be added to a roux to make a "cheese" sauce.
Rice milk	A white beverage used like milk. May be fortified with calcium. Lower in protein than cow's or soy milk. Typically available in a variety of flavors, such as vanilla and carob.
Soy milk	Some brands are fortified with calcium, vitamin D, and riboflavin so that levels equal cow's milk. Some brands are high in iron.
Soy sauce	May be called *shoyu* or *tamari*. Some have wheat added. Reduced-sodium varieties are available.
Tempeh	A cake of whole soybeans with a culture added. Used as a meat substitute.
Tofu	A soft cheese made from soy milk. A high-calcium food if coagulated with a calcium salt. Tofu is high in protein. There are numerous textures, from silken to extra firm, and the protein content varies with the texture.

Nutritional requirements are for essential nutrients, not for specific foods. Do not assume that a diet is inadequate simply because a person chooses to exclude some foods or even food groups. Many people restrict their diet in some way, whether due to religious or ethical food beliefs or simple likes and dislikes. Exhibit 7–1 outlines steps to use in counseling vegetarian children.

Though counseling tools, such as the Vegetarian Food Pyramid (see Figure 7–1), are helpful when counseling vegetarian clients, a thorough diet analysis using a computer nutrient database is best. A diet history and an estimation of key nutrients, such as protein, calcium, and vitamin B_{12}, can also be a useful assessment tool. Simply counting servings from major food groups may severely overestimate or underestimate nutrient composition of the diet. For example, blackstrap molasses would normally be counted as a sweet, yet it contains calcium and iron. Green leafy vegetables would be counted as a vegetable—not a serving of dairy—yet are a good source of calcium. In the example in Exhibit 7–2, one might assume that the meal containing animal foods would have more protein or iron but this is not the case. The vegan breakfast does not contain any foods typically counted as good sources of calcium but contains two-thirds the calcium found in one serving of cow's milk. Substituting one cup of calcium-fortified soy milk and orange juice for the apple juice in the vegan breakfast would give the meal as much calcium as two cups of milk.

Exhibit 7–1 Steps in Dietary Counseling for Vegetarian Children

1. **Caloric intake.** An accurate height and weight measurement can help determine long-term adequacy. Be sure the diet has sufficient caloric density so that the child does not feel full before caloric needs are met.
2. **Calcium.** Calculate the calcium from all sources, including: dairy products; calcium-fortified juices; calcium-fortified soy and rice beverages; low-oxalate vegetables such as collard greens and bok choy; and blackstrap molasses. Inquire whether baked goods are made with either cow's milk or fortified vegetable milks. See Table 7–3 for a listing of plant sources of calcium and Table 7–4 for data on the availability of calcium from vegetarian foods.
3. **Vitamin D.** In southern climates, sunshine can be an adequate source of vitamin D year round. In northern states, there is not adequate sunshine to allow the body to produce adequate vitamin D. Vitamin D synthesis is poorer in people with dark skin and can be blocked by sunscreen. Therefore, a dietary source is recommended for all children. Fluid cow's milk, fortified soy or rice milk, fortified breakfast cereals, or a vitamin supplement can be used as a vitamin D source.
4. **Iron.** Iron deficiency anemia is a common nutritional problem in all children. Look for a good source of dietary iron such as whole grains, beans, or dried fruits. Remind clients that vitamin C enhances non-heme iron absorption and suggest food sources. See Table 7–5 for a listing of the iron content of vegetarian foods.
5. **Vitamin B_{12}.** If the child is vegan, be sure there is a source of vitamin B_{12}. Red Star Brand Nutritional Yeast Vegetarian Support Formula, fortified "milks," meat analogs, and some breakfast cereals are vegan vitamin B_{12} sources. Most children's multivitamins contain vitamin B_{12}. See Table 7–6 for a listing of the vitamin B_{12} content of vegetarian foods.
6. **Protein.** If caloric intake is adequate and the child is not eating an excessive amount of empty calorie foods, chances are that protein intake most likely will be adequate. The frequency of meals in a young child's diet greatly assists in providing a variety of amino acids to be available for protein synthesis throughout the day.
7. **Vitamin and mineral supplements.** Note the supplement, dosage, and how often it is actually consumed by the child.

Key Nutrients in Vegetarian Diets

See Table 7–2 for a check list of nutrient and vegetarian sources.

Calories

Adequate caloric intake is essential to the growth of all children. Vegetarian diets are often high in fiber and bulk. This is a nutritional advantage for adults and the weight conscious yet can be a liability for the young child with a small stomach capacity. The bulk of the diet can easily be reduced so that the young child does not feel full before adequate caloric intake has been achieved. To reduce bulk, some refined grains can replace servings of whole grains; dried and cooked fruits can be substituted for some fresh fruits and vegetables. High fat foods should not be overly restricted. Foods such as seeds, nuts, and nut butters provide a concentrated source of calories as well as necessary minerals and protein.

Protein

Protein needs can be met easily if vegetarian children eat a variety of plant foods and have an adequate intake of calories. Although vegetarian diets tend to be lower in total protein, intake in both lacto-ovo vegetarians and in vegans appears to be adequate.[6]

All plant proteins contain all of the essential amino acids. The question is one of protein qual-

Figure 7-1 Vegetarian Food Guide Pyramid

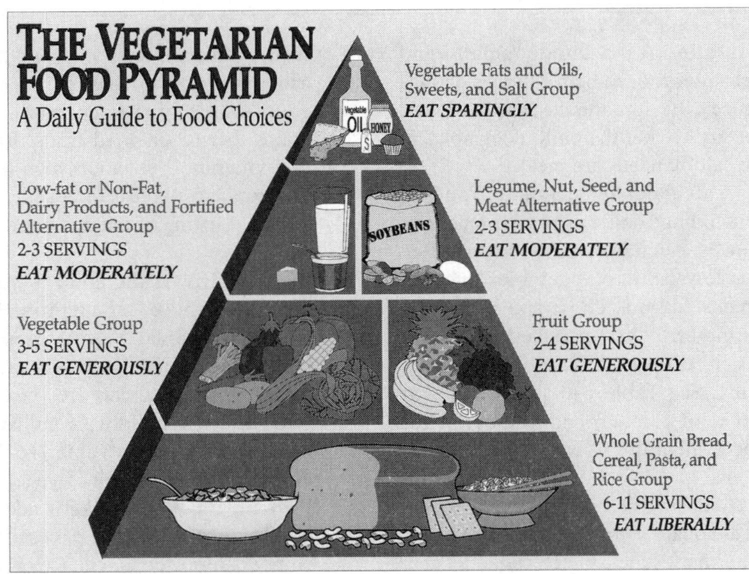

Source: Reprinted with permission from General Conference Nutrition Council, © The Health Connection. Illustration by Merle Poirier. For handouts, posters and other materials, contact The Health Connection, 1-800-548-8700.

Exhibit 7–2 Comparison of Two Vegetarian Breakfasts for a School-aged Child

	Lacto-ovo Vegetarian	Vegan
	1 scrambled egg	1 cup cooked millet with 1 tbsp blackstrap molasses
	1 slice whole wheat toast	1 slice whole wheat toast with 2 tbsp peanut butter
	1 tsp margarine	1 cup apple juice
	8 oz 1% milk	
	TOTAL	
Protein (g)	17	18
Fat (g)	14	19
Iron (mg)	1.7	6.5
Calcium (mg)	353	219

ity, as amino acid patterns may not perfectly match biologic requirements. Protein needs may actually be slightly higher than the Recommended Daily Allowances (RDA) because of the lower quality of some plant proteins.[7] Diets of vegetarian children, whether lacto-ovo or vegan, generally meet or exceed recommendations for protein. It is unnecessary to plan precisely and to complement amino acids within each meal, as the complementary protein theory once suggested.[7] The frequency of meals for children may assist in providing the complement of amino acids for protein synthesis. Legumes, grains, soy products, meat analogs, nut butters, dairy products, and eggs are all concentrated protein sources.

Table 7–2 Vegetarian and Vegan Sources of Nutrients

Nutrient	*Acceptable sources for vegan diets*	*Additional foods acceptable for lacto-ovo vegetarians*
Protein	Whole grains, legumes, and soy-based or wheat-based (gluten) meat analogs. Grains can provide a great deal of protein as several servings are eaten each day.	Dairy and eggs.
Calcium	Fortified soy, rice or other "milks," fortified juices such as apple (usually only 100 mg/serving), orange, and cranberry juice. Dark green low-oxalate vegetables (kale, collard greens).	Cow's milk, goat's milk, other dairy products, supplements derived from dairy products.
Iron	Breast milk, iron-fortified infant formula, some soy milk (such as Pacific Brand), soy products, legumes, whole grains, dried fruits, fortified breakfast cereal, food cooked in cast iron pans. Encourage vitamin C sources at each meal for optimal absorption.	
Riboflavin	Fortified soy milk, legumes, grains, vegetables.	Cow's milk.
Vitamin B_{12}	B_{12}-fortified soy milk, Red Star Nutritional Yeast Vegetarian Support Formula, fortified breakfast cereals, fortified meat analogs, vitamin supplements.	Dairy and eggs.
Zinc	Nuts, legumes, wheat germ.	Dairy and eggs.

When assessing the diet of a vegetarian child, it is important to consider all of the protein in the diet—not just the protein from the concentrated sources. Vegetarian children may get a significant amount of their protein requirement from grains and vegetables simply because of the large number of servings eaten per day.

Calcium

Blood calcium levels are maintained within very narrow limits. When calcium intake is insufficient, blood levels are maintained at the expense of bone. This may lead to inadequate mineralization of bone in the young and osteoporosis in adults, a condition where calcium is lost from bone. The bones become fragile and at increased risk for breakage. Age-appropriate optimal calcium intake for children is given in Appendix K.

Dairy products provide 73% of the calcium in the United States diet.[8] Approximately 30% of the calcium in milk is absorbed.[9] Concern about total dietary fat and saturated fat has led many families to use non-fat or low-fat dairy products. Toddlers need an adequate fat intake for proper growth, and for many, using whole-fat dairy products achieves this goal. On the other hand, some families find it more convenient to purchase only reduced or non-fat dairy products and see to it that young children get fat from other foods. Infants get adequate fat from breast milk or infant formula. Breastfeeding a child during the second year of life helps assure adequate fat intake as well.

Clients should be cautioned that only fluid milk has vitamin D added—other dairy products do not. Also, not every dairy product is necessarily an excellent source of calcium. Some dairy products have extra calcium added. The same product from different manufacturers (chocolate milk or yogurt, for example) can differ by more than 100% in the calcium per serving. Nutritional counselors should encourage careful reading of the nutrition facts label.

Calcium-fortified foods are available in most grocery stores. These include various "milks," such as soy milk, rice milk, and goat milk; fruit juices, such as orange juice, apple juice, and cranberry juice; rice, and breakfast cereals. Careful label reading and brand specificity are important here as different brands within the same category vary widely in the amount of calcium per serving. Calcium-fortified soy milks contain from 200 to 500 mg of calcium per cup. The absorption rate ranges from 50% of the calcium in fortified orange juice to about 30% from other sources.[9]

Low-oxalate green leafy vegetables provide a well-absorbed source of calcium for vegan children (see Table 7–3 for a listing of plant sources of calcium and Table 7–4 for data on the availability of calcium from vegetarian foods). The absorption rate for calcium is about 50–60% for low-oxalate green leafy vegetables such as collard greens, mustard greens, bok choy, turnip greens and kale.[9] These foods can provide an excellent source of calcium. Using these foods in a recipe such as creamed greens or collard green pizza increases the acceptance for some children. Spinach is a poor dietary source of calcium as it is very high in oxalate. The oxalate binds the calcium in the spinach, preventing absorption. Beet greens, rhubarb, and peanuts are also high-oxalate foods.

Although relatively low in calcium, grain products can contribute significant amounts of calcium to the diet, due to the large numbers of servings eaten per day.[10] Many baked goods are made with milk or milk solids, or have calcium added. However, the phytate in cereals can bind calcium and make it unavailable for absorption. Food processing methods such as sprouting grains and adding yeast to bread reduces this effect as phytate is destroyed in the leavening process.[11]

Calcium set tofu, textured vegetable protein, tahini, almonds, blackstrap molasses, legumes, nuts, and seeds can add significant amounts of calcium to the diet. About 20–30% of the calcium in these foods is absorbed.[9] Although soy contains phytate and oxalate—both known to inhibit calcium absorption—the calcium from tofu, soy milk, and soybeans is essentially equivalent to that of cow's milk.[9]

Osteoporosis prevention appears to be enhanced by achieving maximum bone mass in the first years of life. Dietary intake data from the National Health and Nutrition Examination Survey III (NHANES III) show that most people are far from meeting the DRIs through diet alone.[12] Though some calcium supplements, such as calcium citrate, appear to be better absorbed than are other forms of calcium, slightly larger quantities of calcium from other types of calcium supplements, such as calcium carbonate, will make up the difference in absorption.[13]

Calcium supplements are available in capsule, chewable, powder, liquid, and effervescent forms. Liquid or powdered calcium can be easily added to beverages. Powdered calcium can be added to baked goods, from muffins to pizza crust. Powdered milk (from both cow's milk and soy beverages) can also be added to food; these not only boost the calcium but also add protein and other nutrients.

Calcium Balance

The bioavailability of calcium and balance are extremely important. Intake and absorption account for only 25% of variance in calcium bal-

Table 7–3 Plant Sources of Calcium

Food	Calcium Content (mg)	Food	Calcium Content (mg)
Legumes (1 cup, cooked)		**Vegetables** (1/2 cup, cooked)	
Chick peas	78	Bok choy	79
Great Northern beans	121	Broccoli	89
Kidney beans	50	Collard greens	178
Lentils	37	Kale	90
Lima beans	52	Mustard greens	75
Navy beans	128	Butternut squash	42
Pinto beans	82	Sweet potato	35
Black beans	103	Turnip greens	125
Vegetarian baked beans	128	**Fruits**	
Soy foods		Dried Figs (5)	258
Soybeans (1 cup, cooked)	175	Orange	56
Tofu (1/2 cup)	120 to 350*	Raisins (2/3 cup)	53
Tempeh (1/2 cup)	77	Calcium-fortified orange juice	300
TVP (1/2 cup, rehydrated)	85	**Grains**	
Soy milk (1 cup)	84	Corn bread (2-oz piece)	133
Fortified soy milk (1 cup)	250–300	Corn tortilla	53
Soy nuts	252	English muffin	92
Nuts and Seeds (2 tbsp)		Pita bread (1 small pocket)	31
Almonds	50	**Other foods**	
Almond butter	86	Blackstrap molasses (1 tbsp)	187
Brazil nuts	50	Fortified Rice Dream (1 cup)	300
Sesame seeds	176	Vegelicious (1 cup)	300
Tahini	128	Take Care (1 cup)	300

Note: TVP is a trademark of Archer Daniels Midland Company and is textured soy protein.
*Indicates a range of calcium found in different tofu products.

Source: Data from *J.A.T. Pennington Bowes & Church Food Value of Portions Commonly Used.* 16th edition © 1994, Lippincott Williams & Wilkins.

ance, whereas urinary loss accounts for approximately 50%.[10] Optimal calcium balance can be facilitated by adjusting other factors in the diet, such as sodium, oxalate, iron, and protein. Protein and sodium both increase urinary calcium loss. Vegetarian diets are moderate in protein. To increase calcium absorption, moderate the oxalate and phytate in the diet. Note that fiber has not been shown to affect calcium absorption significantly.[9] The potential for calcium supplements to interfere with iron absorption should be noted, especially for populations at increased risk for iron deficiency, such as children.

Iron

Iron deficiency anemia is the most common childhood nutritional problem. Though meat contains heme-iron that is better absorbed than is the nonheme-iron found in plant foods, iron deficiency anemia is no more likely to occur in vegetarian than in non-vegetarian children.[6] Good iron sources for vegetarian children in-

Table 7–4 Availability of Calcium from Plant Foods

*Food Source**	*Calcium Content (mg)*	*Fractional Absorption (%)***	*Estimated Absorbable Calcium (mg)/Serving*
Broccoli	35	52.6	18.4
Brussel sprouts	19	63.8	12.1
Chinese cabbage	79	53.8	42.5
Green cabbage	25	64.9	16.2
Kale	47	58.8	27.6
Milk (one cup)	300	32.1	96.3
Mustard greens	64	57.8	37.0
Pinto beans	44.7	17.0	7.6
Sesame seeds (1 oz)	37	20.8	7.7
Turnip greens	99	51.6	51.1
Tofu, calcium set	258	31.0	80.0

*Serving size equals 1/2 cup unless otherwise indicated.
**Absorption rates were adjusted for load (absolute amount of calcium).

Source: Data from C.M. Weaver and K.L. Plawecki, Dietary calcium: Adequacy of a Vegetarian Diet, American Journal of Clinical Nutrition, vol. 59, pp. 1238–1241, © 1994.

clude whole or enriched grains and grain products, iron-fortified cereals, legumes, green leafy vegetables, and dried fruits (see Table 7–5 for a listing of the iron content of vegetarian foods). Consuming foods rich in vitamin C at the same meal enhances nonheme-iron absorption.

Vitamin B_{12}

All vitamin B_{12} is produced by microorganisms. Vitamin B_{12} is found in foods derived from animals and is made by the microbes that live within them. Lacto-ovo vegetarians obtain dietary B_{12} from eggs and dairy products. Bacteria in the human digestive tract produce B_{12} but the extent to which this is absorbed is unclear, as it seems to be produced in the colon, past the point of B_{12} absorption.[14] Salivary bacteria produce a negligible amount of vitamin B_{12}.

Vegans consume no animal products, so they must consume vitamin B_{12}-fortified foods or supplements. There are several foods that are fortified with a vegetarian (non animal-derived) vitamin B_{12} such as breakfast cereals (eg, Total, Nutri-Grain), nutritional yeast (eg, Red Star Brand Vegetarian Support Formula) nutritional yeast, meat analogs, and some soy milks. Therefore, all types of vegetarians should be able to find an acceptable source of vitamin B_{12}. See Table 7–6 for a listing of the vitamin B_{12} content of vegetarian foods.

Most cases of vitamin B_{12} deficiency are not due to a lack of B_{12} in the diet but to an inability to absorb B_{12}.[14] Most reports of dietary B_{12} deficiency in the literature are in people following a macrobiotic diet.[6] Some foods commonly included in a macrobiotic diet, such as tempeh (a cultured whole soybean product), sea vegetables (kelp, kombu, arame), miso (a fermented soybean paste), algae, and spirulina had been previously reported to contain vitamin B_{12}. Current thinking is that many of these foods actually contain B_{12} analogs and may interfere with active vitamin B_{12} absorption.[14] Because a deficiency risks permanent neurologic damage, it is

Table 7–5 Iron Content of Foods

Food	Iron Content (mg)	Food	Iron Content (mg)
Breads, cereals, grains		**Fruits**	
Bread, white, one slice	0.7	Apricots, 1/4 cup dried	1.5
Bread, whole wheat, one slice	0.9	Prunes, 1/4 cup	0.9
Bran flakes, 1 cup	11.0	Prune juice, 1/2 cup	1.5
Cream of Wheat, 1/2 cup	5.5	Raisins, 1/4 cup	1.1
Oatmeal, instant, one packet	6.3	**Legumes (1/2 cup cooked)**	
Barley, whole, 1/2 cup cooked	1.6	Baked beans, vegetarian	0.7
Pasta, enriched, 1/2 cup cooked	1.2	Black beans	1.8
Rice, brown, 1/2 cup cooked	0.5	Garbanzo beans	3.4
Wheat germ, 2 tbsp	1.2	Kidney beans	1.5
Vegetables (1/2 cup cooked		Lentils	3.2
unless otherwise indicated)		Lima beans	2.2
Acorn squash	0.9	Navy beans	2.5
Avocado, 1/2 raw	1.0	Pinto beans	2.2
Beet greens	1.4	Soybeans	4.4
Brussel sprouts	0.9	Split peas	1.7
Collards	0.9	Tempeh	1.8
Peas	1.2	Tofu	6.6
Pumpkin	1.7	Textured vegetable protein	2.0
Sea vegetables		**Soy milk/vegetable milk**	
Alaria	18.1	Soy milk, 1 cup	1.4*
Dulse	33.1	**Nuts/seeds (2 tbsp)**	
Kelp	42.0	Cashews	1.0
Nori	20.9	Pumpkin seeds	2.5
Spinach	1.5	Tahini	1.2
Swiss chard	1.9	Sunflower seeds	1.2
Tomato juice, 1 cup	1.3	**Other foods**	
Turnip greens	1.5	Blackstrap molasses, 1 tbsp	3.3

*Varies by brand.

Source: Data from *J.A.T. Pennington Bowes & Church Food Value of Portions Commonly Used.* 16th edition, © 1994, Lippincott Williams & Wilkins.

critical to assure a reliable source of this vital nutrient.

The macrobiotic diet generally does not allow the use of fortified foods or supplements.[15] It does allow the use of fish, which can serve as a dietary source of vitamin B_{12}. Some people following a macrobiotic diet would rather remain vegetarian and, therefore, would be inclined to use fortified foods.

Zinc

There is little available information on the zinc content of diets of vegetarian children.[6] Zinc from breast milk is better absorbed than zinc found in infant formula, probably due the presence of zinc-binding proteins in human milk.[16] Phytate has been singled out as the most potent dietary inhibitor of zinc bioavaila-

Table 7–6 Vitamin B12 Content of Foods

Food	Vitamin B12 Content (µg)	Food	Vitamin B12 Content (µg)
Breads, cereals, grains		**Fortified soy milk/vegetable milks** (8 oz)	
Kellogg's Corn Flakes, 3/4 cup	1.5	Better Than Milk (soy milk)	0.6
Grapenuts, 1/4 cup	1.5	Edensoy Extra	3.0
Nutrigrain, 2/3 cup	1.5	Sno E (soy milk)	1.2
Product 19, 3/4 cup	6.0	Soyagen	1.5
Raisin Bran, 3/4 cup	1.5	Take Care (soy milk)	0.9
Total, 1 cup	6.2	Vegelicious (vegetable milk)	0.6
Meat analog (serving sizes are one burger or one serving according to package)		**Animal products**	
		Milk, 1 cup	0.9
Loma Linda "Chicken" Nuggets	3.0	Yogurt, plain, nonfat, 1 cup	0.6
Morningstar Farms Grillers	6.7	Egg, one large	0.6
Loma Linda Sizzle Franks	2.0	**Other**	
Worthington Stakelets	5.2	Nutritional yeast (Red Star brand T6635), 1 tbsp	4.0

Note: Fortification of commercial products can change over time, so that it is always a good idea to check the label.

Source: Data from *J.A.T. Pennington Bowes & Church Food Value of Portions Commonly Used.* 16th edition, © 1994, Lippincott Williams & Wilkins.

bility.[17,18] Food processing, such as sprouting beans and leavening bread (yeast or lactic acid fermentation, such as sourdough), can lower the phytate content of food, thus improving iron and zinc bioavailability.[19,20] High-fiber foods are often associated with diminished zinc absorption. However, refined foods that are low in fiber have less zinc, so total zinc absorption is greater from the high-fiber foods. For example, almost 40% of the zinc in white bread is absorbed, whereas only 17% is absorbed from whole grain bread. However, the total amount of zinc absorbed from whole grain bread is almost 50% more than that absorbed from white bread because whole grain bread contains more than three times the level of zinc found in the white bread.[21] It is estimated that up to 25 g per day of dietary fiber and 1 g per day of phytic acid is unlikely to have a deleterious effect on zinc bioavailability.[22] Professionals should help parents of vegetarian children identify a variety of zinc-rich foods to include in their children's diets, such as whole grain pasta, wheat germ, fortified cereals, cheese, legumes, and peanut butter.

ALTERNATIVE MEDICAL BELIEFS AND THE VEGETARIAN DIET

Ayurveda

Ayurveda is a system of healing originating in India thousands of years ago. Ayurvedic medical therapy prescribes treatments with the goal of achieving or maintaining a balance of three forces called *doshas*.[23] Foods are classified as to whether they increase or decrease (pacify) each dosha within the patient. Ayurvedic dietary prescriptions are generally given in terms of increasing or decreasing the consumption of foods and not necessarily eliminating them from the diet completely. Ayurveda generally recommends a lacto-vegetarian diet.

Fruitarian

A fruitarian diet consists of only fruits. Any plant food that is botanically a fruit or can be obtained without killing or harming the plant is considered a fruit.[6] A popular modification of the diet includes sprouted grains and legumes. Some fruitarian diets are simply vegan diets. That is, they consist of fruits and vegetables (including green leafy vegetables), grains, nuts, and legumes. The additional foods greatly increase the ease in which dietary needs can be met on this type of a diet. Planning a diet that meets all nutritional needs would be very difficult, but not impossible, for the highly motivated. Fortified foods or supplements would be required to meet calcium and vitamin B_{12} needs. Foods such as avocado, nuts, and seeds provide fats. Nuts, seeds, grains, and legumes provide protein and contain needed minerals such as iron, zinc, and calcium. This diet is generally not recommended, especially in the pediatric population.

Macrobiotics

Macrobiotics is a set of beliefs surrounding lifestyle and health.[15] The philosophy is linked loosely to Buddhism, and a strong Chinese influence can be seen, especially surrounding the concept of yin and yang. A macrobiotic diet is generally not totally vegetarian, as fish is included. The diet is based on whole grains, vegetables, fruits, and soups. Most animal products, including dairy products, are generally excluded. The macrobiotic belief eschews the use of vitamin and mineral supplements and fortified foods. Older studies showed that infants on a restrictive macrobiotic diet had poor growth patterns.[6,24] Deficiencies of vitamin B_{12} and low calcium intakes were found. Recently, the macrobiotic community has revised their recommendations and now recommends the inclusion of dairy products to provide calcium and fish to provide a source of vitamin B_{12} in the diet.[25]

VEGETARIAN DIETS THROUGHOUT CHILDHOOD

Diet for Infancy

All infants begin life as vegetarians as meat is generally not introduced into the diet until the latter half of the first year of life. Breastfeeding is the recommended feeding method for infants. Breastfeeding rates among vegetarians are much higher than in the general population; breastfeeding rates above 95% have been reported.[26] In the United States, only 20% of infants in the general population are still being breastfed at age 6 months,[27] whereas studies examining vegan children showed that most were breastfed well into the second year of life.[28] The milk produced by vegetarian mothers is nutritionally adequate, and breastfed infants of well-nourished vegetarian mothers grow and develop normally.[6] Current research indicates that only newly absorbed vitamin B_{12} (as opposed to that stored in the mother's body) is passed through the breast milk. A dietary source of B_{12} for nursing mothers must be established and maintained throughout the nursing period.[29] See Table 7–6 for a list of foods high in vitamin B_{12}. A 1981 report published in the *New England Journal of Medicine* noted that milk from vegetarian mothers had fewer pesticide residues than did milk from mothers in the general population.[30] Vegetarian infants who are not breastfed should receive appropriate cow's milk or soy-based infant formula. Soy formulas are acceptable to most vegan families and support normal growth in infants.[31]

There are few data on the growth of non-macrobiotic vegan infants.[6] Because most vegetarian infants are breastfed, growth should be assessed using tools designed for infants consistent with the feeding method chosen by the parents. Breastfed babies do not follow the same growth patterns as do formula fed infants.[32] Solid foods should be added to the diet, in accordance with normal infant feeding guidelines (see Chapter 4).

Toddlers

Vegetarian toddlers should be expected to have the same nutritional concerns as omnivore toddlers, namely, a dislike of vegetables, "picky" eating habits, and food jags.[33] Raising a child on a vegetarian diet does not assure that the child will like all vegetables. A vegetarian diet planned in accordance with current dietary recommendations can meet the nutritional needs of toddlers and preschoolers, and can aid in the establishment of life-long healthy eating patterns. Young children need more than just three meals a day. Nutritious snacks can add significantly to the nutrient intake of the vegetarian child. See Table 7–7, Exhibit 7–3, and Exhibit 7–4 for meal planning guidelines and tips.

Table 7–7 Meal Planning Guidelines for Vegetarian Children

Food Group	*1–4 years*	*5–6 years*	*7–12 years*	*12–18 years*
Grains	4 servings	6 servings	7 servings	10 servings
Leafy green vegetables	2–4 tsp	1/4 cup	1 serving	1–2 servings
Other vegetables	1/4–1/2 cup	1/4–1/2 cup	3 servings	3 servings
Fruits	3/4–1 1/2 cups	1/2–1 cup	2 servings	4 servings
Legumes	1/4–1/2 cup	1/2–1 cup	2 servings	2 servings
Nuts and seeds	1–2 tbsp	1–2 tbsp	1 serving	1 serving
Milk (breast, soy, or cow's)	3 cups	3 cups	3 cups	3 cups
Fats	3 tsp	4 tsp	5 tsp	4 tsp

Source: Adapted from M. Messina and V. Messina, *The Dietitian's Guide to Vegetarian Diets: Issues and Applications,* © 1996, Aspen Publishers, Inc.

Exhibit 7–3 Meal Planning Tips for Vegetarians

1. Begin with familiar vegetarian foods: peanut butter sandwiches, macaroni and cheese, pasta with vegetables, bean burritos, lentil soup, pizza, vegetables, salads, hot cereal, and breads. The vast majority of foods in any diet should be from the plant foods at the bottom of the food pyramid (grains, fruits, vegetables).
2. Soy and rice milk are used cup for cup like cow's milk in recipes. Choose brands fortified with calcium and vitamin D.
3. Eggs can be replaced with commercial starch-based egg replacers, ground flax seeds, mashed bananas, applesauce, or prune puree, depending on the recipe.
4. Soy or wheat gluten-based meat analogs make familiar-looking main dishes, such as chili, "beef" stew, and "chicken" salad.
5. Many ethnic dishes are not meat based. Stir-fry vegetables with tofu, Indian lentil dishes (dal), and hummus are but a few examples. It may be easier to find vegetarian dishes at ethnic restaurants when eating out.
6. Expand the repertoire. A healthy vegetarian diet does not focus on what is excluded, but on including new grains, vegetables, fruits, and protein sources.
7. There are many excellent vegetarian/vegan cookbooks with step-by-step instructions on replacing animal products in the diet.

Exhibit 7–4 Meal Planning for Those in "Mixed" Families

1. Serve meals that each person assembles themselves. Chef salad served salad-bar style, tacos, etc.
2. Revise dishes currently made with meat. It can be easy to assemble a small nonmeat lasagna alongside a meat-containing one. Chili, pizza, bean soup, and pasta sauce can all be made without meat or using meat analogs.
3. Serve meatless favorites that the entire family enjoys several times a week. Typical meals include cheese pizza, vegetable soup with sandwiches, and bean burritos.
4. Many dishes, such as vegetable and grain casseroles, can serve as the entree for the vegetarian and a side dish for the omnivores.

Table 7–8 Sample Menus for 5-Year-Old and 13-Year-Old Vegan Children

	5-year-old	*13-year-old*
Breakfast		
Oatmeal	1 cup	1 cup
Raisins	1 tsp	2 tsp
Orange juice	1 cup	1 cup
Whole wheat bagel	none	one
Almond butter	none	2 tbsp
Lunch		
Peanut butter and banana sandwich on whole wheat	1 each	1 each
Hummus	3 tbsp	4 tbsp
Baby carrots	9 each	12 each
Fortified soy milk	1 cup	1 cup
Molasses cookie	none	one
Dinner		
Creamy green soup (made with collard greens)	1 cup	1 cup
Crackers	6 each	6 each
Tofu cutlet with gravy	4 oz	4 oz
Baked potato	none	one medium
Fortified soy milk	1 cup	1 cup
Snacks		
Almonds	1 tbsp	3 tbsp
Figs	1/4 cup	1/4 cup
Crackers, whole wheat	none	6
Totals:		
Calories	1,515	2,673
Protein (g)	50	81
Fat (g)	44	88
Vitamin C (mg)	156	188
Iron (mg)	12.6	22.6
Calcium (mg)	894	1,294

School-Aged Children

Many school-aged children have been following a vegetarian diet from birth. However, it is becoming more common for children as young as 7 or 8 years old to choose this diet for themselves. Meal planning and meal preparation tips for "mixed" families can ease this transition. See Table 7–7, Table 7–8, Exhibit 7–3, and Exhibit 7–4 for guidelines and tips.

A common misconception is that vegetarian children will have poor growth. Studies of Seventh Day Adventist children, who follow mostly a lacto-ovo vegetarian diet, show they are slightly taller than omnivores.[34] Other studies have shown growth rates that meet or exceed norms.[28,35]

Most studies of vegan children in the United States have been on children following a macrobiotic diet. One exception is The Farm study.[26] The Farm is a vegan community in Tennessee. A sample of 404 children, vegan from birth, were slightly shorter than controls at ages 1–3 and were comparable in height at age 10.[26] Studies of British vegan (non-macrobiotic) children showed that they were taller than controls and a bit lighter.[36]

Adolescents

Few data are available on the eating habits of vegetarian teenagers. One study noted that female vegetarian teens' diets contained 40% more fiber than diets of omnivores.[37] Vegetarian teens are still teens, and, therefore, common teen eating habits are to be expected. Foods with low nutrient density, such as french fries and nondairy desserts, may be chosen over green leafy vegetables. See Table 7–7, Table 7–8, Exhibit 7–3, and Exhibit 7–4 for guidelines and tips.

Because vegetarian diets are more common among teenagers, as are eating disorders, some health professionals have noted that vegetarian diets are somewhat more common among teens with eating disorders than in the general adolescent population. Recent data suggest that adopting a vegetarian diet does not lead to eating disorders.[38] When counseling any teen, professionals should note clients who greatly limit food choices or exhibit symptoms of eating disorders.[39]

Athletes

Vegetarian diets can meet the needs of the child athlete. Protein needs may be elevated because training increases amino acid metabolism, but vegetarian diets that meet energy needs and include good sources of protein (eg, soy foods, legumes) can provide adequate protein without use of special foods or supplements.[7]

SUMMARY

Many of the concerns and issues that nutrition professionals will encounter when counseling vegetarian families are exactly the same as for all other families. Vegetarian diets can easily meet the nutritional needs of the growing child. The scientific literature shows a positive relationship between vegetarian diets and reduced risk for several chronic diseases and conditions, including obesity, coronary artery disease, hypertension, diabetes mellitus, and some types of cancer.[7] Organizations and recommended publications that clients can use to gather more information on vegetarian diets are listed after the references.

REFERENCES

1. Yankelovich et al. The American vegetarian: coming of age in the 90's—a study of the vegetarian marketplace conditions. *Vegetarian Times*. 1992.
2. Mangels AR. Working with the vegetarian client. *Dietitian Gen Clin Pract*. 1994;12:9–14.
3. Yankelovich, Clancy, Shulman. Survey of adult Americans. *Time Magazine* and *CNN*. April 1992.
4. Finley DA, Dewey KG, Lonnerday B, Grivetti LE. Food choices of vegetarians and nonvegetarians during pregnancy and lactation. *J Am Diet Assoc*. 1985;85:678–685.
5. Johnston PK. Counseling the pregnant vegetarian. *Am J Clin Nutr*. 1988;48:901–905.

6. Messina M, Messina V. *The Dietitian's Guide to Vegetarian Diets: Issues and Applications.* Gaithersburg, MD: Aspen Publishers; 1996.
7. Messina VK, Burke, KI. Position of The American Dietetic Association: Vegetarian diets. *J Am Diet Assoc.* 1997;97:1317–1321.
8. Gerrior S, Bente L. *Nutrient Content of the US Food Supply, 1909–94.* Home Economics Research Report No. 53. Washington, DC: US Department of Agriculture, Center for Nutrition Policy and Promotion; 1997.
9. Weaver CM, Plawecki KL. Dietary calcium: adequacy of a vegetarian diet. *Am J Clin Nutr.* 1994;50(suppl): 1238S–1241S.
10. US Department of Health and Human Services, Public Health Service, National Institutes of Health. *Consensus Development Statement. Optimal Calcium Intake.*1994 June 6–8;12(4):1–31.
11. Weaver CM, Heaney RP, Marin BR, Fitzsimmons ML. Human calcium absorption from whole-wheat products. *J Nutr.* 1991;121:1769–1775.
12. Alaimo K, McDowell MA, Briefel RR, et al. *Dietary Intake of Vitamins, Minerals, and Fiber of Persons Ages 2 Months and Over in the United States; Third National Health and Nutrition Examination Survey, Phase I, 1988–1991.* Advance Data from Vital and Health Statistics; No. 258.
13. Levenson DI, Bockman RS. A review of calcium preparations. *Nutr Rev.* 1994;52:221–232.
14. Herbert V. Vitamin B_{12}: plant sources, requirements, and assay. *Am J Clin Nutr.* 1988;48:852–858.
15. Kushi M, Jack A. *The Book of Macrobiotics: The Universal Way of Health, Happiness and Peace.* New York: Japan Publications; 1986.
16. Cousins RJ. *Zinc.* In: Ziegler EE, Filer LJ Jr, eds. *Present Knowledge in Nutrition.* 7th ed. Washington, DC: ILSI Press; 1996:293–306.
17. Saha PR, Weaver CM, Mason AC. Mineral bioavailability in rats from intrinsically labeled whole wheat flour of various phytate levels. *J Agric Food Chem.* 1994;42:2531–2535.
18. Larsson M, Hulten LR, Sandstrom B, Sandberg A. Improved zinc and iron absorption from breakfast meals containing malted oats with reduced phytate content. *Br J Nutr.* 1996;76:677–688.
19. Kavas A, Sedef NEL. Nutritive value of germinated mung beans and lentils. *J Consumer Studies Home Econ.* 1991;15:357–366.
20. Sandstrom B, Almgren A, Kivisto B, Cederblad A. Zinc absorption in humans from meals based on rye, barley, oatmeal, triticale, and whole wheat. *J Nutr.* 1987;117: 1898–1902.
21. Sandstrom B, Arvidsson, B, Cederblad A, et al. Zinc absorption from composite meals. I. The significance of wheat extraction rate, zinc, calcium and protein content in meals based on bread. *Am J Clin Nutr.* 1980;33: 739–745.
22. Williams CL, Bollella M. Is a high fiber diet safe for children? *Pediatrics.* 1995;96:1014S–1019S.
23. Morrison JH: *The Book of Ayurveda.* New York: Fireside Press; 1995.
24. Dagnelie PC, van Staveren WA. Macrobiotic nutrition and child health: results of a population-based, mixed-longitudinal cohort study in the Netherlands. *Am J Clin Nutr.* 1994;59(suppl):1187S–1196S.
25. Dagnelie PC, van Staveren WA, van den Berg H, Kingjan PG, Hautvast J. High prevalence of rickets in infants on macrobiotic diets. *Am J Clin Nutr.* 1990;51: 202–208.
26. O'Connell JM, Dibley MJ, Sierra J, Wallace B, Marks JS, Yip R. Growth of vegetarian children: the Farm Study. *Pediatrics.* 1989;84:475–481.
27. Ryan AS. The resurgence of breastfeeding in the United States. *Pediatrics.* 1997;99:E12.
28. Sanders TAB, Reddy S. Vegetarian diets and children. *Am J Clin Nutr.* 1994;59(suppl):1176S–1181S.
29. Specker BL, Miller D, Norman EJ, Greene T, Hayes KC. Increased urinary methylmalonic acid excretion in breast-fed infants of vegetarian mothers and identification of an acceptable dietary source of vitamin B_{12}. *Am J Clin Nutr.* 1988;47:89–92.
30. Hergenrather J, Hlady G, Wallace B, Savage E. Pollutants in breast milk of vegetarians. *N Engl J Med.* 1981; 304:792.
31. Committee on Nutrition, Academy of Pediatrics. Soy protein formulas: recommendations for use in infant feeding. *Pediatrics.* 1983;359–363.
32. Garza C. Infancy. In: Brown ML, ed. *Present Knowledge in Nutrition.* 6th ed. Washington, DC: International Life Sciences Institute–Nutrition Foundation; 1990: 320–324.
33. Skinner JD, Carruth BR, Hoouck KS, et al. Longitudinal study of nutrient and food intake of infants aged 2 to 24 months. *J Am Diet Assoc.* 1997;97:496–504.
34. Sabate J, Linsted KD, Harris RD, Sanchez A. Attained height of lacto-ovo vegetarian children and adolescents. *Eur J Clin Nutr.* 1991;45:51–58.
35. Tayter MS, Stanek KL. Anthropometric and dietary assessment of omnivore and lacto-ovo-vegetarian children. *J Am Diet Assoc.* 1989;89:1661–1663.
36. Sanders TAB. Growth and development of British vegan children. *Am J Clin Nutr.* 1988;48:822–825.
37. Donovan UM, Gibson RD. Iron and zinc status of young women aged 14–19 years consuming vegetarian and omnivorous diets. *J Am Coll Nutr.* 1995;14: 463–472.

38. Janelle KC, Barr SI. Nutrient intakes and eating behavior scores of vegetarian and non-vegetarian women. *J Am Diet Assoc*. 1995;95:180–189.

39. O'Connor MA, Touyz SW, Dunn SM, Beaumont PJV. Vegetarianism in anorexia nervosa? A review of 116 consecutive cases. *Med J Aust*. 1987;147:540–542.

RECOMMENDED SOURCES OF VEGETARIAN INFORMATION FOR CLIENTS

The Vegetarian Nutrition Dietetic Practice Group of The American Dietetic Association
216 West Jackson Blvd.
Chicago, IL 60606-6995
(312) 899-0040
http://www.eatright.org

Seventh Day Adventist Dietetic Association
PO Box 75
Loma Linda, CA 92354
(714) 793-8918

Vegetarian Resource Group
PO Box 1463
Baltimore, MD 21203
(410) 366-8343
http://www.vrg.org

The Health Connection
13490 Golden Corn Drive
Highland, MD 20777
(800) 548-8700

RECOMMENDED READING FOR CLIENTS

Coughlin C. *Good News About Good Food.* 2nd ed. Leicester, MA: Cucurbita Moshata; 1999.

Havala S. *Simple Lowfat and Vegetarian.* Baltimore, MD: The Vegetarian Resource Group; 1994.

Krizmanic J. *A Teen's Guide to Going Vegetarian.* New York, NY: Viking Children's Books; 1994.

Messina V, Messina M. *The Vegetarian Way.* New York, NY: Harmony Books; 1996.

Melina V, Davis B, Harrison V. *Becoming Vegetarian.* Summertown, TN: The Book Publishing Company; 1995.

Robertson L, Flinders C, Rupenthal B. *The New Laurel's Kitchen.* Berkeley, CA: Ten Speed Press; 1986.

Chapter 8

Food Hypersensitivities

Lynn Christie

Identification of health problems associated with foods, the mechanism of the problems, and the appropriate treatment has plagued medicine for centuries. Hippocrates was one of the first to report an adverse food reaction to milk, over 2,000 years ago.[1] The National Institutes of Allergy and Infectious Diseases and the American Academy of Allergy, Asthma and Immunology established a common language describing adverse food reactions (see Table 8–1).[1] An adverse food reaction is a clinically abnormal response to an ingested food or food additive. Adverse reactions (food sensitivity) to foods are categorized either as food hypersensitivity (food allergy) or as food intolerance. Food hypersensitivity is caused by an immunologic reaction resulting from the ingestion of a food or food additive. Food intolerance is an abnormal physiologic response to an ingested food or food additive that has not been proven to be immunologic in nature.

There are four types of immune mechanisms (I, II, III, IV) involved in allergies (see Exhibit 8–1).[2] Food hypersensitivity, classically, is an immunoglobulin E (IgE), mast cell-dependent reaction (Type I). After ingestion of a specific food, an IgE-mediated reaction may occur immediately (within 1 hour) and can be followed by late-phase reaction (4–8 hours) inflammation. Type II is an antibody-dependent cytotoxic response, Type III is based on antigen-antibody complexes, and Type IV is cell mediated. A combination of Types II, III, and IV is suspected to play a role in food sensitivities such as food-induced malabsorption syndromes, gluten-sensitive enteropathy, and cow's-milk-associated pulmonary hemosiderosis. Food hypersensitivities are further described in Exhibit 8–2 by their clinical manifestations and whether the disorder is IgE mediated.

Food intolerances proven not to be immunologic in nature are secondary to factors including toxic contaminants, pharmacologic properties of the food, metabolic disorders, and idiosyncratic responses. Exhibit 8–3 provides a differential diagnosis for adverse food reactions.

In one prospective survey,[3] parents reported that approximately 28% of their children experienced adverse food reactions. Only one-third of the possible adverse food reactions could be confirmed by controlled challenges. This study demonstrated that in a pediatric practice of 480 children followed from birth to 3 years of age, physicians or family suspected that 133 (28%) of the children had symptoms produced by ingested foods. When food challenges were performed, 75 (15%) of the children experienced skin rashes and diarrhea following the ingestion of fruits and fruit juices (food intolerance); 56 (12%) of these challenges could be reproduced. Excluding those reactions to fruit and fruit juices, only 37 (8%) of the 480 children had reproducible reactions to foods, usually milk, egg, soy, peanut, chocolate, corn, rice, and wheat. The prevalence

Table 8–1 Categories of Adverse Food Reactions

Term	*Definition*
Adverse food reaction (food sensitivity)	General term applied to any clinically abnormal response resulting from ingestion of food/food additive. Term of choice when underlying causative mechanism(s) is unknown.
Food hypersensitivity (food allergy)	Immunologic hypersensitivity reaction resulting from ingestion of food/food additive.
Food intolerance	General term applied to any abnormal physiologic response resulting from ingestion of food/food additive that is proven not to be immunologically mediated.
Food toxicity (poisoning)	Adverse effect resulting from direct action of food/food additive on host recipient. May involve nonimmune release of chemical mediators. Toxins may be contained in food or released into food by microorganisms present in food.
Food idiosyncrasy	Quantitatively abnormal response to food/food additive. Includes reactions occurring in specific groups of individuals who may be genetically predisposed. May resemble hypersensitivity reaction but does not involve immune mechanisms.
Metabolic food reaction	Result of food/food additive on metabolism of host recipient. Majority of reactions caused by ingestion of average amounts of usually safe food/food additives by individuals who are susceptible because of medications taken, concurrent disease states, malnutrition, inborn errors of metabolism, etc.
Pharmacologic food reaction	Result of naturally occurring or added chemicals that produce a druglike effect in host.

Source: Reprinted from *Adverse Reactions to Foods* (pp 4–6) by JA Anderson and DD Sogn (eds), American Academy of Allergy and Immunology Committee on Adverse Reactions to Foods and National Institutes of Allergies and Infectious Diseases, USDHHS Pub No 84-2442.

Exhibit 8–1 Immune Mechanisms Involved with Adverse Food Reactions

Type I: Immunoglobulin E (IgE), mast-cell-dependent reaction

Type II: Antibody-dependent cytotoxic response

Type III: Antigen-antibody complex

Type IV: Cell-mediated

Exhibit 8–2 Food Hypersensitivity Disorders

Gastrointestinal
- IgE-mediated
  - Oral allergy syndrome (oral and perioral pruritis and angioedema, throat tightness)
  - Gastrointestinal anaphylaxis (nausea, cramping, emesis, diarrhea)
  - Allergic eosinophilic gastroenteritis (subset)
  - Infantile colic (~15% of infants with colic)
- Non–IgE-mediated
  - Food-induced enterocolitis (1–3 hr postingestion: emesis, diarrhea, failure to thrive, and—rarely—hypotension)
  - Food-induced colitis (2–12 hr postingestion; blood in stools)
  - Allergic eosinophilic gastroenteritis (postprandial nausea, emesis, weight loss)
  - Food-induced malsbsorption syndrome ("celiac-like"; nausea, steatorrhea, weight loss)
  - Celiac disease

Cutaneous
- IgE-mediated
  - Acute (common) and chronic (rare) urticaria
  - Atopic dermatitis (pruritic morbilliform rash leading to eczematous lesion)
- Non–IgE-mediated
  - Dermatitis herpetiformis
  - Contact hypersensitivity
  - Contact irritation (especially with acid fruits and vegetables)

Respiratory
- IgE-mediated
  - Rhinoconjunctivitis
  - Laryngeal edema
  - Asthma (both acute wheezing and increased bronchial hyper-reactivity)
- Non–IgE-mediated
  - Heiner's syndrome (rare form of pulmonary hemosiderosis)

Other: Mechanism Unknown
- Migraine (rare)
- Irritability with other symptoms of hypersensitivity
- (?) Arthritis (rare subset)
- (?) Nephritis (rare subset with recurrent glomerulonephritis)

Source: Reprinted with permission from H.A. Sampson, Diagnosing Food Intolerances in Children, in *Current Therapy in Allergy, Immunology, and Rheumatology,* L. M. Lichtenstein and A.S. Fauci, eds., p. 141, © 1996, Mosby-Year Book, Inc.

of immediate food hypersensitivity reactions in the pediatric population is approximately 6–8% in children less than 4 years of age and 1–2% in older children and adults.[4] However, food allergy may be as high as 33% in some groups, such as children with atopic dermatitis.[5] The prevalence of adverse reactions to foods is unknown in the pediatric population.[6]

PATHOPHYSIOLOGY

Interactions between food allergens, the gastrointestinal tract, and the immune system in the

Exhibit 8–3 Differential Diagnosis for Adverse Food Reactions

I. Food additives
   A. Food colors: Azo dye F.D.&C. yellow no. 5 (tartrazine)
   B. Preservatives
      1. Sulfiting agents
      2. Nitrate/nitrite
      3. BHA/BHT
   C. Flavor enhancers: L-monosodium glutamate (MSG)
   D. Sweeteners: aspartame, sorbitol, sucrose
   E. Miscellaneous: antibiotics (penicillin)
II. Unintentional food contaminants
   A. Plant toxins
      1. Cyanogenic compounds: glycosides in fruit pits and cassava
      2. Oxalates: spinach
      3. Solanine alkaloids: potatoes
   B. Microbial toxins
      1. Bacterial
         a. *Staphylococcus aureus, Clostridium botulinum*, etc.
         b. Scromboid poisoning: tuna, mackerel
      2. Fungal (mycotoxins): aflatoxins, ergot
      3. Algal (dinoflagellates)
         a. Ciguatera poisoning: grouper, snapper, barracuda
         b. Saxitoxin: shellfish
   C. Food-borne infectious agents
      1. Bacterial: salmonellosis, *Campylobacter jejuni, Clostridium perfringens*, etc.
      2. Parasitic: *Giardia lambia, Trichinella spiralis*, flukes, etc.
      3. Viral: hepatitis
III. Naturally occurring pharmacologic agents
   A. Methylxanthines: caffeine, theobromine
   B. Biologically active amines: tyramine, phenylethylamine, serotonin, histamine
IV. Gastrointestinal diseases
   A. Structural abnormalities
      1. Gastroesophageal reflux
      2. Hiatal hernia
      3. Pyloric stenosis
      4. Intestinal obstruction
   B. Carbohydrate intolerance
      1. Congenital carbohydrate deficiency: lactase, sucrase, isomaltase, galactose-4-epimerase
      2. Acquired carbohydrate intolerance: lactase, sucrase, isomaltase
   C. Malignancy
   D. Other Conditions
      1. Gastroenteritis
      2. Gastric/duodenal ulcer disease
      3. Cholelithiasis
      4. Pancreatic insufficiency
      5. Irritable bowel syndrome
      6. Inflammatory bowel disease
      7. Mucosal damage secondary to drug therapy

continues

Exhibit 8–3 Continued

V. Other conditions
   A. Malnutrition
   B. Endocrine disorders: hypothyroidism, hyperthyroidism
   C. Eating disorders

Source: Adapted from V. Olejer, Food Hypersensitivities, in *Handbook of Pediatric Nutrition,* P.M. Queen and C.E. Lang, eds., © 1993, Aspen Publishers, Inc.

susceptible individual result in the development of food hypersensitivity. Eggs, milk, peanuts, soybeans, wheat, tree nuts, and fish account for approximately 90% of positive food challenges in children in the United States.[5,7] Any food can cause an allergic reaction. The major food allergens identified are water-soluble glycoproteins, largely heat resistant and acid stable.

Total parenteral nutrition (TPN) is widely used. There are case reports of adults who experienced adverse skin reactions[8,9] and an anaphylactic reaction[10] with TPN. The multivitamin preparation, polysorbate, and chlorhexidine gluconate or the catheter containing the bactericide were suggested as the cause of the reactions.

The gastrointestinal tract is confronted with the largest antigenic load confronting the human immune system. Ingested food is acted upon by stomach acid and pancreatic and intestinal enzymes. Proteins are broken down to small peptides and amino acids, selectively absorbed, and broken down into smaller peptides and nonantigenic fragments by the mucosal endothelial cell lysosomes. Secretory immunoglobulin A (IgA) is the predominant immunoglobulin in the gut lumen that forms complexes with the antigens, preventing their absorption. If antigenic proteins and peptides do cross the endothelial barrier, circulatory IgA may bind foreign protein, thus allowing access to the circulation and leading to its clearing in the bile.[11]

Food antigens are capable of penetrating the physiologic and immunologic barriers of the normal gastrointestinal tract.[12] "Gut-associated lymphoid tissue" and antigen-presenting cells in the reticuloendothelial system play a role in the development of oral tolerance to these proteins.[13] Factors known to affect the amount of antigen absorbed and possibly to alter the timing of symptoms are: the amount of antigen ingested, whether the antigen is consumed alone or with other foods, degree of cooking, the presence of gastrointestinal disturbances that may provide a more permeable mucosal wall, decreased gastric acidity, absence of digestive enzymes, and malnutrition.

The food-specific IgE-mediated response occurs when there is an alteration in the development of oral tolerance and there is production of food-specific IgE in a susceptible individual. After the food allergen crosses the mucosal barrier, it crosslinks with the food-specific IgE antibodies bound to previously exposed mast cells and basophils. This occurs at the end organ sites, such as the skin, respiratory tract, and gastrointestinal tract. The mast cells or basophils release mediators such as histamine, heparin, prostaglandins, and leukotrienes. These mediators will cause vasodilation, smooth muscle contraction, and mucous secretion, producing clinical symptoms of immediate hypersensitivity.[14] Next, the activated mast cells may release a variety of cytokines, which induce the IgE-mediated late-phase response. During the late-phase response (24–48 hours later), neutrophils, eosinophils, lymphocytes, and monocytes also move into the area, are activated, and release inflammatory mediators and cytokines. The lymphocytes and monocytes are thought to be responsible for the chronic inflammatory picture seen with repeated ingestion of a food allergen.[15]

CLINICAL MANIFESTATIONS

IgE-Mediated Food Hypersensitivities

Once foods are ingested, there may be immediate oral symptoms, such as itching and swelling of the lips, palate, tongue, or throat. In the gastrointestinal tract, nausea, cramping, gas, distention, vomiting, abdominal pain, or diarrhea may be experienced. Once the antigen spreads through the bloodstream and lymphatics, degranulation of mast cells may occur in the skin, causing urticaria, angioedema, pruritis, or an erythematous macular rash. Respiratory symptoms include coughing, wheezing, profuse nasal rhinorrhea, sneezing, or laryngeal edema. The eyes may experience edema, tearing, excess mucus, itching, or burning. The role of food hypersensitivity in such conditions as migraine headaches, epilepsy, rheumatoid arthritis, enuresis, or attention deficit hyperactivity disorder is less clear and remains controversial.[16]

Systemic anaphylaxis is an acute and potentially fatal reaction. Anaphylaxis can begin with any of the symptoms mentioned above, as well as with cardiovascular symptoms, including chest tightness, tachycardia, hypotension, and shock. A fatal reaction may begin with mild symptoms and progress to cardiorespiratory arrest and shock over 1–3 hours or may progress more rapidly. The most severe reactions are usually associated with the ingestion of peanuts, tree nuts, fish, and shellfish; whereas milk, egg, and soy are less likely to produce fatal reactions in children. Risk factors for fatal or near-fatal hypersensitivity reactions include children with asthma, adolescent patients, patients who do not receive epinephrine immediately after the reaction begins, extreme atopy, and patients who had a previous serious anaphylactic reaction.[17,18]

Exercise-induced anaphylaxis is associated with the ingestion of a specific food prior to exercise, then during or shortly after exercise, the individual experiences allergic symptoms that may progress to anaphylaxis.[19] This individual can usually ingest this food without any reaction and can exercise without any reaction, as long as the specific food has not been ingested within the past 8–12 hours. Patients with exercise-induced anaphylaxis usually have a positive prick skin test to foods that provoke symptoms. Management requires identifying the food through a challenge with exercise after food ingestion and avoiding the food prior to any expected exercise.

Oral Allergy Syndrome (OAS) is another form of IgE-mediated food allergy.[20] OAS is a complex of clinical symptoms localized to the oral mucosa and pharynx after direct oral contact with an allergic food. There is rapid onset of pruritus and mild angioedema of the lips, tongue, palate and throat, followed by a rapid resolution of symptoms. Fresh fruits and vegetables are most frequently involved in OAS. OAS occurs mainly in patients allergic to pollens. People allergic to birch tree pollen may have symptoms when they eat potatoes, carrots, celery, apples, and kiwi. Those allergic to ragweed may react when they eat watermelon, cantaloupe, honeydew, and bananas. Generally, cooked foods are less likely than raw foods to cause OAS symptoms. To diagnose the IgE-mediated mechanism, a skin prick test is recommended with the "prick + prick" technique, which involves pricking the fresh food first, then the patient's skin with the same lancet.[21] Most individuals are aware of what may happen when they eat a specific food, and because this is a minor reaction, they usually do not require a challenge to confirm OAS. It is important to distinguish the OAS from oropharyngeal symptoms that may precede systemic symptoms, including urticaria, gastrointestinal (GI) symptoms, rhinitis, and anaphylactic shock.

Food hypersensitivities are present in a third of children with atopic dermatitis.[22] The mechanism of this disease involving food hypersensitivity is thought to be a late-phase IgE response.[23,24] A history is not helpful in predicting which foods to suspect.[25] Children with atopic dermatitis who underwent an allergy evaluation, including skin prick test and blinded food challenges, experienced improvement of their disease after avoidance of the identified food.[26] Food hypersensitivity is one of several variables involved in this disease. Other factors play a role in the exacerbation of atopic dermatitis: aeroallergens, temperature extremes, stress, staphylococcal skin infections, and unknown factors.[27]

Infantile colic is a frustrating syndrome occurring in children less than 3 months of age. It is characterized by inconsolable crying, drawing up of the legs, abdominal distention, and excessive gas. A double-blinded, crossover study suggested that an IgE-mediated hypersensitivity to cow's milk whey protein may be a mechanism for about 10–15% of colicky infants.[28]

NON–IGE-MEDIATED FOOD HYPERSENSITIVITY

Food-induced enterocolitis, food-sensitive enteropathy, food-induced or allergic colitis, allergic eosinophilic gastroenteritis, and celiac disease (gluten-sensitive enteropathy) are immunologically mediated food hypersensitivity disorders but are not IgE-mediated.[29] Food-induced enterocolitis usually presents by 6 months of age. Symptoms appear 4–6 hours following ingestion of the food. Symptoms include projectile emesis, diarrhea, dehydration, and/or a "septic" appearance. Diagnosis is confirmed with a food challenge using 0.6 g protein/kg of the suspected food. Cow's milk and soy proteins are usually the offending foods.

Food-sensitive enteropathy is seen in those with an atopic background. The onset of symptoms mimics acute enteritis with transient emesis, anorexia, and protracted diarrhea. Diagnosis through biopsy reveals patchy, subtotal villus injury. The foods commonly associated with food-sensitive enteropathy are cow's milk, soy, chicken, egg, rice, and fish.

Food-induced colitis presents with rectal bleeding within the first few months of life in well-nourished infants. Biopsy of the large intestine reveals eosinophils in the lamina propria. Cow's milk and soy proteins are the usual offending foods.

Food-induced enterocolitis, food-sensitive enteropathy, and food-induced colitis tend to be outgrown by 12–24 months of age, and dietary elimination of the offending foods is the treatment. Eosinophilic gastroenteritis may affect any part of the intestinal tract. Dietary proteins do not appear to play a role in this disease at this time unless there is an IgE reaction upon testing. If a food allergy is diagnosed, elimination of the food is indicated. Otherwise, treatment is with corticosteroids. Celiac disease is an intolerance to gliadin, which is found in wheat, oats, rye, and barley. Diagnosis is made by obtaining a biopsy prior to starting dietary treatment and a follow-up biopsy showing mucosal recovery after a gluten-restricted, gliadin-free diet. Refer to Chapter 16 for more information on celiac disease.

DIAGNOSING FOOD HYPERSENSITIVITY

History

Evaluating a patient with a suspected adverse food reaction requires a thorough medical history and physical examination. Based on the information obtained, a diet diary and various laboratory studies may be helpful. If a food hypersensitivity is suspected, an elimination diet is followed, and food challenges are performed. Incomplete food hypersensitivity work-ups and unorthodox procedures can label one with erroneous food allergies, lead to an incorrect diagnosis, nutrient deficiencies (eg, calcium or vitamin D), and delay treatment for diseases.[30–33]

The medical history may be useful in diagnosing food allergy in acute events (eg, systemic anaphylaxis following the ingestion of peanuts). Historically reported adverse food reactions have been confirmed less than 50% of the time using double-blind placebo-controlled food challenge (DBPCFC).[34,35] The history may be helpful in distinguishing IgE-mediated type food reactions from other forms of adverse food reactions. The history should include:

1. the food suspected to have provoked the reaction

2. the quantity of the food ingested
3. the length of the time between ingestion and development of symptoms
4. a description of the symptoms provoked
5. similar symptoms developed on other occasions when the food was eaten
6. whether other factors (eg, exercise) are necessary
7. the length of time since the last reaction

If the reactions occur within minutes to hours of ingesting a specific food and the symptoms are consistent with those previously mentioned, one should suspect a food hypersensitivity. Adverse food reactions and disorders that mimic food allergic reactions are listed in Exhibit 8–3.

Gastrointestinal symptoms of food hypersensitivity are similar to many structural and enzymatic abnormalities in children. These must be carefully considered in all patients because many of these disorders can also be life-threatening.[36] Lactose intolerance produces symptoms similar to cow's milk allergy. Lactose intolerance is frequently seen after a bacterial or viral gastroenteritis. Toddler's diarrhea or chronic nonspecific diarrhea is aggravated by consumption of simple sugars, especially sorbitol, found in fruits (eg, apple and pear juice), some sugar-free candies, and chewing gums. Gastroenteric complaints can result from consuming legumes, cruciferous vegetables, and prunes.

Older infants and small children may consume pharmacologic amounts of methyl xanthines (eg, caffeine, theobromine) by drinking sodas and iced tea. The side effects are nervousness, excitability, tremor, tachycardia, insomnia, abdominal pain, diarrhea, and nausea.[36] An individual who rarely consumes caffeine is more sensitive than one who consumes caffeine regularly. Toxicity is seen with ≥ 78 mg of caffeine/kg,[37] the equivalent of 26 cans of caffeinated sodas or 5 stimulant pills or weight loss pills for a child that weighs 15 kg. Preservatives, dyes, and other chemicals found in foods are involved in some adverse reactions. Unintentional consumption of food contaminants (infectious organisms and toxins) will result in symptoms similar to an allergic reaction. Naturally occurring pharmacologic agents (eg, histamine, tyramine) may trigger symptoms in highly susceptible individuals.[38]

The physical exam evaluates atopic conditions, such as allergic rhinitis, eczema, and asthma. Anthropometrics, assessment of growth and development, and nutritional status should be performed (see Chapter 2). No specific features of the physical examination will suggest IgE-mediated food hypersensitivity. Abnormal physical findings and a patient's behavior may suggest a diagnosis other than adverse reactions to foods.

Skin Testing and In Vitro Assays

If an IgE-mediated food sensitivity is suspected, epicutaneous skin testing (ie, prick, puncture, scratch) with food extracts will help screen for the responsible food allergens.[34] Glycerated food extracts (1:10 or 1:20) and positive (histamine) and negative (saline) controls are applied by a prick or puncture technique.[39] After 15–20 minutes, the diameter of the wheal is measured. If the wheal (not including erythema) is at least 3 mm greater than the negative control, it is considered positive; anything else is considered negative. A positive skin test indicates the presence of specific IgE to that food. If a food is positive with a skin test, that individual may or may not be hypersensitive to that specific food because the positive predictive accuracy of a positive skin test is less than 50%. A positive skin test should be followed up with a food challenge. A negative skin test confirms the absence of an IgE-mediated reaction. The negative predictive value is greater than 95%. Intradermal skin tests are not recommended because of the increased risk of inducing a systemic reaction.[40]

There are a few exceptions to the above clinical findings to consider when interpreting the skin test results. A child less than 1 year of age may have an IgE-mediated food allergy without a positive skin test, and a child less than 2 years of age may have smaller wheals when tested by the skin prick method.[41] Use of in vitro methods, ie, radioallergosorbent test (RAST), would be indicated in this population. Patients may have positive skin tests long after they have outgrown the food allergy. As mentioned with OAS, IgE-mediated sensitivity to several fruits and vegetables is detected with fresh extracts, not commercial food extracts.[42] Another exception is when a skin test is positive to a food; if that food had been ingested in isolation causing a serious systemic anaphylactic reaction, this scenario may be considered diagnostic. A skin test is not indicated in patients with extensive skin disease, dermatographism, those who cannot be taken off antihistamines, or when exposure to minute amounts resulted in near fatal anaphylaxis. In vitro tests for specific IgE would be indicated in these patients.

RAST is the most commonly used of in vitro assays that detect and quantitate serum-specific IgE antibodies. The test involves placing serum on a solid-phase support, such as 96 well tissue culture plates, glass beads, or paper disk, that contains specific food proteins. The amount of bound IgE antibodies is calculated by adding labeled antihuman IgE antibodies. Like the skin prick test, the RAST has an excellent negative predictive value but a poor positive predictive value for hypersensitivity to foods.[43] RAST provides information similar to skin prick test and is used when a skin prick test is not indicated. This form of testing is more expensive than are skin tests, and results are available within a few days. A recent study with the CAP-RAST system, validated with DBPCFC, has shown that there are specific levels of IgE to several foods (milk, egg, peanuts, soy) that have excellent positive and negative predictive values.[44] Once validated, this system may allow patients with certain specific IgE levels to be considered positive and not require an oral food challenge to diagnose their food allergy. Basophil histamine release assays (BHR) are used in the research setting to determine if they can be used clinically, but the results are no more predictive of clinical sensitivity than are the skin prick test or RAST.[45]

Cross-reactivity occurs when an individual is allergic to more than one food in a plant family. Positive in vivo and in vitro tests for specific IgE suggest that there is a significant amount of cross-reactivity. Clinical reactivity to more than one member of an animal species or botanical family is rare. Several studies have shown that among legumes[46–48] and grains,[49] in vivo or in vitro tests cannot determine the clinical relevance of cross-reactivity between foods. It should be assumed that there is no cross-reactivity unless proven with a food challenge. Otherwise, the patient and family will be unnecessarily avoiding foods. The exception to this is with hypersensitivity to fish,[50,51] crustaceans, and OAS, as mentioned previously.

Diet Diary

A diet diary may be helpful in identifying a relationship between the foods ingested and the symptoms experienced. Families are asked to keep a timed and chronologic record of the amount of formula and/or food ingested for each meal or snack over a specified period of time. The families and other caregivers should record any prescription or over-the-counter medication, including vitamin and mineral supplements or herbal preparations, along with the duration and severity of any symptoms experienced during this time. This experience helps the family pay more attention to who is feeding the child and what the child is actually eating. The diet diary is more accurate and not dependent on a family's memory. The registered dietitian can evaluate the diet for nutritional adequacy. If a food intolerance is responsible for the symptoms, minor dietary changes may be needed, as opposed to elimination diets. Eating out, eating processed foods, and eating prepackaged meals may interfere with the usefulness of this tool.

Elimination Diets

Food elimination, followed by selected food challenges, is important to determine whether a food is responsible for the reported symptoms. The foods to be eliminated and tested by oral food challenge are based on patient history, food diary, skin prick test, and/or RAST results. If the mother is breastfeeding, she should remove the offending foods from her diet.[52] Multiple food allergies are rare, roughly 80–84% of children with positive food challenges react to only one or two antigens,[22,53] approximately 44–48% react to one antigen, and 34–36% react to two antigens. A diet eliminating one food allergen is not as difficult to plan as is the elimination of two or more allergens. The diet can become difficult if the food allergen involves a major food group. Diet education is essential for successful food elimination. The elimination diet used in diagnosing a food allergy may be the same as one needed in treatment of the diagnosed food hypersensitivity. Alternative foods to the foods eliminated should be provided to avoid malnutrition.[33,54,55]

Resolution of symptoms during the elimination phase suggests that the symptoms were triggered by one or more of the eliminated foods. A food challenge is recommended to confirm diagnosis. To diagnose the allergy or intolerance appropriately, the symptoms must be documented after oral ingestion of the suspected food. If improvement of symptoms is not detected within 2 weeks on the elimination diet, there are several possible explanations.

- a food sensitivity is not responsible for the symptoms
- there is poor dietary compliance
- an unrecognized offending food continues to be present in the diet
- other chronic conditions cause flair of symptoms (ie, asthma, atopic dermatitis).

A strict allergen elimination diet is needed in some cases but should be used with caution because it can lead to iatrogenic malnutrition. A strict allergen elimination diet should be followed for less than 6 weeks unless the necessity is confirmed by a DBPCFC. If there is no resolution of symptoms after following the most restrictive oral diet or an elemental diet, it is doubtful that an adverse food reaction is the cause. The following strict allergen elimination diet is recommended by Koerner and Sampson[7] (Each step builds on the previous step as the infant/child gets older.):

- Infants <4 months: casein hydrolysate infant formula (eg, Nutramigen, Alimentum) or amino acid formula (eg, Neocate)
- 4–8 months: infant diet + rice cereal (nonflavored) + pears
- 9–24 months: 4–8 months diet + rice + squash + lamb
- >24 months: 9–24 months diet + fresh lettuce + potato + safflower oil + tea + sugar, or amino acid formula (eg, Neocate One+)

For older children not drinking formula, an elimination diet using fortified rice milk, the foods mentioned above, and other foods may be permitted.[56] In addition, the fruit and fruit juice of apricots, cranberries, peaches, and apples are allowed. Beets, carrots, sweet potatoes, tapioca, white vinegar, olive oil, honey, cane sugar, and salt are also allowed. Through the experience at this center, Arkansas Children's Hospital, these foods are recommended because they are rarely associated with food hypersensitivity. The purpose of the strict allergen elimination diet is to provide a clean baseline. Then, food challenges would begin with the patient's favorite and nutrient dense foods.

If milk protein hypersensitivity is suspected in infants, the Nutrition Committee of the American Academy of Pediatrics[57] recommends a casein-hydrolysate based formula (Alimentum, Nutramigen, or Pregestimil) rather than a soy-based formula (see Table 8–2). Soy sensitivity is more likely to develop when introduced after a reaction to cow's milk protein or gastrointestinal infection. In children with intolerance to milk-based formula, 33–50% cannot tolerate soy formulas.[57] Rarely, infants and children may not tolerate a protein hydrolysate[58,59] and will require an amino acid-based formula (Neocate, Neocate One+, and

Table 8–2 Semi-elemental and elemental hypoallergenic formulas

	Formula					
	*Nutramigen**	*Pregestimil**	*Alimentum†*	*Neocate‡*	*Neocate One +‡*	*Elemental 028 Extra‡*
Energy (kcal/oz)	20	20	20	20	30	25.5
% PRO	11	11	11	12	10	8
% CHO	44	41	41	47	58	48
% FAT	45	50	48	41	32	44
PRO source	Hydrolyzed casein	Hydrolyzed casein	Hydrolyzed casein	Free amino acids	Free amino acids	L-amino acids
CHO source	Glucose polymers, modified corn starch	Glucose polymers, glucose, modified corn starch	Sucrose, tapioca starch	Corn syrup solids	Corn syrup solids	Dried glucose syrup
FAT source	Corn oil	MCT oil (55%), corn oil (20%), soy oil (12.5%), safflower oil (12.5%)	MCT oil (50%), safflower oil (40%), soy oil (10%)	MCT oil (5%), safflower oil (95%)	MCT oil (35%), canola oil (32.5%), safflower oil (32.5%)	MCT oil (35%), canola and safflower oil (65%)
Osmolality, mOsm/kg water	320	320	370	342	610 (powder) 835 (liquid)	502 (unflavored) 636 (flavored)

Note: MCT, medium-chain triglyceride; PRO, protein; CHO, carbohydrate.

Note: These formulas are made by companies that either dedicate their equipment or undergo vigorous cleaning and testing to ensure that there is no cross-contamination.

* Mead Johnson Nutritionals, Evansville, Indiana

† Ross Products Division, Columbus, Ohio

‡ Scientific Hospital Supplies, Gaithersburg, Maryland

for children older than 10 years of age, Elemental 028 Extra).

These formulas are considered expensive and unpalatable, which may be an obstacle in their use. The palatability of these formulas is improved when served chilled, covered and sipped through a straw, or flavored with a hypoallergenic flavor (eg, Vari-Flavors). Titrating the new formula—gradually replacing the old formula over a few weeks with the new formula—may also help with acceptability. The casein hydrolysates are available through the U.S. Department of Agriculture (USDA) Supplemental Food Program for Women, Infants, and Children (WIC) to those who meet the criteria: low-income families, those at nutritional risk, and those in need as substantiated by a physician. The amino acid-based formulas may also be available from WIC (check with local unit for availability) or from a home health agency. States vary in what Medicaid and WIC will provide, and these formulas may be covered. Insurance companies may reimburse for these formulas if a supportive physician is aggressive in communicating medical need for the use of these formulas.

Food Challenges

There are three types of food challenges: open, single-blinded, and double-blinded placebo-controlled. The DBPCFC is considered the "gold standard" for accurately diagnosing food allergies[60] and for examining a wide variety of food-related complaints.[5,61] Open or single-blinded food challenges are useful in the medical practice setting to determine whether symptoms can be reproduced when the food is ingested.

Open Food Challenge

An open, unblinded food challenge means the individual knows what food is consumed. If a patient has no change in symptoms as a result of following an elimination diet, an open challenge is helpful in reintroducing that food into a patient's diet. If a patient has a negative skin test, the history is doubtful, and the patient has been avoiding the food, an open challenge will convince the individual that the food is not responsible for the symptom. Challenges at home should never be performed if there is a remote chance of a severe reaction. If a serious or life-threatening reaction is not suspected, a specific diet can be followed for 2 weeks and new foods added every 2–3 days at home. Open challenges at home are commonly used with adults experiencing food intolerances but rarely with children.

Single-Blinded Food Challenge

In a single-blinded food challenge, the patient and parent do not know what food is being challenged. This procedure is more useful than the open food challenge because it eliminates the bias of the subject and family, and is easily performed in an office setting. The challenge would be performed under the same conditions as a DBPCFC (see following discussion) except the nurse, dietitian, or doctor performing the challenge would know which food is being challenged. The food in question, ie, milk powder (8–10 gm), would be placed in a liquid, like juice, and the placebo, ie, corn starch (8–10 gm), would also be mixed with an equal amount of the same liquid. Increasing doses of either the placebo or test food would be given to the patient every 15 minutes, depending upon expected symptoms, until the total amount is consumed. After 2 hours of observation, the other "juice" is given in the same step-wise fashion. The blinded patient is monitored during the challenge in the doctor's office. Any challenge should be supervised by personnel appropriately trained to recognize and manage any severe food reaction.[62] Multiple positive challenges should be confirmed by a DBPCFC.

Double-Blind, Placebo-Controlled Food Challenge

The DBPCFC has the patient, parent(s), and medical personnel performing the challenge while "blinded" to what substance is being administered—placebo versus food tested. The

DBPCFC is the most objective test and provides the most accurate information. For the DBPCFC or other food challenges to be accurate, suspected foods should be totally eliminated for 10–14 days (or up to 12 weeks in some gastrointestinal disorders) prior to the DBPCFC. The subject should be symptom free during the elimination diet. It might be assumed that once symptoms resolve and the skin tests are positive, a diagnosis could be made. However, less than 50% of histories will be confirmed by a DBPCFC. Certain medications (eg, antihistamines, beta agonist, theophyline, and cromolyn and tricyclic antidepressants) may inhibit food hypersensitivity reactions.[63] Avoidance of medication prior to food challenge may range from 12–96 hours.[64] Children with atopic dermatitis may require aggressive skin care prior to food challenges.

Note of Caution: *If there is a clear history of severe anaphylaxis following an isolated ingestion of a specific food and there is a positive skin test, this patient should* **not** *be challenged.*

Foods to be used in challenges can usually be found locally. Powdered milk, individually packed flours, and baby foods are found in regular and health food stores. Dried whole eggs can be found through bakery suppliers. Camping stores will have freeze-dried foods, including meats, fruits, and vegetables. A vehicle is a type of food or beverage that is used as a carrier of the allergen to be challenged and the placebo. The vehicle should mask the smell, flavor, and texture of the food to be tested. Vehicles to use in food challenges are fruit juices, elemental formulas (with or without flavor packets), baby fruits, hot cereals, and hamburger patties. Placebos can be dextrose, cornstarch, or another grain or baby food meat that is not under suspicion. Dried foods can be administered in colorless No.1 pharmacy capsules. Small children have a difficult time taking capsules containing the food to be challenged or the placebo.

The DBPCFC[56] is administered in the fasting state, starting with a dose not likely to cause symptoms (125–500 mg of dry powder food, 1/20 of the total amount to be consumed). The dose is doubled every 15–60 minutes, depending on the type of reaction that is suspected to occur. Clinical reactivity is generally ruled out once the patient has tolerated 10 g of the dried food or 60–100 g of the wet food blinded without symptoms. Following completion of the challenge, the individual should be observed for 2 hours for food allergic reactions and 4–8 hours for food intolerances. Anyone with suspected GI symptoms should be observed for 4–8 hours. If immediate onset of symptoms is suspected, the DBPCFC can be performed in a day. One series of challenges (active or placebo) is given over 1–2 hours in the morning. In the afternoon, a second series of challenges (opposite of earlier challenge) is performed. If the blinded challenge is negative, the food <u>must</u> be given openly in usual quantities under observation to rule out the rare false-negative challenge. If the open challenge is positive, it may be due to dehydration of the food altering the allergenic epitopes (ie, fish), psychologic factors, or the blinded challenge may not have provided a dose sufficient to cause symptoms. Overall, this method works well except for the delayed- or late-onset reactions. Delayed- or late-onset reactions are either non-IgE food reaction disorders, as mentioned in Exhibit 8–2, or food intolerances listed in Exhibit 8–3. Metcalfe, Sampson, and Simon[16] provide detailed information regarding the diagnosis of these disorders.

Correctly diagnosing a food hypersensitivity can be a long, tedious process. Controversial diagnostic techniques that are not found to be effective in the diagnosing of food allergies are abundant. These include cytotoxic testing, sublingual or subcutaneous provocative challenge, ELISA/ACT, IgG4 antibody food test, lymphocyte activation, food antigen–antibody complexes, and electrodiagnostic devices.

In summary, the medical history identifies possible food hypersensitivity reactions. If IgE-mediated food hypersensitivity is suspected, perform a skin prick test and/or RAST, if indicated. If negative, either stop or consider other possible non-IgE immunologic disorders (Exhibits 8–2, 8–3). If the tests are positive and there is a convincing history of anaphylaxis, restrict the food(s) and stop the work-up. Otherwise, place the child on an elimination diet for the suspected food allergens. If there is improvement, begin the food challenge process. Rarely, an individual is allergic to more than one or two foods. If single-blinded challenges are used and multiple food allergies are identified, a DBPCFC will be needed to clarify the situation. If food protein-induced enteropathy is suspected, do not challenge the patient. If a non-IgE mediated reaction (food intolerance) is suspected, eliminate the suspected offending food from the diet. If symptoms persist, add the foods back and look for other causes. If symptoms improve, add the food(s) back to the diet through open or single-blinded challenges.

THERAPY

Elimination Diets

Once a diagnosis has been made, strict avoidance of the offending allergen(s) is the only proven therapy for food hypersensitivities. Education is the cornerstone for good compliance and a nutritionally adequate diet. This requires extensive education for the patient and family regarding the forms of the food to be avoided, how to read food labels, where the food may be hidden,[65] and alternative food sources for the nutrients that may be eliminated. Trace residues of allergens are potentially fatal to the extremely hypersensitive individual. Symptoms can be produced by inhalation of airborne particles (eg, peanuts) or by kissing the lips of a person who is eating the offending food. Accidental ingestions do occur, and the family must be educated on how to manage an allergic reaction. Some food hypersensitivities can be outgrown.[66] Follow-up with this population involves repeated food challenges to determine whether a child is still hypersensitive to a food and to prevent unnecessary food avoidance.

Milk, egg, peanut, soybean, and wheat are the primary foods responsible for hypersensitivity reactions in children, whereas fish, shellfish, tree nuts, and peanuts are the main culprits of food hypersensitivities in adults.[5,67] If a child is allergic to a single food (eg, peanuts or fish) the nutritional adequacy of the diet may not be compromised. However, the elimination of milk, eggs, soybeans, or wheat can have a major impact on the quality of a diet. These are found in our food supply in many forms, making complete elimination a challenge. If an individual is allergic to more than one food, he or she is at risk of a deficient diet, leading to malnutrition and growth problems.[29,32,65,68] A nutritional assessment (see Chapter 2), including a 3- or 7-day diet record, should be performed twice a year to identify and correct problems.

Labels

Label reading is critical to successfully avoiding a food allergen. The patient and family should read the label every time they shop because ingredients change without warning. One brand may be allergen free but another brand of the same food may not. Patients and families may be deceived by labels. For example, egg substitutes contain egg white, and nondairy creamers contain caseinates. This is why the patient and family need a good command of the terms used by the food industry to detect the presence of a specific food allergen.

Specific ingredients on food labels identify foods that contain a particular food allergen. Exhibit 8–4 contains terms used on labels that indicate the presence of food allergens for milk, egg, soybean, wheat, and peanuts. There are diet manuals and books[7,69,70] available that also have appropriate information regarding the scientific and technical names for foods. Patients and families should look for these terms when reading food labels and should avoid those foods. The diets provide lists of foods to avoid and foods that are safe. The Food Allergy Network (Fairfax, VA) is another valuable resource that provides booklets on guidelines for food allergies and how to work with the schools, as well as cookbooks, newsletters, and wallet-size cards that contain the terms used on labels for the com-

Exhibit 8–4 Label Ingredients that Indicate the Presence of Food Allergens

Milk

artificial butter flavor
butter
casein (rennet casein)
caseinate
calcium caseinate
potassium caseinate
sodium caseinate
cream
cheese
cottage cheese
milk solids (dry)
milk protein
sour cream
whey
yogurt
ghee
lactoalbumin
lactoglobulin
lactose
lactulose
nougat

Label ingredients that MAY indicate the presence of milk protein:

chocolate
flavorings (caramel or natural)
Simplesse
high-protein flour
margarine

Egg

albumin
egg substitutes
livetin
meringue
ovoglobulin
ovomucoid
Simplesse
egg—including white, yolk, dried, powdered, solids
globulin
mayonnaise
ovalbumin
ovomucin
ovovitellin
vitellin

Soybean

miso
shoyo sauce
soy flour, soy grits, soy milk, soy nuts, soy sprouts
soy protein concentrate, soy protein isolate, hydrolyzed soy protein
soy sauce
textured vegetable protein (TVP)
tempeh
tofu (soybean curd)

Label ingredients that MAY indicate the presence of soy protein:

flavorings
hydrolyzed plant protein
vegetable broth, vegetable gum, vegetable starch
hydrolyzed vegetable protein
natural flavoring

continues

Exhibit 8–4 continued

Wheat

bran	bread crumbs	bulgur
cereal extract	couscous	cracker meal
durum flour	enriched flour	farina
gluten	graham flour	high-gluten flour
high protein flour	kamut	spelt
semolina	soft wheat flour	
vital gluten	wheat (bran, germ, gluten, malt, starch)	
whole-wheat berries	whole-wheat flour	

Label ingredients that MAY indicate the presence of wheat protein:

gelatinized starch hydrolyzed	vegetable protein	triticale
modified food starch	modified starch	natural flavoring
soy sauce	starch	vegetable gum or starch

Peanuts

cold pressed, expressed, or expelled peanut oil

mixed nuts	peanut
Nu-Nuts flavored nuts	peanut flour
ground nuts	peanut butter

Label ingredients and foods that MAY indicate the presence of peanut protein:

African, Chinese, and Thai dishes	hydrolyzed plant protein
baked goods (pastries, cookies, etc.)	hydrolyzed vegetable protein
candy	marzipan
chili	nougat
chocolate (candy, candy bars)	egg rolls

Source: Adapted with permission from *How to Read A Label Cards,* © 1990–1995, The Food Allergy Network.

mon individual food allergens. Additional resources for the professional and for families are listed at the end of the chapter.

There are obscure terms on food labels that suggest the presence of a food allergen. Modified food starch, modified starch, vegetable starch, or food starch can be from either corn, tapioca, wheat, soy, potato, or rice. Vegetable gums may be from corn, wheat, soy, or guar. Hydrolyzed plant or vegetable protein may indicate the presence of wheat or soy protein. Caramel is usually from browned sugar but can be made with corn syrup or can contain milk protein. Contacting the individual food companies is the only way to clarify whether a food is safe. If there is any doubt about a food or if the food has no ingredient list, it is best to avoid that food.

The kosher rules and markings may be helpful for those with a milk allergy. The kosher dietary laws prohibit eating dairy products together with meat or fowl. If the word *Parve* or *Pareve* or Rabbinical agency symbols (such as a "K" in a star or triangle or a "U" in a circle) are on the label, the product is identified by a Rabbinical agency as one that does not contain dairy products. Examples of this can be found on the label of La Choy Rice Noodles and Contadina Whole Tomatoes. The food can be considered Pareve and contain very small amounts of milk—always read the ingredient list. A "D" next to a Rabbinical agency symbol indicates that the product contains milk or dairy products that may not be listed in the ingredient statement. Famous Amos Low Fat Iced Gingersnaps have a "U" in a circle with a "D" next to it on the label, and at the bottom of the ingredients list there is a statement "may contain whey, peanuts and tree nuts." If "D.E." (dairy equipment) is on the package, the food has been produced on equipment that was also used to manufacture dairy-containing foods. These foods are not safe for those with milk hypersensitivity.

CROSS-CONTAMINATION

Another major source of hidden allergens is cross-contamination. Packaged and processed foods are at risk because equipment for related products is shared. Failure to clean the equipment satisfactorily between processing of different products can leave allergenic food residues. This may occur with any food, eg, egg-containing and egg-free pastas; breakfast cereals and rice cakes with or without nuts; and juices in final concentration, ready to serve, packaged in quart or half gallon plastic bottles processed in dairy plants. Industry utilizes leftovers by adding what is left over to the next batch; this is called *rework*. For example, ingredients such as nuts may be filtered out of the rework, but the rework contains nut residues and is added to a new batch of nut-free ice cream. Some manufacturers are adding "may contain…" to the label because of potential cross-contamination. Other mistakes are packaging a different, yet similar food in the wrong package, or a formulation error. Consumer advocacy groups such as the Food Allergy Network alert manufacturers of the deadly consequences of these errors and urge them to identify and correct these mistakes.

At the grocery store, cross-contamination can occur in the deli, where meats and cheese are sliced on the same equipment, pastries are side by side, and bulk foods are accidentally mixed. The food service industry has practices that lead to cross-contamination. Cooking utensils, serving utensils, and containers may be shared. Frying oils are used for all deep-fat fried foods (eg, potatoes, fish, foods dipped in egg or milk and battered). The same grill can be used to grill seafood and steaks. Creative or ethnic recipes may contain unexpected ingredients (eg, tree nuts and peanuts).

MILK HYPERSENSITIVITY

If milk is eliminated from the diet, it should be replaced with a soy-based, casein-hydrolysate based, or amino acid-based formula. Caution should be used with a soy-based formula during the first year of life because 33–50% of children with intolerance to milk-based formula do not tolerate soy formulas.[56] Goat's milk is not an alternative to cow's milk because of the potential cross-reactivity with the beta-lactoglobulins in cow's milk,[71] and, if unfortified, it is deficient in folic acid. The vitamin- and mineral-fortified infant casein hydrolysate formulas will provide the calcium, phosphorus, vitamin D, vitamin B_{12}, riboflavin, and pantothenic acid that would be provided by the milk products. Keep infants and children on milk-free formulas as long as they will drink the formula. If the child refuses a formula, fortified soy and fortified rice milk beverages are an acceptable alternative. Some fruit juices are now fortified with calcium but not vitamin D. Calcium and vitamin D supplements may be needed if intake is inadequate. Whole grains, legumes, and nuts can provide alternative sources of other nutrients like phosphorus, riboflavin, and pantothenic acid that are found in milk.

EGG HYPERSENSITIVITY

Nutrients in eggs are easily replaced by other high-protein foods and whole grains. However, eggs are incorporated into breads, pastas, baking mixes, breaded or processed meats, custards, fat substitutes, salad dressings, and sauces. It is the elimination of all of these other foods containing egg that cause problems in providing a nutritionally balanced diet. Families can be taught how to modify recipes at home, providing substitutes for the binding and leavening properties of eggs. Not all egg substitutes are alike. Egg whites are commonly used in most egg substitutes, eg, Egg Beaters has an egg free powder, Egg Replacer. To substitute for eggs in a recipe, substitute one of the following for each egg:[7,69]

- 1 tsp of baking powder + 1 tbsp of water + 1 tbsp of vinegar (add vinegar separately at end)
- 1 tsp of baking soda + 1 tbsp of oil + 2 tbsp of baking powder + 1 tbsp of vinegar (add vinegar separately at end)
- 1 tsp of yeast dissolved in 1/4 cup of warm water
- 1/2 tbsp of water + 1 1/2 tbsp of oil + 1 tsp of baking powder
- 1 tbsp of apricot puree (binder)
- 1 packet of plain gelatin mixed with 1 cup of boiling water. Substitute 3 tbsp of this liquid for each egg. Refrigerate remainder for 1 week, microwave to liquefy (binder).

SOYBEAN HYPERSENSITIVITY

Soybean flour and soybean protein are major ingredients used by the food manufacturers. Soy can be found in processed grains (crackers, cereals, baked goods), processed meats, frozen dinners, sauces, and soups. Soybean oil and soy lecithin are considered safe for soy-allergic individuals because the processing of the oil removes the protein portion. A study using seven soy-allergic individuals who underwent blind food challenges with soy oil found no reactions to the soy oil.[72] Soybeans are legumes, as are peanuts, but being allergic to more than one legume is rare. Peanuts should not be avoided just because of a hypersensitivity to soybeans.

WHEAT HYPERSENSITIVITY

Wheat and wheat products are the foundation of our diets, and they are difficult to eliminate from the diet. They are found in baked products, pastas, cereals, snacks, sauces, soups, and breaded and processed meats. Products made with amaranth, arrowroot, barley, buckwheat, corn, oats, potato, quinoa, rice, rye, or soybean and tapioca flours are suitable wheat alternatives. Specialty food products for individuals with celiac disease (gluten-sensitive enteropathy) are appropriate for those with wheat allergy. These foods and grains can be found in grocery stores, health food stores, and mail-order companies. Wheat flours are fortified in niacin, riboflavin, thiamin, and iron. A child's diet composed of very few grain products may be deficient in these nutrients. Children with a wheat allergy should have their intake evaluated to ensure adequate intake of these and other nutrients.

FISH HYPERSENSITIVITY

An individual may be hypersensitive to one fish and tolerate others[49] but in the marketplace, substituting one fish for another is a common occurrence and one that is dangerous for the fish-allergic individual. It may be prudent for those with a fish allergy to avoid all species of fish. Cross-contamination occurs in restaurants because of shared equipment. Those who are allergic to fish but who can eat shellfish should be aware of Surimi, an imitation shellfish made with fish. Common foods that contain fish are Caesar salad dressing, Worcestershire sauce, and caviar. Nutrients in fish such as vitamin B_6, vitamin B_{12}, vitamin E, niacin, phosphorus, and selenium are also found in meats, grains, and oils.

PEANUT HYPERSENSITIVITY

Peanuts are a legume. Being allergic to peanuts does not automatically make one allergic to other legumes (peas, beans, green beans, and lentils) or tree nuts (pecans, almonds, and walnuts). Peanuts are found in pastries, candies, fruit nut breads, salads, and some ethnic foods (eg, African, Chinese, and Thai). Peanut oil is considered safe for those with peanut allergies.[73] However, peanut oil that has been cold-pressed, expressed, or expelled is not safe for peanut-allergic individuals. Nutrients found in peanuts, such as vitamin E, niacin, magnesium, manganese, and chromium, can also be found in legumes, whole grains, meats, and vegetable oils.

OTHER PRINCIPLES OF MANAGEMENT AND TREATMENT

The Registered Dietitian can play a critical role in working with children with food allergies and their families. Schools need aggressive education for those working with children with peanut and other food allergies. Contact with peanut butter and jelly sandwiches or projects using peanut butter (eg, as part of a bird feeder) can trigger a severe allergic reaction. Thanks to Public Law 93-112, The Rehabilitation Act of 1973, section 504, and the U.S. Department of Agriculture's 7 CFR 15b, schools are required to modify their health services, which include providing menu information, providing substitutions for the foods to be omitted (identified by physician's signed statement), and administering medications at school.[17] The Food Allergy Network[74] has developed a program to assist in managing food allergies at school.

Children and families need continual support as problems arise due to the food elimination diets. The 3- or 7-day diet records can direct suggestions for alternative food sources and recipes that may be needed. If whole foods cannot provide adequate nutrition, a vitamin or mineral supplement can be recommended. Positive behavior modification methods can help families avoid food struggles[75,76] (see Tables 5–5 and 5–6). It may be difficult to determine whether poor growth seen in this population is due to inadequate intake and/or feeding behavior problems.[32,68]

ACCIDENTAL INGESTION

Accidental ingestions do occur, and the patient, family members, and caregivers should be educated regarding signs and symptoms of anaphylaxis and appropriate treatment. Most accidental ingestions that lead to severe systemic anaphylaxis occur when foods are eaten away from home and disguised (eg, sandwiches at a restaurant or hors d'oeuvres at a party). If the allergic reaction is mild (eg, only urticaria or rhinitis) the treatment may be an antihistamine. Antihistamines are never a substitute for epinephrine. Individuals with moderate to severe food hypersensitivities must be taught how to self-inject epinephrine once an allergic reaction is recognized. Epinephrine is available for emergency use in premeasured doses, available by prescription [eg, EpiPen Jr./EpiPen (Center Laboratories, Port Washington, NY) and Ana-Kit/Ana-Guard (Miles Inc., Allergy Products, West Haven, CT)]. Because accidental ingestions commonly occur away from the home, it should be stressed to carry emergency medicine at all times. These devices provide valuable time for transport to the hospital emergency room for observation. No one can predict how a reaction will progress. If epinephrine is given within an hour of exposure of the allergen, it can make the difference between death and near death during a systemic anaphylactic reaction.[77] Emergency medical identification systems (MedicAlert, Turlock, California) may also be indicated.

Preventive therapies using drugs such as antihistamines, corticosteroids, ketotifin, and oral cromolyn sodium may modify symptoms but have minimal efficacy.[15] At this time, the only proven treatment is strict elimination of the offending allergen. Rotation diets (where the offending food is eliminated and rotated back into the diet every few days) are not recommended for children. Strict elimination is needed to outgrow some food allergies, and a rotation diet will keep the individual sensitized, prolonging this process. The effectiveness of subcutaneous neutralization, provocation, or oral desensitization has not been demonstrated. Herbal remedies and nutrition supplements are geared toward boosting the immune system or treating chronic symptoms. Herbal remedies and nutrition supplements do not affect the outcome of a food hypersensitive reaction upon ingestion of the allergen. Atopic individuals should be warned of rare but potential adverse reactions after ingesting some nutrition supplements. Supplements that have been documented through case reports to cause anaphylaxis are bee pollen,[78–80] royal jelly,[81,82] and echinacea.[83] Immunotherapy is a common treatment for environmental allergies but has not been effective with foods. Immunotherapy[84,85] methods are under investigation and may help prevent serious food allergic reactions in the future. Research efforts are directed at identifying the molecular and immunologic mechanisms involved in food allergen-receptor recognition and the cascade of events that leads to an allergic reaction.[86–88] It is hoped this research will provide the foundation for new forms of therapy.

NATURAL HISTORY AND PREVENTION

The general understanding is that most younger children outgrow their food hypersensitivity. Prospective studies evaluating adverse reactions to foods in children demonstrated that 85% of confirmed symptoms were absent by 3 years of age.[3,89] If the correct food allergen is identified and completely eliminated from the diet, approximately one-third of older children[66,90,91] can outgrow their food hypersensitivity within 1–2 years. However, children with peanut, tree nut, fish, or shellfish hypersensitivity will rarely lose their clinical reactivity. Therefore, the allergen responsible for the sensitivity and the compliance with the allergen elimination diet will affect whether one will outgrow the allergic response.[90] Infants with non–IgE-mediated food hypersensitivities also appear to outgrow their food reactivity.[92] Celiac disease is the exception, where gliaden must be avoided for life.

The first step of prevention is to be able to identify those newborn infants who are at high risk. Kjellman[93] found in his population of atopic children that a family history of atopic disease increases the risk of food hypersensitivity during the first 6 years of life. Thirteen percent of young children with no parental history of atopic disease have demonstrated a history of food hypersensitivity, compared with 29% with those with one parent being atopic and 58% of children with both parents having a history of atopic disease.

Delaying exposure to potentially allergenic foods is the primary strategy for preventing or delaying food allergies. What a pregnant woman eats has little to no effect on her child's risk of developing food hypersensitivities.[96] Exposure after birth can affect when and what hypersensitivities develop. Breastfeeding for at least 6 months is recommended. Breastfeeding provides a protective effect through earlier maturation of the gut barrier, contains secretory IgA and immune cells, reduces infections, and reduces exposure to foreign proteins. By excluding the common allergenic foods (milk, egg, and peanuts) from a nursing mother's diet, this benefit is enhanced. If a formula is needed for a high-risk infant, protein hydrolysate formulas (Nutramigen, Alimentum) should be used instead of milk- or soy-based formulas.

Introduction of solid foods should be delayed until 6 months of age. New foods should be introduced one at a time weekly or biweekly. Milk, wheat, corn, citrus, and soy can be added slowly after 1 year of age. Eggs and tree nuts may be added after 2 years of age. Peanuts, fish, and shellfish may be added after 3 years of age. By postponing the introduction of food allergens, the development of food hypersensitivity is delayed in high-risk infants but this does not prevent the disorder.[95]

REFERENCES

1. Anderson JA, Song DD, eds. Adverse reactions to foods. *Am Acad Allergy Immunol*/NIAID: NIH Publ No. 84-2442;1984:1–6.

2. Schwartz RH. Allergy, intolerance, and other adverse reactions to foods. *Pediatr Ann.* 1992;21:654–674.
3. Bock SA. Prospective appraisal of complaints of adverse reactions to foods in children during the first 3 years of life. *Pediatrics.* 1987;79:683–688.
4. Sampson HA. Immediate reactions to foods in infants and children. In: Metcalfe DD, Sampson HA, Simon RA, eds. *Food Allergy: Adverse Reactions to Foods and Food Additives.* 2nd ed. Cambridge, MA: Blackwell Scientific Publications; 1997:169–182.
5. Burks AW, Mallory SB, Williams LW, Shirrell MA. Atopic dermatitis: Clinical relevance of food hypersensitivity reactions. *Pediatrics.* 1988;113:447–451.
6. Young E, Stoneham MD, Petruckevitch A, Barton J, et al. A population study of food intolerance. *Lancet.* 1994;343:1127–1130.
7. Koerner CB, Sampson HA. Diets and nutrition. In: Metcalfe DD, Sampson HA, Simon RA, eds. *Food Allergy: Adverse Reactions to Foods and Food Additives.* 2nd ed. Cambridge, MA: Blackwell Scientific Publications; 1997:461–483.
8. Levy M, Dupuis LL. Parenteral nutrition hypersensitivity. *JPEN.* 1990;14:213–215.
9. Nagata MJ. Hypersensitivity reactions associated with parenteral nutrition: case report with review of the literature. *Annals Pharmacotherapy.* 1993;27:174–177.
10. Nikaido S, Tanaka M, Yamoto M, et al. Anaphylactoid shock caused by chlorhexidine gluconate. *Japanese J Anesthesiology.* 1998;47:330–334.
11. Kleinman RE, Walker WA. Antigen processing and uptake from the intestinal tract. *Clin Rev Allergy.* 1984;2:25–37.
12. Gray I, Walzen M. Studies in absorption of undigested proteins in human beings. VIII. Absorption from the rectum and a comparative study of absorption following oral, duodenal, and rectal administrations. *J Allergy.* 1940;11:245–250.
13. Mowat AM. The regulation of immune responses to dietary protein antigens. *Immunol Today.* 1987;8:93–98.
14. Lemanske RF, Kalinger MA. Late-phase allergic reactions. In: Middleton E, Reed CE, Ellis EF, et al, eds. *Allergy: Principles and Practices.* 3rd ed. St. Louis, MO: CV Mosby;1988:12–30.
15. Sampson HA, Metcalfe DD. Food allergies. *JAMA.* 1992;268:2840–2844.
16. Metcalfe DD, Sampson HA, Simon RA, eds. *Food Allergy: Adverse Reactions to Foods and Food Additives.* 2nd ed. Cambridge, MA: Blackwell Scientific Publications; 1997.
17. Sampson HA, Mendelson L, Rosen JP. Fatal and near-fatal anaphylactic reactions to foods in children and adolescents. *N Engl J Med.* 1992;327:380–384.
18. Smith KJ, Munoz-Furlong A. The management of food allergy. In: Metcalfe DD, Sampson HA, Simon RA, eds. *Food Allergy: Adverse Reactions to Foods and Food Additives.* 2nd ed. Cambridge, MA: Blackwell Scientific Publications; 1997:431–444.
19. Tilles S, Schocket A, Milgrom H. Exercise-induced anaphylaxis related to specific foods. *J Pediatr.* 1995; 127:587–589.
20. Pasterello EA, Incorvaia C, Ortolani C. Mouth and pharynx. *Allergy.* 1995;50:41–44.
21. Dreborg S, Foucard T. Allergy to apple, carrot, and potato in children with birch pollen allergy. *Allergy.* 1983; 36:167–170.
22. Burks AW, James JM, Hiegel A, et al. Atopic dermatitis and food hypersensitivity reactions. *J Pediatr* 1998;132: 132–136.
23. Hannuksela M, Lahti A. Peroral challenge test with food additives in urticaria and atopic dermatitis. *Int J Dermatol.* 1986;25:178–180.
24. Neild VS, Marsden RA, Bailes JA, et al. Egg and milk exclusion diets in atopic eczema. *Br J Dermatol.* 1986; 114:117–123.
25. Sampson HA, Albergo R. Comparison of results of skin test, RAST and double-blind, placebo-controlled food challenge in children with atopic dermatitis. *J Allergy Clin Immunol.* 1984;74:26–33.
26. Sampson HA. The immunopathogenic role of food hypersensitivity in atopic dermatitis. *Acta Derm Venereol.* 1992;176:34–37.
27. Leung DYM. Role of IgE in atopic dermatitis. *Curr Opin Immunol.* 1993;5:956–962.
28. Lothe L, Lindberg T. Cow's milk whey protein elicits symptoms of infantile colic in colicky formula-fed infants: a double-blind cross over study. *Pediatrics.* 1989: 83:262–266.
29. James JM, Burks AW. Food-associated gastrointestinal disease. *Curr Opin Pediatr.* 1996;8:471–475.
30. Lloyd-Still JD. Chronic diarrhea of childhood and the misuse of elimination diets. *J Pediatr.* 1979;95:10–13.
31. Libib M, Gama R, Wright J, et al. Dietary maladvice as a cause of hypothyroidism and short stature. *Br Med J.* 1989;298:232–233.
32. Robertson DAF, Ayres RCS, Smith CL, Wright R. Adverse consequences arising from misdiagnosis of food allergy. *Br Med J.* 1988;297:719–720.
33. Roesler TA, Barry PC, Bock SA. Factitious food allergy and failure to thrive. *Arch Pediatr Adolesc Med.* 1994;148:1150–1155.
34. Bock SA, Lee WY, Remigio LK, et al. Studies of hypersensitivity reactions to foods in infants and children. *J Allergy Clin Immunol.* 1978;62:327–334.
35. Sampson HA. Role of immediate food hypersensitivity in the pathogenesis of atopic dermatitis. *J Allergy Clin Immunol.* 1983;71:473–480.

36. Sampson HA. Differential diagnosis in adverse reactions to foods. *J Allergy Clin Immunol.* 1986;78: 212–219.
37. Chandra RK, Gill B, Kumari S. Food Allergy and atopic disease. *Clin Rev Allergy Immunol.* 1995;13:293–314.
38. Bock SA, Lee WY, Remigio LK, et al. Studies of hypersensitivity reactions to foods in infant and children. *J Allergy Clin Immunol.* 1978;62:327–334.
39. Bock SA, Buckley J, Houst A, May CD. Proper use of skin test with food extracts in diagnosis of food hypersensitivity. *Clin Allergy.* 1978;8:559–564.
40. Menurdo JL, Bousquet J, Rodiere M, et al. Skin test reactivity in infancy. *J Allergy Clin Immunol.* 1985;74: 646–651.
41. Ortoloni C, Ispano M, Partorella EA, et al. Comparison of results of skin prick test (with fresh foods and commercial food extracts) and RAST in 100 patients with oral allergy syndrome. *J Allergy Clin Immunol.* 1989;83:683–689.
42. Sampson HA, Albergo R. Comparison of results of skin test, RAST, and double-blind, placebo-controlled food challenges in children with atopic dermatitis. *J Allergy Clin Immunol.* 1984;74:26–33.
43. Sampson HA, Ho DG. Relationship between food-specific IgE concentrations and the risk of positive food challenges in children and adolescents. *J Allergy Clin Immunol.* 1997;100:444–457.
44. Sampson HA. In vitro diagnosis and mediator assays for food allergies. *Allergy Proc.* 1993;14:259–261.
45. Bock SA, Atkins FM. The natural history of peanut allergy. *J Allergy Clin Immunol.* 1989;83:900–904.
46. Bernhisel-Broadbent J, Sampson HA. Cross-allergenicity in the legume botanical family in children with food hypersensitivity. *J Allergy Clin Immunol.* 1989;83:435–440.
47. Bernhisel-Broadbent J, Taylor SL, Sampson HA. Cross-allergenicity in the legume botanical family in children with food hypersensitivity II. Laboratory correlates. *J Allergy Clin Immunol.* 1989;84:701–709.
48. Jones SM, Magnolfi CF, Cook SK, et al. Immunologic cross-reactivity among cereal grains and grasses in children with food hypersensitivity. *J Allergy Clin Immunol.* 1995;96:341–351.
49. Bernhisel-Broadbent J, Scanlon SM, Sampson HA. Fish hypersensitivity. I. In vitro and oral challenge results in fish allergic patients. *J Allergy Clin Immunol.* 1992;89:730–737.
50. Bernhisel-Broadbent J, Strause D, Sampson HA. Fish hypersensitivity. II. Clinical relevance of altered fish allergenicity caused by various preparation methods. *J Allergy Clin Immunol.* 1992:90:622–629.
51. deBoissieu D, Matarazzo P, Rocchiccioli F. Multiple food allergy: a possible diagnosis in breastfed infants. *Acta Paediatr.* 1997;86:1042–1046.
52. Sampson HA, McCaskill CM. Food hypersensitivity and atopic dermatitis: Evaluation of 113 patients. *J Pediatr.* 1985;107:669–675.
53. Bierman CW, Shapiro GC, Christie DL, et al. Eczema, rickets, and food allergy. *J Allergy Clin Immunol.* 1978;61:119–127.
54. Barratt JA, Summers GD. Scurvy, osteoporosis and megaloblastic anemia due to alleged food intolerance. *BrJ Rheumatol.* 1996;35:701–702.
55. Bock SA, Sampson HA, Atkins FM, et al. Double-blind, placebo-controlled food challenge (DBPCFC) as an office procedure: A manual. *J Allergy Clin Immunol.* 1988;82:986–997.
56. American Academy of Pediatrics Committee on Nutrition. Soy-based formula: Recommendations for use in infant feedings. *Pediatrics.* 1983;72:359.
57. Saylor JD, Bahna SL. Anaphylaxix to casein hydrolysate formula. *J Pediatr.* 1991;118:71–74.
58. deBoissieu D, Matorazzo P, Dupont C. Allergy to extensively hydrolyzed cow milk proteins in infants: Identification and treatment with an amino acid-based formula. *J Pediatr.* 1997;131:744–747.
59. Sampson H. Immunologically mediated food allergy: importance of food challenge procedures. *Ann Allergy.* 1988;60:262–269.
60. Bernstein M, Day JH, Welsh A. Double-blind food challenge in the diagnosis of food sensitivity in the adult. *J Allergy Clin Immunol.* 1982;70:205–210.
61. Executive Committee of the Academy of Allergy and Reactions Caused by Immunotherapy with Allergic Extracts (position statement). *J Allergy Clin Immunol.* 1986;77:271–273.
62. Bock SA. In vivo diagnosis: Skin testing and oral challenge procedures. In: Metcalfe DD, Sampson HA, Simon RA, eds. *Food Allergy: Adverse Reactions to Foods and Food Additives.* 2nd ed. Cambridge, MA: Blackwell Scientific Publications; 1997:151–166.
63. Sampson HA. Diagnosing food intolerances in children. In: Lichtenstein LM, Fauci AS. *Current Therapy in Allergy, Immunology, and Rheumatology.* 5th ed. St. Louis, MO: Mosby; 1996:140–145.
64. Steinman HA. "Hidden" allergens in foods. *J Allergy Clin Immunol.* 1996;98:241–250.
65. Bock SA. The natural history of food sensitivity. *J Allergy Clin Immunol.* 1982;69:173–177.
66. Sampson HA. Food allergy. *J Allergy Clin Immunol.* 1989;84:1062–1067.
67. Price CE, Rona RJ, Chinn S. Height of primary school children and parents' perceptions of food intolerance. *Br Med J.* 1988;296:1696–1699.
68. Nelson JK, Moxness KE, Jensen MD, Gastineau CF, eds. *Mayo Clinic Diet Manual: A Handbook of Nutrition Practices.* 7th ed. St. Louis, MO: Mosby-Year Book; 1994.

69. Williams CP, ed. *Pediatric Manual of Clinical Dietetics*. American Dietetic Association; 1998:219–234.
70. Juntunen K, Backman A. Goat's milk: A substitute for cow's milk? In: *Proceedings of the 2nd International Symposium of Immunological Clinical Problems of Food Allergy*. Milan, Italy: 1982.
71. Bush RK, Taylor CL, Nordlee JA, Busse WW. Soybean oil is not allergenic to soybean-sensitive individuals. *J Allergy Clin Immunol.* 1985:76:242–245.
72. Taylor SL, Busse WW, Sachs MI, et al. Peanut oil is not allergenic to peanut-sensitive individuals. *J Allergy Clin Immunol.* 1981;68:372–375.
73. Munoz-Furlong A. *The School Food Allergy Program*. Fairfax, VA: The Food Allergy Network; 1995.
74. Taylor JF, Latta RS. *Why Can't I Eat That? Helping Kids Obey Medical Diets*. 2nd ed. Saratoga, CA: R & E Publishers; 1993.
75. Satter E. *How to Get Your Child to Eat...But Not Too Much*. Palo Alto, CA: Bull Publishing Company; 1987.
76. Sampson HA, Mendelson L, Rosen J. Fatal and near-fatal anaphylactic reactions to foods in children and adolescents. *N Engl J Med.* 1992;327:380–386.
77. Geyman JP. Anaphylactic reaction after ingestion of bee pollen. *JABFP*. 1994;7:250–252.
78. Mansfield LE, Goldstein GB. Anaphylactic reaction after ingestion of local bee pollen. *Annals of Allergy*. 1981;47:154–156.
79. Cohen SH, Yunginger JW, Rosenberg N, Fink JN. Acute allergic reaction after composite pollen ingestion. *J Allergy Clin Immunol.* 1979;64:270–274.
80. Leung R, Ho A, Chan J, et al. Royal jelly consumption and hypersensitivity in the community. *Clin Exp Allergy*. 1997;27:333–336.
81. Thien FC, Leung R, Baldo BA, et al. Asthma and anaphylaxis induced by royal jelly. *Clin Exp Allergy*. 1996; 26:216–222.
82. Mullins RJ. Echinacea-associated anaphylaxis. *Med J Australia*. 1998;168:170–171.
83. Opperheimer JJ, Nelson HS, Bock SA, et al. Treatment of peanut allergy with rush immunotherapy. *J Allergy Clin Immunol.* 1992;90:256–262.
84. Nelson HS, Conkling C, Areson J, et al. Treatment of patients anaphylactically sensitive to peanuts with injections of peanut extract. *J Allergy Clin Immunol.* 1994; 93:211–217.
85. Stanley JS, King N, Burks AW, et al. Identification and mutational analysis of the immunodominant IgE binding epitopes of the major peanut allergen Ara h 2. *Arch Biochem Biophys.* 1997;342:244–253.
86. Burks AW, Shin D, Cockrell G, Stanley JS, et al. Mapping and mutational analysis of the IgE binding epitopes on Ara h 1, a legume vicilin protein and a major allergen in peanut hypersensitivity. *Eur J Biochem Biol.* 1997; 245:334–339.
87. Helm R, Cockrell G, Burks AW, Bannon GA. Cellular and molecular characterization of a major soy allergen. *Int Arch Allergy Appl Immunol.* 1998 (in press).
88. Host A. Cow's milk protein allergy and intolerance in infancy. *Pediatr Allergy Immunol.* 1994;5:5–36.
89. Sampson HA, Scanlon SM. Natural history of food hypersensitivity in children with atopic dermatitis. *J Pediatr*. 1989;115:23–27.
90. Businco L, Benincori N, Contani A, et al. Chronic diarrhea due to cow's milk allergy. A 4- to 10-year follow-up study. *Ann Allergy*. 1985;55:844–847.
91. Sampson HA. Food allergy. *JAMA*. 1997;278:188–189.
92. Kjellman N-IM. Development and prediction of atopic allergy in childhood. In: Bostrom H, Ljungstedt N, eds. *Skandia International Symposia: Theoretical and Clinical Aspects of Allergic Diseases*. Stockholm: Almqvist and Wickell; 1983:55–73.
93. Falth-Magnussom K, Kjellman NI. Allergy prevention by maternal elimination diet during late pregnancy: A 5-year follow-up of a randomized study. *J Allergy Clin Immunol.* 1992;89:709–713.
94. Zeiger R, Heller S. The development and prediction of atopy in high risk children: Follow-up at age seven years in a prospective randomized study of combined maternal and infant food allergen avoidance. *J Allergy Clin Immunol.* 1995;95:1179–1190.
95. Sigurs V, Hattevig G, Kjellman B. Maternal avoidance of eggs, cow's milk, and fish during lactation: Effect on allergic manifestations, skin-prick test, and specific IgE antibodies in children at age 4 years. *Pediatrics.* 1992; 89:735–737.

RESOURCES

Allergy and Asthma Network/Mothers of Asthmatics, Inc.
3554 Chain Bridge Road, Suite 200
Fairfax, Virginia 22030
(800)878-4403
Web site: http://npin.org/reswork/workorgs/allasthm.html

American Academy of Allergy Asthma & Immunology
611 East Wells Street
Milwaukee, Wisconsin 53202
(800)822-2762
Web site: http://www.aaaai.org

Asthma/Allergy Information Association
30 Eglinton Avenue West, Suite 750
Mississauga, Ontario CANADA L5R 3E7
(905)712-2242

Asthma and Allergy Foundation of America
1125 15th Street, NW, Suite 502
Washington, DC 20056
(800)7-ASTHMA

The American Dietetic Association
216 West Jackson Boulevard
Chicago, Illinois 60606-6995
Web site: http://www.eatright.org

Celiac Sprue Association/United States of America, Inc.
PO Box 31700
Omaha, Nebraska 68131-0770
(402)558-0600

The Food Allergy Network
10400 Eaton Place, Suite 107
Fairfax, Virginia 22030-2208
(800)929-4040
(703)691-2713
Web site: http://www.foodallergy.org

International Food Information Council Foundation
1100 Connecticut Avenue, NW, Suite 430
Washington, DC 20036
(202)296-6540
Web site: http//ificinfo.health.org

National Jewish Center for Immunology and Respiratory Medicine
1400 Jackson Street
Denver, Colorado 80206
(800)222-lung
(303)388-4461

Ener-G Foods, Inc.
5960 1st Avenue, South
PO Box 84487
Seattle, Washington 98124-5787
(206)767-6660
Web site: http://www.ener-g.com

The Gluten-Free Pantry
PO Box 840
Glastonbury, Connecticut 06033
(800)291-8386
Web site: http://www.glutenfree.com

Mead Johnson Nutritionals
Bristol-Myers Squibb Company
2400 West Lloyd Expressway
Evansville, Indiana 47721
(800)BABY-123

Ross Products Division
Abbott Laboratories
625 Cleveland Avenue
Columbus, Ohio 43216
(800)227-5767

Novartis Nutrition
5100 Gamble Drive
St. Louis Park, Minnesota 55416
(800)999-9978

Scientific Hospital Supplies
PO Box 117
Gaithersburg, MD 20884
(800)365-7354

CHAPTER 9

Childhood Obesity

Karen A. Weaver and Ann Piatek

Obesity is an excess accumulation of adipose tissue containing stored fat in the form of triglycerides. This chapter defines and describes obesity among children and adolescents, and offers suggestions for its assessment, diagnosis, and treatment.

Childhood obesity has become the most prevalent pediatric nutritional problem in the United States.[1,2] It affects as many as 15%–30% of grade-school children and adolescents, depending on the standards used to define obesity.[3,4] The prevalence rate has been rising steadily, increasing since 1965, with a relative increase of 20% in children aged 6–11 years and 18% in adolescents from 1976 to 1991.[1] There are variations in the prevalence of obesity among different ethnic groups. Among school-aged children, there is a higher occurrence of obesity in Black, Native American, Puerto Rican, Mexican, and Native Hawaiians.[5] Children are also becoming obese at younger ages. This increased prevalence is problematic because obesity that occurs early in life and persists throughout childhood is more difficult to treat. If obesity continues into adolescence, it is unlikely that he or she will outgrow it.[6,7]

RISKS ASSOCIATED WITH CHILDHOOD OBESITY

Obesity in childhood and adolescence presents significant health risks. Overweight in adolescence is associated with elevated health risks in adulthood, such as increased morbidity from coronary heart disease, atherosclerosis, colorectal cancer, gout, and arthritis.[2] Obesity that persists through childhood and adolescence into adulthood leads to hypertension and increased incidence of ischemic heart disease.[8] Thus, childhood obesity poses a significant public health problem. The greatest problem accompanying chronic childhood obesity is the emotional distress and subsequent loss of self-esteem caused by the stigma of being "too fat."[9] In the United States, children are regarded as responsible for their weight, with obesity being viewed as a sign of weakness and/or lack of self-control.[10] Among adolescents, obesity and an intense preoccupation with appearance may lead to a poor self-image, social isolation, delayed psychosocial development, and difficulty relating to family and peers. Compared with adolescents who were of normal weight, women who were overweight as teens had higher poverty rates, less household income, fewer completed years of school, and were less likely to be married.[11]

DEFINITION AND MEASUREMENT

Three commonly used methods for measuring obesity in children are: triceps skinfold thickness, weight for height by age and sex, and body mass index (BMI) (weight in kilograms divided by height in square meters). There is no single level of fatness in children that demarcates a higher or lower mortality rate.[12] For this reason, we must rely purely on statistical definitions of obesity.

Standards Used and Measurement Techniques

The Expert Committee on Clinical Guidelines for Overweight in Adolescent Preventive Services has recently defined the criteria for overweight to be used for routine screening of adolescents. They recommended BMI as the standard measure of obesity in adolescents.[13] Rosner et al[14] have developed tables for the distributions of BMI that are age-, race-, and gender-specific for children 5–17 years of age (Appendix E). BMI is consistently the best simple measure to evaluate obesity and is highly correlated with other estimates of fatness. Possibly, BMI will become the most commonly used standard for clinical and public health purposes. Obesity can also be measured by triceps skinfold thickness (Appendix H) and/or weight for height, using established procedures and standardized reference charts. The recommended standard for assessing physical growth of children in the United States is the National Center for Health Statistics (NCHS) percentile curves. Using the NCHS growth charts, obesity in children is defined as a weight for height above the 90th percentile, or weight in excess of 120% of the median weight for height. A weight greater than 140% of the median weight for a given height is defined as superobesity. Using skinfold thickness, obesity is defined by a measure greater than the 85th percentile and superobesity at a measure above the 95th percentile.[15]

ETIOLOGY

Ultimately, obesity represents an imbalance between energy intake and expenditure. The causes of obesity are multifactorial. There is a tendency to blame childhood obesity on overeating alone. The NHANES III data indicate that energy intakes among most age groups did not increase, compared with the previous decade, whereas the incidence of obesity increased.[16] Data on the physical activity of children are sparse, but the trend seems to be toward decreasing activity and exercise. The factors controlling the growth, development, and metabolism of adipose tissue are complex and are related to both genetics and environment. Animal studies show that food intake, metabolic rate, and physical activity have genetic components.[17,18] Some evidence suggests that thermogenesis may be impaired in human obesity. Twin and adoption studies point to evidence of a genetic factor for fatness.[19–21]

Although, a genetic susceptibility may be present, it is difficult to separate its effect from social and environmental factors.[22,23] In contrast to the genetic predispositions that drive hunger, appetite is a learned phenomenon. Caregiver food preferences, eating habits, and behaviors may present conditions that support appetite overriding hunger and satiety.[24] Environmental factors that likely contribute to obesity include abundant food availability, opportunities for decrease in energy expenditures through modern transportation, decreased urbanization, decreased physical activity curriculum in schools, labor-saving devices, and modern technology.[25] Evidence supporting these environmental and social factors include studies that show variance in obesity with population density, season, and geographic region, as well as with socioeconomic status, parental education, ethnicity, and parent marital status.[26] Parent marital status has been associated with the incidence of obesity, as well as with rate of weight loss in children in a treatment program. Children in single-parent families are at greater risk to be overweight and are less likely to be successful when they attempt treatment.[26]

LONGITUDINAL PERSPECTIVE ON CHILD AND ADOLESCENT OBESITY

To better understand the relationship of early and later fatness, it is useful to have a longitudinal overview. With this information, we can more precisely determine the relative risk of obesity at a particular age and focus prevention and treatment efforts on those children who are at the greatest risk for chronic obesity. Table 9–1 highlights the ages of children at which obesity is associated with an increased risk of continuing to be obese.

Infant Fatness and Later Obesity

High birth weights and fatness in early infancy have been examined as a potential cause of later obesity, due to excessive fat cell proliferation. Brown fat (adipose tissue) is present in small quantities in newborn infants for the purpose of maintaining thermogenesis. A perplexing phenomenon is that in childhood obesity, there is an increase in both the amount and size of the adipose tissue. In adult obesity, there is an increase only in cell size. However, there appears to be more than a causal relationship between obesity in infancy and later obesity.[27,28] Although larger maternal weight gains may result in heavier-for-date babies, these babies are not necessarily more likely to be obese later in life.[28] With regard to infant feeding methods, obesity is related to a greater energy intake but not to type of milk feeding, method of feeding, breast versus bottle feeding, or timing of the introduction of solids. Infant obesity in the first year is not significantly related to fatness in early childhood.[29] With regard to infancy, it is important to consider the magnitude of the expected and required growth during the first year; the accumulation of fat tissue is considered normal. The Committee on Nutrition of the American Academy of Pediatrics[30] states that the correlation between obesity in late childhood, adolescence, and adulthood is considerably stronger than that between obesity in infancy and in adulthood.

Fatness in Preschool and School-Aged Children

In children of normal weight, percentage of body fat increases in both boys and girls until about age 4. However, excessive fatness during the later preschool years is a good predictor of later childhood obesity.[27] For example, there is some relationship between fatness in the second year of life and later fatness, but excessive fatness at around age 5 is a stronger predictor of adolescent obesity. Between the ages of 4 and 11, the amount of body fat is stable in children who are close to their ideal body weight.[31] A small but continuous intake of calories beyond what is needed for growth may result in a gradual increase in excess body fat. Studies show that childhood obesity increases the risk of obesity in adulthood, but for children younger than 13 years, predictions are only questionable.[6]

The highest-risk group is obese children between ages 3 and 10 years who have one or more obese parent. Their risk of becoming obese can be as high as 60%.[6] Recent data show that about 33% of obese preschool children and 42% of obese school-aged children were also obese as adults.[5] Because parents influence both their child's intake and activity at this age, intervention designed to slow down the child's rate of weight gain over a period of months or years

Table 9–1 Relationship between Early and Later Obesity

Obesity at 0–1 years of age and adult obesity	Weak
Obesity at 3–5 years of age and adult obesity	Stronger
Obesity in adolescence and adult obesity	Strongest

Source: Reprinted from R. Crocker, Childhood Obesity, in *Handbook of Pediatric Nutrition,* P.M. Queen and C.E. Lang, eds., © 1993, Aspen Publishers, Inc.

may help to reduce the potential for obesity in adolescence and adulthood.

Adolescent Fatness and Later Obesity

Adolescence is a vulnerable time for the development of obesity. Early adolescence is frequently characterized by transient fatness in both boys and girls. Among females, percentage of body fat increases until approximately age 16, then plateaus for a period of time before it begins to increase again. Among males, percentage of body fat increases until age 16, then decreases.[31] Teenage obesity often persists into adulthood, especially for the older adolescent. For the 18-year-old with a BMI >60th percentile, chances of being overweight at age 35 are 36%.[32] The consequences of adolescent obesity are problematic and may include inactivity, overeating, social isolation, decreased self-esteem, depression, and more weight gain. The Expert Committee on Clinical Guidelines for Overweight in Adolescent Preventive Services[13] recommend a screening program for teens based on BMI. Adolescents with BMIs > 95th percentile of age and sex should be referred for medical evaluation and treatment. Adolescents with BMIs between the 85th and 95th percentiles should be referred for a second-level screen that identifies other risk factors. Figure 9–1 gives schematic representation of the committee's recommended screening protocol.

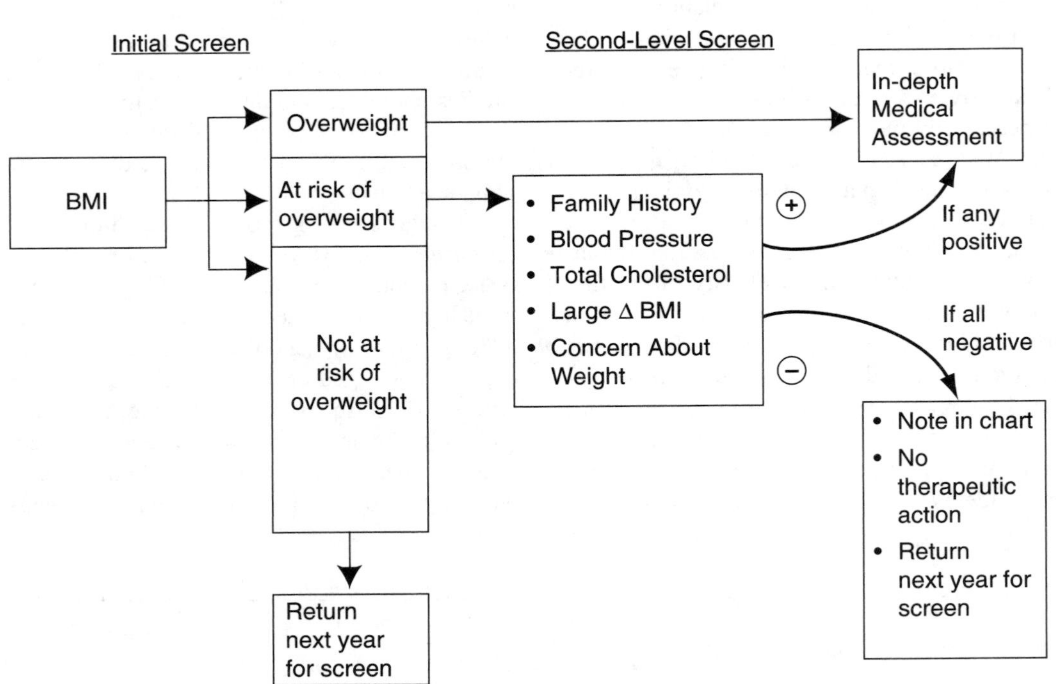

Figure 9–1 Schematic representation of recommended overweight screening in adolescence. *Source:* Reprinted with permission from J. Hines and W. Dietz, Guidelines for overweight in adolescent preventive services: recommendations from an expert committee, *American Journal of Clinical Nutrition,* Vol. 59, pp. 307–316, © 1994, American Society for Clinical Nutrition.

ASSESSMENT AND DIAGNOSIS

The assessment of the obese child is critical in the treatment of childhood obesity. Persistence of the condition is based on a wide variety of factors, including age, sex, family history of obesity, developmental stage, ethnicity, and social environment. Each of these factors will influence the treatment goal, the selection of type of treatment, and the course of therapy. Obesity is a complex disease and, even with excellent adherence to treatment recommendations, progress may be slow. Because of the extended time that children may need to be in treatment, the assessment must include a careful review of family lifestyle patterns and the child's social environment. The first step, however, is the physical assessment. This will establish whether the obesity is accompanied by any other disorder and whether the child has any physical limitations that will be affected by an exercise program.

Physical Assessment

Each overweight child should be given a complete physical examination by a pediatrician or a pediatric nurse practitioner. Table 9–2 provides a summary of the physical findings or symptoms associated with specific disorders that can cause childhood obesity. The physical should begin with the child's neonatal and birth history, with a view toward the possibility of an undiagnosed developmental disability. For example, a history of congenital hypotonia followed by failure to thrive in the first few months of life may suggest a rare condition such as Prader-Willi syndrome. Other symptoms associated with various developmental disabilities include cold intolerance and constipation associated with hypothyroidism, and headaches or vision changes related to Cushing's syndrome.

Height may be increased above that expected and should be measured carefully. Surges in height are frequently seen in children and adolescents who have experienced rapid and excessive weight gain. A child with less than expected height with respect to average parental height or expected linear growth must be evaluated for endocrine disorders or one of the rare congenital syndromes. The skin may show white stretch marks (striae), which are not unexpected, even in moderately obese children. Purplish striae may indicate Cushing's syndrome. Acanthosis nigricans, a blackish pigmentation around the neck that suggests hormonal imbalance or insulin resistance, may also be found.[33,34]

The child's rate and pattern of weight gain should also be carefully assessed. A rapid and excessive weight gain in recent months may be due to a lifestyle change or an emotional reaction to a significant event. If the events paralleling the weight gain have not been resolved, these children and their families may need psychologic counseling before weight control is initiated, to prevent failure in a weight control program.

Table 9–2 Medical Causes of Obesity

Genetic Syndromes	Possible Symptoms or Physical Findings
Prader-Willi syndrome	Congenital hypotonia, failure to thrive, developmental delay
Rare congenital syndromes	Short stature, developmental delay
Endocrine Disorders	
Hypothyroidism	Cold intolerance, constipation
Insulin resistance	Acanthosis nigricans
Cushing's syndrome	Headaches, vision changes, purple striae

Source: Adapted from R. Crocker, Childhood Obesity, in *Hanbook of Pediatric Nutrition,* P.M. Queen and C.E. Lang, eds., © 1993, Aspen Publishers, Inc.

Medical Complications Related to Obesity

Table 9–3 lists the physical and metabolic problems related to childhood obesity. Obese children may experience orthopedic problems, such as a slipped capital femoral epiphysis, Blount's disease, or bowed femurs. They may also develop respiratory problems, such as in increased incidence of infection or sleep apnea. Obstructive sleep apnea is an obstruction of the airway during sleep caused by an increase in peripharnygeal fat and large tonsils. It should be suspected in obese children who snore at night and are sleepy during the day. This condition is thought to be the major cause of Pickwickian syndrome, a condition rarely found in children but having a mortality rate of 25% in children with the syndrome.[33]

Obese children should be assessed for hyperlipidemia, hypercholesterolemia, hypertension, and abnormal glucose metabolism. Hypertension is more prevalent among obese children than in normal-weight children. Although the cause of hypertension in obese children is not clear, there is frequently an immediate reduction in blood pressure following the initiation of a hypocaloric diet.[33] Finally, the risk of obesity into adulthood and the increased morbidity and mortality associated with adult obesity is substantial.

Social Assessment

Psychosocial factors influence the etiology and maintenance of obesity.[35,36] A detailed social assessment, including a family interview at the onset of treatment, should be a key component of any weight control program designed for children. Parents, grandparents, siblings, and others who are involved in caring for the child should attend. The purpose of the family interview is to gather as much information as possible about daily life in the family and to explore attitudes and beliefs about obesity and obesity treatment. Exhibit 9–1 lists sample questions that might be asked by the interviewer during the family interview. Questions such as, "How much weight should the child lose?" are aimed at exploring areas of agreement and conflicts between parents. Parents who agree on child-rearing practices and have a good marital relationship usually have children who are more successful in a weight control program.[37]

Another goal of the family interview is to open communication lines among family members and to establish a collaborative atmosphere. The interview may provide the family with their first experience of discussing the problem as a family unit. The tone of the interview must be exploratory and nonjudgmental. Some family members may have strong feelings that weight

Table 9–3 Medical Complications of Obesity

Acute
Sleep apnea with Pickwickian syndrome
Slipped capital femoral epiplysis
Blount's disease
Glucose intolerance
Hypertension (also long term)

Chronic
Hyperlipidemia
Hypercholesterolemia
Hypertension
Diabetes

Exhibit 9–1 Sample Questions for Family Interview

Who prepares food in the family?
Who shops, organizes meals?
Are special foods prepared on holidays, at family events?
How often does the family eat together?
What does the family do for recreation?
Who else in the family has a weight problem?
Do parents feel that the obese child has a weight problem or that he or she will "grow out of it"?
How much weight should the child lose?
What if the child doesn't lose weight?
Have there been previous attempts to lose weight?
Who makes the rules about child behavior in the family?
Who enforces them?
What caused the child to become obese?
Is there obesity elsewhere in your family (other relatives)?
How close do you live to grandparents and other relatives?
Who is the most independent member of your family?
Who is the most dependent member of your family?
Which words best describe your family?

Source: Reprinted from R. Crocker, "Childhood Obesity," in *Handbook of Pediatric Nutrition,* P.M. Queen and C.E. Lang, eds., ©1993, Aspen Publishers, Inc.

loss should be immediate and dramatic, even when this may not be necessary or appropriate. Such beliefs should be addressed and corrected, but only after all of the family members have responded and shared their views. Emphasis should stay on the family members by encouraging them to respond to one another. This will yield the greatest amount of information about parenting style, lifestyle patterns, achievement of family development tasks, and social and economic resources.

Nutrition and Physical Activity Assessment

Food intake in childhood obesity has been the subject of much controversy. Although it is widely believed that obesity is caused by excessive calorie intake, several investigators have reported that they could find no difference between the food intakes of lean children and those of obese children.[38–41] One recent study did show that lower baseline intakes of fat, as well as decreased intakes of kilocalories from fat, were correlated with a decrease of BMI in preschoolers.[42] Variations in food selection are related to patterns of physical and social activities, and to consistency in timing of meals and snacks. Individuals may also vary their intake in response to changes in appetite.[43]

A detailed dietary history will yield important information about diet content, eating patterns, and where and with whom the child eats. Determining who shops for the family's food and how often they shop is also important. Often, children eat meals with several different family members at different times of the day, for various reasons. It is very useful to begin the dietary assessment by asking the child what time he or she awakens, what is the first thing that he or she has to eat or drink, and proceed with questions about the day. After the basic framework of the child's eating pattern is established, information about nonschool days, weekends, and holidays can be gathered. All dietary information should be collected in a neutral manner and atmosphere, reserving any suggestions for modifications until a complete picture of the child's food habits has been established. Keeping a positive and professional tone is beneficial, especially when parents attempt to make a child "confess" to overeating or to consuming a particular food. Parents are often uncomfortable about discussing food and their overweight child. Every effort should be made to help parents feel comfortable and to support them as capable and competent parents.

It is also effective to collect information about activity patterns of both the child and family while gathering dietary information. Decreased physical activity has been found in children of obese parents.[44] Usually, children's food and activity patterns are intertwined. They often associate activities with food: getting ice cream at the mall, ordering nachos at the ballpark, stopping at the snack bar at the swimming pool, or having pizza after a sports event. The interviewer must listen for places where changes can be made when individualizing treatment recommendations.

Developing a Treatment Method

The development of a working hypothesis about the needs of the child and the family is a crucial step in treatment. In some cases, the obesity treatment may be deferred, based on evidence that, although necessary, it is not appropriate at that time. This is often the case when there is severe parental conflict or when the child is not ready, or has attended weight control programs without success. Patients may be referred for family counseling if deemed necessary. An obese child in a dysfunctional family is often identified as the family problem to distract them from addressing more painful family issues. Obese children of divorced or separated parents may find that weight control attempts help superficially to hold their parents together. In both cases, children are more likely to fail at weight control.[45] Five fundamental interaction factors that have been associated with chronic obesity in children and failure of a pediatric weight control program are:

- Chronic, unresolved marital discord;
- Exclusion of one parent from an overinvolved parent–child relationship;
- An overprotective orientation by one or both parents;
- Encouragement to overeat and to avoid exercise;
- Overinvolvement of child in parental problems.

TREATMENT

A conservative approach to weight management treatment is recommended for obese children of all ages. Appetite depressants and other substances of this nature should not be used by children and adolescents, due to the risks associated with them. Many teenagers use over-the-counter diet aids and are not familiar with the risks and ineffectiveness of these products. An exception is the severely obese child who needs to achieve significant weight loss, but obesity is secondary to other medical problems. Included in this group are children with Prader-Willi syndrome, steroid-induced obesity, or morbid obesity in the presence of other serious medical problems, such as sleep apnea. The protein-sparing modified fast (PSMF), a low-calorie, low-carbohydrate, high-protein diet has been used with success in these children.[46,47] Close medical supervision is necessary because these diets require supplementation with potassium, magnesium, and calcium. These patients also need to be in a behavioral-based treatment program to have continued success when the PSMF program is complete. Current research is underway to evaluate the use of antidepressants in the treatment of severe obesity. Again, these treatments are for only the small group of children and adolescents with life-threatening obesity.

Treatment of obesity for children and adolescents requires a comprehensive program. Components of a successful weight management program include modified energy intake, decreased fat intake, increased physical activity, parental participation, and behavior modification for the parent and child.[48,49] Careful attention must be paid to monitoring linear growth, and protein intake must remain adequate to protect lean body mass. The goal of treatment is twofold. First, weight gain should be stopped or slowed until the child grows into an appropriate weight for height and age. If the patient is an obese adolescent, weight loss may be necessary. Second, weight loss or weight maintenance should be monitored carefully to ensure that fat is being lost while linear growth is continuing normally and lean body mass is maintained.

Modifications in energy and fat intake can be achieved without severe restrictions, exchange diets, or other defined meal plans. Teaching parents and children how to eat a healthy diet should substantially reduce their calorie and fat intake. This can be achieved by using such tools as the food guide pyramid and by reading food labels, eating low-fat foods, and following guidelines for dining out and snacking. Tables 9–4 and 9–5 provide examples of simple tools that can be used to initiate nutrition education. After completing a weight management program, families should understand that there are no "good" or "bad" foods, but rather that all foods are acceptable. Limiting low-nutrient, calorically dense foods is a healthier alternative. Food intake should be based on listening to your body's needs and not your "head" or emotions.[51] Exhibit 9–2 is an example of a tool that can be used to achieve eating based on appropriate internal cues versus external inappropriate cues.[50]

Obese children are often less physically active. Decreased physical activity and increased television viewing are also associated with increased obesity.[44] Physical activity is a necessary component of a successful weight management and weight maintenance program. Children should add 30 minutes of continuous movement per day. Exercise not only burns calories, but it increases lean body mass, which increases the basic metabolic rate, decreases body fat, helps control appetite, and may improve self-esteem. The exercise program might include information on warm-up and cool-down exercises, energy expenditure for various activities, endurance and strengthening exercises, aerobic activity, identification of exercises that require little space or equipment, and time management for exercise (see Table 9–6). The exercise component of a weight management program is a must. Both the parent and child or teen should be included, and they should establish a goal and reward system. The goal could be earning weekly tokens to cash in for a special treat. Depending on the treat, the cost may vary (one, two, or more tokens). The participant keeps a daily activity record and earns a token at the end of each week that included at least 5 days of 30-minute continuous activity. The reward could be treating the child or teen to a special activity, such as a movie, play, or trip to the mall, or allowing the child or teen to skip a chore.

Behavior modification includes techniques such as self-monitoring, social reinforcement, stimulus control, and modeling.[48–51] There is a good correlation between self-monitoring and weight loss and maintenance. Recording eating and activity habits allows for the evaluation of behavior with established goals (see Exhibit 9–3 and Exhibit 9–4 for an example of a daily recording tool and guidelines for completing food records). This can allow for dialogue between the parent and child regarding progress and setbacks. Feedback to the family is a good tool for the weight management instructor. Social reinforcement is achieved by allowing for parental support through contingency management. It involves praise and rewards for behavior change. This technique works best when the rewards are defined by the child and are frequent (weekly versus monthly). This reward system can be applied to the parents, as well as to the child.

Stimulus control is classic behavior modification. It is the modification of factors that serve as cues for decreasing inappropriate eating behaviors or increasing desirable physical activity behaviors. Stimulus control might include keeping problem foods out of the house, making meal times last 20 minutes or longer, using smaller

Table 9–4 Fast Food Tidbits

Green Light Choices		Red Light Choices
extra lettuce and tomato	vs.	bacon, mayonnaise, and "special sauces"
plain hamburger or roast beef sandwich or broiled chicken sandwich	vs.	fried fish or fried chicken sandwich, or chicken nuggets, or super-sized hamburger
mashed potatoes or an ear of corn	vs.	french fries
whole-wheat, rye, or pita bread	vs.	croissant or biscuits
crisp, crunchy vegetables	vs.	creamy salads, such as potato or macaroni salads
low-fat milk, fruit juice, diet soda, or water	vs.	shakes and regular soda
thin-crust pizza with mushrooms, green peppers, or other vegetables	vs.	thick-crust pizza with extra cheese, sausage, or pepperoni
plain baked potato with chili topping or with cottage cheese, a small amount of grated cheese or vegetables from the salad bar	vs.	french fries or baked potato with sour cream, bacon, butter/margarine, cheddar or Swiss cheese
fruit muffin, low-fat frozen yogurt, sorbet, small ice cream cone, fresh fruit from home, plain cake, English muffin, bagel	vs.	fruit pie, fruit turnovers, danish pastries, cookies
chocolate spinkles or fruit toppings	vs.	hot fudge, chocolate, caramel, or butterscotch sauces, nuts or whipped toppings
soft tacos, tostados, bean burritos, nonfried items, rice, Mexican pizza	vs.	hard-shell tacos, nachos, deluxe burritos, refried beans, pinto beans with cheese
extra tomatoes, lettuce, and salsa	vs.	sour cream and guacamole

dishes and glasses, etc. It may also include removing barriers to achieving desirable behavior, such as moving the TV out of the kitchen or moving exercise equipment from the basement to the family room. Modeling involves parents making an effort to avoid eating and exercise behaviors that they don't want their child to mimic and practicing the behaviors that they wish to see in their children.

Much of the literature on treatment of obesity in children suggests that intervention is unsuccessful. It is imperative that any attempt to inter-

Table 9–5 Healthy Snacks for Hungry Kids (Includes examples of appropriate single serving size)

Angelfood cake (1/16 of cake)
Applesauce—unsweetened (1 cup)
Bagel (1)
Bread stick (6–8)
Cereal, low-sugar, low-fat (1 1/2 cup)
Cheese, low-fat (1–2 slices)
Cottage cheese, low-fat (1/2 cup)
Crackers, low-fat (6–12)
English muffin (1)
Fresh fruit (1–2 pieces)
Fruit, canned in own juice (1/2–1 cup)
Frozen fruit juice bars
Ginger snaps (6)
Graham crackers (2–4 sq)
Pretzels (30 sticks)
Rice cakes (2–3)
Sorbet (3/4 cup)
Vanilla wafers (6–8)
Vegetables—fresh with fat-free dip
Yogurt, nonfat (1 cup)

vene not result in failure and leave a child with even less self-esteem than they had before seeking treatment. Studies do show that comprehensive programs are beneficial.[48,52,53] When dealing with an obese child and family, one must avoid implying that the obesity is from self-indulgence. One must also not simply suggest a low-calorie diet and increased exercise. Health care providers must become familiar with reliable treatment centers in the area, making sure that the program is comprehensive and includes all of the necessary components, as discussed. Some nationally available programs that facilitate behavior change are SHAPEDOWN, Body Shop, KidShape, LESTER, and Committed to Kids. These programs vary in length, educational tools available, such as books, videos, etc., number of professional staff, nutritional and exercise approach, and cost. Before purchasing a program, it is wise to compare all of the features. Some features to look for in weight loss programs are:

1. Program includes diet modification, exercise, and behavior modification;
2. There is multidisciplinary expertise available (medical, nutritional, psychologic, exercise);
3. The diet component includes variety and flexibility and does not require special foods;
4. The program ideally should be at least 8 weeks and include a maintenance component.

CONCLUSION

Pediatric obesity is a chronic and increasing problem. The relationship between childhood obesity and adult obesity increases as children grow older. Obesity is a major risk factor for increased adult morbidity for many chronic diseases, including heart disease and cancer. Childhood obesity is a public health problem.

Exhibit 9–2 Weight Management: Traditional Diets vs. the Nondiet Approach

	DIET PARADIGM	NONDIET PARADIGM
WEIGHT	Achieving ideal weight (or as close as possible), used as measure of success.	Body will seek its natural weight as individual eats in response to physical cues of hunger, fullness, and sense of well-being, as well as taste.
HUNGER	Attempt to suppress or ignore hunger. Transgressions associated with lack of will power or "giving in." Physical and emotional hunger confused.	Physical cues to eat are valuable and relied upon. Responding to physical hunger and fullness (with occasional emotional eating) will bring about natural weight.
EXERCISE	Reaching and maintaining goal weight dependent on exercise, which is often dropped when individual falls off diet. It is seen as a "have to" or "should." It is common to develop exercise resistance.	Physical activity, listening to body, seeking play and natural movement are explored. Not connected to weight loss or change of body size or shape.
FOOD	Moralized as good/bad, legal/illegal, should/shouldn't, on/off diet. Variety, quantity, calories, fat grams, etc., determined by external source, ie, the diet, program, and/or staff.	Neutralized. All food is acceptable. Quantity, quality, and frequency are determined by individual exploring and responding to physical cues, sense of well-being, taste, and medical values ie, blood glucose levels. It is self-regulated, internally cued, nonrestrained.
SELF-ESTEEM/ SIZE ACCEPTANCE	Individual typically gains a false sense of power and control with weight loss, adherence to diet, and exercise plan. Self-esteem and body acceptance rarely improve. This goal is elusive as one can usually get thinner and/or more toned.	Increase in self-esteem/personal power from self-determined eating style and movement. Bodies come in all sizes and are naturally beautiful. Cultural standards are hazardous; pursuit of these standards can interfere with quality of life.
TRUST/ DISTRUST IN SELF AND BODY	Individual may come to distrust body and sense of judgment, especially with history of failure. Trust typically is placed primarily in diet or staff.	Trust develops in self and body by discerning physical cues and freely responding to them without judgment or criticism.

Source: Reprinted with permission from N. King, *Moving Away from Diets,* Helm Publishing, ©1995, Nancy L. King, MS, RD, CDE.

Table 9–6 Components of an Exercise Program

Warm-Up and Cool-Down Exercises	
Breathing	
Head Rolls	
Side Bends	
Hamstring Stretch	
Endurance Exercises	**Strengthening Exercises**
Biking	Push-ups
Swimming	Sit-ups
Dancing	Bridges
Stair-Stepping	Leg Lifts
Walking	Leg Extensions
Jogging	Weight Training
Skating	
Finding Time-Out for Exercise	
Pick a time of day	
Keep a written exercise activity record	
Plan a substitution for an outdoor activity ahead of time, in case of inclement weather	
Keep exercise equipment or clothing in plain view	

Exhibit 9–3 How To Fill Out the Daily Food Record

_______ Write down everything you eat or drink.

You might find it helpful to write down foods eaten immediately after they are eaten.

_______ List foods by meals or snacks.

_______ Write down how much of everything you eat.

Example: *1 cup skim milk*
small banana
2 slices of American cheese
3 tablespoons peanut butter

_______ Include all additions to foods.

Example: *Margarine or butter*
Salad dressing
Gravy
Jelly
Sugar

Remember, by writing down what you eat and drink, you take charge of your food habits and weight control!

Exhibit 9–4 Daily Food and Exercise Diary

Name ____________________
Week ____________________

Weekly Exercise Goal
Warm-up/Cool Down _______ x/week
Endurance _______ x/week
Strengthening_______ x/week

	Day 1					Day 2					Day 3				
Please write down food or drink eaten and amount	**Breakfast**					**Breakfast**					**Breakfast**				
	Lunch					**Lunch**					**Lunch**				
	Afternoon Snack					**Afternoon Snack**					**Afternoon Snack**				
	Dinner					**Dinner**					**Dinner**				
	Evening Snack					**Evening Snack**					**Evening Snack**				
Daily Nutrition Summary															
Food Pyramid Food Group	MK	Mt	F/V	G	O	MK	Mt	F/V	G	O	MK	Mt	F/V	G	O
# Serving Consumed															
	Key: Daily Servings:		MK=Milk 3		Mt=Meat 2–3		F/V=Fruits/Vegetables 3–5			G=Grain 6–11		O=Other use sparingly			
Daily Exercise Summary	Warm-up/Cool Down ______ Endurance ______ Strengthening ______					Warm-up/Cool Down ______ Endurance ______ Strengthening ______					Warm-up/Cool Down ______ Endurance ______ Strengthening ______				

(continued)

Exhibit 9–4 Continued

Weekly Exercise Summary

Day 4	Day 5	Day 6	Day 7
Breakfast	**Breakfast**	**Breakfast**	**Breakfast**
Lunch	**Lunch**	**Lunch**	**Lunch**
Afternoon Snack	**Afternoon Snack**	**Afternoon Snack**	**Afternoon Snack**
Dinner	**Dinner**	**Dinner**	**Dinner**
Evening Snack	**Evening Snack**	**Evening Snack**	**Evening Snack**

MK	Mt	F/V	G	O	MK	Mt	F/V	G	O	MK	Mt	F/V	G	O	MK	Mt	F/V	G	O

Key: Daily Servings:	MK=Milk 3	Mt=Meat 2–3	F/V=Fruits/Vegetables 3–5	G=Grain 6–11	O=Other use sparingly

Warm-up/Cool Down ________ Endurance ________ Strengthening ________	Warm-up/Cool Down ________ Endurance ________ Strengthening ________	Warm-up/Cool Down ________ Endurance ________ Strengthening ________	Warm-up/Cool Down ________ Endurance ________ Strengthening ________

Source: Courtesy of Health & Wellness Child/Teen Weight Management Program, Cardinal Glemon Children's Hospital, St. Louis, Missouri.

Genetic and metabolic studies are offering new insights in the causes of obesity, which may eventually lead to new treatment options. For now, treatment depends on lowering energy intake and increasing energy output. Many treatment programs have poor success rates, and physicians are reluctant to refer children to treatment programs because of the risk of psychologic distress associated with failure. The treatment of all overweight children should be age-appropriate, and management of the obese child and family must be approached with sensitivity and awareness of the tremendous complexity of the disease.

REFERENCES

1. Troiano RP, Flegal KM, Kuczmarski RJ, Campbell SM, Johnson CL. Overweight prevalence and trends for children and adolescents. *Arch Pediatr Adolesc Med.* 1995; 149:1085.
2. Must A, Jacques PF, Dallal GE, Bajema CJ, Dietz WH. Long-term morbidity and mortality of overweight adolescents. *N Engl J Med.* 1992;327:1350.
3. Kuczmarski RJ, Flegal KM, Campbell SM, et al. Increasing prevalence of overweight among US adults. *JAMA.* 1994;272:205–210.
4. Gortmaker SL, Must A, Suho AM, et al. Television viewing as a cause of increasing obesity among children in the United States. *Arch Pediatr Adolesc Med.* 1996; 150:356–362.
5. Kumanyika S. Ethnicity and obesity development in children. *Ann NY Acad Sci.* 1993;699:81–86.
6. Serdula MK, Ivery D, Coates RJ, et al. Do obese children become obese adults? *Prev Med.* 1993;22:167–176.
7. Whitaker RC, Wright JA, Pepe MS, Seidel KD, Dietz WH. Predicting obesity in young adulthood from childhood and parental obesity. *N Engl J Med.* 1997;337: 869–873.
8. Gunnell DJ, Frankel SJ, Nanchahal K, et al. Childhood obesity and adult cardiovascular mortality: A 57-yr follow-up study based on the Boyd Orr cohort. *Am J Clin Nutr.* 1998;67:1111–1118.
9. Lloyd JK, Wolff OH. Overnutrition and obesity. In: Falkner F, ed. *Prevention in Childhood of Health Problems in Adult Life.* Geneva: World Health Organization; 1980.
10. Striegel-Moore R, Rodin J. Prevention of obesity. In: Rosen JC, Solomon LJ, eds. *Prevention in Health Psychology.* London: University Press; 1985.
11. Gortmaker SL, Must A, Perrin JM, Sobol AM, Dietz WH. Social and economic consequences of overweight in adolescence and young adulthood. *N Engl J Med.* 1993;329:1008–1012.
12. Garn SM. *Continuities and Changes in Fatness from Infancy Through Adulthood.* Chicago, IL: Year Book Medical Publishers; 1985.
13. Himes JH, Dietz WH. Guidelines for overweight in adolescent preventive services: Recommendations from an expert committee. *Am J Clin Nutr.* 1994;59:307–316.
14. Rosner B, Prineas R, Loggie J, Daniels SR. Percentiles for body mass index in U.S. children 5 to 17 years of age. *J Pediatr.* 1998;132:211–221.
15. Schonfeld-Warden N, Warden CH. Pediatric obesity: An overview of etiology and treatment. *Pediatric Clin North Am.* 1997;44:339–361.
16. IFIC Foundation. Moving to prevent childhood obesity. *Fd Insight.* 1997;4:1–4.
17. Leibel RL, Rosenbaum M, Hirsch J. Changes in energy expenditure resulting from altered body weight. *N Engl J Med.* 1995;332:621–624.
18. Friedman JM, Leibel RL. Tackling a weighty problem. *Cell.* 1992;69:217–220.
19. Chau SC, Leibel RL. Molecular genetic approaches to obesity. In: Bouchard C, ed. *The Genetics of Obesity.* Boca Raton, FL: CRC Press; 1994:213–222.
20. Bogardus C, Lillioja S, Ravussin E, et al. Familial dependence of the resting metabolic rate. *N Engl J Med.* 1986;315:96–100.
21. Bouchard C, Tremblay A, Despres JP, et al. The response to long-term overfeeding identical twins. *N Engl J Med.* 1990;322:1477–1482.
22. Dietz WH, Gortmaker SL. Factors within the physical environment associated with childhood obesity. *Am J Clin Nutr.* 1984;39:619.
23. Gortmaker SL, Must A, Perrin JM. Social and economic consequences of overweight in adolescence and young adulthood. *N Engl J Med.* 1993;329:1008–1012.
24. Dietz WH. Therapeutic strategies in childhood obesity. *Horm Res.* 1993;39(suppl 3):86–90.
25. Lytle L, Achterberg C. Changing the diet of America's children: What works and why? *J Nutr Ed.* 1995;27(s): 250–260.
26. McGinnis JM. The public health burden of a sedentary lifestyle. *Med Sci Sports Exercise.* 1992;24(s):196–200.
27. Yeung D. Obesity in infancy and early childhood: Any relationship? Presented at the Fourth International Congress on Obesity, New York: October 5–8, 1983.
28. Rosenbaum M, Leibel RL. Pathophysiology of childhood obesity. *Adv Pediatr.* 1988;35:73–138.

29. Leibel RL, Hirsch J. Diminished energy requirements in reduced-obese patients. *Metabolism.* 1984;33:164–170.
30. Committee on Nutrition. Nutrition aspects of obesity in infancy and childhood. *Pediatrics.* 1981;68:880–885.
31. Engle MA. Hypertension. In: Hoekelman RA, ed. *Primary Pediatric Care.* St. Louis, MO: CV Mosby; 1987.
32. Guo SS, Roche AF, Chumlea WC, Gardner JD, Siervogel RM. The predictive value of childhood body mass index values for overweight at age 35 years. *Am J Clin Nutr.* 1994;59:810–819.
33. Dietz WH. Nutrition and obesity. In: Grand RJ, Sutphen JL, Dietz WH, eds. *Pediatric Nutrition: Theory and Practice.* Boston, MA: Butterworths; 1987.
34. Rimm I, Rimm AA. Association between juvenile onset obesity and severe adult obesity in 73,532 women. *Am J Public Health.* 1976;66:479.
35. Lissau I, Sorensen TI. Parental neglect during childhood and increased risk of obesity in young adulthood. *Lancet.* 1994;343:324–327.
36. Lissau-Lund-Sorenson I, Sorenson TI. Prospective study of the influence of social factors in childhood on risk of overweight in young adulthood. *Int J Obes Relat Metab Disord.* 1992;16:169–175.
37. Huenemann R. Environmental factors associated with preschool obesity. *J Am Diet Assoc.* 1974;64:480.
38. Huenemann RL, Shapiro LR, Hampton MC, et al. Food and eating practices of teenagers. *J Am Diet Assoc.* 1968;53:17.
39. Mayer J. *Overweight.* Englewood Cliffs, NJ: Prentice-Hall; 1968.
40. Leon GR, Chamberlain K. Comparison of daily eating habits and emotional state of overweight persons successful or unsuccessful in maintaining a weight loss. *J Consult Clin Psychol.* 1973;41:108.
41. Cohen E, Gelfand DM, Dodd DK, et al. Self-control practices associated with weight loss maintenance in children and adolescents. *Behav Ther.* 1980;11:26.
42. Klesges RC, Klesges LM, Eck LH, Shelton ML. A longitudinal analysis of accelerated weight gain in preschool children. *Pediatrics.* 1995;95:126–130.
43. Frankle RT. Obesity a family matter: Creating new behavior. *J Am Diet Assoc.* 1985;85:597.
44. Klesges RC, Eck LH, Hanson CL, Haddock CK, Lesges LM. Effects of obesity, social interactions, and physical environment on physical activity in preschoolers. *Health Psychol.* 1990;9:435–449.
45. Dietz WH, Gortmaker SL. Do we fatten our children at the television set? Obesity and television viewing in children and adolescents. *Pediatrics.* 1985;75:807.
46. Buckmaster L, Brownell KD. Behavior modification: The state of the art. In: Frankle R, Yang M, eds. *Obesity and Weight Control.* Gaithersburg, MD: Aspen Publishers; 1988.
47. Brownell KD, Stunkard AJ. Behavioral treatment of obesity in children. *Am J Dis Child.* 1978;132:403.
48. Epstein LH. Family-based behavioral intervention for obese children. *Int J Obesity.* 1996;20:S14–S12.
49. Epstein LH, Valoski AM, Kalarchian MA, McCurley J. Do obese children lose and maintain weight easier than adults: A comparison of child and parent weight changes from six months to ten years. *Obese Res.* 1995;3:411–418.
50. King NL, Hayes D, Kratina K. In: *Moving Away From Diets.* Lake Dallas, TX: Helm Pub;1996.
51. Foreyt JP, Goodrick GK. *Living Without Dieting.* Houston, TX: Harrison Pub;1992.
52. Mellin LM, Slinkard LA, Irwin CE. Adolescent obesity intervention: Validation of the SHAPEDOWN program. *J Am Diet Assoc.* 1987;87:162–167.
53. NIH Technology Assessment Conference Panel. Methods for voluntary weight loss and control. *Ann Int Med.* 1993;119:764–770.

Chapter 10

Eating Disorders

Andrea Bull McDonough

Eating disorders can start as early as the age of 9 years or before puberty.[1] Girls are predominantly affected, but approximately 5% of all cases are males.[1] Anorexia nervosa, bulimia nervosa, and binge eating disorders are complex, multidimensional disorders having psychologic, medical, sociocultural, and nutritional components.[2] An interdisciplinary team approach with clinicians experienced in these varied areas is the treatment model of choice. It is critical for dietitians to define their role on the team. Dietitians will assess nutritional status, implement a nutrition care plan, coordinate their treatment goals with those of other team members, and monitor progress of the treatment.[3] Most often, these clinical activities are pursued in the context of a counseling relationship. It should be borne in mind that, owing to the psychologic disturbances frequently at work in eating disorders, the conduct of the therapeutic relationship is no less important for treatment success than is monitoring concrete data, such as height, weight, calorie intake, or energy expenditure.

Apart from actual involvement with eating-disordered patients, the dietitian has a role to play in the prevention of eating disorders. Alarming statistics support the need for serious prevention efforts.

- 30–50% of 8- and 9-year-old American girls report feeling "too fat," and 20–40% are dieting
- Over 50% of 14-year-old girls have dieted during the 8th grade year
- In high school, 40–60% of girls feel overweight and are dieting.[4]

The genesis of disordered eating behaviors typically includes the use of unsafe diets and unproven diet products, and obsession with arbitrary standards of ideal weight. The American Dietetic Association position paper on eating disorders warns against promoting dieting strategies to youngsters coming for help with weight loss.[3] Alternatively, dietitians should focus their counseling on normalization of eating, increased connection with hunger and fullness, body image issues, and how to stop the pursuit of thinness. Helping a child grow into his or her size while exploring in a nonjudgmental way the genetic, environmental and behavioral contribution to his or her weight status may be the best combination of prevention and nutrition counseling. This chapter presents information about the etiology, incidence, and prognosis of anorexia nervosa, bulimia nervosa, and binge eating disorders, and their clinical treatment guidelines relevant to the in-patient and outpatient dietitian's role.

DEFINITIONS

Exhibit 10–1 gives the definitions of anorexia nervosa, bulimia nervosa, and binge eating disorders, according to the fourth edition of *The Diagnostic and Statistical Manual of Mental*

Disorders.[5] For a diagnosis to be made, all features of the eating disorder must be met. Although the eating disorders are defined separately, common characteristics are shared by both:

1. A fear of becoming fat and a drive to be or become thin
2. An obsession with food, weight, calories, and dieting
3. The use and abuse of eating or not eating to cope with emotional discomfort, stressful life events, and developmental challenges
4. An increased incidence of depression, obesity, substance abuse, and eating disorders in the families of the sufferers
5. A world view valuing external appearance over personal integrity.[1]

ETIOLOGY

Anorexia Nervosa

It is believed that underlying developmental disturbances are the primary antecedents of anorexia nervosa.[2] Some time before the illness manifests itself, girls have felt helpless and ineffective in conducting their own lives, and severe discipline over their bodies represents their paramount effort to ward off panic about being completely powerless. This serious illness occurs in individuals who, according to family and school reports, have been unusually good, successful, and gratifying children. With the onset of the disorder, marked changes in behavior appear. A previously compliant girl becomes negativistic, angry, and distrustful. Help and care is stubbornly rejected by the girl, who claims not to need it and insists on the right to be as thin as she wants to be.[2]

Bulimia Nervosa

Bulimia nervosa can begin after a distressing life event (loss of a close relationship), a major disappointment (not making a team), a perceived personal failure (not sticking to a rigid diet), or memories of child abuse. Body weight and shape become the primary focus and the emotional distress gets pushed aside. Very often, a cycle of restricting calories becomes the primary goal to achieve good feelings, and any "mistakes" are "corrected" through purging (vomiting, laxatives, diuretics, excessive exercise, and starvation).[6]

Three major factors are believed to encourage development of bulimia.[6] The first is a biologic vulnerability or predisposition, which supports the etiologic role of genetics, physiology, the endocrine system, and biochemical mechanisms. Next are psychologic predispositions, such as early negative experiences and family interactions that result in psycho-developmental problems. Lastly, sociocultural influences are involved, such as the cultural bias toward thinness and conflicting messages of female success that seem to push independence at the expense of authentic, intimate relationships.

Binge Eating Disorder

Only recently has binge eating disorder (BED) been recognized as a distinct condition; therefore, few studies are available to explain the etiology of this eating disorder.[7] Many people with BED report a history of depression and connect the desire to binge with experiencing negative emotions. Severe food restriction associated with dieting may have an impact on developing BED. Early research suggests that about half of all people with BED had binge episodes before they started to diet. Other areas of research include how brain chemicals and metabolism effect binge eating.

INCIDENCE AND PREVALENCE

Definitive statements as to "the real prevalence of eating disorders" are unwarranted. The research is beset by problems with sampling, methods of assessment, definitions of key concepts such as "*case*" and "*binge*," and the fact that eating disorders are probably underreported,

Exhibit 10–1 Diagnostic Criteria for Eating Disorders

Anorexia Nervosa (Diagnostic Code 307.10)

A. Refusal to maintain body weight at or above a minimally normal weight for age and height, e.g., weight loss leading to maintenance of body weight less than 85% of that expected; or failure to make expected weight gain during period of growth, leading to body weight less than 85% of that expected.

B. Intense fear of gaining weight or becoming fat, even though underweight.

C. Disturbance in the way in which one's body weight, size, or shape is experienced, undue influence of body weight or shape on self-evaluation, or denial of the seriousness of the current low body weight.

D. In postmenarcheal females, amenorrhea, i.e., the absence of at least three consecutive menstrual cycles. (A woman is considered to have amenorrhea if her periods occur only following hormone, e.g., estrogen, administration.)

Specify type:

Restricting Type: during the current episode of Anorexia Nervosa, the person has not regularly engaged in binge-eating or purging behavior (i.e., self-induced vomiting or the misuse of laxatives, diuretics, or enemas)

Binge-Eating/Purging Type: during the current episode of Anorexia Nervosa, the person has regularly engaged in binge-eating or purging behavior (i.e., self-induced vomiting or the misuse of laxatives, diuretics, or enemas)

Bulimia Nervosa (Diagnostic Code 307.51)

A. Recurrent episodes of binge eating (rapid consumption of a large amount of food in a discrete period of time).

B. A feeling of lack of control over eating behavior during the eating binges.

C. The person regularly engages in self-induced vomiting, use of laxatives or diuretics, strict dieting or fasting, or vigorous exercise in order to prevent weight gain.

D. A minimum average of two binge eating episodes a week for at least three months.

E. Persistent overconcern with body shape and weight.

Binge Eating Disorder (Research Criteria)

A. Recurrent episodes of binge eating. An episode of binge eating is characterized by both of the following:
(1) eating, in a discrete period of time (e.g., within any 2-hour period), an amount of food that is definitely larger than most people would eat in a similar period of time under similar circumstances
(2) a sense of lack of control over eating during the episode (e.g., a feeling that one cannot stop eating or control what or how much one is eating)

B. The binge-eating episodes are associated with three (or more) of following:
(1) eating much more rapidly than normal
(2) eating until feeling uncomfortably full
(3) eating large amounts of food when not feeling physically hungry
(4) eating alone because of being embarrassed by how much one is eating
(5) feeling disgusted with oneself, depressed, or very guilty after overeating

C. Marked distress regarding binge eating is present.

D. The binge eating occurs, on average, at least 2 days a week for 6 months.
Note: The method of determining frequency differs from that used for Bulimia Nervosa; future research should address whether the preferred method of setting a frequency threshold is counting the number of days on which binges occur or counting the number of episodes of binge eating.

E. The binge eating is not associated with the regular use of inappropriate compensatory behaviors (e.g., purging, fasting, excessive exercise) and does not occur exclusively during the course of Anorexia Nervosa or Bulimia Nervosa.

Source: Reprinted with permission from the *Diagnostic and Statistical Manual of Mental Disorders,* Fourth Edition,

due to their connection with secretiveness and shame.[8] In general, a conservative estimate of the postpubertal females affected by eating disorders is 5–10%. Girls are at least 9 times more likely than boys to develop any sort of eating disorder. Some researchers believe the incidence of eating disorders is on the rise and that the age of onset continues to decline.[9] Eating disorders have been described as a "wealthy person's disease," implying that only families from the upper income brackets are susceptible to them. Today, male and female patients from all socioeconomic and cultural backgrounds are being diagnosed and treated.[9]

MEDICAL, PSYCHOLOGIC, AND BEHAVIORAL CHANGES

People with eating disorders are at medical risk (see Table 10–1). The complications of anorexia nervosa are primarily a result of starvation. In bulimia, it is the purging behavior that places the person at greatest medical risk. The psychologic and behavioral changes associated with anorexia nervosa are similar to those caused by starvation. In a landmark 1950 study[10] on the long-term effects of a semi-starvation diet on 36 male volunteers, none of the men had an eating disorder prior to joining the study, and they were healthy and psychologically well adjusted. The following parallel features were noticed with these men as they relate to starvation. The same features are evident in patients with food-restrictive bulimia nervosa.[6]

1. obsessions about food and weight
2. unusual eating and drinking habits
3. emotional disturbance
4. social withdrawal
5. binge eating[10]

Table 10–1 Medical Risks Associated with Eating Disorders

Cardiovascular Complications
- Sudden death
- Arrhythmias
- Congestive heart failure
- Cardiac tamponade

Fluid and Electrolyte Disturbances
- Dehydration
- Overhydration
- Hypokalemia
- Hypernatremia

Gastrointestinal Problems
- Esophageal tear (from vomiting)
- Delayed gastric emptying
- Constipation
- Altered bowel function

Reproductive Problems
- Amenorrhea

Musculoskeletal Problems
- Osteoporosis

Endocrine Disturbances
- Hypothyroidism

Dental and Salivary Abnormalities
- Loss of tooth enamel (vomiting)

PROGNOSIS

Do people recover from eating disorders? Recovery is an individual experience. For some, recovery means being symptom free, whereas for others, it means that 10% and not 90% of their lives revolve around their eating-disordered behaviors and attitudes. Understandably, research outcomes on the prognosis of eating disorders are varied. A review of reports on anorexia finds that younger patients represent a higher percentage of recovered patients and have reduced mortality, in comparison with older patients.[9] The general consensus of outcome studies is as follows: 40% of all patients totally recover, 30% are improved, and 30% are chronically afflicted. Approximately 5% of chronically afflicted patients with anorexia nervosa will die as a result of the illness.

The prognosis for bulimia nervosa and BED has not been investigated as thoroughly. Outcome studies show that 85% of patients recover in 5 years or less.[7] Overall, the effects of different treatment approaches on long-term outcome have not been studied. Given that a longer duration of illness is associated with a lesser chance of recovery, earlier intervention may boost the chances of a better outcome. Therefore, the earlier the intervention, the better the prognosis.[9]

TREATMENT

The Counseling Relationship

The role of the dietitian treating eating disorders has evolved into one with a nutrition therapy focus. Eating disorder patients have underlying psychologic disturbances that range from mild depression to severe personality disorders.[11,12] The dietitian must have specialized counseling skills, including the psychotherapeutic model of counseling, to effectively blend the nutrition and psychologic issues inherent in working with this patient population. Counseling skills can be acquired through professional supervision, conferences, and continuing education.[13–16] Ongoing supervision from a mental health professional or an experienced nutrition therapist can enhance the dietitian's effectiveness. Dietitians have also become licensed professional counselors and mental health counselors.

The Initial Interview

The initial interview provides the dietitian with the first opportunity to develop a therapeutic alliance with the patient while gathering information critical to the assessment. Developing an alliance with the patient is important in building a trusting relationship. Ensuring an atmosphere of acceptance during the interview allows the patient to feel comfortable and to share openly. Exhibit 10–2 lists the topics to cover during the initial interview. In addition to the information gathered from the initial interview, a nutrition assessment should include—at a minimum—the data listed in Exhibit 10–3.

Treatment Goals

Strategies to implement nutrition rehabilitation goals include

1. education about food, weight, body composition, and normal growth and development;
2. cognitive-behavioral therapy; and
3. psychoeducation.

Treatment areas to consider are

1. understanding what areas of concern the patient is interested in changing,
2. implementing goals to challenge and change maladaptive behaviors and thoughts, and
3. exploring the patient's readiness for change.[16]

When developing a treatment plan, it is important to view change as a process and not as a single event. Behavior change expert James Prochaska, PhD, developed a six-

Exhibit 10–2 Important Topics for Initial Interviews

1. *Background information*
   - Diagnosis
   - Age and age of onset
   - Treatment history: treaters, time in treatment
   - Weight: premorbid and current
   - Height
   - Menstruation history: last menstrual period, typical cycle
2. *Food/dieting/exercise history*
   - "Usual" intake prior to diagnosis
   - Typical day's intake or food frequency or 24-hour recall
   - Safe and forbidden foods
   - Food likes and dislikes
   - Weight loss techniques employed
   - Exercise and activity level: current and premorbid
3. *Weight history*
   - History of weight conflicts
   - Weight high/low
   - Patient's goal weight
4. *Binge/purge activity*
   - Frequency of binges
   - Method of purging
   - Frequency of purging
   - Subjective report on severity of bingeing/purging
5. *Family history*
   - Family members at home
   - Food/dieting/exercise/weight conflicts among other members
   - Heights and weights of family members
   - History of psychiatric illness, especially affective illness
   - General health status of family members
6. *Social history*
   - School and grade
   - Overall school performance: current and premorbid
   - Peer interactions: current and premorbid
7. *Physical status*
   - General observations: hair loss; dry, flaking skin; swollen parotid glands; calluses on knuckles
   - Reported clinical effects of starvation: decreased tolerance to cold, poor sleep habits, increased moodiness
8. *Medication and substance use*
   - Prescription medication
   - Over-the-counter medication, including laxatives, diuretics, and vomiting agents, such as ipecac
   - Alcohol use
   - Other substance use

stage model of behavior change to identify and specify what an individual needs and does at various points in the change process.[16]

The six stages of behavior change are:

- Precontemplation—patient has no intention of taking action within the next 6 months
- Contemplation—patient intends to take action within the next 6 months

Exhibit 10–3 Additional Data Needed for the Initial Assessment

1. *Growth data*
   - Frame size
   - Height
   - Weight
   - Weight-for-length (when appropriate for age)
   - Ideal body weight range for height (using National Center for Health Statistics tables or the Metropolitan Life Insurance tables)
   - Percent ideal body weight for height
2. *Energy*
   - Basal energy expenditure for ideal body weight for height
   - Requirement for weight gain (BEE × 1.5)
3. *Body composition data (if available)*
   - Triceps skinfold measurement
   - Electrical impedance calibration
4. *Biochemical data with nutritional implications*
   - Electrolyte balance
   - Calcium status (bone scan when indicated)
   - Lipid status (cholesterol level elevated with starvation)
   - Phosphorus status
   - Thiamin status
   - Urine specific gravity

- Preparation—patient intends to take action within the next 30 days and has taken some behavioral steps in this direction
- Action—patient has adopted this behavior for less than 6 months
- Maintenance—patient has adopted this behavior for more than 6 months
- Termination Phase—patient behavior pattern is now habitual and requires little conscious thought

Prochaska's Model of Change is helpful to dietitians in assessing where patients fall along a behavioral continuum, which, in turn, can help establish appropriate nutrition rehabilitation goals.

An important team goal is to determine the rules concerning communication between the clinician and the patient under 18, as well as the patient's parent(s). As parents are responsible for the health of their child, they need to be privy to certain information. Deciding what information from the patient gets shared with parents must be determined at the onset of treatment. Without these guidelines, it may be difficult to establish an alliance, which depends on trust and confidentiality. Consulting with other team members may help in establishing these guidelines.

Hospitalization

The success of outpatient nutrition counseling depends in part on establishing a long-term collaborative relationship between the patient and dietitian.[13] However, some patients will require hospitalization. The decision to hospitalize a patient is based on team findings of signs of medical and/or psychologic crisis. These may include a drop in weight (eg, >40% loss of premorbid weight or >30% loss within a 3-month period), severe metabolic disturbances, severe depression or suicide risk, severe bingeing and purging, psychosis, or family crisis.[2,17]

Inpatient and Outpatient Treatment Strategies

This section will include treatment options for patients needing weight rehabilitation (for anorexia nervosa and low-weight bulimia) and management of the binge/purge cycle or bingeing (for BED).

Three key areas of nutrition intervention will be discussed:

1. Weight status and nutritional rehabilitation
2. Normalization of eating patterns
3. Education; nutrition, and psychoeducation

Weight Status and Nutritional Rehabilitation

The physical, behavioral, and psychologic effects of starvation on humans were studied by Keys et al in the 1940s.[10] It was determined that weight loss and malnutrition due to food deprivation promote unusual eating behaviors (prolongation of meals, increased use of seasonings and spices, secretive and ritualized eating, food hoarding, and obsessive thoughts). Additional effects secondary to starvation were social isolation, impaired concentration, apathy, and mood swings. Improving nutritional status reversed these consequences, although for some, bingeing behavior erupted. In outpatients maintaining low body weights despite eating calorie levels adequate for weight gain, increased physical activity is likely to account for the lack of weight change.[18] Nutrition intervention to relieve the effects of starvation is accepted as a necessary prerequisite to successful psychiatric intervention in the anorexia nervosa patient.[19]

Determining the calorie amount necessary for weight gain in patients with anorexia nervosa is a primary concern of the dietitian. Great variation is found in this population when the caloric cost of weight gain is quantified. In a study conducted by Dempsey, the excess calories necessary to gain 1 kg of body weight ranged from 5,569 to 15,619 kcal; the mean was 9,768 kcal/week.[20] Another study found that 34 kcal/lb of current body weight is a beginning estimate for weight restoration in anorexia nervosa.[21] It is important to note that long-term weight changes during nutritional rehabilitation in anorexia nervosa are meaningful indicators of caloric balance, but short-term weight changes (daily, weekly) are not.[20] On any given day, body weight in healthy, young women can fluctuate by 0.5–1 kg.[22] When a patient first starts on a nutritional rehabilitation program, rapid weight gain can occur. This is a result of increased retention of water through expansion of the extracellular compartment, retention of electrolytes, and restoration of liver and muscle glycogen.[19] Weight gain that is too rapid can precipitate congestive heart failure, gastric dilation, and malabsorption.[18] A recent study found that increasing a 4-day weight gain criterion from 0.8 to 1.2 pounds using behavior-contracting intervention was associated with an increase in the rate of weight gain without an accompanying increase in the complications associated with refeeding.[23] Studies looking at the metabolic effects of the "refeeding" process show that physiologic disturbances contribute to the maintenance of weight after patients complete a weight restoration program. Kaye[24] looked at weight gain in non-bulimic and bulimic anorexics. Nonbulimic anorexics require 30–50% more calories than do bulimic anorexics to maintain a stable weight. This finding was noted at low weights and at intervals after weight restoration.[24]

Body composition changes after refeeding are difficult to quantify, due to the marked shifts in fluid balance. Although difficult to measure accurately, levels of body fat at the end phase of feeding may be an important component of physiologic outcome. A critical amount of body fat may be necessary for return of menses, which is often used as an indicator of normal physiologic function and, presumably, for improved calcium balance and bone status.[19]

Normalization of Eating Patterns: Refeeding and Rethinking

The refeeding period often marks the beginning of normalized eating patterns. Patients with severe cachexia and electrolyte imbalance may receive peripheral hyperalimentation or nasogastric tube feedings.[3,20] Because of the increased medical and psychologic risks associated with these refeeding methods, they are recommended for acute interventions only. Refeeding with food and oral supplements are the treatments of choice. Meals should consist of adequate amounts of carbohydrate, protein, and fat. The dietitian helps the patient to select acceptable food, thereby starting the process of relearning how to eat normally. A critical balance exists between allowing gradual, small changes in a patient with very restricted eating patterns and ensuring adequate nutrition and weight gain. Reminding the patient that the treatment team does not want the patient's weight gain to be out of control but reflective of physiologic changes may soothe fears about adding new foods and increasing the amount of calories consumed. Specific principles for nutritional intervention for anorexia nervosa were developed by Rock:[25]

1. Provide a nutritionally balanced diet (this may be varied according to patient preferences, eg, vegetarian).
2. Provide multivitamin-mineral supplements at Recommended Dietary Allowance (RDA) levels.
3. Provide dietary fiber from grain sources to enhance elimination.
4. Whenever possible, permit small, frequent feedings to reduce sensation of bloating.
5. Use liquid supplements (eg, Boost, Instant Breakfast, etc.) when the patient cannot achieve goal intake via foods.
6. Provide cold or room-temperature food to reduce satiety sensations.
7. Reduce caffeine intake if appropriate.

Bulimic patients of normal or excess body weight often present with a history of attempts to control weight through severe caloric restriction.[12] Foods become categorized as "good" and "bad" or "safe" and "forbidden." Low-fat foods (eg, fruits, vegetables, rice cakes, nonfat yogurt) become the staples at meals, leading to decreased satiety at meals and an increased vulnerability to bingeing. Food intake patterns are usually quite rigid, and the patient often believes that this seemingly controlled intake is healthy and is the only way to eat to lose or maintain weight. These unrealistic diet restrictions need to be met with clear guidelines that promote satiety, thereby reducing the risk of bingeing. Specific recommendations for nutrition intervention are as follows:[24]

1. Provide well-balanced diets and meals to increase satiety.
2. Increase the variety of foods consumed.
3. Include warm foods rather than cold or room-temperature foods to increase meal satiety.
4. Choose high-fiber foods to increase satiety and aid in digestion.
5. Plan meals and snacks.

Additionally, other areas need to be addressed, such as the patient's:

1. attitudes about food and weight
2. understanding of his or her eating patterns and the physiologic, behavioral, and emotional role of food
3. ability to disconnect weight status from self-esteem

Self-monitoring tools can be helpful in revealing to the patient his or her food beliefs and eating patterns. Through recognition of certain harmful or self-defeating thoughts and behaviors, choices can be made to find alternatives.[14] Records or journals should include facts, state of mind, and some reflection about his or her emotional world, for example:

1. type and amount of food eaten
2. time of day
3. degree of hunger (low, medium, high) and fullness (low, medium, high)
4. binge/purge activity
5. self-talk (positive and negative)
6. affective changes (feelings, thoughts, concerns).

Reviewing these journals with a patient can help to identify problems and to quantify progress toward the patient's goals.

Education: Psychoeducation and Nutrition

It is commonly believed that patients with eating disorders know more about nutrition than does the average person. Although this may be true, the manner in which they practice their knowledge does not keep them healthy. Nutrition education is a critical component of treatment. For the hospitalized patient, specialized nutrition classes may be implemented to address concerns. Group classes create an environment in which patients may feel freer to discuss difficult emotional issues related to weight and food, and information regarding nutrition facts and fallacies may be efficiently imparted. The dietitian should instruct outpatients with the same information in individual counseling sessions. Topics to cover in meetings include the following:

1. sociocultural influences on weight and body image
2. the physiologic, behavioral, and emotional effects of food restricting
3. facts about metabolism, weight gain, and body composition
4. food and eating beliefs
5. body image
6. core minimums of daily food groups
7. micro- and macronutrient needs for health (growth, menses, bone development, etc.)

The psychoeducational component of patient education expands on nutrition topics by including information about how cultural factors and emotional responses to weight regulation and dieting affect one's thinking about self and self-worth.[24] A list of recommended reading on the sociocultural issues surrounding eating disorders is found at the end of the chapter. The information in these publications will help the clinician develop a useful framework in which to impart the psychoeducational treatment component.

CASE STUDY: ANOREXIA NERVOSA

Sarah is a 15 1/4-year-old female presenting with rapid weight loss over the past 4 months. She meets all criteria for anorexia nervosa. She denies any laxative or diuretic use or vomiting. This is her second hospitalization. Nutrition intervention during the first hospitalization consisted of 1,500 kcal of liquid supplement per day and bed rest. When discharged, she continued to lose weight. At the time of this admission, Sarah had not received any psychiatric intervention. When Sarah is asked about her understanding of why she is in the hospital, she acknowledges that it is because of her low weight, although she sees nothing wrong with it: "I know I would look and feel better if I could lose more weight." Four months earlier, a girl on the track team introduced Sarah to the benefits of eating a low-fat diet. Sarah took the information to heart and vehemently began a rigid diet with no fat. Her usual weight was 122 lb (height 5 feet, 4 inches), and she had never before dieted to lose weight. She could not remember growing up feeling fat but did remember her father commenting after her returning from a physical, "How could you weigh that much?" Sarah's current daily intake is less than 1,000 kcal/day. During the day, she runs 4 miles, completes a 1-hour aerobics tape, and walks whenever she gets the chance. She will not allow herself any fat and eats the same thing every day. Before the anorexia, Sarah was interested in every type of food and was known to occasionally "chow" (eat large quantities of food). Sarah's last menstrual period was 3 months ago, at a weight of 109 pounds. She reports an increased intolerance to cold, difficulty sleeping, irritability, and some hair loss. Sarah's parents want her to "get it together" and get better: "She's so smart, why can't she beat this thing?" "You will be missing out on so much if you stay sick." Neither parent can understand why their daughter is starving herself.

Clinical Parameters

- Height: 5 feet, 4 inches
- Weight: 96 lb
- Frame size: medium
- Ideal body weight range:[24] 113–128 lb
- Premorbid body weight: 122 lb
- Calories required for weight gain: 96 × 34 kcal/lb=3,264 and/or basal energy expenditure (BEE) × 1.5, using the average kcal/day as a goal

Recommendations for Refeeding

Start calorie level at 1250 kcal/day (composition: carbohydrate 55%, protein 20%, fat 25%). Provide a multivitamin with minerals. Increase calories in a stepwise fashion up to caloric requirement for weight restoration to within 5% of ideal body weight range for height. For each day that weight does not increase by 0.2 kg, 500-calorie supplements should be given. The weekly weight gain goal is 1.2 kg; if it is not reached, the daily calorie ration is to increase by 500 kcal. Meals should consist of a variety of foods from all food groups. Develop meal plans reflecting a variety of calorie levels. Use American Diabetic Association exchange lists to develop meals. Have the patient choose meals, emphasizing a variety of foods; limit patient dislikes to three foods. Time parameters must be set for completion of meals; for example, 30 minutes per meal. When calories are increased, the dietitian may choose to add snacks (250- or 500-kcal snacks at 10 AM, 2 PM, or 8 PM). Review nutritional guidelines for addressing delayed gastric emptying: provide dietary fiber from grain sources and small, frequent feedings when possible. Providing cold or room-temperature foods may decrease satiety sensations.

Activity

Exercise should be limited; specific recommendations should be made. For example, the patient may be allowed to stretch 30 minutes per day for first week, add 30-minute walks per day during the second week (depending on weight gain and mental status), and increase exercise up to a healthy, "normalized" level with progress in treatment.

Education

See recommendations in "Education: Nutrition and Psychoeducation" section, earlier in this chapter.

Family Work

Meetings with the family members, especially parents, are an important component of treatment. These meetings can provide a time to discuss anorexia nervosa, the varied effects of starvation, and calorie and nutrient needs. Meetings with parents should be arranged to review changes, progress with treatment, and plans for outpatient work. Parents need to understand the food plan, even though they are not often responsible for monitoring intake. The medical doctor should be responsible for the patient's weight status and should inform the dietitian of the need for increasing caloric intake when there is weight loss. Ultimately, patients need to be responsible for their own food intake and their overall health.

CASE STUDY: BULIMIA NERVOSA

Jen is a 14 1/2-year-old presenting with bulimia nervosa. The bingeing and purging started 1 year ago, then ended for 3 months. Jen was symptom-free until the fall, when she started at a new school and her parents had separated. She started dieting and lost 15% of her usual weight. At this point, her mother took her to a therapist, and she stopped dieting. The bulimic symptoms returned when she started gaining back the weight she had lost. Jen has never been hospitalized. Jen is the youngest of three children; she has two sisters, aged 19 and 21. Her oldest sister is somewhat overweight, and the middle sister exercises excessively and has shown signs of bulimia. Jen's father is a successful businessman and has always been a bit overweight but relies on exercise to keep in shape. Jen's mother is starting her own food business, has a "perfect" body, and follows a low-fat meal plan to keep her shape. Jen's peer relations have varied over the years, due to school changes. She talks about being lonely for friends but at the same time "puts down" the kids at her school. Jen is an average student, maintaining a high C average. Her parents de-emphasize grades and emphasize interpersonal relationships. Although part of her wants to stop the bulimia, she believes that the only way she can control her weight is to vomit. Her daily intake is as follows: no breakfast, no lunch, snack food before tennis practice, a big dinner, and bingeing all night. Jen throws up once before she goes to bed. Bulimia is her biggest secret, and at one point, she said, "If you only knew how bad it was."

Clinical Parameters

- Height: 5 feet, 7 inches
- Weight: 143 lb
- Frame size: medium
- Ideal body weight range: 125–140 lb
- Percent body fat: 17% (quite muscular, due to sports and inherited body type from father)
- BEE: 1,386 requirement; for maintenance, BEE × 30%=1,800 kcal

Treatment Plan

- weekly visits with psychiatrist
- weekly visits with dietitian
- periodic meetings with parents and dietitian
- family therapy
- medical follow-up

Recommendations for Normalization of Eating Patterns

Establish patient goals for "normal" eating. Set the calorie level for weight maintenance to model weight control and to reduce the risk of increased hunger and increased vulnerability to bingeing. Develop a meal plan with the following in mind: The patient should develop a list of "safe" and "forbidden" foods. Most often, the "safe" foods are not adequate for meeting nutrient needs and creating satiety. Therefore,

1. find out why certain foods are forbidden and dispel any myths, and
2. slowly negotiate adding foods from forbidden list to meal plan.

Ensure that the patient eats at least three regular meals per day. Consider implementing small, frequent meals, if that would help. Use food records to monitor eating patterns and follow changes. (However, for a variety of reasons, some patients are not able to complete food records; therapeutically, it is best to work with what the patient feels comfortable doing.) Help the patient to recognize internal and external cues for bingeing and purging behavior and to develop alternative behaviors when cues occur.

Activity

Develop exercise guidelines that support moderation and are achievable.

Education

The patient needs to learn how to eat in a way that promotes emotional and physical health. Dispelling diet myths, eliminating food rules, and letting go of value judgments associated with eating or not eating certain foods are crucial for recovery. Strict meal plans and weekly weigh-ins are counterproductive for this process. The patient needs to be reminded that people are not good or bad because of the food they eat. Food has such power over the patient that it becomes a barometer for self-esteem. Helping the patient to feel he or she has choices and can make choices, gives back a sense of control.

REFERENCES

1. Levine M. *How Schools Can Combat Student Eating Disorders: Anorexia Nervosa and Bulimia*. Washington, DC: National Education Association; 1987.
2. Garner D, Garfinkel P. *Handbook of Psychotherapy for Anorexia Nervosa and Bulimia Nervosa*. New York: Guilford Press; 1985.
3. American Dietetic Association. Position of the American Dietetic Association: Nutrition intervention in the treatment of anorexia nervosa, bulimia nervosa and binge eating. *J Am Diet Assoc*. 1994;94:902–907.
4. Smolak L, Levine M. Toward an empirical basis for primary prevention of eating problems with elementary school children. *Eating Disord.* 1994;2:19.
5. American Psychiatric Association. *Diagnostic and Statistical Manual of Mental Disorders*. 4th ed. Washington, DC: American Psychiatric Association; 1994.
6. Johnson C, Connors M. *The Etiology and Treatment of Bulimia Nervosa*. New York: Basic Books; 1987.
7. US Dept HHS *Public HealthService*, NIH Pub. No. 94-3589, Nov; 1993:2.
8. Levine M. The prevalence of eating disorders: some tentative facts. *Eating Disord Awareness Prevent*. Fact sheet. 1996.
9. Berg F. *Afraid to Eat: Children and Teens in Weight Crisis*. Hettinger, ND: Healthy Weight Publishing Network;1997:69.
10. Keys A, Brozek J, Henshel A, et al. *The Biology of Human Starvation*. Minneapolis, MN: University of Minnesota Press; 1950.
11. Garfinkel P, Garner D. *Anorexia Nervosa: A Multidimensional Perspective*. New York: Brunner Mazel; 1982.
12. Swift W, Andrews D, Barklage NE. The relationship between affective disorder and eating disorders: a review of the literature. *Am J Psychiatry*. 1989;149:290–299.
13. Snetselaar L. *Nutrition Counseling Skills*. 2nd ed. Gaithersburg, MD: Aspen Publishers; 1989.
14. Reiff D, Lampson R. *Eating Disorders: Nutrition Therapy in the Recovery Process*. Gaithersburg, MD: Aspen Publishers; 1992.
15. Kratina K, King NL, Hayes D. *Moving Away from Diet*. Lake Dallas, TX: Helm Seminars; 1996.
16. Helm KK, Klawitter B. *Nutrition Therapy: Advanced Counseling Skills*. Lake Dallas, TX: Helm Seminars; 1995:3–15.
17. Prochaska J, Norcross J, DiClemente C. *Changing for Good.* New York: William Morrow Company; 1994.
18. Herzog D, Copeland P. Eating disorders. *N Engl J Med.* 1985;313:295–303.
19. Rock CL, Curran-Calantano J. Nutritional disorders of anorexia: a review. *Int J Eating Disord.* 1994:15:187–203.
20. Dempsey DT, Crosby LO, Pertschuk MJ, et al. Weight gain and nutritional efficacy in anorexia nervosa. *Am J Clin Nutr.* 1984;39:236–242.
21. Walker J, Roberts SL, Halmik KA, et al. Caloric requirements for weight gain in anorexia nervosa. *Am J Clin Nutr*. 1979;32:1396–1400.
22. Robinson M, Watson P. Day-to-day variations in body weight of young women. *Br J Nutr*. 1965;19:225–235.
23. Solanto M, Jacobson M, Heller L, Golden N, Hertz, S. Rate of weight gain of inpatients with anorexia nervosa under two behavioral contracts. *Pediatrics*. 1994;93: 989–991.
24. Kaye WH, Gwirtsman HE, Obarzanek E, et al. Caloric intake necessary for weight maintenance in anorexia nervosa: nonbulimics require greater caloric intake than bulimics. *Am J Clin Nutr*. 1986;44:435–443.
25. Rock CL, Yager J. Nutrition and eating disorders: a primer for clinicians. *Int J Eating Disord*. 1987;6:267–279.

RECOMMENDED READINGS

Agras WS and Apple R. *Overcoming Eating Disorders: Therapist's Guide*. 1997.

Cash, TF. *The Body Image Workbook: An 8-Step Program for Learning to Like Your Looks*. New Harbinger Publications; 1997.

Garner DM and Garfinkel PE, eds. *Handbook of Treatment for Anorexia Nervosa and Bulimia*, 2nd ed. Guilford Press; 1997.

Kratina K, King NL, Hayes D. *Moving Away from Diet*. Lake Dallas, TX: Helm Seminars; 1996.

Werne J, ed. *Treating Eating Disorders*. San Francisco: Jossey-Bass, 1996.

ASSOCIATIONS

Eating Disorders Awareness and Prevention, Inc. (EDAP)
603 Stewart Street, Suite 803
Seattle, WA 98101
206-382-3587
http://members.aol.com/edapinc
Provides extensive resources and educational materials for clinicians and the public.

Massachusetts Eating Disorders Association (MEDA)
92 Pearl Street
Newton, MA 02458
617-558-1881
Masseating@aol.com

American Anorexia/Bulimia Association, Inc.
165 W. 46th Street
Suite 1108
New York, NY 10036
212-575-6200
amanbu@aol.com

National Association of Anorexia Nervosa and Associated Disorders
P.O. Box 7
Highland Park, IL 60035
847-831-3438
Anad20@aol.com

EDUCATIONAL MATERIALS

See EDAP web site for "Resources for the Prevention of Eating Disorders."

Gurze Books
P.O. Box 2238
Carlsbad, CA 92018
800-756-7533
http://gurze.com

CHAPTER 11

Sports Nutrition for Children and Adolescents

Nancy L. Nevin-Folino

PHYSICAL ACTIVITY

Activity should be encouraged for every child in order to initiate lifetime habits of physical exercise.[1] Physical involvement could determine the long-term health of the population to come. Benefits directly associated with physical activity include reduced incidence of coronary heart disease and other degenerative diseases, maintenance of desired weight for height, and lessened symptoms of anxiety and depression.[2,3] Exercise also provides children opportunities for developing basic communication skills and social interaction, which improves self-esteem and confidence.[3] Table 11–1 outlines a variety of different levels of activity for children and adolescents, with age recommendations, associated dietary comments, fluid needs, and appropriate health assessments.

Attitudes about physical activity and an active lifestyle are often formed in the first ten years of life.[4] Children's health fitness is associated with the physical behaviors of parents; therefore, family fitness should be promoted.[5]

PHYSIOLOGIC EFFECTS OF EXERCISE

Exercise and training produce many physiologic effects in children. Sports participation should be enjoyable and beneficial to the child and can be so if the healthy child is matched correctly to the sport.

Cardiorespiratory exercise is important for children and adolescents because of the associated lifelong benefits.[1] Some of the effects of cardiorespiratory exercise on the child are as follows:[3–7]

- improves strength and flexibility
- conditions the cardiorespiratory system
- increases endurance
- develops power, agility, and speed
- aids in development of muscles
- exercises neuromuscular skill
- controls percentage of body fat
- provides mental well-being

To achieve cardiorespiratory benefits, the exercise should be at least 20 minutes in duration, use large muscles, produce mild perspiration, and cause the heart to beat at 60–80% of maximum rate.[6,7] A cardiorespiratory activity is recommended three to five times a week. See Table 11–2 for heart beat rates for different ages.

Deleterious consequences of exercise can be prevented. Assessment from a physician and health professionals before exercise or sport involvement is strongly recommended.[8] For training and participation in competitive sports, determination of the match of maturation age with the sport, injury risk, and general health status should be done prior to participation by a pediatrician or a physician trained in sports medicine.[8,9] Education on proper training, diet, and injury prevention should also be given.[7] Coaches

Table 11–1 Exercise Levels with Age, Nutrition, Fluid, and Health Assessment Guidelines

Definitions	*Examples (Not Inclusive)*	*Recommended Age*	*Nutrition Comments*	*Fluid Intake*	*Recommended Health Assessment*
1. ROUTINE: The duration of the activity is less than 20 min, and it may or may not reach 60% of maximum heart beat rate.	Recess play, casual walking, recreational noncontinual sport (i.e., T-ball, volleyball)	Minimum activity level for any age	Normal nutrition for age from the basic food groups	Normal for age	Yearly routine exam from a pediatrician or physician for all ages of children.
2. HEALTH FITNESS: 60%–80% of maximum heart beat rate is achieved for greater than 20 min at least three times per week for a minimum of 6 months. The activity should involve muscular strength and flexibility.	Brisk walking, jogging, running, cycling, hiking, swimming, dancing	Preferred level for any age	Normal nutrition for age from the basic food groups. If desired weight for height, possibly more calories.	Good hydration, especially in adverse weather. Normal requirements for age and replacement of lost fluid from activity.	Yearly routine exam from a pediatrician or physician for all ages of children. Education from a physician or health professional on healthy practices (diet, fluid, injury prevention, warm-up and cool-down techniques, etc.). Immediate attention from an appropriate health professional for an injury or insult.
3. COMPETITIVE SPORTS: An activity less than or equal to 6 months that consists of team involvement, preseason training, and competing either as a team member	Swimming, gymnastics, diving, volleyball, wrestling, sprinting, relay,	Junior high age and above	Nutrition assessment, recommendations, and education, preferably from a registered dietitian, for an individual's season intake to	Pre-event, event, and postevent (or prepractice and postpractice) hydration. Good hydration at other times.	Preparticipation assessment by a health team consisting of a physician, dietitian, nurse or nurse practitioner, and

Source: Data from references 4, 5, 9, 17, 26, and 38 to 40.

or individually at an intramural or interschool level.	football, soccer, basketball, tennis, field hockey, cross country.		achieve weight and body composition for the sport. Recommendations will be dependent on type of activity, duration, and intensity.	Electrolyte replacement may be needed if heavy sweating occurs or in adverse weather conditions.	possibly a physical therapist. Examination as well as education should be given to students at this time. Immediate attention from an appropriate health professional for any injury or insult during the sports season.
3a. Competitive < 6 months: Short endurance—intense activity that lasts for 20 min or less.	As above	Junior high age and above	2 g pro/kg for growing athletes ≥ 1 g pro/kg for mature athletes		
3b. Competitive <6 months: Long endurance—activity, intense or nonintense, that lasts for longer than 20 min.	As above	High school age and above	May need carbohydrate during the event if long in duration (> 4 h). Modified carbohydrate loading (normal diet, intense exercise 7–4 days before, high carbohydrate diet 3–1 days before event) no more than 2–3 times per year.	Electrolyte replacement needs assessed and replacement given if necessary.	

Table 11–1 continued

Definitions	*Examples (Not Inclusive)*	*Recommended Age*	*Nutrition Comments*	*Fluid Intake*	*Recommended Health Assessment*
4. COMPETITIVE SPORTS: Longer than 6 months. Same as Competitive, above, but usually involved at a personal level other than school.	Same as 3, above, but may include state or national competition	High school age and above	Same as 3, above	Same as 3, above	As above. It is very important that a physician determine that the maturation age of the participant is appropriate for the sport.
4a. Competitive ≥ 6 months: Short endurance—same as above.	As above				
4b. Competitive ≥ 6 months: Long endurance—same as above.	As above				
5. PERFORMING: An activity that requires dedicated practice (several times a week) to perform with a group or individually a routine lasting anywhere from 5 min to 1 hr (or longer) in competition or performance.	Ballet, dance, or gymnastics	Junior high age and above as determined by a physician	Nutrition assessment, recommendations, and education provided, preferably by a registered dietitian due to the usually restricted intake to achieve desired weight for performance.	Normal hydration and replacement of lost fluids from practice or performance	Preparticipation assessment by a physician, dietitian, and possibly an orthopedist or physical therapist. Injury attention as in competitive sports.

6. MARCHING BAND: Involvement with a band that competes or performs in marching or choreographed performance. Includes preseason training as well as competition or performance.	High school marching or competing bands	Junior high age and above	Nutrition assessment, recommendations, and education, preferably from a registered dietitian in a group setting, or individually if necessary.	As in 3a, 3b, above	Same as in 2 or 3a, 3b, above. Nutrition attention by a registered dietitian if the participant is less than 85% or greater than 120% of desired weight for height.
7. SEASONAL: Intramural involvement with a team or individual activity not based heavily on winning but just participation. Practice required. May or may not last longer than 20 min three or more times a week, but activity is not sustained longer than 2 or 3 months.	Soccer, softball, swimming lessons	All ages	As in 2, above	As in 3a, 3b, above	Preparticipation assessment by a pediatrician or physician, as in 2, above. Nutrition attention by a registered dietitian if the participant is less than 85% or greater than 120% of desired weight for height.

Table 11–2 Suggested Training Heart Rates*

	Heart Rate (beats/min)		
Age (yr)	*Maximum*	*80%*	*60%*
5–8	220	176	132
10	210	168	126
11	209	167	125
12	208	166	125
13	207	165	124
14	206	165	123
15	205	164	123
16	204	163	122
17	203	162	122
18	202	162	121

*These numbers are taken from a variety of sources and are suggested guidelines initially developed for training athletes. Individuals will vary. If target heart rate seems too hard to maintain, accept a lower one, and conversely, if the target rate does not seem high enough to make one perspire, work harder.

Source: Adapted with permission from *Pediatrics in Review,* Vol. 10, pages 141–148, 1988.

and trainers should be conscious of the health consequences of sports and refer team members who develop risks during the season to the appropriate health professional (physician, dietitian, orthopedist, physical therapist, etc.). See Table 11–1 for preparticipation health assessment recommendations.

NUTRITIONAL CONCERNS

Nutritional needs of children involved in routine exercise or sports are for adequate energy supplies that come from the recommended dietary intake for age (see Appendix K). This should include a variety of food products emphasizing a normal, balanced diet. If extra calories are needed, they should come from healthful food choices within the Food Guide Pyramid.[10–12] (See Appendix L.) Fluid needs include the amount required for normal hydration for age and weight plus extra for training, participation, and cool-down activity.[13–16] It is imperative that the school-age athlete is given education on how the young body uses fluid, when the body needs more fluid, and why fluid needs for children are different. Dehydration and its symptoms should be discussed in detail.[14–16]

There is no indication that there are increased needs for any other nutrient beyond the Recommended Dietary Allowances (RDAs), although some teens may need more protein during periods of rapid growth (see Chapter 5). In this instance, protein needs should be evaluated on an individual basis by a registered dietitian. If, in the initial diet review, deficiencies in intake are identified—calcium, iron, or any other nutrient—the child or teen athlete should receive individualized nutrition counseling. Independent and arbitrary use of vitamins and minerals is discouraged in youth. Over-the-counter supplements should be evaluated carefully.

Guidelines for base calorie needs are outlined in the RDAs.[17] (See Appendix K.) The need to increase calorie allotments for an activity will depend on the child's age, sex, present weight, desired weight, particular sport, and level of involvement. Many factors for calorie needs vary with each child. Achieving desired weight and maintaining the weight will be the indicators of adequate calories (see Table 11–3). Because of the variance in the age of sexual development for children and the connection of body fat composition to development, body fat measurement should not be used as a qualification of weight status or goal, as it is in adults.[10,11] Percent of fat content of the child's body can be monitored for changes throughout a sports season, but the importance of the change is emphasized here because of the connection to maturation.[14] A skilled professional should do body fat measurements to ensure accurate measurements and evaluation. Instructors and students need guidance in altering weight to ensure that safe practices are followed. Frequent monitoring is recommended if weight change is desired to prevent too rapid a weight gain or loss. Rapid body changes can and will affect performance, so weight changes should be started prior to the sports season.[15,16]

Fluid requirements should be emphasized to the growing athlete so that performance is not compromised by dehydration.[15] (See Table 11–4.) Table 11–5 compares beverages frequently consumed and available to youths. This chart also includes data on sports nutritional supplements. The need for so much instruction provides an excellent opportunity for the registered dietitian to be involved prior to training season as a consultant to groups sponsoring organized sports or activities and to the participating youth.[10,11]

EXERCISE RECOMMENDATIONS IN SPECIFIC GROUPS

Newborns to Age 3

An appropriately stimulating environment for infant activity sets the stage for regular exercise as the child grows. Unstructured, safe play without special exercise equipment can provide all that the infant needs for healthy development.[19] Playpens and walkers restrict babies from exploring and from fully using their muscles or developing their coordination and are not recommended for play time.

Ages 3–8 Years

Exercise interest should be piqued during these years to develop habits of routine participation in enjoyable physical activity.[5] Parental habits will be mimicked, so, ideally, the entire family should be committed to physical activity.[1,4] Group as well as unorganized play also fosters normal physical and social development of children. At this age, it is vital that the activities offered focus on participation and not on the end-all goal of winning. Caution should be used so that organized sports at this age are for the children, not extended zealousness of the parents.[12]

Ages 8–12 Years

The foundations of health should be established at this formative age to help the child begin a lifelong pattern of regular exercise using the cardiorespiratory system. Activity programs should consist of exercise that can be carried into adulthood.[6] School-age children should be encouraged to participate in casual, unorganized activity, school-sponsored competitive sport, or community sport leagues.[1] School-age children accrue the same psychosocial and physical benefits of sports that younger children gain.

If a child is considering serious sports involvement and/or competition, his or her maturation level should be determined by a health professional.[8,13,14] The vast range of pubertal development is remarkable at this age, and the early maturer will excel in a sport because of his or her maturity-associated skill and muscular level. This advantage does not always continue as the child gets older.[20] Matching an early maturer with a late maturer could cause the latter to lose interest in sports permanently. Explanation

Table 11–3 Calorie Requirements*

	Recommended Daily Allowances kcal/lb/d				Competitive‡			Long Endurance§		
Age	*Low Calorie*	*Median Calorie*	*High Calorie*	*Health Fitness*†	*Weight Loss*	*Weight Stable*	*Weight Gain*	*Weight Loss*	*Weight Stable*	*Weight Gain*
4–6	30	41	52	+3	—	—	—	—	—	—
7–10	27	39	54	+3	—	+8	+16	—	—	—
Males										
11–14	20	27	37	+2	+2	+7	+12	+19	+24	+29
15–18	14	19	27	+2	+1	+5	+8	+13	+16	+20
Females										
11–14	15	22	30	+2	+0	+5	+10	+14	+19	+24
15–18	10	17	25	+1½	+0	+4	+8	+12	+16	+20

*Note: The amounts listed are given in ranges to account for variability of body build and maturational level within an age group. For additional calorie needs for sports to achieve weight maintenance, add figures listed to the daily calorie needs per pound per day. Weight loss or gain is based on 1-lb change per week, with the object of losing body fat or gaining lean muscle mass. These figures are estimates and may need to be adjusted for the individual. Competitive and long-endurance sports are not recommended for 4- to 10-year-olds.

† Based on an average amount of calories expended for four 30-minute periods of exercise per week.

‡ Based on an average amount of calories expended for six 2-hour practices per week.

§ Based on an average amount of calories expended for seven 3.5-hour practices per week plus three 4-hour competitive events per month.

Table 11–4 Fluid Needs*

Age	*Fluid per Day*†	*Fluid Needs to Replace for Activity*	*Pre-Event*	*Competitive Event*	*Post Event*	*Preferred Fluid for Exercise Hydration*	*Electrolyte Replacement Above Normal Diet*
4–6	26–50 oz	Normal hydrations. Drinking preferred before and after an activity.				Cold water or diluted beverage	Not necessary
7–10	40–56 oz	As above	12–15 oz 2 hr before; 4–8 oz 15 min before	2–4 oz per 15 min	Weight before minus weight after times 16 oz	Cold water or diluted beverage	Not necessary unless long-endurance activity or profuse sweating. Individual assessment needs to be done, with salt, potassium, and/or chloride to be contained in the diet or a diluted fluid.§
Males 11–15	52–70 oz	As above	15–20 oz 2 hr before; 8–12 oz 15 min before	4 oz per every 15 min	As above	Cold water. Sport beverage if needed for long endurance activity.	As above
Females 11–15	48–64 oz	As above	As above	As above	As above	As above	As above
Males 16–18	60–80 oz	As above	As above	As above	As above	As above	As above
Females 16–18	52–69 oz	As above	As above	As above	As above	As above	As above

* Given in minimum amounts, and individual needs may vary.

† Data in this column from reference 18 .

§ The American College of Sports Medicine recommends 10 mEq sodium and 5 mEq potassium for adults.

Source: Data from references 41 to 44.

Table 11–5 Fluid Comparison

Beverage	*Serving Size*	*Cal*	*CHO*	*Na+*	*Minerals mg K+*	*Cl−*	*Osmolality (mOsm/kg H_2O)*	*Recommended Dilution**
Municipal water	8 oz	0	—	7	1	NA	2	None
Apple juice	8 oz	116	29 g	7	296	NA	718†	1 oz juice, 7 oz water
Kool-aid	8 oz	98	20 g	8	1	NA	243†	1 oz Kool-aid, 7 oz water
Gatorade	8 oz	50	14 g	110	30	45	NA	1½ oz Gatorade, 6½ oz water
Cola	8 oz	100	27 g	6	0	NA	709†	1 oz cola, 7 oz water
Noncola	8 oz	95	24 g	31	1	NA	691†	1 oz noncola, 7 oz water
Sports beverages								To be used as intended by manufacturer for long endurance events
POWERaDE (Coca Cola Company)	8 oz	70	19 g	55	30	45	NA	None
10-K (Suntory Water Group Inc.)	8 oz	60	15 g	55	30	45	NA	None
All Sport (Pepsi Co Carbonated)	8 oz	70	19 g	55	55	45	NA	None

NA, not available.
* Dilute to provide 2.5 g carbohydrate per 100 mL.
† Measured in the Children's Medical Center Laboratory, Dayton, Ohio, by the Advanced Digimatic Osmometer, model 3DII Freezing Point.

Source: Data from J.A.T. Pennington, *Bowes and Church Food Values of Portions Commonly Used,* 17th edition, © 1997, Lippincott Williams & Wilkins, and product label information.

of physiologic changes that occur during puberty should be given to budding athletes to prevent unsafe practices aimed at changing body composition for sports participation or appearances.[14,15,21]

Ages 13–18 Years

At this age, physical activity should be incorporated into the lifestyle to yield enjoyment from either participation or accomplishments in a sport or activity. This pleasure will be the motivating force in a child's continued participation in exercise.[22] Exercise should be a year-around activity, not just during a sports season. Problems may occur in the many children of this age who are immersed in competitive sports or performing arts, to the exclusion of other interests. These children should be helped to develop other, complementary interests, so that sports or dance are not the only arenas for exercise and social interaction.

Eating habits of teens usually consist of meal-skipping or erratic eating, snacking, reliance on fast foods, and unfounded rituals (see Chapter 5). Normal nutrition education should be emphasized with this group, either in school classes or in conjunction with a sport. Often, students are willing to change their eating behaviors for the outcome of better performance and appearance.[23]

Competitive or Performing Sports

Many of today's youth participate in competitive sports, dance, or gymnastics at the grade-school age. It is important to provide them with an assessment by appropriate health care professionals.[8,11] An efficient way to accomplish group assessment to aspiring competitors at one time is to set up a mobile clinic situation in a large room and provide stations for each type of assessment needed. The stations can be staffed with the appropriate professionals. Table 11–1 gives recommendations for the type of health professional that should be included in checkups for various types of activities. The diet of a participant will give medical information, as well as a prediction of health status and potential. A registered dietitian should collect diet and intake data and make diet change recommendations, if needed.[10,11] Exhibit 11–1 shows a sample of a preparticipation nutrition assessment form. The nutrition assessment questionnaire can be completed by the participant prior to the health assessment. This will allow individual instruction at the time of the assessment. Adequate nutrition is of major importance for the budding athlete, and education on nutrition needs and safe nutrition practices should begin early.[22–24] The registered dietitian should also instruct coaches, dance teachers, parents, and students on normal diet needs for age, healthful diet practices for competition, and normal body changes, if necessary. This should help to combat the food fads and quackery often practiced by school-age athletes.

Skinfold measurements, midarm circumference measurements, or body mass index should be used to assess body fat.[14] (See Chapters 1 and 2 for additional information.) Registered dietitians are trained to measure body fat composition. Body fat results should be used judiciously per individual athlete and should never be used as a criterion for sports participation or classification.[10,11,14]

Calcium and iron should be checked in all females participating[25] and in males of low socioeconomic status because of frequent deficiencies in these population groups. Extra protein needs for the young growing athlete can be easily met in the normal diet that contains milk products and meat/protein servings. The dietitian should individually counsel children who choose to be vegetarian. (See Chapter 7.)

Complex carbohydrates are important to the young athlete, not just for health, but also for performance. This nutrient can efficiently fuel the body before, during, and after sports events or competition. Timing of carbohydrate ingestion is important.[12] Prior to events, meals should consist of complex carbohydrates, low-fat protein, and fluids. See Table 11–6 for timing and food selections. Often, parents or trainers need

Exhibit 11–1 Preparticipation Nutrition Assessment Questionnaire Form

1. Have you ever been on a diet before? ________ If yes, why and for how long? ______________
   Has anyone in your immediate family ever been on a diet for (circle appropriate answer/s)
   Blood Pressure Cholesterol Diabetes If so, who? ____________________
2. Do you take a vitamin/mineral supplement? If yes, what and how often? ______________
3. Have you ever tried to (circle the appropriate answer) gain or lose weight before? If yes, how much? _____ lbs

---

1. Do you drink milk? Yes No If yes, how often (circle appropriate answer)
   4 glasses/day 1–3 glasses/day 4–6 glasses/week 1–3 glasses/week
2. Do you eat (circle foods eaten) cheese, yogurt, or cottage cheese? How often?
   1 or more times/day 4–6 times/week 1–3 times/week
3. Do you eat meat or protein foods? Yes No How often?
   2 or more times/day 1 time/day 4–6 times/week 1–3 times/week
   List the types of meat or protein foods you eat: ____________________
4. Do you eat vegetables? Yes No How often?
   2 or more times/day 1 time/day 4–6 times/week 1–3 times/week
   List the types of vegetables you eat: ____________________
5. Do you eat fruits or drink 100% fruit juice? Yes No How often?
   2 or more times/day 1 time/day 4–6 times/week 1–3 times/week
   List the types of fruits you eat or juice you drink: ____________________
6. Do you eat (circle foods eaten) bread, cereal, pasta, potatoes, or crackers? How often? (total for foods circled)
   6 or more times/day 1–4 times/day 4–6 times/week 1–3 times/week
7. Do you drink water? Yes No How many glasses per day? ______Size glass? ______
8. Check the foods or beverages you eat or drink and fill in how often in the space provided.
   __ Chips _____ __ Diet pop _____ __ Candy _____
   __ Pop _____ __ Cakes, pies _____ __ Cookies _____

---

1. Are you satisfied with your current weight? Yes No If no, what would you like to weigh? __________ lbs
2. Are you satisfied with your present body composition? Yes No If no, how would you like to change it? ____________________
3. Have you ever not eaten or drunk anything for up to a day before weigh in to make weight?
   Yes No If yes, how often? ____________________
4. Do you ever get so hungry that you eat two–five times more than you usually do and then regret it? Yes No If yes, have you ever not eaten the next day or taken laxatives because you felt guilty or did not want to gain weight? ____________________

Dietitian's Information
Student's Name __________________ Age _____ Sex _____ Intended sport ___________
Height: _____ %tile _____ Weight: _____ %tile _____ Comments: ______________
If indicated: Hct/Hgb _____ Cholesterol _____ Blood Pressure _____/_____ Other ______
% Desired weight for height _____% % Fat _____% Means of measurement ____________
Weight change needed ________________ % Body fat change needed ______________
Calorie level ________/day ± ________ Milk Products ± ________ Meat/protein servings
Recommended fluid amounts _____ oz. ± _____ Fruit/vegetable ± _____ Grain group
Exercise time/day needed for weight change __________________
Other diet needs: ____________________
Comments: ____________________
Recommended body measurement: ________________ How often? ______________

information about pre-event meals. Meals should be 3–4 hours before the event. Easily digested food high in carbohydrate but low in protein and fat can be eaten. Adequate fluid should be provided, as suggested in Table 11–4. If scheduling of events precludes time for a meal or nervousness makes eating unpleasant, a liquid meal replacement can be considered. Table 11–5 gives an example of sports nutrition supplements. Products such as Ensure (Ross Laboratories), Boost (Mead Johnson), or sports bars also may be used. These supplements can be purchased at drug or grocery stores. Complex carbohydrates should be offered approximately 2 hours after events to replenish glucose stores. Suggested choices are bagels, grain muffins low in fat, fruit, yogurt, or fruit juice.[14] Table 11–7 gives several training and competition scenarios, and suggested eating regimes.

Electrolyte losses in sweat from moderate activity can be easily recovered in a postevent meal. However, if a participant sweats profusely, is involved with a very long endurance event, or participates in adverse weather, electrolyte replacement is recommended.

Some female athletes may need individual counseling because of their tendency to restrict caloric intake.[26] Poor nutrition could affect their performance and their iron and calcium levels, as previously mentioned. A very low body fat status may interfere with normal menstrual cycles. Amenorrhea should be assessed by a physician to determine its cause.

It is beyond the scope of this chapter to provide nutrition guidance for those who have chosen to dedicate their time to long endurance or in-depth training for competition at a national or worldwide level. These children need instruction on physical conditioning, nutrition, and training practices similar to what is given to college-age or adult athletes.

Obese Children

Calorie intake of obese children is not significantly different from that of normal-weight children, but their activity level may be very low. Obese children and their family members should be encouraged to participate in appropriate forms of physical activity, as approved by a

Table 11–6 Eating During Competition

3 or More Hours Before	*2–3 Hours Before*	*1–2 Hours Before*	*2–3 Hours After*
Fruit or vegetable juice	Fruit or vegetable juice	Fruit or vegetable juice	Bagel
Fresh fruit	Fresh fruit	Fresh fruit (low fiber such as plums, melons, cherries, peaches)	Pretzels
Bread, bagels	Bread, bagels	Sports drink	Fruit yogurt
English muffins	English muffins		Large banana
Peanut butter, lean meat, low-fat cheese	No margarine or cream cheese		Cranapple juice
Low-fat yogurt			Apple juice
Baked potato			Orange juice
Cereal with low-fat (1%) milk			
Pasta with tomato sauce			

Source: Adapted from D.S. Jennings and S.N. Steen, *Play Hard, Eat Right: A Parent's Guide to Sports Nutrition for Children*, © 1995, John Wiley & Sons, Inc. Adapted with permission of John Wiley & Sons, Inc.

Table 11–7 Eating Well While in Training and Competition

Situation	*Suggestion*
Middle school or high school student eats lunch at 10:30 a.m. and must compete at 4:00 p.m.	Eat a large lunch: lots of variety; get a quick after-school snack that won't irritate, such as nutri-grain bars, bagels, banana, as well as plenty of fluid.
The same situation but one where the athlete cannot tolerate any food in stomach just prior to competition.	Definitely eat more lunch and include a little more fat in the meal; good situation for a sports bar, if possible, or a drink in between classes.
Student of any age who has a ball game at 8 or 9 a.m. on a Saturday morning.	Eat a good dinner the night before with lots of carbohydrates. Get to bed a little early and get up a few minutes earlier to eat. Depending on the event, perhaps dry cereal, toast with jelly, and a juice drink may help. Milk and orange juice may not be easily digested.
A track, gymnastics, or swimming athlete who competes at 9 a.m., 1 p.m., and again at 3 p.m. on Saturday.	Eat a good dinner the night before competing. Be prepared. Take a small cooler with foods and fluids. Use foods easily digested such as bagels, bananas and oranges, cheese and crackers, granola bars, and pretzels. Stay away from all chips, greasy fries, and hot dogs. Food choices depend on individual preferences.
An athlete too nervous on game day to eat.	May eat better if in a group; provide favorite finger-foods; periodic snacking is great; pre-event visualization also helps.
A 5- to 10-year old who has to play in hot, humid weather.	Drink flavored fluids 2 hr before event and water (~1 C) within 1 hr of event. Drink fluids during warm-ups and coach's talk. Studies reveal that grape flavoring in fluids resulted in more fluid consumption in kids. Have Popsicles and more fluids afterwards.
An athlete who is exhausted after practice every night and falls asleep before eating dinner or while studying.	If poor nutrition is suspected, consult an RD. Have favorite foods more available—fresh fruit and cut-up veggies with low-fat dip; pack food for after school and before practice; provide favorite juices, meats, carbohydrates, and dairy products. Step up efforts to support nutrition throughout the season.
An athlete who is very concerned about weight gain and refuses to eat lunch or eats only an apple.	Needs at least some education; consult RD. Help athlete by noting calories and fat content; demonstrate healthy choices.
Athletes attending away games.	If no prior arrangements are made, pack a small cooler with a well-balanced meal, plenty of variety, and plenty of fluids.

Source: Reprinted with permission from D. Habash and J. Buell, *Nutrition...A Communique to Health and Education Professionals*, Vol. 2, No. 3, © 1998, The Ohio State University Extension.

trained sports physician.[27,28] Family support helps the heavy child to continue with exercise and reinforces fitness as a healthful goal. All health professionals seeing school-age children should address an obesity problem by including exercise in the treatment plan.[27] Physical activity for obese children can serve as a cure for boredom, increase metabolism, and improve feelings of self-esteem and accomplishment, just as it can for other children.[29] The exercise should be cardiorespiratory and calorie burning in nature. This can be accomplished by walking, swimming, or biking three to five times a week for 30 minutes or longer.

Children with Special Health Care Needs

For the child with a developmental disorder or delay resulting in physical limitations, physical activity at an appropriate level should be encouraged to help the child develop self-esteem and to obtain the benefits of exercise. Regular physical exercise will help to combat the obesity that often comes in later years for children with special health care needs. An appropriate physical activity that can be carried out at accessible facilities with professional guidance should be prescribed for children with special needs.

RECOGNITION AND TREATMENT OF NUTRITION DISORDERS RELATED TO SPORTS

The identification of eating disorders is a responsibility of all professionals involved with sports programs. Preparticipation assessments may single out some students who have eating disorder symptoms or who are at risk for them because of bizarre eating or exercise rituals. Students with anorexia nervosa or bulimia nervosa can concomitantly have a compulsive exercise addiction.[30] (See Chapter 10.) Anyone who is identified, either in preparticipation assessments or during the sports season, to have problems associated with food or exercise control should be referred to an appropriate professional.[31] Some of the unhealthful practices associated with efforts to influence weight and body composition changes can be eliminated if a protocol for safe body changes is established by a coach or a registered dietitian at the beginning of the weight training season, with an appropriate time frame to achieve the changes.

ERGOGENIC AIDS AND DRUGS

The drugs abused by young athletes range from steroids and amphetamines to street drugs. These drugs—particularly steroids—have detrimental health effects on the adolescent athlete, and their use is condemned by the American Academy of Pediatrics.[32,33] The physician screening athletes, as well as the coach, should be asking in-depth questions about drug use. Giving preventive education at early ages is most helpful to establish safe practices.[34] If drug abuse is suspected or identified, referral to appropriate professionals is required.

High intakes of caffeine prior to sports events to hype the athlete is to be discouraged in the school-age population because of its side effects and the illegality of the practice in international competition. Caffeine is widely available, and coaches or sponsors may not be aware of this abuse. The sports participant should be educated about caffeine's effects and the dangers or side effects of high doses.[35]

Ergogenic aids are becoming popular with adult and endurance athletes, and the use of over-the-counter ergogenic aids to increase performance or muscle ability during prolonged activity is a concern in the pediatric population. These aids have not been tested with pediatric athletes. Many of the products have not had reproducible scientific studies of the initial and/or extrapolated data to make any conclusions as to added benefit. The manufacturers of ergogenic aids advertise miracle changes in performance or endurance, and these must be evaluated for truth, as with any other media promotion.[36] An example is dehydroepiandrosterone (DHEA) that is touted as the "youth hormone" and promoted to improve vigor, health, and well-being.

There is a claim that DHEA can be converted to testosterone in the body, which would give some young athletes the notion that the supplement could increase their endurance and strength. Side effects of DHEA are possible acne flare-ups, unwanted hair growth, irritability, and rapid heart beat with larger doses. The studies on DHEA have shown no beneficial effect on body composition or energy expenditure, and DHEA use has been banned by the U.S. Olympic Committee.[36] Unscrupulous use of this product by adolescents could be useless, expensive, and potentially harmful. Mega-doses of specific nutrients or ergogenic aids can be deleterious to health and should not be promoted by coaches or professional athletes to school-age sports participants.

Advertisement and word of mouth tend to be the biggest promoters of ergogenic aids and nutritional supplements. These products fall under the Dietary Supplement and Education Act (DSHEA) and do not require the rigorous testing required for sale, as do additives or drugs.[36] There are many ergogenic aids available, and questions should be asked as to their use. Table 11–8 lists ergogenic aids, advertisers' claims, and available scientific evidence. The coach and/or health professional working with the team should educate the athletes on the risks and evaluation process of ergogenic aids.

Table 11–8 Ergogenic Aids: Advertisers' Claims and Scientific Evidence

Ergogenic Aid	*Claim of Advertiser*	*Scientific Evidence*
Protein powders	Facilitates muscle growth, weight gain.	Usual dietary intake provides extra amount needed.
Glutamine	Restores energy to working muscle; increases protein synthesis.	Needs further research.
BCAA's (Branched-Chain Amino Acids)	Energy source during exercise; delays central fatigue.	May be helpful to include a protein source in meals after exercise. Needs further research.
Taurine	Increases protein synthesis.	Needs further research.
Individual amino acids: lysine/arginine, aspartates ornithine/tyrosine	Stimulates release of human growth hormone (HGH) and insulin, which facilitates muscle growth.	Serum HGH may increase; no proof that muscle growth is stimulated.
Creatine	Increases use of fat; spares muscle glycogen; increases endurance.	Some evidence for ability to perform repeated high-intensity work with sufficient rest; no evidence of effectiveness for long-term exercise. More research needed.

Source: Data from Kanter M et al, Ergogenic aids: the scientist's perspective. Gatorade Sports Science Institute. *Sports Science Exchange Roundtable,* Winter 1991; Benardot D, ed., *Sports nutrition: a guide for the professional woking with active people.* 2nd ed. Chicago, IL: American Dietetic Association, 1993; Kris-Etherton PM, The facts and fallacies of nutritional supplements for athletes. Gatorade Sports Science Institute. *Sports Science Exchange,* August 1989; Williams MH, Nutritional supplements for strength trained athletes. Gatorade Sports Science Institute, *SportsScience Exchange,* 1993; and Williams MH, Nutritional ergogenics in athletics, J Sports Sci, 1995;13:S63.

Table 11–8 Continued

Ergogenic Aid	*Claim of Advertiser*	*Scientific Evidence*
Inosine	Increases oxygen delivery; improves strength.	No data to support claim.
Chromium	Assists insulin; increases lean mass.	Most research inconsistent; need controlled studies.
Magnesium	Increases muscle growth and strength.	No data to support claim.
Boron	Increases testosterone and growth.	No proof of increased growth.
Vitamin B_{12}	Stimulates muscle growth.	No studies completed.
Antioxidants (vitamins C, E, beta carotene)	Prevents muscle damage from high-intensity exercise.	Some data to support claim; need controlled studies.
Medium chain triglycerides	Increases thermic effect and fat loss.	No data to support claim.
Omega-3 fatty acids	Stimulates HGH; increases muscle.	No data to support claim.
High-fat diet	Spares use of muscle glycogen.	Insufficient data.
Glycerol	Induces hyperhydration.	Controlled research needed.
CoEnzyme Q10 (CoQ10)	Boosts ATP production.	Limited supportive data.
Dihydroxyacetone pyruvate	Enhances endurance time.	Limited supportive data.
Phosphates	Increases endurance.	Need controlled research.
Ginseng	Need controlled research.	Data inconsistent; more research needed.
Yohimbine and gamma oryzanol	Plant extracts that stimulate testosterone and HGH release.	No data to support claim.
Smilax	Increases serum testosterone; increases muscle growth/ strength.	No data to support claim.
Caffeine	Improves high-intensity effort.	Data still inconsistent; can dehydrate.
Sodium bicarbonate	Buffers lactic acid; delays fatigue.	Some supportive data.

continues

Table 11–8 Continued

Ergogenic Aid	*Claim of Advertiser*	*Scientific Evidence*
Bee pollen	Mix of bee saliva/plant nectar/ pollen; increases energy/fitness.	No data to support claim.
Brewer's yeast	Product of beer brewing used to increase energy.	No data to support claim.
Gelatin	Protein from collagen; improves muscle contraction.	No data to support claim.
Kelp	Vitamin/mineral increases energy.	No data to support claim.
Pangamic acid	Increases delivery of oxygen.	No data to support claim.
Octacosanol	Alcohol isolate from wheat germ; increases energy and performance.	No data to support claim.
Royal jelly	Substance fed to queen bee by worker bees; increases strength.	No data to support claim.
Superoxide dismutase	Enzyme to decrease peroxidation.	No data to support claim.
DHEA (Dehydroepiandrosterone)	Increases strength, lean body mass, and protein synthesis.	No data to support claim; research is ongoing.
HMB (Hydroxymethylbutyrate)	Slows muscle breakdown after workout.	No data to support claim.
Vanadyl sulfate	Builds muscle and lean mass.	No data to support claim.

EXERCISE PROGRAM RECOMMENDATIONS

All sectors of society should be involved in physical activity the year around.[6] Efforts should be made to provide education opportunities to the public through school systems or community resources about exercise safety, nutrition requirements, and the importance of achieving cardiorespiratory benefits.

REFERENCES

1. *Healthy Children 2000 National Health Promotion and Disease Prevention Objectives Related to Mothers, Infants, Children, Adolescents, and Youth;* 1991. US De-

partment of Health and Human Services DHHS Publication No. HRSA-M-CH-91-2.

2. Physical activity and fitness risk reductions objective 1.3. In: *Healthy Children 2000.* US Department of Health and Human Services; 1991:10.
3. Berg FM. *Afraid to Eat, Children and Teens in Weight Crisis.* Hettinger, ND: Healthy Weight Publishing Network; 1997.
4. Birrer RB, Levine R. Performance parameters in children and adolescent athletes. *Sports Med.* 1987;4:211–227.
5. Ross JG, Gilbert GG. A summary of findings. (The National Children and Youth Fitness Study). *J Phys Educ Recreation Dance.* 1985;56:1–48.
6. Physical activity and fitness risk reduction objective 1.4. In: *Healthy Children 2000.* US Department of Health and Human Services; 1991:11–12.
7. Sady SP. Cardiorespiratory exercise training in children. *Clin Sports Med.* 1986;5:493–514.
8. Emery HM. Considerations in child and adolescent athletes. *Rheum Dis Clin North Am.* 1996:22(3):499–513.
9. Goldberg B, Saraniti A, Witman P, Gavin M, Nicholas JA. Pre-participation sports assessment: an objective evaluation. *Pediatrics.* 1980;66:736–745.
10. American Dietetic Association. Timely statement of the American Dietetic Association: nutrition guidance for child athletes in organized sports. *J Am Diet Assoc.* 1996;6:610–611.
11. American Dietetic Association. Timely statement of the American Dietetic Association: nutrition guidance for adolescent athletes in organized sports. *J Am Diet Assoc.* 1996;6:611–61.
12. Jennings DS, Nelson S. *Play Hard Eat Right.* Minneapolis, MN: Chronimed Publishing; 1995.
13. Spear BA. Nutrition management of the child athlete. In: Williams CP, ed., *Pediatric Manual of Clinical Dietetics.* Chicago: The American Dietetic Association; 1998:139–1448.
14. Steen SN. Nutrition for the school-age child athlete. In: Berning JR, Steen S, eds. *Nutrition for Sport and Exercise.* 2nd ed. Gaithersburg, MD: Aspen Publishers; 1998:199.
15. Paul PH. Childhood. In: Benardot D, ed. *Sports Nutrition A Guide for the Professional Working with Active People.* Chicago: The American Dietetic Association; 1993:107–112.
16. Schoonen JC. Adolescence. In: Benardot D, ed. *Sports Nutrition A Guide for the Professional Working with Active People.* Chicago: The American Dietetic Association; 1993:113–121.
17. Food and Nutrition Board. Recommended Dietary Allowances. 9th ed. Washington, DC: National Academy of Sciences; 1989.
18. Nelson WE, Behrman RE, Vaughan VC. *Nelson Textbook of Pediatrics.* 15th ed. Philadelphia, PA: WB Saunders Company; 1995.
19. Committee on Sports Medicine 1986–1988. Infant exercise programs. *Pediatrics.* 1988;82(5):800.
20. Rarick GL. The significance of normal patterns of behavior and motor development as important determinants of participation in sports programs. In: *Sports Medicine for Children and Youth, Report of the Tenth Ross Roundtable on Critical Approaches to Common Pediatric Problems.* Columbus, OH: Ross Products, a division of Abbott; 1979.
21. Rogoi AD. Effects of endurance training on maturation. *Consultant.* 1985;25:68–83.
22. Douglas PD, Douglas JG. Nutrition knowledge and food practices of high school athletes. *J Am Diet Assoc.* 1984;84:1198–1202.
23. Berning J. Fueling their engines for the long haul: teaching good nutrition to young athletes. *J Am Diet Assoc.* 1998;98:418.
24. Lewis M, Brun J, Talmage H, Rashev S. Teenagers and food choices: the impact of nutrition education. *J Nutr Educ.* 1988;20:336–340.
25. Benson JE, Geiger CJ, Eiserman PA, Wardlaw GM. Relationship between nutrient intake, body mass index, menstrual function, and ballet injury. *J Am Diet Assoc.* 1989;89:58–63.
26. Benardot D, Schwarz M, Heller DW. Nutrient intake in young, highly competitive gymnasts. *J Am Diet Assoc.* 1989;89:401–403.
27. Korsten-Reck U, Bauer S, Keul J. Sports and nutrition—an out-patient program for adipose children (long-term experience). *Int J Sports Med.* 1994;15:242–248.
28. Physical activity and fitness risk reductions objective 1.7. In: *Healthy Children 2000.* US Department of Health and Human Services; 13–14.
29. International Food Information Council. *Food Insight. The Fight for Fit and Trim Kids.* Washington, DC: International Food Information Council; 1989.
30. Berg FM. *Afraid to Eat, Children and Teens in Weight Crisis,* Hettinger, ND: Healthy Weight Publishing Network; 1997.
31. Marston AR, Jacobs DF, Singer RD, Widaman KE, Little TD. Characteristics of adolescents at risk for compulsive overeating on a brief screening test. *Adolescence.* 1988;23:59–65.
32. Committee on Sports Medicine 1986–1988. Anabolic steroids and the adolescent athlete. *Pediatrics.* 1989; 83:127–128.
33. Cheung S. Issues in nutrition for the school-age athlete. *J School Health.* 1985;55:35–37.
34. Goldberg L, Elliot DL, Clarke GN, et al. The Adolescents Training and Learning to Avoid Steroids (AT-

LAS) prevention program. Background and results of a model intervention. *Arch Pediatr Adolesc Med.* 1996; 150(7):713–721.

35. O'Neil FT, Hynak-Hankinson MT, Gorman J. Research and application of current topics in sports nutrition. *J Am Diet Assoc.* 1986;86:1007–1015.
36. Burke ER. Nutritional ergogenic aids. In: Berning JR, Steen S, eds. *Nutrition for Sports and Exercise.* 2nd ed. Gaithersburg, MD: Aspen Publishers; 1998.
37. Pennington JAT. Bowes and Church Food Values of Portions Commonly Used. 17th ed. Philadelphia, PA: JB Lippincott Co, 1997.
38. Rogoi A. Effects of endurance training on maturation. *Consultant.* 1985;25:68–83.
39. Benson J, Gillien DM, Bourdet K, Luosli AR. Inadequate nutrition and chronic calorie restriction in adolescent ballerinas. *Phys Sports Med.* 1985;13:79–90.
40. Harvey JS. Nutritional management of the adolescent athlete. *Clin Sports Med.* 1984;3:671–678.
41. Hecker AL. Nutritional conditioning for athletic competition. *Clin Sports Med.* 1984;3:567–582.
42. O'Neil FT, Hynak-Hankinson MT, Gorman J. Research and application of current topics in sports nutrition. *J Am Diet Assoc.* 1986;86:1007–1015.
43. Manjarrez C, Birrer R. Nutrition and athletic performance. *Am Fam Phys.* 1983;28:105–115.
44. Narins DM, Belkengren RP, Sapala S. Nutrition and the growing athlete. *Pediatr Nurs.* 1983;9:163–168.

Chapter 12

Community Nutrition

Luz Gómez Pardini

Community and public health nutritionists play an increasingly important role in promoting and protecting the health of children. Public and community health agencies should consider the importance of the nutritional health of children when setting priorities for services. Community nutritionists assess the community's needs, plan appropriate interventions, implement them, and evaluate their success. They are also sensitive to the issues affecting the populations they serve, including socio-economic, ethnic, cultural, linguistic, and political factors.

It is critical that nutritionists and other health care providers be aware of the numerous nutrition programs available for children in their communities. Referring eligible families to all appropriate programs will help to assure their nutritional health. Because our system of health care is so rapidly changing, health care providers should be aware of national public health initiatives, the importance of advocacy, the key role of data (health statistics), and the need for creative funding strategies. Serving the nutritional needs of the community is a responsibility shared by all health care workers, especially community dietitians and public health nutritionists.

COMMUNITY NUTRITION SERVICES AND PROGRAMS FOR CHILDREN

There are many organizations and programs that provide nutrition services for children, including federal programs, state health departments, local health agencies such as city and county health departments, community health centers, health maintenance organizations (HMOs), hospitals, and clinics. Dietitians in private practice, schools, volunteer organizations, businesses, and industries also provide nutrition services and information.[1]

This section summarizes some of the available community nutrition resources, describing their scope of benefits, eligibility, and participation levels, as well as their sponsorship. These resources are not available in all communities. Information on their availability can be obtained from the local health department or public health nursing service.

FEDERAL FOOD AND NUTRITION EDUCATION RESOURCES

Food and Nutrition Service

The Food and Nutrition Service (FNS), formerly known as the Food and Consumer Service, administers the nutrition assistance programs of the U.S. Department of Agriculture (USDA).[2] The mission of FNS is to provide children and needy families improved access to food and a more healthful diet through its food assistance programs and comprehensive nutrition education efforts. In addition to providing access to nutritious food, FNS also works to empower program participants with knowledge of the link between diet and health.

The agency was established in 1969, but many of the food programs originated long before FNS existed as a separate agency. The Food Stamp Program, now the cornerstone of USDA's nutrition assistance, was begun in its modern form in 1961, but it had its origins in the Food Stamp Plan to help the needy in the 1930s. The National School Lunch Program also has its roots in Depression-era efforts to help low-income children. The Needy Family Program, which has evolved into the Food Distribution Program on Indian Reservations, was the primary means of food assistance during the Great Depression.

FNS works in partnership with the states in all its programs. States determine most administrative details regarding distribution of food benefits and eligibility of participants, and FNS provides funding to cover most of the administrative costs of the states.

FNS administers the following nutrition assistance programs that benefit children (and adults):

Food Stamp Program

The Food Stamp Program is the foundation of the USDA nutrition assistance programs. Initiated as a pilot program in 1961 and made permanent in 1964, the program issues monthly allotments of coupons that are redeemable at retail food stores or provides benefits through electronic benefit transfer (EBT). Eligibility and allotments are based on household size, income, assets, and other factors.

The Food Stamp Program has been closely scrutinized because of its size and importance. USDA has the authority to examine retailers' records and to remove those who violate program rules. State food stamp agencies oversee the authorization of individual food stamp recipients and can revoke the eligibility of those who violate the rules.

All of the states are converting their food stamp issuance to EBT systems. The welfare reform act of 1996 requires all states to convert to EBT issuance by the year 2002. EBT allows food stamp customers, using a plastic card similar to a bank card, to buy groceries by transferring funds directly from a food stamp benefit account to a retailer's account. As of 1998, 32 states and the District of Columbia were using EBT to issue at least part of their food stamp benefits. All others were in some stage of planning or implementing EBT.

The welfare reform law of 1996 also made major changes in food stamp eligibility requirements, most notably, by limiting benefits to legal immigrants and to able-bodied adults without dependents. The law also changed some eligibility and income criteria and scaled back benefits across the board.

The Food Stamp Program served an average of 22.9 million people in fiscal year (FY) 1997, and average benefits were more than $71 per person per month. The federal government pays for the benefits issued through the Food Stamp Program and shares with the states the cost of administrative expenses.

Special Supplemental Nutrition Program for Women, Infants, and Children (WIC)

Established as a pilot program in 1972, WIC became permanent in 1974. Formerly known as the Special Supplemental Food Program for Women, Infants, and Children, WIC's name was changed under the Healthy Meals for Healthy Americans Act of 1994 to emphasize its role as a nutrition program.

WIC's goal is to improve the health of low-income pregnant women, postpartum women (breastfeeding and non-breastfeeding), and infants and children up to 5 years old who are at nutritional risk. WIC provides supplemental foods, nutrition education, and access to health services. Participants receive vouchers that are redeemable at retail food stores for specific foods that are rich sources of the nutrients frequently lacking in the diet of low-income mothers and children.

The WIC program encourages mothers to breastfeed their babies. A greater variety and quantity of food is offered to breastfeeding participants than to postpartum participants who are not breastfeeding. In addition, since 1992, breastfeeding mothers who elect not to receive infant formula through WIC for their infants receive an enhanced food package.[3]

The foods provided are high in protein, calcium, iron, and vitamins A and C. These are the nutrients frequently lacking in the diets of the target population of the program. WIC foods include iron-fortified infant formula and infant cereal, iron-fortified adult cereal, vitamin C-rich fruit or vegetable juice, eggs, milk, cheese, and peanut butter or dried beans or peas.

Nutritional risk may be either medically based (ie, anemia, underweight, maternal age, history of pregnancy complications, or poor pregnancy outcomes), or diet-based (such as inadequate dietary pattern). Health professionals such as physicians, nutritionists, or nurses determine nutritional risk based on federal guidelines.

To be eligible for WIC participation, applicants' income must fall below 185% of the U.S. Poverty Income guidelines (approximately $29,700 for a family of four in 1998). Families that participate in certain other benefit programs, such as the Food Stamp Program or Medicaid, automatically meet the income eligibility requirement.

WIC is effective in improving the health of pregnant women, new mothers, and their infants. A 1997 study[2] showed that women who participated in the program during their pregnancies had lower Medicaid costs for themselves and their babies than did women who did not participate. WIC participation was also linked with longer gestation periods, higher birth weights, and lower infant mortality. In the five states studied, savings in Medicaid dollars ranged from $1.77 to $3.13 for each dollar spent in prenatal WIC benefits. WIC participation averaged more than 7.4 million people each month in FY 1997.

National School Lunch Program

The National School Lunch Program provides cash reimbursements and commodity foods to help support non-profit food services in elementary and secondary schools, and in residential child care institutions. Every school day, more than 26 million children in 94,000 schools across the country eat a lunch provided through the National School Lunch Program. More than half of these children receive the meal free or at a reduced price.

The USDA has the responsibility to provide school meals that meet nutrition objectives. Regulations require school meals to meet nutritional standards and to comply with the Dietary Guidelines for Americans, the federal policy on what constitutes a healthful diet.

Encouraging needy families to participate in this program is crucial in local efforts to prevent hunger-related nutrition disorders, including iron-deficiency anemia.

School Breakfast Program

Some 6.9 million children in more than 68,000 schools participated in the School Breakfast Program every day in 1997. As in the school lunch program, low-income children may qualify to receive school breakfast free or at a reduced price, and states are reimbursed according to the number of meals served in each category. Meals must meet nutritional standards similar to those in the National School Lunch Program.

Local communities would greatly benefit from encouraging school districts not currently serving breakfast to implement the School Breakfast Program, especially in low-income areas. Studies have shown that this program enables students to perform better in school and that it reduces behavioral problems associated with hunger.

Summer Food Service Program (SFSP)

More than 2 million low-income children receive meals during school vacation periods through the SFSP. All SFSP meals are free, and the federal government reimburses local sponsoring organizations for meals served.

For many low-income families, school meals represent most of the caloric intake of their children during school months. By encouraging local organizations to sponsor the SFSP, local communities can decrease the incidence of hunger during off-school periods. The program can serve a small geographic area (determined by percentage of households below the poverty level in certain census tracts) where all children under 18 years of age can participate for free. It can also serve a larger area where income eligibility must be demonstrated by participants.

The Emergency Food Assistance Program (TEFAP)

TEFAP provides commodity foods to states for distribution to households and to soup kitchens and food banks. First initiated in 1981 as the Temporary Emergency Food Assistance Program, TEFAP was designed to reduce inventories and storage costs of surplus commodities through distribution to needy households. Though some surplus food is still distributed through TEFAP, Congress since 1989 has appropriated funds to purchase additional commodities for households.

Child and Adult Care Food Program (CACFP)

This program provides cash reimbursements and commodity foods for meals served in child and adult day care centers, and in family and group day care homes for children. In March 1998, CACFP provided meals to 2.6 million children and 58,000 adults. There are new income eligibility guidelines. Meals must meet certain nutritional requirements and patterns to qualify for reimbursement.

WIC Farmers' Market Nutrition Program

The Farmers' Market Nutrition Program was established in 1992 to provide WIC participants with increased access to fresh produce. WIC participants are given coupons to purchase fresh fruits and vegetables at authorized local farmers' markets. The program is funded through a legislatively mandated set-aside in the WIC program appropriation. As of 1998, this program is offered in 32 states.

Commodity Supplemental Food Program (CSFP)

A direct food distribution program with a target population similar to WIC, CSFP also serves the elderly. As in WIC, food packages are tailored to the nutritional needs of participants. Average monthly CSFP participation in 1997 was more than 370,000 people.

Special Milk Program

Children in schools, summer camps, and child care institutions that have no federally supported meal program receive milk through the Special Milk Program. In 1997, more than 140 million half-pints of milk were served through this program.

Food Distribution Program on Indian Reservations

This program provides commodity foods to low-income families who live on Indian reservations and to Native American families who live near reservations. The program evolved from the Needy Family Program, which was the primary source of federal food assistance to needy people during the Great Depression of the 1930s. More than 123,000 people participated in the program each month in 1997.

Homeless Children Nutrition Program

The Homeless Children Nutrition Program reimburses providers for nutritious meals served to homeless preschool-age children in emergency shelters. First established as a demonstration project in 1989, the Homeless Children Nutrition Program was made permanent in 1994. Congress appropriated $3.4 million for the program for FY 1998.

Nutrition Education

The Food and Nutrition Service operates the Nutrition Education and Training (NET) Program to support nutrition education in the food assistance programs for children. The Secretary of Agriculture allocates NET funds to states each year in the form of grants.

Through its Team Nutrition, FNS also provides schools with nutrition education materials and other support for children, technical assistance for food service professional staffs, and nutrition education materials for other food assistance programs, such as food stamps and WIC.

OTHER FOOD RESOURCES IN THE COMMUNITY

Food Pantries and Soup Kitchens

Certain churches and community organizations provide hot meals or bags of food to the hungry. They receive food from local food banks, food drives, and other donations. Unfortunately, too many families with children are starting to use these services on a regular basis. Food pantries and soup kitchens serving large metropolitan areas are faced with the challenge of meeting the increased demand. Often, families are limited to one food bag per month or to one meal per day or week.

Food Cooperatives

Self Help and Resource Exchange (SHARE), a national food cooperative, is helping many families "stretch" their food dollars. By purchasing a food package for approximately $15 at the beginning of the month, people can receive a box of nutritious food worth twice to three times as much at the end of the month, a time when needy families tend to run out of food. Sponsoring organizations and volunteers make the program work. Recipients agree to volunteer two hours of their time in their communities every month that they participate. Local food banks, health departments, or community organizations typically know how to contact SHARE sites.

NUTRITION COMPONENTS AND SERVICES IN FEDERAL PROGRAMS

Medicaid

This federal health insurance program provides health care for low-income pregnant women and children. States can opt to provide nutrition assessment and counseling as a benefit. The U.S. Department of Health and Human Services (USDHHS) administers the program at the federal level, whereas state health and/or welfare agencies administer it locally. Income eligibility and benefits vary by state. Access to health care providers has been an issue for many years, but recently there has been a trend to provide Medicaid services through managed care plans in an effort to increase access and decrease cost. Health care providers should help needy families understand their benefits and navigate the increasingly complex system of health care delivery.

Early and Periodic Screening, Diagnosis, and Treatment (EPSDT)

This is a federally mandated program created to identify and treat health conditions in low-income children early to prevent long-term health problems. The program has set guidelines that require providers of EPSDT services to conduct wellness exams according to a periodicity schedule from birth to age 21. The wellness exam should be comprehensive: history and physical, nutritional assessment, health education and anticipatory guidance, dental assessment, hearing and vision screening, hemoglobin/hematocrit testing, etc. Conditions identified should be referred for treatment, including nutrition-related conditions. Case management is an essential component of the program. A designated agency administers the program at the state level (typically, social services or health and welfare agencies). Local county agencies then deliver the administrative and case management services and conduct quality assurance.

State Program for Children with Special Health Care Needs (CSHCN)

The USDHHS and a designated state agency administer this program. The program provides case management, diagnosis, and treatment for eligible children with special health care needs.

University Affiliated Programs (UAP)

Administered locally by institutions of higher learning/universities, this USDHHS program provides assessment and development of a treatment plan for mentally handicapped/chronically ill children as needed, in an effort to support the training of health professionals. The programs stress multidisciplinary team approaches that typically include a registered dietitian with special training. Major teaching research hospitals around the country may have an affiliated program.

Early Intervention Program

This program of the U.S. Department of Education is administered locally by a designated state agency. It provides necessary health services to enable handicapped newborns to 5-year-olds to benefit from education and to prevent or minimize developmental delay. Nutrition consultation may be available to families.

Head Start

Head Start[4] is a national program that provides comprehensive developmental services for America's low-income, preschool children aged 3–5 years and social services for their families.[4] Specific services for children focus on education, socio-emotional development, physical and mental health, and nutrition.

Head Start began in 1965 in the Office of Economic Opportunity as an innovative way in which to serve children of low-income families and is now administered by the Administration for Children and Families. In 1995, almost 751,000 children were enrolled in over 37,000 Head Start classrooms. About 13% of the enrollees were children with disabilities.

The cornerstone of the program is parent and community involvement—which has made it one of the most successful preschool programs in the country. Approximately 1,400 community-based non-profit organizations and school systems develop unique and innovative programs to meet specific needs.

Major Components of Head Start

- *Education*—Head Start's educational program is designed to meet the needs of each child, the community served, and its ethnic and cultural characteristics. Every child receives a variety of learning experiences to foster intellectual, social, and emotional growth.
- *Health*—Head Start emphasizes the importance of the early identification of health problems. Every child is involved in a comprehensive health program, which includes immunizations; medical, dental, and mental health; and nutritional services.
- *Parent Involvement*—An essential part of Head Start is the involvement of parents in parent education, program planning, and operating activities. Many parents serve as members of policy councils and committees and have a voice in administrative and managerial decisions. Participation in classes and workshops on child development and staff visits to the home allow parents to learn about the needs of their children and about educational activities that can take place at home.
- *Social Services*—Specific services are geared to each family after its needs are determined. They include community outreach, referrals, family need assessments, recruitment and enrollment of children, and emergency assistance and/or crisis intervention.

Early Head Start

In 1994, the Head Start Reauthorization Act established a new program for low-income pregnant women and families with infants and toddlers. The program recognizes the powerful research evidence that the period from birth to age 3 years is critical to healthy growth and development and to later success in school and in life.

The purpose of this program is to enhance children's physical, social, emotional and cognitive development; to enable parents to be better caregivers of and teachers to their children; and to help parents meet their own goals, including that of economic independence.

Either directly or through referrals, the program provides early, continuous, intensive, and comprehensive child development and family support services to low-income families with children under the age of 3 years. Projects must coordinate with local Head Start programs to ensure continuity of services for children and families. Depending on family and community needs, programs have a broad range of flexibility in how they provide these services.

The services provided by Early Head Start programs are designed to reinforce and respond to the unique strengths and needs of each child and family. Nutrition services are a part of these services. Community nutritionists are involved in the implementation of nutrition guidelines in Early Head Start.

As of 1996, 142 agencies in 42 states have been selected to serve more than 10,000 children and families. Program sponsors include Head Start grantees, school systems, universities, colleges, community mental health centers, city and county governments, Indian tribes, community action agencies, child care programs, and other non-profit agencies.

STATE AND LOCAL NUTRITION SERVICES

Public Health Nutrition Services

Public health nutritionists provide a wide range of nutrition services in local government agencies such as health departments and migrant health centers. They also work in community health centers and certain community-based organizations.

A wide range of services may be available, depending on the state or local agency involved. Typical services include nutrition assessments and counseling; nutrition education on general topics, such as health promotion and weight management; and topics for special target groups, such as pregnant women, parents of young children, or individuals with chronic diseases or HIV infection. Public health nutritionists also provide professional and paraprofessional training and participate in program planning and implementation.

Public Health Nursing Services

State and local health departments employ public health nurses to provide many services, including home visiting, case management of special conditions, pre- and postnatal classes for parents, or community outreach for issues related to lead exposure, immunizations, tuberculosis, etc. These nursing services are a valuable resource to local community nutritionists.

School Health, Nursing Services, and Occupational/Physical Therapy

Local school systems assist school staff and food services to meet students' special needs. These services may include nutrition counseling, and they can target teens or parenting teens. Partnerships between schools and local health departments can bring more nutrition services to school children.

Schools also assist children with special health care needs. They assist children with feeding problems, food modification needs, adaptive feeding equipment, and special feeding techniques. Nutrition consultation may be available at the district or state levels.

Private Dietitian Services and Hospital Outreach Programs

Dietitians in private practice offer nutritional assessment and counseling to private patients and often offer nutrition education classes for groups. They provide medical nutrition therapy

(MNT) when prescribed by a physician. There is a need for more pediatric dietitians in private practice and for simpler reimbursement mechanisms when working with Medicaid children.

Hospitals are increasingly using nutrition services to improve their revenues and serve their communities, HMOs are recognizing the value of preventive services, and nutrition education classes are surfacing in medical centers frequently. Private health insurance plans now reimburse for more nutrition services than ever before, a testament to the potential cost-savings of these services.

OTHER NUTRITION EDUCATION RESOURCES

Table 12–1 lists other important resources to consider when looking for ways to educate the community. Some of these resources are free of charge.

THE ROLE OF COMMUNITY NUTRITIONISTS IN PUBLIC HEALTH PROGRAMS

Public health agencies have a mandate to promote and protect the health of the public. The goal of public health nutrition is to improve the nutritional status of the population served by the public health agency. The public health nutritionist is responsible for identifying the nutrition problems and needs in the community and for developing solutions to the problems.[5,6] This requires a thorough understanding of the effect of economic, social, and political issues on health, as well as on the community as a whole, and their effect on community resources.

Today's community nutritionists should be aware of cultural factors that can impact nutritional status. Practices such as using home remedies that contain lead in some Middle-Eastern cultures or the use of lard when cooking in some Latino cultures can seriously affect a family's health. Recognizing how language presents a potential barrier is also important. Though it is not a requirement, learning a second language is useful in today's health care environment. Thankfully, it is now easier to find interpreters for a variety of languages in larger metropolitan areas.

As health care costs continue to rise, administrators are looking for ways to maximize their potential by hiring staff that is able to multi-task. Nutritionists with additional training in lactation services, smoking cessation, diabetes education, alcohol and drug issues, social marketing, or community organizing become stronger assets to the health care agency.

There are several levels of responsibility for public health nutritionists:

The entry level nutritionist

- counsels consumers/clients
- educates the public
- coordinates nutrition services within the agency

The experienced nutritionist

- sets standards
- plans, develops, and manages services
- implements and evaluates services, and ensures quality
- locates and maximizes resources and financing
- provides expert consultation and educates health professional colleagues
- advocates for nutrition services
- informs decision and policy makers of service needs
- coordinates nutrition services with other agencies

The nutritionist at an advanced level of practice

- participates in agency strategic and operational planning
- establishes policy
- supervises staff
- manages personnel and financing
- may conduct applied research[7]

Advocacy, one of the traditional roles of community nutritionists, is becoming increasingly important in today's political and economic cli-

Table 12–1 Nutrition Education Resources

Program/Service	*Assistance Provided*	*Sponsor*
Cooperative extension home economics services	Education in home economics, food and nutrition, child care, food preservation, food purchasing, menu planning, weight control	US Department of Agriculture (USDA), land grant colleges
Expanded Food and Nutrition Education Program (EFNEP)	Education by supervised paraprofessionals in nutrition, food preparation, money management, shopping, housekeeping, sanitation, child rearing, family relations; for low-income families	USDA, Cooperative Extension Service
Nutrition Education and Training (NET)	Teaches fundamentals of nutrition to children, parents, educators, and food service personnel	USDA, state agency
Dairy Council	Nutrition education materials for individuals, teachers, health professionals; nutrition education for preschool and school-age children, pregnant women	National Dairy Council and local affiliates
Heart Association	Educational materials and classes on prevention and control of heart disease for the public, individuals, and health professionals	American Heart Association and state and local affiliates
Cancer societies	Education materials on prevention and control of cancer for the public, individuals, and health professionals	American Cancer Society and state and area affiliates
Diabetes Association	Educational materials and classes on control of diabetes for the public, individuals, and health professionals	American Diabetes Association and affiliates and chapters
Red Cross	Educational materials and classes on nutrition, child care, prenatal care, menu planning, food service	American Red Cross and local chapters
March of Dimes	Educational materials, and classes on maternal and infant nutrition	March of Dimes Birth Defects Foundation national headquarters and local chapters

Source: Adapted from M. Caldwell, Community Nutrition in *Handbook of Pediatric Nutrition,* P.M. Queen and C.E. Lang, eds., © 1993, Aspen Publishers, Inc.

mate. It is often through advocacy that programs are funded, awareness is raised, and policies are changed. Strategies for effective advocacy are discussed later in this chapter.

Figure 12–1 illustrates various levels of nutrition services that a public health system could provide.[8]

PROVIDING COMMUNITY NUTRITION SERVICES IN A CHANGING ENVIRONMENT

The public health professional in today's health care environment should consider increasingly complex issues in planning and

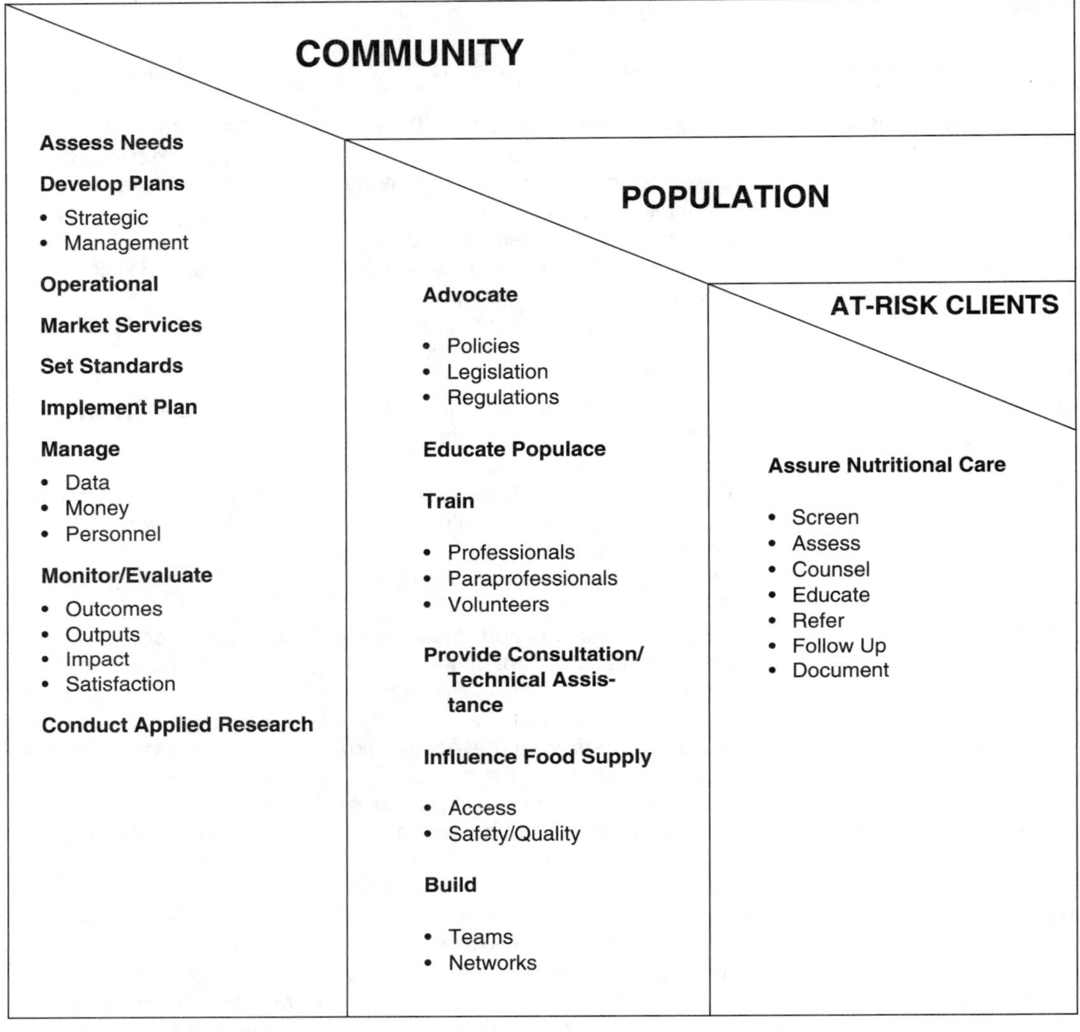

Figure 12–1 Nutrition Services to Reach the Public. *Source:* Adapted from M. Kaufman, *Nutrition in Public Health: A Handbook for Developing Programs and Services,* p. 11. © 1990. Aspen Publishers, Inc.

implementing nutrition services for children. There are national public health initiatives, such as Healthy People 2000 and 2010,[9] that contain nutrition related objectives, as well as national nutrition surveillance data sources, such as the Pediatric Nutrition Surveillance System (PedNSS),[10] that can guide decision making. Effective public health departments emphasize *collaboration*—this includes community-oriented planning, coalition building, and resource leveraging. Community nutritionists should learn program planning and grant writing. They should understand the implications of health care reform and "managed care," and they should know how to use the latest technologies, including the Internet.

The Importance of Data/Information

To plan and implement nutrition programs for children or to assess the needs of the target population, relevant data are necessary. Some sources of information on nutrition problems and needs are outlined in Table 12–2.

Program Planning and Grant Writing

Program planning is a critical activity in all health care settings. Establishing a program plan for nutrition services encompasses many of the activities involved in developing a grant application. Grant funds help to develop, expand, or retain services to meet the nutritional needs of the population. Both tasks involve the functions described below.

Needs Assessment: What Are the Nutrition Problems or Needs in the Community?

Assessing the community involves[11,12]

- identifying health problems that have implications for nutrition
- identifying resources available to solve or prevent the nutrition problems
- identifying gaps in needed services
- characterizing the population by culture, ethnicity, religion, education, socioeconomic status, age, sex, marital status, housing, schools, hospitals, group care settings and other institutions, health care providers, values, disease patterns, food supply, and marketplaces.

Identifying resources available to meet the needs of the population involves contacting health, nutrition, social service, and education agencies, organizations, and institutions to identify available nutrition and food programs and financial resources that can pay for nutrition services. See the "Community Nutrition Services and Programs for Children" section earlier in this chapter for information about food and nutrition programs and resources found in many communities.

Goals and Objectives: Establishing and Setting Priorities

Goals are statements of the long-range mission or purpose of a program[13] or broad ideals derived from values.[11] Objectives, on the other hand,

- are specific, measurable statements of what is to be accomplished by a given point in time
- should emphasize results or outcomes
- must be feasible within the available resources
- must be clearly related to the program goals

Objectives can often be stated by using the following formula: By (a specified date), (some condition) will be reduced/modified by (a specific percent or amount). In other words, "*who is going to do how much of what, when.*"

Priorities must be established among objectives as resources are finite. They should consider the

- impact and severity of the problem
- size and nature of the problem (ie, number affected)
- effect of intervention (great or small, certain or uncertain)
- feasibility of accomplishment (ie, politically or economically feasible)

Methods: Establishing a Course of Action

This involves identifying and stating the activities that will be used to reach the objectives. Steps in defining the methodology include[11]

- determining the activities that must be carried out and their order of accomplishment
- determining a schedule or time line for completing the activities

Table 12–2 Some Sources of Information on Nutrition Problems and Needs

The Community Profile	
Population	Census Bureau (most recent data)
	Health departments
	Social service departments
	Universities and colleges—programs in nutrition, medicine, urban health, allied health, community health, nursing
	Offices of congressional, state, and local representatives
	Federal, state, and local bureaus of labor, statistics, or commerce
	Department of Aging
	Board of Education
	City/county government offices
Housing	Same as above and, in addition, departments of housing, Department of Housing and Urban Development
Food marketing facilities	Local offices for supermarket chains
	Local office of consumer affairs or markets
	Local association of food stores or farmers' markets
	Local newspapers and advertisements
Health statistics	Regional, state, and municipal health/hospital departments
	State and local health agencies
	State health and local universities and colleges, community medicine, population studies, health planning
	Health systems agencies
	Data from the National Center for Health Statistics and the Health and Nutrition Examination Survey
Community and mental health care programs	Local hospitals, nursing homes, home health care agencies
	Local health and social services departments
	Local prepaid health care groups
	Local programs for the elderly, handicapped, and special groups
	Community health centers
	Migrant health centers
	Indian health clinics
	School health services for data on pregnant teenagers
Community agencies	Local United Fund or equivalent
	Local telephone directory
	Local health, social services department, and education agencies
	Local March of Dimes
	Local community action and/or legal services organizations
	Local Agricultural Extension Service
	Local community colleges, universities, and professional schools
	Local home health care agencies
	Local heart, cancer, and similar associations
	Local courthouse
Food and nutrition programs	State and local health departments, social services
	State or local board of education
	Local community action groups

continues

Source: Adapted from M.D. Simko, C. Cowell, and J.A. Gilbride, *Nutrition Assessment: A Comprehensive Guide for Planning Intervention,* 2nd ed. pp. 64 and 65, © 1991, Aspen Publishers, Inc.

Table 12–2 continued

Nutrition education programs	County, city health departments Board of education Social services departments Local extension or Farm Bureau office Local office of the Dairy Council and similar interest groups
Educational facilities	Local board of education State commissioner of education
Nutrition training programs	Local educational institutions, universities, and colleges Community colleges and vocational (trade) schools National, state, and local organizations of dietitians and nutritionists Local school food service office

- specifying the tasks in each activity
- determining the resources needed to carry out activities and tasks, including the amount and type of personnel and other resources needed and related costs
- assigning responsibility for each activity and task

Evaluation: Establishing Monitoring Methods

Evaluation determines to what extent program objectives are met and whether program resources are used in a cost-effective manner. The most common types of evaluation are process and outcome evaluations. Planners should decide ahead of time what type of information will be most useful to them and what type of evaluation is realistic to undertake. Monitoring determines success in carrying out the identified activities.

Evaluation and monitoring

- should be considered and methods determined at the time each objective and activity is written
- involves determining data items, including cost data, to be used in evaluation
- identifies mechanisms to obtain, compile, and summarize the data in a timely fashion
- places responsibility for obtaining data and establishes time frames for this activity
- are used for program control
- requires a feedback mechanism so that an ineffective or inefficient activity can be identified and changed while the program continues

Cost/benefit analysis, which involves converting all costs of and benefits from the program into monetary terms, and cost-effectiveness analysis, which measures the cost involved in attaining some desirable health-related outcome, are often used in program evaluation. Cost/benefit analysis allows for comparison of different types of projects, whereas cost-effectiveness analysis allows for comparison of only those projects sharing similar outcomes.[12,14,15]

Budgeting: Determining Needed Financial Resources

Financial resources needed to carry out the program plan include direct and indirect costs. Direct costs include personnel salaries and benefits; equipment; office and clinic supplies; counseling and educational materials; reference materials; and travel, phone, and correspondence costs. Indirect costs include administrative overhead, clinic and office space, maintenance, depreciation, central supplies, bookkeeping, and data processing.[13] If the personnel needed to carry out the activities and tasks were identified while establishing the course of action, direct personnel costs can be readily determined. Time involved by each type of worker should be translated into man-days or full- or part-time employee equivalents. Employee benefit costs, which are often substantial, can usually be obtained from the business office.

Other material resource needs should similarly have been identified while planning the activities. Data collection and analysis costs may involve personnel costs and use of equipment or administrative charges or fees for data processing. If subcontracts are used, costs of administering these contracts must be included along with the costs of the contract itself.

Reviewing the budgets of similar programs is useful in identifying costs that are often overlooked. It is often wise to draft the budget and have it reviewed by experienced administrators and fiscal managers.

Advocating for Programs and Services

Meeting the needs of a community often involves obtaining more resources than are presently available and advocating for additional resources. The advocacy target may be an agency supervisor or policy maker; another public or private agency, organization, or foundation; or the city, state, or federal legislature.

Advocacy involves[11]

- being well informed about the need for the program by having sound statistics on the severity of the problem, the numbers of people affected, and the disadvantages of not having the program
- understanding views of opponents and being prepared to address them
- knowing alternate funding sources, ways of making the program self-supporting, or other financing mechanisms if financing is a major issue
- obtaining support for the program from appropriate sources, such as other program directors, other agencies, professional organizations or civic groups, influential citizens, or constituents
- building a coalition with those with similar interests, particularly those with a track record of successful advocacy
- communicating effectively with the potential resource on a substantial basis, providing written documentation for your position, and being available to answer questions or to problem solve
- understanding the legislative process if the advocacy target is a legislature, so that verbal and written comment can be appropriate, timely, and adequately prepared
- knowing when hearings are to be held on related regulations or guidelines so that testimony can be presented to include appropriate nutrition services

Financing Nutrition Services

Potential sources for financing nutrition services include[16]

- federal, state, and local governmental agencies, block, or project grants or contracts
- private sector funding sources, such as foundation or corporate grants or contracts, civic organizations, not-for-profit health-related organizations, or associations
- fees for services
- income from sale of products such as educational materials

Major sources of information on funding resources include

- Federal health, education, and agriculture agencies, especially the U.S. Public Health Service and the USDA. Nutrition personnel of the federal agencies can provide information on specific federal support applicable to nutrition services
- The Federal Register, which contains requests for applications (RFAs) on programs funded by the federal government

- the Federal Office of Management and Budget, which disseminates information through the Catalog of Federal Domestic Assistance
- the Maternal and Child Health Clearinghouse, which can provide information on projects that have been funded through Maternal and Child Health grants
- state health, mental health, education, and social service agencies, whose employees can identify potential sources of financial support, including reimbursement for services
- corporations or foundations, which often have a department to deal with corporate giving
- the Foundation Center, with libraries in New York City, Cleveland, Washington, DC, and San Francisco, and a nationwide network of reference collections with information on foundation grants and workshops for individuals seeking grants
- private and public insurers, which can provide information on coverage of specific nutrition services

Providing Client Nutrition Services

Direct provision of nutrition services to clients served by public agencies is sometimes a responsibility of local public health nutritionists. These services include traditional clinical nutrition services:

- performing a nutrition assessment (see Chapter 2)
- providing nutrition counseling and education (see Chapter 6)
- developing and monitoring the nutrition care plan
- utilizing all available resources needed by the client
- ensuring quality care and evaluation services
- providing case management when nutrition problems are a major concern of the client

Community nutrition practice will continue to expand and change as the community does. Responding to new and emerging needs is a challenge and an opportunity that makes the work of community nutrition incredibly rewarding. Staying informed, staying connected, and bringing diverse skills to the job are essential to truly serve the community.

REFERENCES

1. Committee on Nutrition, American Academy of Pediatrics. *Pediatric Nutrition Handbook*, 3rd ed. Elk Grove Village, IL: American Academy of Pediatrics; 1993.
2. United States Department of Agriculture (USDA), Food and Nutrition Service. *1998 Electronic Information Pages*. http://www.usda.gov/fcs/about/fnsunf~1.htm (date of access 10/16/98).
3. Baydar N, McCann M, et al. *WIC Infant Feeding Practices Study*. USDA, Food and Nutrition Service, Office of Analysis and Evaluation. November 1997.
4. United States Department of Health and Human Services, Administration for Children, Youth and Families, Head Start Fact Sheet. *1998 Electronic Information Pages*. www.acf.dhhs.gov/programs/hsb/hsgen.htm (date of access 10/16/98).
5. *Guide for Developing Nutrition Services in Community Health Programs*. Rockville, MD: US Department of Health, Education, and Welfare Public Health Service. DHEW Pub No. (HSA) 78-5103; 1978.
6. Dodds JW, Kaufman M, eds. *Personnel in Public Health Nutrition for the 1990s*. Washington, DC: US Department of Health and Human Services; 1991. Officials Foundation; 1982.
7. Frankle RT, Owen AL. *Nutrition in the Community. The Art of Delivering Services*. 3rd ed. St. Louis, MO: Mosby-Year Book; 1993.
8. Kaufman M, ed. *Nutrition in Public Health: A Handbook for Delivering Programs and Services*. Gaithersburg, MD: Aspen Publishers; 1990.
9. Public Health Service. *Healthy People 2000: National Health Promotion and Disease Prevention Objectives*. Full report. Washington, DC: U.S. Department of Health and Human Services; 1990.
10. CDC Pediatric Nutrition Surveillance System—United States, 1980–1991. In: CDC Surveillance Summaries, Nov 27, 1992. *MMWR*. 1992;41(55-7):1–24.
11. Owen AY, Frankle RT. *Nutrition in the Community. The Art of Delivering Services*. St Louis, MO: Mosby; 1986.

12. Simko MD, Cowell C, Gilbridge JA. *Assessing Nutritional Needs of Groups. A Handbook for the Health Care Team*. New York, NY: Department of Human Economics and Nutrition, New York University; 1980.

13. Kaufman M, ed. *Quality Assurance in Ambulatory Nutrition Care*. Chicago: American Dietetic Association; 1983.

14. Disbrow D, Bertram K. *Cost Benefit Cost Effectiveness Analysis. A Practical Step-by-Step Guide for Nutrition Professionals*. Modesto, CA: Bertram Nutrition Associates; 1984.

15. Splett P, Caldwell M. *Costing Nutrition Services. A Workbook*. Chicago, IL: Region V Public Health Service, US Department of Health and Human Services; 1985.

16. Office of Disease Prevention and Health Promotion. *Locating Funds for Health Promotion Projects*. Washington, DC: US Department of Health and Human Services, Public Health Service; 1993.

Part II

Therapeutic Pediatric Nutrition

CHAPTER 13

Nutrition Support of Inborn Errors of Metabolism

Phyllis B. Acosta

Nutrition support of infants and children with inborn errors of metabolism requires in-depth knowledge of metabolic processes, the science and application of nutrition, growth and development, and food science. When providing nutrition support for patients with inborn errors, the specific nutrient needs of each patient, based on individual genetic and biochemical constitution, must be considered. Nutrient requirements established for normal populations[1,2] may not apply to individuals with inborn errors of metabolism.[3,4] Some chemical compounds, normally not considered essential because they can be synthesized de novo, may not be synthesized in patients with a metabolic defect. Consequently, dependent on the inborn error, the subsequent organ damage that accrues, and the rate of loss of specific chemicals from the body, several compounds may become conditionally essential. Among these are the amino acids arginine,[5] carnitine,[6] cystine,[7] and tyrosine,[8] and the "vitamins" coenzyme Q10,[9] lipoic acid,[9] and tetrahydrobiopterin.[10] Failure to adapt nutrient intake to the individual needs of each patient can result in mental retardation, metabolic crises, neurologic crises, growth failure, and, with some inborn errors, death.[4] Quality care is best achieved by an experienced team of specialists in a genetic/metabolic center.

This chapter addresses principles and practical considerations in nutrition support of inborn errors of metabolism; nutrition support of selected inborn errors of amino acid, nitrogen, carbohydrate, lipid, and mineral metabolism; selected areas needing further research; and roles and functions of the dietitian in nutrition support of inborn errors of metabolism. For a detailed guide to nutrition support, see *Nutrition Support Protocols*.[11]

PRINCIPLES AND PRACTICAL CONSIDERATIONS IN NUTRITION SUPPORT

Principles of Nutrition Support[3]

A number of approaches to nutrition support of inborn errors of metabolism are discussed here. The appropriate approach is dependent on the biochemistry and pathophysiology of disease expression. Several therapeutic strategies may be used simultaneously:

1. Enhancing anabolism and depressing catabolism: This involves the use of high-energy feeds, appropriate amounts of amino acid mixtures, and administration of insulin, if needed. Fasting should be prevented. This therapeutic maneuver is important to all inborn errors involving catabolic pathways.
2. Correcting the primary imbalance in metabolic relationships: This correction reduces, through dietary restriction, accumulated toxic substrate(s). Examples are phenylke-

tonuria, maple syrup urine disease, and galactosemia, where phenylalanine, leucine, isoleucine, valine, and galactose are limited.

3. Providing alternate metabolic pathways to decrease accumulated toxic precursors in blocked reaction sequences: For example, innocuous isovalerylglycine is formed from accumulating isovaleric acid if supplemental glycine is provided to drive glycine-N-transacylase. Isovalerylglycine is excreted in the urine.
4. Supplying products of blocked primary pathways: Some examples are arginine in most disorders of the urea cycle,[12] cystine in homocystinuria,[7] tyrosine in PKU,[8] tetrahydrobiopterin in biopterin synthesis defects,[10] and ether lipids[13] and docosahexaenoic acid[14] in patients with some peroxisomal disorders.
5. Supplementing conditionally essential nutrients: Examples are carnitine, cystine, and tyrosine in secondary liver disease[15] or with excess excretion of carnitine in organic acidemias.[6]
6. Stabilizing altered enzyme proteins: The rate of biologic synthesis and degradation of holoenzymes is dependent on their structural conformation. In some holoenzymes, saturation by a coenzyme increases their biologic half-life and, thus, overall enzyme activity at the new equilibrium. This therapeutic mechanism is illustrated in homocystinuria and maple syrup urine disease. Pharmacologic intake of pyridoxine in homocystinuria and of thiamine in maple syrup urine disease increases intracellular pyridoxal phosphate and thiamine pyrophosphate, respectively, and increases the specific activity of any functional cystathionine ß-synthase and branched-chain α-ketoacid dehydrogenase complex, respectively.[16,17]
7. Replacing deficient cofactors: Many vitamin-dependent disorders are due to blocks in coenzyme production and are "cured" by pharmacologic intake of a specific vitamin precursor. This mechanism presumably involves overcoming a partially impaired enzyme reaction by mass action. Impaired reactions required to produce methylcobalamin and/or adenosylcobalamin result in homocystinuria and/or methylmalonic aciduria. Daily intakes of appropriate forms of milligram quantities of vitamin B_{12} may cure the disease.[18]
8. Inducing enzyme production: If the structural gene or enzyme is intact but suppressor, enhancer, or promoter elements are not functional, abnormal amounts of enzyme may be produced. The structural gene may be "turned on" or "turned off" to enable normal enzymatic production to occur. In the acute porphyria of type I tyrosinemia, excessive Δ-aminolevulinic acid (ALA) production may be reduced by suppressing transcription of the Δ-ALA synthase gene with excess glucose.[19]
9. Supplementing nutrients that are inadequately absorbed or not released from their apoenzyme: Examples are zinc in acrodermatitis enteropathica[20] and biotin in biotinidase deficiency.[21]

Practical Considerations in Nutrition Support

Nutrients

Diet restrictions required to correct imbalances in metabolic relationships usually require the use of chemically defined or elemental medical foods. These medical foods are normally supplemented with small amounts of intact protein that supply the restricted amino acid(s). Intact protein seldom supplies more than 50%, and often much less,[22] of the protein requirements of patients with disorders of amino acid or nitrogen metabolism. Other nitrogen-free foods that provide energy are limited in their range of nutrients. Consequently, care must be taken to provide nutrients previously considered to be food contaminants because their essentiality has been demonstrated through long-term use of total parenteral nutrition.[23] Thus, in addition to nutrients for which recommended dietary allowances (RDAs)[1] are established, other nutrients must be supplied in adequate amounts. These include the trace minerals chromium, copper, manganese, and molybdenum, and the vitamins biotin, pantothenic acid, choline, and inositol. Other possible conditionally essential nutrients for patients with phenylketonuria have been described.[24]

Osmolality

Elemental medical foods consist of small molecules that may result in an osmotic load greater than the physiologic tolerance of the patient. Abdominal cramping, diarrhea, distention, nausea, or vomiting may result from use of hyperosmolar feeds. Aside from gastrointestinal distress, more serious consequences can occur in infants, such as hypertonic dehydration, hypovolemia, hypernatremia, and death. Osmolalities of several medical foods intended for use in treating inherited diseases of amino acid metabolism have been published.[11,25] A mathematic formula for estimating approximate osmolarity of medical food mixtures is given in *Nutrition Support Protocols*.[11] The neonate should not be fed an elemental formula that contains greater than 450 mOsm/kg water.[11]

Maillard Reaction

Medical foods for inborn errors of amino acid or nitrogen metabolism are formulated from L-amino acids or hydrolysates, carbohydrate, and, often, fat. The Maillard reaction is a complex group of chemical reactions in foods in which reacting amino acids, peptides, and protein condense with sugars, forming bonds for which no digestive enzymes are available. The Maillard reaction is accelerated by heat and is characterized in its initial stage by a light brown color, followed by buff yellow and dark brown in the intermediate and final stages. Caramel-like color and roasted aromas develop. Those who prepare medical foods must be able to recognize the Maillard reaction because it causes loss of some sugars and amino acids. For this reason, medical foods should not be heated beyond 100°F.

Introduction of Puréed Foods

Puréed foods (beikost) should be introduced into the diet at about 4 months of age if the infant shows developmental readiness by a decrease in tongue thrust. Beikost is important in the diet as sources of unidentified nutrients, to provide fiber, to enhance the infant's acceptance of a variety of tastes and textures, and, when table foods are eaten, to develop jaw muscles important for speech. (See the section on weaning and feeding progression in Chapter 4.)

Changes in Nutrition Support Prescription

As soon as nutrition support is well established in an infant or child, the prescription should be fine-tuned routinely and frequently. The frequency depends on the age of the child; infants require at least weekly changes in prescription, whereas children who are growing more slowly may not require a diet change more than monthly or every 2–3 months. Small, frequent changes in prescription prevent "bouncing" of plasma amino acid, glucose, organic acid, or ammonia concentrations and allow the intake to grow with the child, thus precluding the child's "growing out of the prescription."[11]

Monitoring

Successful management of inborn errors of metabolism requires frequent monitoring. Frequent monitoring gives the physician and dietitian data that verify the adequacy of the nutrition support prescription. These data are also useful in motivating patient/parent compliance with the prescription. Patients with insulin-dependent diabetes often monitor blood glucose concentrations three times daily, so frequent monitoring of plasma amino acid concentrations or other indicated analytes should pose no major problem. Premature and full-term infants to at least 6 months of age require twice weekly monitoring. Thereafter, weekly monitoring may be adequate if the patient is compliant with the diet prescription.

Some centers may wish to draw blood when the patient is fasting to monitor plasma amino acid concentrations. Prolonged fasting (> 8 hours) may cause spurious elevations of plasma amino acid concentrations that could lead to unwarranted diet changes,[26] and blood drawn 15 minutes to 1 hour after a meal may also yield spuriously high values.[27]

INBORN ERRORS OF AMINO ACID METABOLISM

The problem of ensuring adequate nutrition for infants and children with inborn errors of metabolism may be decreased by the use of a protocol or plan for treatment.[11] Each patient requires individualized medical and nutrition care. Information in Table 13–1 describes various inborn errors, nutrients to modify, vitamin responsiveness, and medical foods available. Data in Table 13–2 outline recommended nutrient intakes for beginning therapy,[11] whereas Table 13–3 provides information on nutrition support during acute illness, medications and nutrient interactions, and nutrition assessment parameters.

When specific amino acids require restriction, total deletion for 1–2 days only is the best approach to initiating therapy. Longer-term deletion or overrestriction may precipitate deficiency of the amino acid(s).[11] The most limiting nutrient determines growth rate, and overrestriction of an amino acid, nitrogen, or energy will result in further intolerance of the toxic nutrient. Results of amino acid and nitrogen deficiencies are described in Table 13–4. Data outside the parentheses in Table 13–2 describe amounts of amino acids with which to begin nutrition support. For some disorders, in which the initial concentration(s) of toxic amino acid is 14–20 times the upper limit of the normal reference range, after 2–3 days of 0 intake of the amino acid, the amino acid should be introduced with the lowest recommended amount for age in parentheses.[11] Data within the parentheses indicate the possible range of amino acid requirements, depending on the gene mutation and extent of the enzyme deficit.[28] Only frequent monitoring of plasma concentrations of amino acids and other analytes, nutrient intake, and growth can verify the adequacy of intake.[11]

Protein requirements of infants and children with inborn errors of amino acid metabolism are normal if liver or renal function is not compromised. However, the form in which the protein is administered must be altered to restrict specific amino acids. Consequently, medical foods formulated from L-amino acids, or specially treated protein hydrolysate, must be used with very small amounts of intact protein to provide amino acid and nitrogen requirements.[11, 22] Because nitrogen retention from L-amino acid mixes differs somewhat from use of amino acids derived from intact protein,[29,30] recommended protein intakes of infants and children with inborn errors of amino acid metabolism are 125–150% greater than National Academy of Sciences/National Research Council (NAS/NRC) RDAs.[1] Medical food with intact protein should be given 4–6 times daily to enhance nitrogen retention.[29,30]

Energy intakes of infants and children with inborn errors of metabolism must be adequate to support normal rates of growth. Provision of apparently adequate amino acids and nitrogen without sufficient energy will lead to growth failure. Pratt et al[31] suggested that energy requirements are greater than normal when L-amino acids supply the protein equivalent. Maintenance of adequate energy intake is essential for normal growth and development, and to prevent catabolism. If NAS/NRC RDAs[1] for energy cannot be achieved through oral feedings, nasogastric, gastrostomy, or parenteral feedings must be employed. Amino acid solutions designed for specific metabolic defects may be obtained from PharmaThera (Memphis, TN)[32] if parenteral alimentation is required.

Major, trace, and ultratrace mineral and vitamin intakes should meet or exceed NAS/NRC RDAs and Safe and Adequate Daily Dietary Intakes[1] for age. If the medical food mixture fails to supply 100% of requirements for the infant and at least 80% of the requirement for children, appropriate supplements should be given.

The Infant Formula Act (IFA)[33] specifies minimum and maximum concentrations of

Table 13–1 Nutrition Support of Inborn Errors of Metabolism

Inborn Error and Defect	*Nutrient(s) to Modify*	*Vitamin-Responsive*	*Medical Foods Available*
INBORN ERRORS OF AMINO ACID METABOLISM			
Aromatic Amino Acids			
Phenylketonuria and hyperphenylalaninemia (phenylalanine hydroxylase)[102]	Restrict PHE, increase TYR[3,11,102] (see Table 13–2); Maintain protein intake greater than NAS/NRC RDA. See Chapters 4 and 5 for other nutrient needs.	No	Periflex Lofenalac Phenex-1, -2 Phenyl-Free PKU1, 2, 3 XP Analog, Maxamaid, Maxamum
Hyperphenylalaninemia (dihydropteridine reductase) GTP cyclohydrolase I; (6-pyruvoyltetrahydropterin synthase)[102]	Same as for phenylketonuria.[103]	Yes. Tetrahydrobiopterin 2 mg/kg/d[10]	Same as for phenylketonuria
Tyrosinemia type I (fumarylacetoacetate hydrolyase)[104]	Restrict PHE and TYR; restrict MET if plasma MET concentration is above normal.[11,104] Provide greater than normal protein and energy intakes. (See Table 13–2). See Chapters 4 and 5 for other nutrient needs.	No	Tyromex-1 Tyrex-2 XPHEN, TYR, MET Analog, Maxamaid
Tyrosinemia type II (tyrosine aminotransferase)[104]	Restrict PHE and TYR (see Table 13–2).[3,11,104] Maintain protein intake greater than NAS/NRC RDA. See Chapters 4 and 5 for other nutrient needs.	No	Low-PHE/TYR Diet Powder TYR1, 2 Tyrex-2 XPHEN, TYR, Analog, Maxamaid

continues

Table 13–1 continued

Inborn Error and Defect	*Nutrient(s) to Modify*	*Vitamin-Responsive*	*Medical Foods Available*
	Branched-Chain Amino Acids		
Maple syrup urine disease (branched-chain ketoacid dehydrogenase complex)[105]	Restrict ILE, LEU and VAL (See Table 13–2).[3,11,103,105] Maintain protein and energy intakes above NAS/NRC RDA for age. See Chapters 4 and 5 for other nutrient needs.	Yes. Thiamine-responsive if any residual enzyme activity.[16] Response to thiamine inadequate to alleviate need for restriction of BCAAs.[115] 300 mg *oral* thiamine/d.[16]	Ketonex-1, -2 MSUD1, 2 MSUD Diet Powder MSUD Maxamaid, Maxamum
Isovaleric acidemia (isovaleryl-CoA dehydrogenase);[106] ß-methylcrotonylglycinuria (3-methylcrotonyl-CoA carboxylase);[106]	Restrict LEU; supplement with L-carnitine and GLY[11,106,107] (see Table 13–2). Maintain protein and energy intakes above NAS/NRC RDA for age. See Chapters 4 and 5 for other nutrient needs.	No	I-Valex-1, -2 XLEU Analog, Maxamaid
	Sulfur Amino Acids		
Homocystinuria, pyridoxine-nonresponsive (cystathionine-ß-synthase)[108]	Restrict MET,[3,11] increase CYS,[7] supplement folate betaine (see Table 13–2).[109,110] Maintain protein and energy intakes at or above NAS/NRC RDA for age.	No	HOM1, 2 Hominex-1, -2 Low Methionine Diet Powder XMET Analog, Maxamaid, Maxamum
Homocystinuria, pyridoxine-responsive (cystathionine-ß-synthase)[17,108]	See Chapters 4 and 5 for other nutrient needs	Yes; 25 to 1,000 mg of *oral* pyridoxine daily. Use smallest amount that results in biochemical normalcy because excess causes peripheral neuropathy.[111]	None indicated

	Other Inborn Errors of Amino Acid Metabolism		
Glutaric aciduria type I (glutaryl-CoA dehydrogenase);[112] Ketoadipic aciduria (2-ketoadipic acid dehydrogenase);[112]	Restrict LYS and TRP,[16,113] supplement L-carnitine[114] (see Table 13–2). Maintain protein and energy intakes at or above NAS/NRC RDA for age. See Chapters 4 and 5 for other nutrient needs.	Yes. Some patients have a partial response to *oral* riboflavin, 100–300 mg daily.[115]	Glutarex-1, -2 XLYS, TRY Analog, Maxamaid, Maxamum
Methylmalonic acidemia (methylmalonyl-CoA mutase ^{0} or $^{-}$)[18]	Restrict ILE, MET, THR, VAL,[11] long-chain unsaturated fatty acids,[116] supplement L-carnitine[117] (see Table 13–2). Provide greater than normal protein and energy intakes. See Chapters 4 and 5 for other nutrient needs.	No	Propimex-1, -2 OS1, 2 XMET, THRE, VAL, ISOLEU Analog, Maxamaid, Maxamum
Methylmalonic acidemia (cobalamin reductase; adenosyltransferase)[18]	Minimum restriction of ILE, MET, THR, VAL; supplement L-carnitine (see Table 13–2). See Chapters 4 and 5 for other nutrient needs.	Yes. 1–2 mg hydroxycobalamin daily.[18]	None indicated
Propionic acidemia[18] (propionyl-CoA carboxylase)	Restrict ILE, MET, THR, VAL,[11] and long-chain fatty acids.[116] Provide greater than normal protein and energy intakes for age. Supplement L-carnitine[117] (see Table 13–2). See Chapters 4 and 5 for other nutrient needs.	Questionable. Some clinicians supplement with 5–10 mg *oral* D-biotin daily.[118]	Propimex-1, -2 OS1, 2 XMET, THRE, VAL, ISOLEU Analog, Maxamaid, Maxamum
	INBORN ERRORS OF NITROGEN METABOLISM		
Carbamylphosphate synthetase deficiency; Ornithine transcarbamylase deficiency[119]	Restrict protein,[3,11 12] supplement with EAAs,[12] L-carnitine,[120] L-citrulline;[12] provide greater than normal energy intake (see Table 13–2). See Chapters 4 and 5 for other nutrient needs.	No	Cyclinex-1, -2 Pro-Phree Protein-Free Diet Powder UCD1, 2 UCD Maxamaid

continues

Table 13–1 continued

Inborn Error and Defect	*Nutrient(s) to Modify*	*Vitamin-Responsive*	*Medical Foods Available*
Citrullinemia (argininosuccinate synthetase)[119] Argininosuccinic aciduria (argininosuccinate lyase)[119]	Restrict protein;[3,11] supplement with EAAs,[12] L-arginine,[12] L-carnitine;[120] provide greater than normal energy intake (see Table 13–2). See Chapters 4 and 5 for other nutrient needs.	No	Cyclinex-1, -2 Pro-Phree Protein-Free Diet Powder UCD1, 2 UCD Maxamaid
Argininemia (arginase)[119]	Restrict protein;[3,11,12] supplement with EAAs,[12] L-carnitine;[120] provide greater than normal energy intake (see Table 13-2). See Chapters 4 and 5 for other nutrient needs.	No	Cyclinex-1, -2 Pro-Phree Protein-Free Diet Powder UCD1, 2 UCD Maxamaid
INBORN ERRORS OF CARBOHYDRATE METABOLISM			
Galactosemias			
Epimerase deficiency[121]	Delete galactose. Add specific known amount of galactose[122,123] (see Table 13–2). Maintain normal energy and protein intakes for age. See Chapters 4 and 5 for other nutrient needs.	No	Isomil Next Step Soy ProSobee RCF
Galactokinase deficiency[121]	Delete galactose.[121] Maintain normal energy and protein intakes for age. See Chapters 4 and 5 for other nutrient needs.	No	Isomil Next Step Soy ProSobee RCF
Galactose-1-phosphate uridyl transferase deficiency	Delete galactose.[121] Maintain normal energy intake for age. See Chapters 4 and 5 for other nutrient needs.	No	Isomil Next Step Soy ProSobee RCF

	Glycogen Storage Disease		
Type Ia (glucose-6-phosphatase) Type Ib (defective glucose-6-phosphate transport)[124]	Modify type of carbohydrate and frequency of feedings[64] (see Table 13–2). Maintain normal energy and protein intakes for age. Avoid lactose, fructose, and sucrose.[124] See Chapters 4 and 5 for other nutrient needs.	No	ProViMin RCF Uncooked cornstarch
Type III (amylo-1, 6-glucosidase)[124]	Provide high protein[64], supplement with L-ALA,[69] modify type of carbohydrate[64] and frequency of feedings[64] (see Table 13–2). Avoid lactose, fructose, and sucrose.[124] Provide normal energy intake for age. See Chapters 4 and 5 for other nutrient needs.	No	ProViMin RCF Uncooked cornstarch
Type IV (α-1, 4-glucan: α-1, 4-glucan 6-glucosyltransferase)[124]	Provide high protein unless cirrhosis present; modify type of carohybrate and frequency of feedings[64] (see Table 13–2). Provide normal energy intake for age. See Chapters 4 and 5 for other nutrient needs.	No	ProViMin RCF
Type V[124]	Provide high protein;[64] supplement L-ALA[69] (see Table 13–2). Provide normal energy intake for age. See Chapters 4 and 5 for other nutrient needs.	No	Mono- and Disaccharide-Free Diet Powder ProViMin RCF
	Hereditary Fructose Intolerance		
Hereditary fructose intolerance (aldolase B)[125]	Restrict fructose;[126] restrict protein if liver damage[51] (see Table 13–2). Maintain energy intake at NAS/NRC RDA for age. See Chapters 4 and 5 for other nutrient needs.	No	Enfamil ProViMin, RCF; or whole cow's milk for children Similac

continues

Table 13–1 continued

Inborn Error and Defect	*Nutrient(s) to Modify*	*Vitamin-Responsive*	*Medical Foods Available*
	INBORN ERRORS OF LIPOPROTEIN METABOLISM		
Abetalipoproteinemia and hypobetalipoproteinemia (absence and decrease in apoβ)[72]	Restrict triglycerides with long-chain fatty acids; supplement with vitamins A, D, E, K[72,76] (see Table 13–2). Maintain protein and energy intakes at NAS/NRC RDAs for age. See Chapters 4 and 5 for other nutrient needs.	No	MCT ProViMin
Lecithin: cholesterol acyltransferase deficiency (LCAT)[73]	Restrict fat[73,76] (see Table 13–2). Maintain protein and energy intakes at NAS/NRC RDA for age. See Chapters 4 and 5 for other nutrient needs.	No	MCT ProViMin
	Hyperlipoproteinemias		
Type I (extrahepatic lipoprotein lipase; apo CII absent or decreased)[71]	Restrict triglycerides with long-chain fatty acids[71,76] (see Table 13–2). See Chapters 4 and 5 for other nutrient needs.	No	MCT ProViMin
Type IIa (LDL receptors absent or defective)[74]	Restrict cholesterol, saturated fat;[74,76,77] increase PUFAs (see Table 13–2). Maintain normal protein and energy intakes. See Chapters 4 and 5 for other nutrient needs.	No	Enfamil ProViMin RCF Similac
Type IIb[74]	Restrict cholesterol, saturated fat, mono- and disaccharides, alcohol; increase fiber and PUFAs[74,76,77] (see Table 13–2). Maintain normal protein and energy intakes. See Chapters 4 and 5 for other nutrient needs.	No	Mono- and Disaccharide-Free Diet Powder ProViMin RCF

Type III (hepatic lipoprotein lipase; homozygous for abnormal apo-E2; remnant receptor defect)[75]	Restrict cholesterol, saturated fat; mono- and disaccharides, alcohol. Increase PUFAs and fiber (see Table 13–2). Restrict energy if patient is overweight.[75,76] Maintain normal protein intake. See Chapters 4 and 5 for other nutrient needs.	No	Enfamil ProViMin RCF Similac
INBORN ERRORS OF MINERAL METABOLISM			
Acrodermatitis enteropathica (defect in intestinal zinc absorption)[20]	Give zinc supplements[20] (see Table 13–2). Maintain normal protein and energy intakes. See Chapters 4 and 5 for other nutrient needs.	No	None indicated
Wilson's disease Hepatolenticular degeneration (excessive accumulation of copper)[78,79]	Restrict dietary copper (see Table 13–2). Maintain normal protein and energy intakes. See Chapters 4 and 5 for other nutrient needs.	No	None indicated

Note: ALA, alanine; BCAAs, branched-chain amino acids; CYS, cystine; EAAs, essential amino acids (includes conditionally essential cystine and tyrosine); GLY, glycine; GTP, guanosine triphosphate; ILE, isoleucine; IM, intramuscular; LEU, leucine; LYS, lysine; MCT, medium-chain triglycerides; MET, methionine; MSUD, maple syrup urine disease; PHE, phenylalanine; PUFAs, polyunsaturated fatty acids; THR, threonine; TRP, tryptophan; TYR, tyrosine; VAL, valine.

Table 13–2 Recommended Nutrient Intakes (with Ranges) for Beginning Therapy

Nutrients to Modify	*Age (years)* 0.0 < 0.5	0.5 < 1.0	1 < 4	4 < 7	7 < 11	11 < 19
INBORN ERRORS OF AMINO ACID METABOLISM						
Aromatic Amino Acids						
Phenylketonuria and hyperphenylalaninemia [3, 4, 11]						
PHE (mg)	55 (70–20)/kg	30 (50–15)/kg	325 (200–450)/d	425 (225–625)/d	450 (250–650)/d	500 (300–750)/d
TYR (mg)	195 (210–180)/kg	185 (200–170)/kg	2800 (1400–4200)/d	3150 (1750–4550)/d	3500 (2100–4900)/d	3850 (2100–5600)/d
Protein (g)	3.5–3.0 kg	3.0–2.5/kg	≥ 30/d	≥ 35/d	≥ 40/d	50–65/d
Energy (kcal)	120/kg	110/kg	900–1800/d	1300–2300/d	1650–3300/d	1500–3300/d
Tyrosinemia type I [3, 11]						
PHE (mg)	75 (95–45)/kg	55 (75–30)/kg	600 (500–700)/d	650 (550–750)/d	700 (600–800)/d	800 (700–900)/d
TYR (mg)	75 (95–45)/kg	55 (75–30)/kg	400 (300–500)/d	450 (350–550)/d	500 (400–600)/d	550 (450–650)/d
MET (mg)	40 (50–20)/kg	30 (40–20)/kg	300 (200–400)/d	350 (250–450)/d	400 (300–500)/d	400 (300–500)/d
Protein† (g)	3.5–3.0/kg	3.5–3.0/kg	30/d	35/d	40/d	50-65/d
Carbohydrate	60–80% of calories					
Energy	100–120% of NAS/NRC RDA for age					
Tyrosinemia type II [3, 11]						
PHE (mg)	100 (125–65)/kg	80 (105–45)/kg	450 (400–500)/d	500 (450–550)/d	550 (500–600)/d	600 (550–700)/d
TYR (mg)	75 (100–40)/kg	55 (80–20)/kg	400 (350–450)/d	450 (400–500)/d	500 (450–550)/d	475 (400–550)/d
Protein (g)	3.5–3.0/kg	3.0–2.5/kg	≥ 30/d	≥ 35/d	≥ 40/d	50–65/d
Energy (kcal)	120/kg	110/kg	900–1800/d	1300–2300/d	1650–3300/d	1500–3300/d
Branched-Chain Amino Acids						
Maple syrup urine disease [3, 4, 11]						
ILE (mg)	60 (90–30)/kg	50 (70–30)/kg	50 (70–20)/kg	25 (30–20)/kg	25 (30–20)/kg	25 (30–10)/kg
LEU (mg)	80 (100–40)/kg	55 (75–40)/kg	55 (70–40)/kg	50 (65–35)/kg	45 (60–30)/kg	40 (50–15)/kg
VAL (mg)	70 (95–40)/kg	55 (80–30)/kg	50 (70–30)/kg	40 (50–30)/kg	28 (30–25)/kg	22 (30–15)/kg
Protein (g)	3.5–3.0/kg	3.0–2.5/kg	≥ 30/d	≥ 35/d	≥ 40/d	50–65/d
Energy	100–125% OF NAS/NRC RDA for age					

Isovaleric acidemia and beta-methylcrotonyl glycinuria [3, 11, 117, 118]						
LEU (mg)	95 (110–65)/kg	75 (90–50)/kg	975 (800–1150)/d	1275 (1050–1500)/d	1445 (1190–1700)/d	1955 (1610–2300)/d
L-carnitine (mg)	300–100/kg	300–100/kg	300–100/kg	300–100/kg	300–100/kg	300–100/kg
GLY (mg)	125 (150–100)/kg	125 (150–100)/kg	125 (150–100)/kg	15 (150–100)/d	125 (150–100)/kg	125 (150–100)/kg
Protein (g)	3.5–3.0/kg	3.0–2.5/kg	≥ 30/d	≥ 35/d	≥ 40/d	50–65/d
Energy	100–125% OF NAS/NRC RDA for age					
Sulfur Amino Acids						
Homocystinuria, cystathionine-ß-synthase deficiency (pyridoxine nonresponsive) [3, 11, 103, 109, 110]						
MET (mg)	35 (50–20)/kg	28 (40–15)/kg	20 (30–10)/kg	15 (20–10)/kg	15 (20–10)/kg	15 (20–10)/kg
CYS (mg)	300–250/kg	250–200/kg	150 (200–100)/kg	150 (200–100)/kg	150 (200–100)/kg	75 (60–50)/kg
Betaine[110] (g)	1–3 d		3–6 d			
Folate (mg)	0.5–1.0/d		1–3/d			
Protein (g)	3.5–3.0/kg	3.0–2.5/kg	≥ 30/d	≥ 35/d	≥ 40/d	≥ 50–65/d
Energy (kcal)	120/kg	115/kg	900–1800/d	1300–2300/d	1650–3300/d	1500–3300/d
Other Amino Acids						
Glutaric aciduria type I and ketoadipic aciduria [11, 94, 96, 100, 103, 114, 115, 127, 128]						
LYS (mg)	85 (100–70)/kg	65 (90–40)/kg	55 (80–30)kg	50 (75–25)/kg	45 (65–25)/kg	40 (60–20)/kg
TRP (mg)	25 (40–10)/kg	15 (30–10)/kg	12 (16–8)/kg	12 (16–8)/kg	8 (10–5)/kg	6 (8–4)/kg
L-carnitine (mg)	300–100/kg					
Riboflavin (mg)	300–100/d, administer orally					
Protein (g)	3.5–3.0/kg	3.0–2.5/kg	≥ 30/d	≥ 35/d	≥ 40/d	≥ 50–65/d
Energy (kcal)	120/kg	115/kg	900–1800/d	1300–2300/d	1650–3300/d	1500–3300/d
Propionic acidemia and methylmalonic acidemia [11, 18, 116–118]						
ILE (mg)	95 (120–60)/kg	70 (90–40)/kg	610 (485–735)/d	795 (630–960)/d	900 (715–1090)/d	1215 (956–1470)/d
MET (mg)	35 (50–15)/kg	25 (40–10)/kg	330 (275–390)/d	435 (360–510)/d	495 (410–580)/d	665 (550–780)/d
THR (mg)	90 (135–50)/kg	55 (75–20)/kg	505 (415–600)/d	660 (540–780)/d	745 (610–885)/d	1010 (830–1195)/d

continues

Table 13–2 continued

Nutrients to Modify	*Age (years)* 0.0 < 0.5	*0.5 < 1.0*	*1 < 4*	*4 < 7*	*7 < 11*	*11 < 19*
VAL (mg)	85 (105–60)/kg	55 (75–30)/kg	690 (550–830)/d	900 (720–1080)/d	1020 (815–1225)/d	1380 (1105–1655)/d
D-Biotin (mg)	5–10/d for propionic acidemia					
Hydroxycobalamin (mg)	1–2/d for cobalamin-responsive methylmalonic acidemia					
L-Carnitine (mg)	300–100/kg	300–100/kg	300–100/kg	300–100/kg	300–100/kg	300–100/kg
Protein† (g)	3.5–3.0/kg	3.0–2.5/kg	≥ 30/d	≥ 35/d	≥ 40/d	50–65/d
Energy	100–125% OF NAS/NRC RDA for age					
INBORN ERRORS OF NITROGEN METABOLISM						
Citrullinemia; Argininosuccinic aciduria [3, 5, 11, 12, 119, 120]						
ARG (mg)	700–350/kg	700–350/kg	500–250/kg	500–250/kg	500–250/kg	400–200/kg
Protein‡ (g)	2.2–1.15/kg	1.15–1.0/kg	8.0–12.0/day	12.0–15/day	14.0–17.0/day	20.0–32.0/day
L-carnitine (mg)	100–50/kg	100–50/kg	100–50/kg	100–50/kg	100–50/kg	100–50/kg
Energy	125–150% OF NAS/NRC RDA for age					
Carbamylphosphate synthetase deficiency; Ornithine transcarbamylase deficiency [3, 5, 11, 12, 119, 120]						
CIT (mg)	700–350/kg	700–350/kg	500–250/kg	500–250/kg	500–250/kg	400–200/kg
Protein‡ (g)	2.2–1.15/kg	1.15–1.0/kg	8.0–12.0/d	12.0–15/d	14.0–17.0/d	20.0–32.0/d
L-carnitine (mg)	100–50/kg	100–50/kg	100–50/kg	100–50/kg	100–50/kg	100–50/kg
Energy	125–150% OF NAS/NRC RDA for age					
Argininemia [3, 5, 11, 12, 119, 120]						
Protein‡ (g)	2.2–1.15/kg	1.15–1.0/kg	8–12/d	12–15/d	14–17/d	20–32/d
L-carnitine (mg)	100–50/kg	100–50/kg	100–50/kg	100–50/kg	100–50/kg	100–50/kg
Energy	125–150% of NAS/NRC RDA for age					
INBORN ERRORS OF CARBOHYDRATE METABOLISM						
Galactosemias						
Epimerase deficiency [11, 122, 123]						
Galactose (mg)	1000–1500/d		500–1000/d			
Protein (g)	≥ 2.2/kg	≥ 2.0/kg	≥ 23/d	≥ 30/d	≥ 35/d	45–65/d
Energy (kcal)	120/kg	115/kg	900–1800/d	1300–2300/d	1650–3300/d	1500–3300/d

Galactokinase deficiency [129]						
Galactose (mg)	< 50/d	< 50/d	< 100/d	< 100/d	< 100/d	< 100/d
Protein (g)	≥ 2.2/kg	≥ 2.0/kg	≥ 23/d	≥ 30/d	≥ 35/d	≥ 45-65/d
Energy (kcal)	120/kg	115/kg	900–1800/d	1300–2300/d	1650–3300/d	1500–3300/d
Galactose-1-phosphate uridyl transferase deficiency [55, 129]						
Galactose (mg)	< 50/d	< 50/d	< 100/d	< 100/d	< 100/d	< 100/d
Protein (g)	≥ 2.2/kg	≥ 2.0/kg	≥ 23/d	≥ 30/d	≥ 35/d	≥ 45–65/d
Energy (kcal)	120/kg	115/kg	900–1800/d	1300–2300/d	1650–3300/d	1500–3300/d
Glycogen Storage Disease						
Glucose-6-phosphatase deficiency (von Gierke's disease, type Ia); type Ib [62-68]						
Carbohydrate	60–70% of calories. Provide at least 50% of carbohydrate as uncooked cornstarch every 4 hours during the day and via continuous tube feeding at night. During the first 3 months of life, feed every 2 hours and use Polycose instead of uncooked cornstarch; gradually change to raw cornstarch over 3 months.					
Protein† (g)	≥ 2.2/kg	≥ 2.0/kg	≥ 23/d	≥ 30/d	≥ 35/d	≥ 45–65/d
Energy (kcal)	120/kg	115/kg	900–1800/d	1300–2300/d	1650–3300/d	1500–3300/d
Amylo-1, 6-glucosidase deficiency (Cori's disease, type III) [64]						
Protein (g)	4.4/kg	4.0/kg	4.0/kg	3.5/kg	3.0/kg	2.5/kg
L-Alanine (mg)	500–400/kg	400–300/kg	300–200/kg	200–100/kg	200–100/kg	200–100/kg
Carbohydrate	40–50% of calories. Provide about one-half as uncooked cornstarch every 6 hours during the day and night. During the first 3 months of life, feed every 2 hours and use Polycose instead of uncooked cornstarch; gradually change to raw cornstarch over 3 months.					
Energy (kcal)	120/kg	115/kg	900–1800/d	1300–2300/d	1650–3300/d	1500–3300/d
α-1, 4-glucan:α-1, 4-glucan 6-glucosyltransferase deficiency (Anderson's disease, type IV) [64]						
Protein	High protein as for type III unless cirrhosis present					
Carbohydrate	Uncooked cornstarch every 4–5 hours to maintain normoglycemia. See under type III					
Energy (kcal)	120/kg	115/kg	900–1800/d	1300–2300/d	1650–3300/d	1500–3300/d

continues

Table 13–2 continued

Nutrients to Modify	*Age (years)* 0.0 < 0.5	0.5 < 1.0	1 < 4	4 < 7	7 < 11	11 < 19
Muscle phosphorylase deficiency (McArdle's disease type V)						
Protein (g)	High protein as for type III					
L-Alanine (mg)	Same as for type III					
Energy (kcal)	120/kg	115/kg	900–1800/d	1300–2300/d	1650–3300/d	1500–3300/d
Hereditary Fructose Intolerance[11, 126, 130]						
Fructose (mg)	< 10/kg	< 10/kg	< 10/kg	< 20/kg	< 30/kg	< 40/kg
Protein	Restriction only with liver damage					
Energy (kcal)	120/kg	115/kg	900–1800/d	1300–2300/d	1650–3300/d	1500–3300/d
INBORN ERRORS OF LIPID METABOLISM						
Abetalipoproteinemia and hypobetalipoproteinemia[72, 131]						
Long-chain triglycerides	13–15% of energy					
Linoleic acid	3% of energy					
α-Linolenic acid	1% of energy					
Vitamin A	Use water-miscible form to supplement					
Vitamin E (mg)	1000–2000/day		5000–10,000/d			
Vitamin K (mg)	Supplement with water-miscible form if bruising, bleeding, or hypothrombinemia present					
Protein (g)	≥ 2.2/kg	≥ 2.0/kg	≥ 23/d	≥ 30/d	≥ 35/d	44–65/d
Energy (kcal)	120/kg	115/kg	900–1800/d	1300–2300/d	1650–3300/d	1500–3300/d
LCAT deficiency[71, 131]						
Long-chain triglycerides	13–15% of energy					
Linoleic acid	3% of energy					
α-linolenic acid	1% of energy					
Protein (g)	≥ 2.2/kg	≥ 2.0/kg	≥ 23/d	≥ 30/d	≥ 35/d	≥ 44–65/d
Energy (kcal)	120/kg	115/kg	900–1800/d	1300–2300/d	1650–3300/d	1500–3300/d

Hyperlipidemias

Type I[71, 76]						
Long-chain triglycerides	< 15% of energy					
Linoleic acid	3% of energy					
α-linolenic acid	1% of energy					
Protein (g)	≥ 2.2/kg	≥ 2.0/kg	≥ 23/d	≥ 30/d	≥ 35/d	≥ 44-65/d
Energy (kcal)	120/kg	115/kg	900–1800/d	1300–2300/d	1650–3300/d	1500–3300/d
Type IIa[74, 76]						
Total fat	< 30% of energy					
Cholesterol (mg)	< 100/1000 kcal. Never > 300/d					
Saturated fat	< 10% of energy					
PUFAs	< 15% of energy					
MUFAs	< 10% of energy					
Protein (g)	≥ 2.2/kg	≥ 2.0/kg	≥ 23/d	≥ 30/d	≥ 35/d	≥ 44–65/d
Energy (kcal)	120/kg	115/kg	900–1800/d	1300–2300/d	1650–3300/d	1500–3300/d
Type IIb[74]						
Cholesterol (mg)	< 100/1000 kcal. Never > 300/d					
Total fat	< 30% of energy					
Saturated fat	< 10% of energy					
PUFAs	< 15% of energy					
MUFAs	< 10% of energy					
Fiber	Increase					
Mono- and diglycerides	Restrict					
Protein (g)	≥ 2.2/kg	≥ 2.0/kg	≥ 23/d	≥ 30/d	≥ 35/d	≥ 44–65/d
Energy (kcal)	120/kg	115/kg	900–1800/day	1300–2300/d	1650–3300/d	1500–3300/d

continues

Table 13–2 continued

Nutrients to Modify	*Age (years)* 0.0 < 0.5	0.5 < 1.0	1 < 4	4 < 7	7 < 11	11 < 19
Type III[75–77]						
Cholesterol (mg)	< 100/1000 kcal. Never > 300/d					
Saturated fat	< 10% of energy					
PUFAs	< 15% of energy					
Fiber	Increase					
Protein (g)	≥ 2.2/kg	≥ 2.0/kg	≥ 23/d	≥ 30/d	≥ 35/d	≥ 44–65/d
Energy	Restrict					
INBORN ERRORS OF MINERAL METABOLISM						
Acrodermatitis enteropathica[20]						
Zinc (mg)	35–100/d elemental zinc; give in 2 or 3 doses					
Protein (g)	≥ 2.2/kg	≥ 2.0/kg	≥ 23/d	≥ 30/d	≥ 35/d	≥ 45–65/d
Energy (kcal)	120/kg	115/kg	900–1800/d	1300–2300/d	1650–3300/d	1500–3300/d
Wilson's disease[78–80]						
Copper (mg)	0.3/d	0.4/d	0.5/d	0.8/d	1.0/d	1.0/d
Zinc (mg)	20/d	20/d	20/d	30/d	30/d	30/d
Protein (g)	≥ 2.2/kg	≥ 2.0/kg	≥ 23/d	≥ 30/d	≥ 35/d	≥ 45–65/d
Energy (kcal)	120/kg	115/kg	900–1800/d	1300–2300/d	1650–3300/d	1500–3300/d
Pyridoxine (mg)	25/d					

Note: ARG, arginine; CIT, citrulline; CYS, cystine; GLY, glycine; ILE, isoleucine; LCAT, lecithin:cholesterol acyl transferase; LEU, leucine; LYS, lysine; MET, methionine; MUFA, monounsaturated fatty acid; PHE, phenylalanine; PUFA, polyunsaturated fatty acid; THR, threonine; TRP, tryptophan; TYR, tyrosine; VAL, valine.

†Protein may need to be decreased 5–10% if liver damage with hyperammonemia is present.

‡Total protein intake may be somewhat greater with the use of drugs that enhance waste nitrogen loss.

Table 13–3 Nutrition Support during Acute Illness; Medications and Nutrient Interactions and Nutrition Assessment Parameters

Inborn Error and Defect	*Nutrition Support during Acute Illness*	*Medications and Nutrient Interaction*	*Nutrition Assessment Parameters*
	INBORN ERRORS OF AMINO ACID METABOLISM **Aromatic Amino Acids**		
Phenylketonuria and Hyperphenylalaninemia (phenylalanine hydroxylase)	Delete dietary PHE 1–2 days **only**. For infant, offer Pedialyte to maintain electrolyte balance if needed. Give fruit juices and sugar-sweetened, caffeine-free soft drinks with added Polycose or Moducal if tolerated to maintain energy intake at 100% RDA for age. If necessary, give IV glucose, lipid and L-amino acids free of PHE to maintain anabolism. Return to oral medical food and complete diet as rapidly as tolerated.[11]	No medication required with early and continuing therapy throughout life.	Plasma PHE and TYR; dietary intake of PHE, TYR, protein, energy, minerals, vitamins.[11] See Chapter 2 for other routine assessment parameters and standards.
Hyperphenylalaninemia (dihydropteridine reductase; GTP cyclohydrolase I; 6-pyruvoyltetrahydropterin synthase)	Same as above.	L-DOPA, 5-hydroxytryptophan carbidopa.[10]	Plasma PHE and TYR; dietary intake of PHE, TYR, protein, energy, minerals, vitamins. See Chapter 2 for other routine assessment parameters and standards.
Tyrosinemia type I (fumarylacetoacetate hydrolyase)	Delete dietary PHE, TYR, MET, 1–2 days **only**. For infant, offer Pedialyte to maintain electrolyte balance if needed. Give fruit juices and sugar-sweetened, caffeine-free soft drinks with added Polycose or Moducal if tolerated to maintain energy intake at 120–130% RDA for age. Return to oral medical food and complete diet as rapidly as tolerated.[11]		Plasma PHE, TYR, MET; plasma bicarbonate, phosphate, potassium, plasma alkaline phosphatase, electrolytes; liver enzymes; urinary succinylacetone; dietary intake of PHE,

continues

Table 13–3 continued

Inborn Error and Defect	*Nutrition Support during Acute Illness*	*Medications and Nutrient Interaction*	*Nutrition Assessment Parameters*
			TYR, MET, protein, energy, minerals, vitamins. Liver imaging studies.[3, 11] See Chapter 2 for other routine assessment parameters and standards.
Tyrosinemia type II (tyrosine aminotransferase)	Delete dietary PHE, TYR, 1–2 days **only**. For infant, offer Pedialyte to maintain electrolyte balance if needed. Give fruit juices and sugar-sweetened, caffeine-free soft drinks with added Polycose or Moducal if tolerated to maintain energy intake at 100% RDA for age. If necessary, give IV glucose, lipid and L-amino acids free of PHE and TYR to maintain anabolism. Return to oral medical food and complete diet as rapidly as tolerated.		Plasma PHE and TYR; urinary N-acetyl-tyrosine, p-tyramine, p-hydroxyphenylorganic acids; dietary intake of PHE, TYR, protein, energy, minerals, vitamins. See Chapter 2 for other routine assessment parameters and standards.
Branched-Chain Amino Acids			
Maple syrup urine disease (branched-chain ketoacid dehydrogenase complex)	Delete dietary BCAAs 1–2 days **only**. For infant, offer Pedialyte to maintain electrolyte balance if needed. Give fruit juices and sugar-sweetened, caffeine-free soft drinks with added Polycose or Moducal if tolerated to maintain energy intake at 100–125% of RDA for age. If necessary, give IV glucose, lipid and L-amino acids free of BCAAs. Return to oral medical food and complete diet as rapidly as tolerated.	Anticonvulsants if seizures occur. Phenobarbital and phenytoin lead to accelerated metabolism of vitamin D and vitamin D deficiency that responds to 1,25-dihydroxyvitamin D.[132]	Plasma BCAAs, ALA, ALLO; urine ketoacids of BCAAs; bone radiographs of lumbar vertebrae; cation/anion gap; dietary intakes of BCAAs, protein, energy, minerals, vitamins.[11] See Chapter 2 for other routine assessment parameters and standards.

Isovaleric acidemia (isovaleryl-CoA dehydrogenase); ß-methylcrotonylglycinuria (3-methylcrotonyl-CoA carboxylase)	Delete dietary LEU 1–2 days **only**.[133] Increase GLY and L-carnitine. For infant, offer Pedialyte to maintain electrolyte balance if needed. Give fruit juices and sugar-sweetened, caffeine-free soft drinks with added Polycose or Moducal if tolerated to maintain energy intake at 100–125% of RDA for age. If necessary, give IV glucose, lipid and L-amino acids free of LEU. Return to oral medical food and complete diet as rapidly as tolerated.	Benzoates, salicylates are contraindicated.[106]	Plasma BCAAs, L-carnitine, GLY; isovalerylglycine; CBC/differential; bone radiographs of lumbar vertebrae; urinary isovalerylglycine, beta-hydroxyisovaleric acid; cation/anion gap; dietary intakes of LEU protein, energy, minerals, vitamins.[11] See Chapter 2 for other routine assessment parameters and standards.
Sulfur Amino Acids			
Homocystinuria, pyridoxine-nonresponsive (cystathionine-ß-synthase)	Delete dietary MET 1–2 days **only**. For infant, offer Pedialyte to maintain electrolyte balance if needed. Give fruit juices and sugar-sweetened, caffeine-free soft drinks with added Polycose or Moducal if tolerated to maintain energy intake at 100% of RDA for age. If necessary, give IV glucose, lipid and L-amino acids free of MET. Return to oral medical food and complete diet as rapidly as tolerated.[3,11]	Anticonvulsants if seizures occur. Phenobarbital and phenytoin lead to accelerated metabolism of vitamin D and cause vitamin D deficiency that responds to1,25-dihydroxyvitamin D.[132]	Plasma MET, CYS, HOMOCYS; erythrocyte folate; bone radiographs of lumbar vertebrae; dietary intake of MET, CYS, protein, energy, minerals, vitamins.[11] See Chapter 2 for other routine assessment parameters and standards.

continues

Table 13–3 continued

Inborn Error and Defect	*Nutrition Support during Acute Illness*	*Medications and Nutrient Interaction*	*Nutrition Assessment Parameters*
	Other Inborn Errors of Amino Acid Metabolism		
Glutaric aciduria type I (glutaryl-CoA dehydrogenase) Ketoadipic aciduria (2-ketoadipic acid dehydrogenase)	Delete LYS and TRP 1–2 days **only**. For infant, offer Pedialyte to maintain electrolyte balance if needed. Increase L-carnitine. Give fruit juices and sugar-sweetened, caffeine-free soft drinks with added Polycose or Moducal if tolerated to maintain energy intake at 100% of RDA for age. If necessary, give IV glucose, lipid and L-amino acids free of LYS and TRP. Return to oral medical food and complete diet as rapidly as tolerated.[11]	Baclofen-Geneva Generics, Inc. Valproic acid depresses appetite, causes an increase in plasma glycine, and loss of carnitine.	Plasma LYS, TRP, free-carnitine; urinary glutaric acid; dietary intake of LYS, TRP, protein, energy, minerals, vitamins. See Chapter 2 for other routine assessment parameters and standards.
Propionic acidemia (propionyl-CoA carboxylase)	Delete ILE, MET, THR, VAL 1–2 days **only**. Increase L-carnitine. For infant, offer Pedialyte to maintain electrolyte balance if needed. Give fruit juices and sugar-sweetened, caffeine-free soft drinks with added Polycose or Moducal if tolerated to maintain energy intake at 100–125% of RDA for age. If necessary, give IV glucose, lipid and L-amino acids free of ILE, MET, THR and VAL to maintain anabolism. Return to oral medical food and complete diet as rapidly as tolerated.[11]	Sodium benzoate during acute illness if accompanied by elevated blood ammonia,[134] supplement folate, pantothenate, pyridoxine, and vitamin B_{12} at 3–5 times RDA for age when phenylbutyrate is used.	Plasma ILE, MET, THR, VAL, GLY, carnitine (free); blood ammonia; cation/anion gap; urinary metabolites of propionate or methylmalonate; CBC/differential; plasma prealbumin or RBP; bone radiographs of lumbar vertebrae; dietary intake of ILE, MET, THR, VAL, protein, energy, minerals, vitamins.[11] See Chapter 2 for other routine assessment parameters and standards.

	INBORN ERRORS OF NITROGEN METABOLISM		
Urea cycle disorders	Blood NH_3 > 200 µmol/L. Delete protein 1–2 days **only**. Increase L-ARG or L-CIT if not arginase deficient. Give fruit juices and sugar-sweetened, caffeine-free soft drinks with added Polycose or Moducal if tolerated to maintain energy intake at 125–150% of RDA for age. If necessary, give IV L-ARG or L-CIT, glucose, and lipid to maintain energy intake.[135] Return to oral medical food and complete diet as rapidly as tolerated.	UCEPHAN; phenylbutyrate: folate, niacin, pantothenate, pyridoxine,vitamin B_{12} (administer at 3–5 times RDA for age). Anticonvulsants for seizures. Phenobarbital and phenytoin lead to accelerated metabolism of vitamin D and vitamin D deficiency that responds to1,25-dihydroxy-vitamin D.[132]	Plasma amino acids, blood ammonia; plasma prealbumin or RBP; plasma triglycerides; urinary pyroglutamic acid,[46] 3-methyl-histidine;[46]; dietary intake of protein, energy, minerals, vitamins. See Chapter 2 for other routine assessment parameters and standards.
	INBORN ERRORS OF CARBOHYDRATE METABOLISM		
	Galactosemias		
Epimerase deficiency	Same as for normal infant. Avoid drugs containing galactose or lactose.		Erythrocyte galactose-1 phosphate and UDP-galactose;[121–123] dietary intake of galactose, protein, energy, minerals, vitamins. See Chapter 2 for other routine assessment parameters and standards.

continues

Table 13–3 continued

Inborn Error and Defect	*Nutrition Support during Acute Illness*	*Medications and Nutrient Interaction*	*Nutrition Assessment Parameters*
Galactokinase deficiency	Same as for normal infant. Avoid drugs containing galactose or lactose.		Urinary galactose; routine eye examinations for cataracts.[121] See Chapter 2 for other routine assessment parameters and standards.
Galactose-1-phosphate uridyl transferase deficiency	Same as for normal infant. Avoid drugs containing galactose or lactose.		Erythrocyte galactose-1 phosphate; and UDP-galactose;[121–123] routine eye examinations for cataracts; liver enzymes;[121] dietary intake of galactose, protein, energy, minerals, vitamins. See Chapter 2 for other routine assessment parameters and standards.
Glycogen Storage Disease			
Type 1a, III, IV	Give oral carbohydrate and/or IV glucose to maintain normoglycemia.		Blood glucose; liver enzymes; dietary intake of carbohydrate,[64, 68] protein, energy, minerals, vitamins. See Chapter 2 for other routine assessment parameters and standards.

INBORN ERRORS OF LIPOPROTEIN METABOLISM			
Abetalipoproteinemia and hypobetalipoproteinemia (absence and decrease in apoß)	Same as for normal individual except restrict fat.		Plasma concentrations of retinol; RBP; tocopherol; 1,25-dihydrocholecalciferol; clotting time;[72] dietary intake of energy, protein, linoleic and α-linolenic acids, total fat, minerals, vitamins.[77] See Chapter 2 for other routine assessment parameters and standards
Lecithin: cholesterol acyltransferase deficiency	Same as for normal individual except restrict fat.		Plasma lipoproteins; plasma albumin;[73] dietary intake of energy, protein, linoleic and α-linolenic acids, total fat, minerals, vitamins.[77] See Chapter 2 for other routine assessment parameters and standards.

continues

Table 13–3 continued

Inborn Error and Defect	*Nutrition Support during Acute Illness*	*Medications and Nutrient Interaction*	*Nutrition Assessment Parameters*
	Hyperlipoproteinemias		
Type I	Same as for normal individual except restrict fat.		Plasma chylomicrons (triglycerides);[71] dietary intake of energy, protein, linoleic and α-linolenic acids, total fat, minerals, vitamins. See Chapter 2 for other routine assessment parameters and standards.
Type IIa, IIb	Same as for normal individual except restrict cholesterol, saturated fat. Increase PUFAs.	Cholestyramine, colestipol, lovastatin. Cholestyramine and colestipol cause fecal loss of fat, fat-soluble vitamins, folate, vitamins B_{12} and iron.[43, 76]	Plasma LDL cholesterol; plasma ferritin, erythrocyte B_{12} and folate, plasma RBP; dietary intake of energy, protein, total fat, PUFAs, MUFAs, fiber, mono- and diglycerides, minerals, vitamins.[73,74] See Chapter 2 for other routine assessment parameters and standards.
Type III	Same as for normal individual except restrict cholesterol, saturated fat. Increase PUFAs.	Nicotinic acid, clofibrate, gemfibrozil, mevinolin.[76]	Plasma LDL, VLDL, and cholesterol; blood glucose, uric acid; dietary intake of energy, protein, total fat, PUFAs,

			mono- and diglycerides, minerals, vitamins.[75,77] See Chapter 2 for other routine assessment parameters and standards.
INBORN ERRORS OF MINERAL METABOLISM			
Acrodermatitis enteropathica (defect in intestinal zinc absorption)	Same as for normal individual.		Plasma neutrophil or urinary zinc;[20] dietary intake of energy, protein, minerals, vitamins. See Chapter 2 for other routine assessment parameters and standards.
Wilson's disease Hepatolenticular degeneration (excessive accumulation of copper)	Dependent on etiology of acute illness.	D-penicillamine binds other divalent minerals, such as zinc, and causes excess excretion.[78] D-penicillamine increases the pyridoxine requirement to 25 mg/d.[79,80]	Plasma copper, ferritin, prealbumin;[78,79] dietary intake of energy, protein, copper, zinc, other minerals, vitamins. See Chapter 2 for other routine assessment parameters and standards.

Note: ARG, arginine; BCAAs, branched-chain amino acids; CBC, complete blood count; CIT, citrulline; CYS, cystine; GLY, glycine; GTP, guanosine triphosphate; HOMOCYS, homocystine; ILE, isoleucine; LCAT, lecithin:cholesterol acyltransferase; IV, intravenous; LEU, leucine; LDL, low-density lipoprotein; LYS, lysine; MET, methionine; MUFA, monounsaturated fatty acid; PHE, phenylalanine; PUFA, polyunsaturated fatty acid; RBP, retinol-binding protein; THR, threonine; TRP, tryptophan; TYR, tyrosine; UDP, uridine diphosphate; VAL, valine; VLDL, very low-density lipoprotein.

Table 13–4 Results of Amino Acid and Nitrogen Deficiencies

Amino Acid	*Manifestations of Deficiency*
Arginine	Elevated blood ammonia Elevated urinary orotic acid Generalized skin lesions Poor wound healing Retarded growth
Carnitine	Fatty myopathy Cardiomyopathy Depressed liver function Neurologic dysfunction Defective fatty acid oxidation Hypoglycemia Hypertriacylglycerolemia
Citrulline	Elevated blood ammonia
Cysteine	Impaired nitrogen balance Impaired sulfur balance Decreased tissue glutathione Hypotaurinemia
Isoleucine	Weight loss or no weight gain Redness of buccal mucosa Fissures at corners of mouth Tremors of extremities Decreased plasma cholesterol Decreased plasma isoleucine Elevations in plasma lysine, phenylalanine, serine, tyrosine, and valine Skin desquamation, if prolonged
Leucine	Loss of appetite, apathy, irritability Weight loss or poor weight gain Decreased plasma leucine Increased plasma isoleucine, methionine, serine, threonine, and valine
Lysine	Weight loss or poor weight gain Impaired nitrogen balance
Methionine	Decreased plasma methionine Increased plasma phenylalanine, proline, serine, threonine, and tyrosine Decreased plasma cholesterol Poor weight gain

Source: Data from references 5 to 8, 11, 15, 31, and 85 to 101.

continues

Table 13–4 continued

Amino Acid	*Manifestations of Deficiency*
Phenylalanine	Weight loss or poor weight gain Impaired nitrogen balance Aminoaciduria Decreased serum globulins Decreased plasma phenylalanine Mental retardation Anemia
Taurine	Impaired visual function Impaired biliary secretion
Threonine	Arrested weight gain Glossitis and reddening of the buccal mucosa Decreased plasma globulin Decreased plasma threonine
Tryptophan	Weight loss or no weight gain Impaired nitrogen retention Decreased plasma cholesterol
Tyrosine	Impaired nitrogen retention Catecholamine deficiency Thyroxine deficiency
Valine	Poor appetite, drowsiness Excess irritability and crying Weight loss or decrease in weight gain Decreased plasma albumin
Nitrogen	No or decreased weight gain Impaired nitrogen retention

selected nutrients per 100 kcal of infant formula in the form prepared for consumption (Table 13–5). However, IFA does not address amounts of chromium, molybdenum, and selenium that should be present per 100 kcal, and IFA specifications often differ from those of the NAS/NRC RDAs.[1] Consequently, an infant formula may meet IFA requirements but fail to supply some nutrients in amounts specified by NAS/NRC RDAs[1] (Table 13–5). Data in Table 13–6 describe formulations and major nutrient composition of medical foods for inborn errors of metabolism.

INBORN ERRORS OF NITROGEN METABOLISM

The urea cycle normally contributes large amounts of arginine to the body arginine pool. When the urea cycle is nonfunctional, arginine becomes an essential amino acid.[5] Consequently, arginine supplements must be administered in all disorders of the urea cycle except arginase deficiency (Tables 13–1 and 13–2). In carbamyl phosphate synthetase (CPS) or ornithine transcarbamylase (OTC) deficiency, L-citrulline may be given in place of L-arginine.

Table 13–5 Comparison of Nutrient Specifications in Infant Formula Act (IFA) and 1989 Recommended Dietary Allowances (RDAs)

Nutrients	*IFA (per 100 kcal)*	*RDAs (per 100 kcal)*
Protein (g)	1.8–4.5	2.0
Fat (g)	3.3–6.0	NG
Linoleic acid (mg)	300	NG
Arginine (mg)	NG	NG
Cystine (mg)	NG	See (MET + CYS)
Histidine (mg)	NG	26
Isoleucine (mg)	NG	65
Leucine (mg)	NG	148
Lysine (mg)	NG	95
Methionine (mg)	NG	53 (MET + CYS)
Phenylalanine (mg)	NG	115 (PHE + TYR)
Threonine (mg)	NG	80
Tyrosine (mg)	NG	See (PHE + TYR)
Tryptophan (mg)	NG	16
Valine (mg)	NG	86
Minerals		
Calcium (mg)	60	62
Chloride (mg)	55–150	40
Chromium (μg)	NG	1.54
Copper (μg)	60	62
Iodine (μg)	5–75	6
Iron (mg)	0.15–3.0	0.92
Magnesium (mg)	6	6.15
Manganese (μg)	5	46
Molybdenum (μg)	NG	2.3
Phosphorus (mg)	30	46
Potassium (mg)	80–200	51
Selenium (μg)	NG	1.54
Sodium (mg)	20–60	17
Zinc (mg)	0.50	0.77
Calcium/phosphorus ratio	1.1–2.0	1.3
Vitamins		
A (IU)	250–750	192
D (IU)	40–100	46
E (IU)	0.7	0.68
K (μg)	4	0.76
B_1 (μg)	40	46
B_2 (μg)	60	62
B_6 (μg)	35	46
B_{12} (μg)	0.15	0.046
Biotin (μg)	1.5	1.5

Source: Reprinted with permission from *Recommended Dietary Allowances,* 10th revised edition. Copyright © 1989 by the National Academy of Sciences. Courtesy of the National Academy Press, Washington, DC.

continues

Table 13–5 continued

Nutrients	*IFA (per 100 kcal)*	*RDAs (per 100 kcal)*
C (mg)	8	4.6
Choline (mg)	7	NG
Folacin (μg)	4	3.8
Inositol (mg)	4	NG
Niacin (μg)	250	769 NE
Pantothenic acid (μg)	300	307

Note: CYS, cystine; MET, methionine; NE, niacin equivalent; NG, none given; TYR, tyrosine.

When administered in adequate amounts, these amino acids also enhance waste nitrogen excretion.[12]

Protein (nitrogen) restriction has been the primary approach to prevention of elevated blood ammonia (Tables 13–1 and 13–2). Protein quality is determined by its essential amino acid content. Protein synthesis and nitrogen utilization are more efficient when all essential amino acids are present in appropriate amounts. Severe restriction of intact protein leads to inadequate intake of several essential and conditionally essential amino acids. Because of this, medical foods consisting of essential and conditionally essential amino acids have been devised (Table 13–6). Carnitine, cystine, taurine, and tyrosine may not be synthesized in adequate amounts when liver parenchymal cells are damaged, as reported with some urea cycle enzyme defects.[34,35] Thus, any medical food used for therapy of urea cycle disorders should contain carnitine, cystine, taurine, and tyrosine. Overrestriction of an essential amino acid or nitrogen leads to decreased protein synthesis or body protein catabolism and increased blood ammonia. Thus, to provide adequate amounts of essential amino acids in the protein-restricted diet, about one-half to two-thirds of the protein prescription should be supplied by medical food.

Bachmann and Colombo[36] reported that elevated blood ammonia enhances brain uptake of tryptophan. The resulting enhanced serotonin synthesis appears to decrease appetite, which can account for inadequate energy intake that results in body protein catabolism.[37] Unless blood ammonia can be maintained in the normal range, tryptophan content of medical foods designed for urea cycle disorders should be on the low side of normal requirements.

Protein quality of medical foods must also be evaluated based on their mineral and vitamin content because intact protein sources (dairy products, meat, fish and other seafood, and poultry) normally supply large amounts of minerals and vitamins. Intracellular minerals are important for protein synthesis. Medical foods devised for patients with urea cycle disorders must supply all minerals and vitamins not contributed by the small quantities of low-protein breads/cereals, fruits, fats, and vegetables the patient may ingest. The medical foods UCD1 and 2 contain no added chromium, magnesium, or selenium. UCD2 is low in all added minerals and vitamins[38] (Table 13–6).

Because protein intake is severely restricted, energy (kcal) intake should be increased to prevent use of muscle protein for energy purposes, thereby preventing catabolism of body protein (Table 13–2). Energy is the first requirement of the body, and inadequate energy intake for protein synthesis and other needs will lead to elevated blood ammonia concentration.[3,12]

Waste nitrogen excretion is enhanced through treatment with sodium benzoate, sodium phenylacetate, or sodium phenylbutyrate.[39] Sodium benzoate is conjugated with glycine, pri-

Table 13–6 Formulation, Nutrient Composition, and Sources of Medical Foods for Selected Inborn Errors of Metabolism[11]

Disorder and Medical Food	*Modified Nutrient(s) (mg/100 g)*	*Protein Equivalent (g/100 g), source*	*Fat (g/100 g), source*	*Carbohydrate (g/100 g), source*	*Energy (g/100 g)*	*Minerals Not Added*
			Aromatic Amino Acids			
PKU and Hyperphenylalaninemia						
Lofenalac*	PHE-80; TYR-800; TRP-195; L-carnitine, taurine added	15 Enzymatically hydrolyzed casein, L-amino acids	18 Corn oil	60 Corn syrup solids, modified tapioca starch	460	Chromium Molybdenum
Periflex‡	PHE-0; TYR-1850; TRP-270; L-carnitine-20; added taurine	20 L-amino acids	17 Canola oil, hybrid safflower oil, fractionated coconut oil	40.5 corn syrup solids	395	None
Phenex-1†	PHE-0; TYR-1500; TRP-170; L-carnitine-20; added taurine	15 L-amino acids	23.9 Palm oil, hydrogenated coconut oil, soy oil	46.3 Hydrolyzed cornstarch	480	Chromium§ Molybdenum§
Phenex-2†	PHE-0; TYR-3000; TRP-340; L-carnitine-40; added taurine	30 L-amino acids	15.5 Palm oil, hydrogenated coconut oil, soy oil	30 Hydrolyzed cornstarch	410	Chromium§ Molybdenum§
XP Analog‡	PHE-0; TYR-1370; TRP-300; L-carnitine-10; added taurine	13 L-amino acids	20.9 Peanut oil, refined lard, hydrogenated coconut oil	59 Corn syrup solids	475	None
XP Maxamaid‡	PHE-0, TYR-2650, TRP-570; L-carnitine-20; added taurine	25 L-amino acids	< 1.0 None added	62 Sucrose, hydrolyzed corn starch	350	None

XP Maxamum‡	PHE-0; TYR-4030; TRP-890; L-carnitine-20; added taurine	39 L-amino acids	< 1.0 None added	34 Sucrose, hydrolyzed corn starch	301	None
Phenyl-Free*	PHE-0; TYR-2000; TRP-280; L-carnitine, taurine added	19.8 L-amino acids	6.6 Corn and coconut oils	66 Sucrose, corn syrup solids, modified tapioca starch	410	Chromium Molybdenum
PKU 1*	PHE-0; TYR-3400; TRP-1000; no L-carnitine, taurine	50 L-amino acids	0 None added	19 Sucrose	280	Chromium Selenium
PKU 2*	PHE-0; TYR-4500; TRP-1400; no L-carnitine, taurine	67 L-amino acids	0 None added	7 Sucrose	300	Chromium Selenium
PKU 3*	PHE-0; TYR-6000; TRP-1400; no L-carnitine, taurine	68 L-amino acids	0 None added	3 Sucrose	290	Chromium Selenium
Tyrosinemia Types I, Ib						
Tyromex-1†	PHE-0; TYR-0; MET-0; L-carnitine-20; added taurine	15 L-amino acids	23.9 Palm oil, hydrogenated coconut oil, soy oil	46.3 Hydrolyzed cornstarch	480	Chromium§ Molybdenum§
Tyrex-2†	PHE-0; TYR-0; L-carnitine-40; added taurine	30 L-amino acids	15.5 Palm oil, hydrogenated coconut oil, soy oil	30 Hydrolyzed cornstarch	410	Chromium§ Molybdenum§

continues

Table 13–6 continued

Disorder and Medical Food	*Modified Nutrient(s) (mg/100 g)*	*Protein Equivalent (g/100 g), source*	*Fat (g/100 g), source*	*Carbohydrate (g/100 g), source*	*Energy (g/100 g)*	*Minerals Not Added*
XPHEN, TYR, MET Analog‡	PHE-0; TYR-0; MET-0; L-carnitine-10; added taurine	13 L-amino acids	20.9 Peanut oil, refined lard, hydrogenated coconut oil	59 Corn syrup solids	475	None
XPHEN, TYR Maxamaid†	PHE-0; TYR-0; L-carnitine-20; added taurine	25 L-amino acids	< 1.0 None added	62 Sucrose, hydrolyzed corn starch	350	None
Tyrosinemia Types II, III						
Low PHE/TYR Diet Powder*	PHE-75; TYR-38; L-carnitine, taurine added	15 Enzymically hydrolyzed casein, L-amino acids	18 Corn oil	60 Corn syrup solids, modified tapioca starch	460	Chromium Molybdenum
TYR 1*	PHE-0; TYR-0; no L-carnitine, taurine	47 L-amino acids	0 None added	21 Sucrose	270	Chromium Selenium
TYR 2*	PHE-0; TYR-0; no L-carnitine, taurine	63 L-amino acids	0 None added	12 Sucrose	300	Chromium Selenium
Tyrex-2†	PHE-0; TYR-0; L-carnitine-40; added taurine	30 L-amino acids	15.5 Palm oil, hydrogenated coconut oil, soy oil	30 Hydrolyzed cornstarch	410	Chromium§ Molybdenum§
XPHEN, TYR Analog‡	PHE-0; TYR-0; L-carnitine-10; added taurine	13 L-amino acids	20.9 Peanut oil, refined lard, hydrogenated coconut oil	50 Corn syrup solids	475	None

XPHEN, TYR Maxamaid‡	PHE-0; TYR-0; L-carnitine-20; added taurine	25 L-amino acids	< 1.0 None added	62 Sucrose, hydrolyzed corn starch	350	None
		Branched-Chain Amino Acids				
Maple Syrup Urine Disease, ß-Ketothiolase Deficiency						
Acerflex‡	ILE-0; LEU-0; VAL-0	20 L-amino acids	17 Canola oil, hybrid safflower oil, fractionated coconut oil	40.5 Corn syrup solids	395	None
Ketonex-1†	ILE-0; LEU-0; VAL-0; L-carnitine-100; added taurine	15 L-amino acids	23.9 Palm oil, hydrogenated coconut oil, soy oil	46.3 Hydrolyzed cornstarch	480	Chromium§ Molybdenum§
Ketonex-2†	ILE-0; LEU-0; VAL-0; L-carnitine-200; added taurine	30 L-amino acids	15.5 Palm oil, hydrogenated coconut oil, soy oil	30 Hydrolyzed cornstarch	410	Chromium§ Molybdenum§
MSUD 1*	ILE-0; LEU-0; VAL-0; L-carnitine-0; taurine-0	49 L-amino acids	0 None added	29 Sucrose	280	Chromium Selenium
MSUD 2*	ILE-0; LEU-0; VAL-0; L-carnitine-0; taurine-0	54 L-amino acids	0 None added	22 Sucrose	310	Chromium Selenium

continues

Table 13–6 continued

Disorder and Medical Food	*Modified Nutrient(s) (mg/100 g)*	*Protein Equivalent (g/100 g), source*	*Fat (g/100 g), source*	*Carbohydrate (g/100 g), source*	*Energy (g/100 g)*	*Minerals Not Added*
MSUD Analog[‡]	ILE-0; LEU-0; VAL-0; L-carnitine-10; added taurine	13 L-amino acids	20.9 Peanut oil, refined lard, hydrogenated coconut oil	59 Corn syrup solids	475	None
MSUD Diet Powder*	ILE-0; LEU-0; VAL-0; added L-carnitine, taurine	8.8 L-amino acids	20 Corn oil	63 Corn syrup solids, modified tapioca starch	470	Chromium Molybdenum
MSUD Maxamaid[‡]	ILE-0; LEU-0; VAL-0; L-carnitine-10; added taurine	25 L-amino acids	< 1.0 None added	62 Sucrose, hydrolyzed cornstarch	350	None
MSUD Maxamum[‡]	ILE-0; LEU-0; VAL-0; L-carnitine-20; added taurine	39 L-amino acids	< 1.0 None added	45 Sucrose, hydrolyzed cornstarch	340	None
Isovaleric Acidemia						
I-Valex-1[†]	ILE-430; LEU-0; TRP-170; VAL-480; L-carnitine-900; GLY-1000; added taurine	15 L-amino acids	23.9 Palm oil, hydrogenated coconut oil, soy oil	46.3 Hydrolyzed cornstarch	480	Chromium[§] Molybdenum[§]
I-Valex-2[†]	ILE-860; LEU-0; TRP-340; VAL-960; L-carnitine-1800; GLY-3020; added taurine	30 L-amino acids	15.5 Palm oil, hydrogenated coconut oil, soy oil	30 Hydrolyzed cornstarch	410	Chromium[§] Molybdenum[§]

XLEU Analog[‡]	ILE-400; LEU-0; TRP-260; VAL-450; GLY-2500; L-carnitine-10; added taurine	13 L-amino acids	20.9 Peanut oil, refined lard, coconut oil, soy oil	59 Corn syrup solids	475	None
XLEU Maxamaid[‡]	ILE-780; LEU-0; TRP-500; VAL-870; GLY-3990; L-carnitine-20; added taurine	25 L-amino acids	< 1.0 None added	62 Sucrose, hydrolyzed cornstarch	350	None
			Sulfur Amino Acids			
Homocystinuria, Pyridoxine-nonresponsive						
HOM 1*	MET-0; CYS-2500; L-carnitine-0; taurine-0	52 L-amino acids	0 None added	18 Sucrose	280	Chromium Selenium
HOM 2*	MET-0; CYS-3400; L-carnitine-0; taurine-0	69 L-amino acids	0 None added	5 Sucrose	300	Chromium Selenium
Hominex-1[†]	MET-0; CYS-450; L-carnitine-20; added taurine	15 L-amino acids	23.9 Palm oil, hydrogenated coconut oil, soy oil	46.3 Hydrolyzed cornstarch	480	Chromium[§] Molybdenum[§]
Hominex-2[†]	MET-0; CYS-900; L-carnitine-40; added taurine	30 L-amino acids	15.5 Palm oil, hydrogenated coconut oil, soy oil	30 Hydrolyzed cornstarch	410	Chromium[§] Molybdenum[§]

continues

Table 13–6 continued

Disorder and Medical Food	*Modified Nutrient(s) (mg/100 g)*	*Protein Equivalent (g/100 g), source*	*Fat (g/100 g), source*	*Carbohydrate (g/100 g), source*	*Energy (g/100 g)*	*Minerals Not Added*
XMET Analog‡	MET-0; CYS-390; L-carnitine-10; added taurine	13 L-amino acids	20.9 Peanut oil, refined lard, hydrogenated coconut oil	59 Corn syrup solids	475	None
XMET Maxamaid‡	MET-0; CYS-750; L-carnitine-20; added taurine	25 L-amino acids	< 1.0 None added	62 Sucrose, hydrolyzed cornstarch	350	None
XMET Maxamum‡	MET-0; CYS-1180; L-carnitine-20; added taurine	39 L-amino acids	< 1.0 None added	45 Sucrose, hydrolyzed cornstarch	340	None
Other Amino Acids						
Glutaric Aciduria Type I, Ketoadipic Aciduria						
Glutarex-1†	LYS-0; TRP-0; L-carnitine-900, added taurine	15 L-amino acids	23.9 Palm oil, hydrogenated coconut oil, soy oil	46.3 Hydrolyzed cornstarch	480	Chromium§ Molybdenum§
Glutarex-2†	LYS-0; TRP-0; L-carnitine-1800, added taurine	30 L-amino acids	15.5 Palm oil, hydrogenated coconut oil, soy oil	30 Hydrolyzed cornstarch	410	Chromium§ Molybdenum§
XLYS, TRY Analog‡	LYS-0; TRP-0; L-carntine-10, added taurine	13 L-amino acids	20.9 Peanut oil, refined lard, hydrogenated coconut oil	59 Corn syrup solids	475	None

XLYS, TRY Maxamaid‡	LYS-0; TRP-0; L-carnitine-20, added taurine	25 L-amino acids	< 1.0 None added	62 Sucrose, hydrolyzed cornstarch	350	None
XLYS, TRY Maxamum‡	LYS-0; TRP-0; L-carnitine-20, added taurine	39 L-amino acids	< 1.0 None added	45 Sucrose, hydrolyzed cornstarch	340	None
<u>Propionic and Methylmalonic Acidemias</u>						
OS1*	ILE-0; MET-0; THR-0; VAL-0; L-carnitine-0, taurine-0	42 L-amino acids	0 None added	29 Sucrose	280	Chromium Selenium
OS21*	ILE-0; MET-0; THR-0; VAL-0; L-carnitine-0, taurine-0	56 L-amino acids	0 None added	20 Sucrose	300	Chromium Selenium
Propimex-1†	ILE-120; MET-0; THR-100; VAL-0; L-carnitine-900; added taurine	15 L-amino acids	23.9 Palm oil, hydrogenated coconut oil, soy oil	46.3 Hydrolyzed cornstarch	480	Chromium§ Molybdenum§
Propimex-2†	ILE-240; MET-0; THR-200; VAL-0; L-carnitine-1800; added taurine	30 L-amino acids	15.5 Palm oil, hydrogenated coconut oil, soy oil	30 Hydrolyzed cornstarch	410	Chromium§ Molybdenum§
XMET, THRE, VAL, ISOLEU Analog‡	ILE-0; MET-0; THR-0; VAL-0; L-carnitine-10; added taurine	13 L-amino acids	20.9 Peanut oil, refined lard, hydrogenated coconut oil	59 Corn syrup solids	475	None

continues

Table 13–6 continued

Disorder and Medical Food	*Modified Nutrient(s) (mg/100 g)*	*Protein Equivalent (g/100 g), source*	*Fat (g/100 g), source*	*Carbohydrate (g/100 g), source*	*Energy (g/100 g)*	*Minerals Not Added*
XMET, THRE, VAL, ISOLEU Maxamaid‡	ILE-0; MET-0; THR-0; VAL-0; L-carnitine-20, added taurine	25 L-amino acids	< 1.0 None added	62 Sucrose, hydrolyzed cornstarch	350	None
		Fatty Acid Oxidation Defects				
ProViMin	Fat	73.0 Casein, L-amino acids	1.4 Coconut oil	2.0 None added	312	Chromium
<u>Urea Cycle Enzyme Defects</u>						
Cyclinex-1†	Non-essential amino acids-0; L-carnitine-190; added taurine	7.5 L-amino acids	27 Palm oil, hydrogenated coconut oil, soy oil	52 Hydrolyzed cornstarch	515	Chromium§ Molybdenum§
Cyclinex-2†	Non-essential amino acids-0; L-carnitine-370; added taurine	15 L-amino acids	20.7 Palm oil, hydrogenated coconut oil, soy oil	40 Hydrolyzed cornstarch	480	Chromium§ Molybdenum§
UCD 1*	Non-essential amino acids-0; No L-carnitine, taurine	67 L-amino acids	0	8 Sucrose	260	Chromium Magnesium Selenium
UCD 2*	Non-essential amino acids-0; No L-carnitine, taurine	67 L-amino acids	0	6 Sucrose	290	Chromium Magnesium Selenium

Pro-Phree†	Protein-0; L-carnitine-25; added taurine	0		31.0 Palm oil, hydrogenated coconut oil, soy oil	60.0 Hydrolyzed cornstarch	520	Chromium§ Molybdenum§
Protein-Free Diet Powder*	Protein-0; L-carnitine, taurine added	0		23.0 Corn oil	72.0 Corn syrup solids, modified tapioca starch	500	Chromium Molybdenum

*Mead Johnson Nutritional Division, Evansville, IN; 1/800-457-3550.

†Ross Products Division, Abbott Laboratories, Columbus, OH; 1/800-551-5838.

‡Scientific Hospital Supplies, North American Division, Gaithersburg, MD; 1/800-365-7354.

§Ingredients contain adequate naturally occurring chromium and molybdenum.

Note: Values listed, although accurate at time of publication, are subject to change. The most current information may be obtained by referring to product labels.

marily in hepatic and renal cell mitochondria, to form hippurate, which is cleared by the kidney.[40] Sodium phenylacetate conjugates with glutamine in kidney and liver cells to form phenylacetylglutamine, which is excreted by the kidney.[40,41] Phenylacetic acid conjugates with taurine in the kidney.[42]

Concerns with the Use of Sodium Benzoate and Sodium Phenylacetate

Chronic exposure of mammalian cortical neuronal cultures with 0.6 mmol phenylacetate has a detrimental effect on their growth and function. Detrimental effects may be mediated by deficiencies of pantothenate, niacin, folate, and vitamin B_{12}, which are all required for conjugation reactions by cytochrome P-450 systems.[43]

The synthesis of hippurate from benzoate and glycine requires adenosine triphosphate (ATP) and coenzyme A (CoA).[44] If glycine is inadequate, benzoyl CoA will accumulate and can impair hepatic gluconeogenesis and lipogenesis,[45] possibly due to CoA sequestration. An oral dose of 4 g sodium benzoate given to healthy adults depleted the metabolic pool of glycine, as indicated by an increased urinary excretion of pyroglutamic acid (5-oxoproline).[46] Inadequate available glycine for heme and glutathione synthesis could have serious pathologic effects. Cyr et al[47] found that benzoyl CoA accumulated in isolated hepatocytes when incubated with benzoate. Synthesis of urea and orotate were depressed in this system. The authors suggested that benzoate potentiates ammonia toxicity by blocking the urea cycle through sequestration of CoA. Batshaw et al[48] and Hyman and coworkers[37] reported that sodium benzoate increased tryptophan uptake by the brain and increased serotonin flux. The suggestion was made that clinical symptoms of sodium benzoate intoxication are related to this alteration in serotonin metabolism.

Glycine is readily made from serine. Tetrahydrofolate (FH_4) is required for this reaction to occur. Glycine can also be synthesized from glutamate. Pyridoxal phosphate (PLP) and an aldolase are required for this set of reactions. Because of the several coenzymes required to maintain serine, nicotinamide-adenine dinucleotide (NAD), PLP, and glycine (FH_4) pools, and the use of CoA in synthesis of hippurate, folate, pantothenate, pyridoxine, and niacin should be administered at three to five times their RDAs for age when sodium benzoate is given therapeutically.

INBORN ERRORS OF CARBOHYDRATE METABOLISM

Galactosemias and Hereditary Fructose Intolerance

Deletion of galactose in most forms of galactosemia and fructose in hereditary fructose intolerance must be accompanied by adequate intakes of protein, energy, minerals, and vitamins (Tables 13–1 and 13–2). Both galactose and fructose bind with phosphate in patients with galactosemia and hereditary fructose intolerance.[49–52] This intracellular sequestering of phosphorus, in combination with excess urinary phosphate loss (Fanconi syndrome), suggests the need for phosphorus intake greater than RDA[1] for age. If the patient with galactose-1-phosphate uridyl transferase or aldolase B deficiency has any residual enzyme activity, pharmacologic doses of folic acid may extend the enzymes' half-life[53] and provide for better outcomes.

Therapy of galactosemia due to galactose-1-phosphate uridyl transferase deficiency, though lifesaving, has resulted in less than optimum outcomes.[54] Poor outcomes may be the result of small but significant intakes of naturally occurring galactose in fruits, vegetables, grains, legumes, and other foods[55] or from ongoing deficiencies of riboflavin,[56] phosphorus,[57] and inositol.[58] On the other hand, in vivo synthesis of galactose[59] may be partially responsible for long-term complications in patients with gene mutations resulting in no enzyme activity.[60] Infant formulas made from soy protein isolate without added lactose contain significantly less galactose[61] than do formulas made from hydrolyzed casein.[61] One such formula (Next Step Soy, Mead Johnson Nutritionals, Evansville, IN) may be used in the long term after Isomil or ProSobee is discontinued as a source of protein, minerals, and vitamins. Milk products and organ meats must be eliminated. Careful label reading for the presence of lactose, casein, or whey and examination of all drug ingredients should be practiced before suggesting the use of any food or drug. Patients with no enzyme activity may also require deletion of some fruits, vegetables, and legumes from the diet.[55]

Glycogen Storage Diseases

Outcomes of patients with glycogen storage disease have been significantly improved by two recent therapeutic approaches.[62,63] These are continuous nasogastric feeding and administration of raw cornstarch (Table 13–1).[64,65] Both therapeutic modalities aim at maintaining normal blood glucose at all times.[66–68] High-protein diets and L-alanine supplements[64–69] have been found to be beneficial in muscle phosphorylase deficiency (Table 13–2).

INBORN ERRORS OF LIPOPROTEIN METABOLISM

Abetalipoproteinemia, hypobetalipoproteinemia, lecithin:cholesterol acyl tranferase (LCAT) deficiency, and type I hyperlipoproteinemia all require stringent restriction of dietary triglycerides with long-chain fatty acids.[70–73] In all four disorders, adequate linoleic and α-linolenic acids must be provided to prevent deficiency (Table 13–2). Medium-chain triglycerides (MCT) may be used as an energy source. In the abeta- and hypobetalipoproteinemias, all the fat-soluble vitamins require supplementation.[70–72] In particular, pharmacologic dosesof vitamin E are necessary to prevent myopathy and neurologic degeneration[72] in abetalipoproteinemia.

Restriction of total dietary fat, cholesterol, and saturated fat[74,75] is used to treat types IIa, IIb, and III hyperlipoproteinemia. Natural fiber in the form of whole grains, legumes, fruits, and vegetables should be increased in the diets of children with types IIb and III hyperlipoproteinemias. Mono- and disaccharides are restricted in the diets of patients with type IIb and type III hyperlipoproteinemias.[76] When cholestyramine or colestipol is used, total dietary fat, fat-soluble vitamins, vitamin B_{12}, and iron may need to be increased in the diet.[43] Great care must be taken to ensure an adequate diet because growth failure and nutritional dwarfing may otherwise result.[77]

INBORN ERRORS OF MINERAL METABOLISM

Acrodermatitis enteropathica, characterized by mental depression, circumoral and acral dermatitis, alopecia, diarrhea, failure to thrive, and death, is a rare inherited disorder affecting zinc absorption.[20] Large supplements of zinc given two to three times daily cure all the symptoms of this disorder (Table 13–2).

Wilson's disease is a rare disorder that results in accumulation of copper in the brain, liver, and kidneys, resulting in neurologic deterioration and liver and renal failure.[78] Therapy includes restriction of foods high in copper and the use of D-penicillamine (Table 13–3). Zinc and pyridoxine supplements should be administered when D-penicillamine is used.[79,80]

AREAS REQUIRING FURTHER RESEARCH

In 1988, the National Institutes of Health recognized the need for research on nutrition therapy of inborn errors of metabolism by issuing a request for applications (RFA).[81] The goals listed in the RFA were (1) to improve the effectiveness of currently utilized nutrition therapies of inborn errors by making them safer, more palatable, and less likely to lead to secondary deleterious consequences and (2) to develop new rational diet therapies based on knowledge of pathogenesis. Research approaches outlined in

Table 13–7 were identified for support, and investigations utilizing these approaches were encouraged. Other approaches for meeting the goals of the RFA were not excluded.

FUNCTIONS OF THE DIETITIAN IN NUTRITION SUPPORT OF PATIENTS WITH AN INBORN ERROR OF METABOLISM

The roles of the dietitian in nutrition support of patients with an inborn error of metabolism are outlined in Table 13–8.[82] Because of the dietitian's central role in therapy, he or she is often the case manager,[83] coordinating clinic care and acting as liaison with the public health nutritionist[84] or home health agency. The crucial role of the dietitian in long-term management of the patient with an inborn error of metabolism mandates excellent interpersonal skills, as well as a knowledge base far in excess of entry level requirements. Without this knowledge and the capability to transmit this knowledge to patients, parents, and professionals, outcomes may be poor, or death may occur.

Table 13–7 Research Approaches to Nutrition Therapy of Inborn Errors of Metabolism

1. Investigations of how vitamins may affect active cofactor concentrations and activate specific deficient enzymes.
2. Studies of the pathogenesis of the clinical manifestations of inborn errors, designed to develop rationale for better diet therapy.
3. Longitudinal studies of the adequacy of nutrition therapies in maintaining normal growth and development while maximizing therapeutic response.
4. Studies of the development of secondary nutrient deficiencies in patients in therapeutic diets, due to interference with the availability of other nutrients, such as trace elements.
5. Investigation of possible injurious effects of specific components of therapeutic diets.
6. Attempts to improve nutrition therapies of inborn errors to eliminate metabolic problems not completely controlled, such as hyperlipidemia and hyperuricemia in glycogen storage disease, carnitine wasting in renal Fanconi syndrome, or the organic acidemias.
7. Development of methods for improving the palatability or acceptability of nutrition therapy, such as by the substitution of specific amino-acid-deficient peptides for amino acid mixtures.
8. Development of animal models for the study of nutrition therapies of inborn errors, either by a search for heterozygotes or through use of recombinant DNA methods.
9. Investigations of how vitamins may affect active cofactor concentrations and activate specific deficient enzymes.
10. Studies of the pathogenesis of the clinical manifestations of inborn errors, designed to develop rationale for better diet therapy.

Source: Data from E.Y. Levin and F. de la Cruz, *Nutritional Therapy of Inborn Errors of Metabolism RFA: 89-HD/DK-01,* 1988, National Institute of Child Health and Human Development.

Table 13–8 Functions of the Dietitian in Nutrition Support of Patients with Inborn Errors of Metabolism

During Diagnosis
- Evaluate nutrient intake
- Implement nutrition support plan
- Prepare nutrition support plan
- Evaluate nutrition support plan
- Evaluate nutrition status
- Record in medical record
- Adjust amino acid prescription (eg, glycine)
- Adjust selected medications (eg, sodium benzoate)

During Critical Illness
- Recommend composition of feedings
- Develop tube feedings when needed
- Monitor nutrition support
- Record in medical record
- Recommend amount to feed per hour
- Recommend continuous or intermittent feedings
- Recommend route of alimentation
- Recommend laboratory tests
- Recommend peripheral or central line feeding
- Recommend size of feeding tube

During Long-Term Care
- Formulate diet prescription/nutrition care plan
- Record in medical record
- Monitor for diet compliance
- Revise nutrition care plan as needed
- Evaluate effectiveness of nutrition care plan
- Coordinate with other agencies
- Prepare sample menus
- Modify diet prescription during illness
- Prescribe medical food
- Prescribe very-low-protein foods
- Recommend methods of feeding
- Evaluate research findings and apply to clinical care
- Fill diet prescription
- Monitor for gastrointestinal complications
- Refer to other specialists
- Monitor potential nutrient–drug interactions
- Prepare patient-specific food lists
- Prepare shopping lists
- Review grocery receipts

REFERENCES

1. Committee on Dietary Allowances, *Food and Nutrition Board. Recommended Dietary Allowances*. 10th revised ed. Washington, DC: National Academy of Sciences; 1989.
2. FAO/WHO/UNU. *Expert Consultation. Energy and Protein Requirements*. Geneva: World Health Organization; 1985.
3. Elsas LJ, Acosta PB. Nutrition support of inherited metabolic diseases. In: Shils ME, Olson JA, Shike M, eds. *Modern Nutrition in Health and Disease*. 9th ed. Philadelphia: Lea & Febiger, 1999.
4. Martin SB, Acosta PB. Nutrition support of phenylketonuria and maple syrup urine disease. *Top Clin Nutr*. 1987;2:9–24.
5. Goldblum OM, Brusilow SW, Maldonado YA, Farmer ER. Neonatal citrullinemia associated with cutaneous manifestations and arginine deficiency. *J Am Acad Dermatol*. 1986;14:321–326.
6. Borum PR, Bennett SG. Carnitine as an essential nutrient. *J Am Col Nutr*. 1986;5:177–182.
7. Sansaricq C, Garg S, Norton PM, Phansalkar SV, Snyderman SE. Cystine deficiency during dietotherapy of homocystinemia. *Acta Paediatr Scand*. 1975;64: 215–218.
8. Laidlaw SA, Kopple JD. Newer concepts of the indispensable amino acids. *Am J Clin Nutr*. 1987;46:593–605.
9. Przyrembel H. Therapy of mitochondrial disorders. *J Inher Metab Dis*. 1987;10:129–146.
10. Blau N. Inborn errors of pterin metabolism. *Ann Rev Nutr*. 1988;8:185–209.
11. Acosta PB, Yannicelli S. *Nutrition Support Protocols*, 3rd ed. Columbus, OH: Ross Products Division, Abbott Laboratories; 1997.
12. Batshaw ML, Monahan PS. Treatment of urea cycle disorders. In: Tada K, Colombo JP, Desnick RJ, eds. *Recent Advances in Inborn Errors of Metabolism*. New York: Karger; 1987:242–250.
13. Holmes RD, Wilson GN, Hajra A. Oral ether lipid therapy in patients with peroxisomal disorders. *J Inher Metab Dis*. 1987;10(suppl 2):239–241.
14. Martinez M. Docosahexaenoic acid therapy in docosahexaenoic acid-deficient patients with disorders of peroxisomal biogenesis. *Lipids*. 1996;31(suppl): S145–S152.
15. Rudman DA, Feller A. Evidence for deficiencies of conditionally essential nutrients during total parenteral nutrition. *J Am Col Nutr*. 1986;5:101–106.
16. Elsas LJ, Danner D, Lubitz D, Fernhoff P, Dembure P. Metabolic consequences of inherited defects in branched chain α-ketoacid dehydrogenase: Mechanism of thiamine action. In: Walser M, Williamson JR, eds. *Metabolism and Clinical Implications of Branched Chain Amino and Ketoacids*. New York: Elsevier Science; 1981:369–382.
17. Barber GW, Spaeth GL. Pyridoxine therapy in homocystinuria. *Lancet*. 1967;1:337–340.
18. Rosenberg LE, Fenton WA. Disorders of propionate and methylmalonate metabolism. In: Scriver CR, Beaudet AL, Sly WS, Valle D, eds. *The Metabolic and Molecular Bases of Inherited Disease*. 7th ed. New York: McGraw-Hill; 1995:1423–1449.
19. Bonkowsky HL, Magnussen CR, Collins AR, Donerty JM, Ress RA, Tschudy DP. Comparative effects of glycerol and dextrose on porphyrin precursor excretion in acute intermittent porphyria. *Metabolism*. 1976;25: 405–414.
20. Aggett PJ. Acrodermatitis enteropathica. *J Inher Metab Dis*. 1983;6(suppl 1):39–43.
21. Wolf B. Disorders of biotin metabolism. In: Scriver CR, Beaudet AL, Sly WS, Valle D, eds. *The Metabolic and Molecular Bases of Inherited Disease*. 7th ed. New York: McGraw-Hill; 1995:3151–3177.
22. Stepnick-Gropper S, Acosta PB, Clarke-Sheehan N, Wenz E, Cheng M, Koch R. Trace element status of children with PKU and normal children. *J Am Diet Assoc*. 1988;88:459–465.
23. Chipponi JX, Bleier JC, Santi MT, Rudman D. Deficiencies of essential and conditionally essential nutrients. *Am J Clin Nutr*. 1982;35:1112–1116.
24. Acosta PB, Stepnick-Gropper S. Problems related to diet management of maternal phenylketonuria. *J Inher Metab Dis*. 1986;9(suppl 2):183–201.
25. Martin SB, Acosta PB. Osmolalities of selected enteral products and carbohydrate modules used to treat inherited metabolic disorders. *J Am Diet Assoc*. 1987;87:48–52.
26. Guttler F, Olesen ES, Wamberg E. Diurnal variations of serum phenylalanine in phenylketonuric children on low phenylalanine diet. *Am J Clin Nutr*. 1969; 22:1568–1570.
27. Stepnick-Gropper S, Acosta PB. The effect of simultaneous ingestion of L-amino acids and whole protein on plasma amino acid concentrations and urea nitrogen concentrations in humans. *J Parenter Enter Nutr*. 1991; 5:48–53.
28. Guttler F, Guldberg P. Mutations in the phenylalanine hydroxylase gene: Genetic determinants for the phenotypic variability of hyperphenylalaninemia. *Acta Paediatr*. 1994;407(suppl):49–56.
29. Hermann ME, Broesicke HG, Keller M, Moench E, Helge H. Dependence of the utilization of a phenylalanine-free amino acid mixture on different amounts of

single dose ingested. A case report. *Eur J Pediatr.* 1994;153:501–503.

30. Schoeffer A, Hermann ME, Broesicke HG, Moench E. Effect of dosage and timing of amino acid mixtures on nitrogen retention in patients with phenylketonuria. *J Nutr Med.* 1994;4:415–418.
31. Pratt EL, Snyderman SE, Cheung MW, Norton P, Holt LE. The threonine requirement of the normal infant. *J Nutr.* 1955;56:231–251.
32. *PharmaThera.* 1785 Nonconnah Blvd, Suite 118, Memphis, TN 88132.
33. Young FE, Heckler MM. Nutrient requirements for infant formulas. *Fed Reg.* 1985;50:45106–45108.
34. LaBrecque DR, Latham PS, Riely CA, Hsia YE, Klatskin G. Heritable urea cycle enzyme deficiency: Liver disease in 16 patients. *J Pediatr.* 1979;94:580–587.
35. Zimmerman A, Baumgartner R. Severe liver fibrosis in argininosuccinic aciduria. *Arch Pathol Lab Med.* 1986; 110:136–140.
36. Bachmann C, Colombo JP. Increased tryptophan uptake into the brain in hyperammonemia. *Life Sci.* 1983; 33:2417–2424.
37. Hyman SL, Porter CA, Page TJ, Iwata BA, Kissel R, Batshaw ML. Behavior management of feeding disturbances in urea cycle and organic acid disorders. *J Pediatr.* 1987;111:558–562.
38. Mead Johnson Nutritionals. *Dietary Management of Metabolic Disorders.* Evansville, IN: Mead Johnson Nutritionals; 1994.
39. Brusilow SW. Treatment of urea cycle disorders. In: Desnick RJ, ed. *Treatment of Genetic Diseases.* New York: Churchill Livingstone; 1991:79–94.
40. Moldave K, Meister A. Synthesis of phenylacetylglutamine by human tissue. *J Biol Chem.* 1957;229: 463–476.
41. Ambrose AM, Power FW, Sherwin CP. Further studies on the detoxication of phenylacetic acid. *J Biol Chem.* 1933;101:669–675.
42. James MO, Smith RL, Williams RT, Reidenberg M. The conjugation of phenylacetic acid in man, subhuman primates and some non-primate species. *Proc R Soc Lond.* 1972;182:25–35.
43. Zeman FJ. Drugs and nutritional care. In: *Clinical Nutrition and Dietetics*, 2nd ed: New York: Macmillan Publishing USA; 1991:86–116.
44. Gatley SJ, Sherratt HSA. The synthesis of hippurate from benzoate and glycine by rat liver mitochondria. *Biochem J.* 1977;166:39–47.
45. McCune SA, Durant PJ, Flanders LE, Harris RA. Inhibition of hepatic gluconeogenesis and lipogenesis by benzoic acid, p-tert-butylbenzoic acid and a structurally related hypolipidemic agent SC-33459. *Arch Biochem Biophys.* 1982;214:124–133.
46. Jackson AA, Badaloo AV, Forrester T, et al. Urinary excretion of 5-oxo-proline (pyroglutamic aciduria) as an index of glycine insufficiency in normal man. *Br J Nutr.* 1987;58:207–214.
47. Cyr DM, Maswoswe SM, Trembloy GC. Inhibition of the urea cycle and de novo pyrimidine biosynthesis by sodium benzoate. *J Inher Metab Dis.* 1987;10(suppl 2):308–310.
48. Batshaw ML, Hyman SL, Coyle JT, Bachmann C. Effect of sodium benzoate (SB) on brain serotonin (5-HT) metabolism in experimental hyperammonemia (HA). *Pediatr Res.* 1986;20:326A.
49. Komrower GM. Galactosaemia: Thirty years on. The experience of a generation. *J Inher Metab Dis.* 1982; 5(suppl 2):96–104.
50. Sardharwalla IB, Wraith JE. Galactosemia. *Nutr Health.* 1987;5:175–188.
51. Odievre M, Gentil C, Gautier M, Alagille D. Hereditary fructose intolerance in childhood. *Am J Dis Child.* 1978;132:605–608.
52. Kogut MD, Roe TF, Ng W, Donnell GN. Fructose-induced hyperuricemia: observations in normal children and in patients with hereditary fructose intolerance and galactosemia. *Pediatr Res.* 1975;9: 774–778.
53. Rosensweig NS, Herman RH, Stifel FB, Herman YF. Regulation of human jejunal glycolytic enzymes by oral folic acid. *J Clin Invest.* 1969;48:2038–2042.
54. Waggoner DD, Buist NRM, Donnell GN. Long-term prognosis in galactosaemia: Results of a survey of 350 cases. *J Inher Metab Dis.* 1990;13:802–818.
55. Acosta PB, Gross KC. Hidden sources of galactose in the environment. *Eur J Pediatr.* 1995;154(suppl 2): S87–S92.
56. Prchal JT, Conrad ME, Skalka HW. Association of presenile cataracts with heterozygosity for galactosaemic states and with riboflavin deficiency. *Lancet.* 1978;1: 12–13.
57. Pennington JS, Prankerd TAJ. Studies of erythrocyte phosphate ester metabolism in galactosemia. *Clin Sci.* 1958;17:385–391.
58. Wells WW, McIntyre JP, Schlichter DJ, Wacholtz MC, Spieker SE. Studies on myo-inositol metabolism in galactosemia. *Ann NY Acad Sci.* 1969;165:599–608.
59. Berry GT, Nissim I, Lin Z, Mazur AT, Gibson JG, Segal S. Endogenous synthesis of galactose in normal men and patients with hereditary galactosaemia. *Lancet.* 1995; 346:1073–1074.
60. Elsas LJ, Fridovich-Keil JL, Leslie ND. Galactosemia: A molecular approach to the enigma. *Intl Pediatr.* 1993;8:101–109.
61. Mead Johnson Nutritionals. *Galactosemia in Infancy.* Evansville, IN: Mead Johnson Nutritionals; 1976:1–15.

62. Greene HL, Slonim AE, Burr IM, Moran JR. Type I glycogen storage disease: Five years of management with nocturnal intragastric feeding. *J Pediatr*. 1980; 96:590–595.

63. Ullrich K, Schmidt H, van Teeffelen-Heithoff A. Glycogen storage disease type I and III and pyruvate carboxylase deficiency: results of long-term treatment with uncooked cornstarch. *Acta Pediatr Scand*. 1988; 77:531–536.

64. Parker PH, Ballew M, Greene HL. Nutritional management of glycogen storage disease. *Ann Rev Nutr*. 1993; 13:83–109.

65. Wolfsdorf JI, Crigler JF. Cornstarch regimens for nocturnal treatment of young adults with type I glycogen storage disease. *Am J Clin Nutr*. 1997;65:1507–1511.

66. Chen YT, Cornblath M, Sidbury JB. Cornstarch therapy in type I glycogen-storage disease. *N Engl J Med*. 1984;310:171–175.

67. Chen YT, Leinhas J, Coleman RA. Prolongation of normoglycemia in patients with type I glycogen storage disease. *J Pediatr*. 1987;111:567–570.

68. Schwenk WF, Haymond MW. Optimal rate of enteral glucose administration in children with glycogen storage disease type I. *N Engl J Med*. 1986;314:682–685.

69. Slonim AE, Schiff MJ. Alanine is an effective fuel in McArdle's disease. *Clin Res*. 1989;37:461A.

70. Assmann G, von Eckardstein A, Brewer HB. Familial high density lipoprotein deficiency. In: Scriver CR, Beaudet AL, Sly CS, Valle D, eds. *The Metabolic and Molecular Bases of Inherited Disease*. 7th ed. New York: McGraw-Hill; 1995:2053–2072.

71. Brunzell JD. Familial lipoprotein lipase deficiency and other causes of the chylomicronemia syndrome. In: Scriver CR, Beaudet AL, Sly CS, Valle D, eds. *The Metabolic and Molecular Bases of Inherited Disease*. 7th ed. New York: McGraw-Hill; 1995:1913–1932.

72. Kane JP, Havel RJ. Disorders of the biogenesis and secretion of lipoproteins containing the ß-lipoproteins. In: Scriver CR, Beaudet AL, Sly CS, Valle D, eds. *The Metabolic and Molecular Bases of Inherited Disease*. 7th ed. New York: McGraw-Hill; 1995:1897–1912.

73. Gjone E, Norum KR, Glomset JA, Assmann G. Lecithin: Cholesterol acyltransferase deficiency, including fish eye disease. In: Scriver CR, Beaudet AL, Sly CS, Valle D, eds. *The Metabolic and Molecular Bases of Inherited Disease*. 7th ed. New York: McGraw-Hill; 1995:1933–1951.

74. Goldstein JL, Hobbs HH, Brown MS. Familial hypercholesterolemia. In: Scriver CR, Beaudet AL, Sly CS, Valle D, eds. *The Metabolic and Molecular Bases of Inherited Disease*. 7th ed. New York: McGraw-Hill; 1995:1981–2030.

75. Mahley RW, Rall SC. Type III hyperlipoproteinemia. In: Scriver CR, Beaudet AL, Sly CS, Valle D, eds. *The Metabolic and Molecular Bases of Inherited Disease*. 7th ed. New York: McGraw-Hill; 1995:1953–1980.

76. Schaefer EJ, Levy RI. Pathogenesis and management of lipoprotein disorders. *N Engl J Med*. 1985;312: 1300–1310.

77. Lifshitz F, Moses N. Growth failure: A complication of dietary treatment of hypercholesterolemia. *Am J Dis Child*. 1989;143:537–542.

78. Danks D. Disorders of copper transport. In: Scriver CR, Beaudet AL, Sly CS, Valle D, eds. *The Metabolic and Molecular Bases of Inherited Disease*. 7th ed. New York: McGraw-Hill; 1995:2211–2235

79. Walshe JM. Hudson memorial lecture: Wilson's disease: genetics and biochemistry—their relevance to therapy. *J Inher Metab Dis*. 1983;6(suppl 1):51–58.

80. *Physicians' Desk Reference*. Des Moines, IA: Edward R. Barnhart; 1996:1675.

81. Levin EY, de la Cruz F. *Nutritional Therapy of Inborn Errors of Metabolism*. RFA: 89-HD/DK-01. Bethesda, MD: National Institute of Child Health and Human Development; 1988.

82. Acosta PB, Ryan AS. Functions of dietitians providing nutrition support to patients with inherited metabolic disorders. *J Am Diet Assoc*. 1997;97:783–786.

83. Belsten LM, Rarback S, Wellman NS. The metabolic nutritionist as a team member and case manager. *Top Clin Nutr*. 1987;2:76–81.

84. Stephens-Hitchcock E, Walker EJ. The public health approach to the treatment and follow-up of children with metabolic disorders. *Top Clin Nutr*. 1987;2:82–86.

85. Snyderman SE, Boyer A, Phansalkar SV, Holt LE. Essential amino acid requirements of infants: Tryptophan. *Am J Dis Child*. 1961;102:163–167.

86. Snyderman SE, Norton PM, Fowler DI, Holt LE. The essential amino acid requirements of infants: Lysine. *Am J Dis Child*. 1959;97:175–185.

87. Barbul A. Arginine: biochemistry, physiology and therapeutic implications. *J Parenter Enter Nutr*. 1986; 10:227–238.

88. Milner JA. Metabolic aberrations associated with arginine deficiency. *J Nutr*. 1985;115:516–523.

89. Visek WJ. Arginine needs, physiological state and usual diets. A reevaluation. *J Nutr*. 1986;116:36–46.

90. Visek WJ, Shoemaker JD. Orotic acid, arginine, and hepatotoxicity. *J Am Col Nutr*. 1986; 5:153–166.

91. Zieve L. Conditional deficiencies of ornithine or arginine. *J Am Col Nutr*. 1986;5:167–176.

92. Gilbert EF. Carnitine deficiency. *Pathology*. 1985; 17:161–169.

93. Rebouche CJ, Paulson DJ. Carnitine metabolism and function in humans. *Ann Rev Nutr*. 1986;6:41–66.

94. Snyderman SE, Roitman E, Boyer A, Norton PM, Holt LE. The essential amino acid requirements of infants. IX. Isoleucine. *Am J Clin Nutr*. 1964;15:313–321.

95. Snyderman SE, Roitman E, Boyer A, Holt LE. The essential amino acid requirements of infants: Leucine. *Am J Dis Child.* 1961;102:157–162.
96. Snyderman SE, Boyer A, Norton PM, Roitman E, Holt LE. The essential amino acid requirements of infants. X. Methionine. *Am J Clin Nutr.* 1964;15:322–330.
97. Snyderman SE, Pratt EL, Cheung MW, et al. The phenylalanine requirement of the normal infant. *J Nutr.* 1955;56:253–263.
98. Ament ME, Geggel HS, Heckenlively JR, Martin DA, Kopple J. Taurine supplementation in infants receiving long-term total parenteral nutrition. *J Am Col Nutr.* 1986;5:127–135.
99. Sturman JA, Wen GY, Wisniewski HM, Neuringer MD. Retinal degeneration in primates raised on a synthetic human infant formula. *Int J Dev Neurosci.* 1984; 2:121–129.
100. Snyderman SE, Holt LE, Smellie F, Boyer A, Westall RG. The essential amino acid requirements of infants: valine. *Am J Dis Child.* 1959;97:186–191.
101. Snyderman SE, Holt LE, Dancis J, Roitman E, Boyer A, Balis ME. "Unessential" nitrogen: A limiting factor for human growth. *J Nutr.* 1962;78:57–72.
102. Scriver CR, Kaufman S, Woo SLC. The hyperphenylalaninemias. In: Scriver CR, Beaudet AL, Sly WS, Valle D, eds. *The Metabolic and Molecular Bases of Inherited Disease.* 7th ed. New York: McGraw-Hill; 1995:1015–1076.
103. Acosta PB. The contribution of therapy of inherited amino acid disorders to knowledge of amino acid requirements. In: Wapnir RA, ed. *Congenital Metabolic Diseases.* New York: Marcel Dekker; 1985:115–135.
104. Mitchell GA, Lambert M, Tanguay RM. Tyrosinemia and related disorders. In: Scriver CR, Beaudet AL, Sly WS, Valle D, eds. *The Metabolic and Molecular Bases of Inherited Disease.* 7th ed. New York: McGraw-Hill; 1995:1077–1106.
105. Chuang DT, Shih VE. Disorders of branched chain amino acid and ketoacid metabolism. In: Scriver CR, Beaudet AL, Sly WS, Valle D, eds. *The Metabolic and Molecular Bases of Inherited Disease.* 7th ed. New York: McGraw-Hill; 1995:1239–1278.
106. Sweetman L, Williams JC. Branched chain organic acidurias. In: Scriver CR, Beaudet AL, Sly WS, Valle D, eds. *The Metabolic and Molecular Bases of Inherited Disease.* 7th ed. New York: McGraw-Hill; 1995: 1387–1422.
107. Itoh T, Ito T, Ohba S et al. Effect of carnitine administration on glycine metabolism in patients with isovaleric acidemia: Significance of acetylcarnitine determination to estimate the proper carnitine dose. *Tohoku J Exp Med.* 1996;179:101–109.
108. Mudd SH, Levy HL, Skovby F. Disorders of transsulfuration. In: Scriver CR, Beaudet AL, Sly WS, Valle D, eds. *The Metabolic and Molecular Bases of Inherited Disease.* 7th ed. New York: McGraw-Hill; 1995:1279–1328.
109. Carey MC, Fennelly JJ, Fitzgerald O. Homocystinuria II. Subnormal serum folate levels, increased folate clearance and effects of folic acid therapy. *Am J Med.* 1968;45:26–31.
110. Wilcken DEL, Wilcken B, Dudman NPB, Tyrell PA. Homocystinuria: The effects of betaine in the treatment of patients not responsive to pyridoxine. *N Engl J Med.* 1983;309:448–453.
111. Schaumburg H, Kaplan J, Windebank A, et al. Sensory neuropathy from pyridoxine abuse. A new megavitamin syndrome. *N Engl J Med.* 1983;309:445–448.
112. Goodman SI, Frerman FE. Organic acidemias due to defects in lysine oxidation: 2-ketoadipic acidemia and glutaric acidemia. In: Scriver CR, Beaudet AL, Sly WS, Valle D, eds. *The Metabolic and Molecular Bases of Inherited Disease.* 7th ed. New York: McGraw-Hill; 1995:1451–1460.
113. Warman ML, Levy HL, Perry TL. Clinical and biochemical studies in three sibs with glutaric aciduria type I: Response to dietary therapy. *Am J Hum Genet.* 1988; 43:A17.
114. Seccombe DW, James L, Booth F. L-carnitine treatment in glutaric aciduria type I. *Neurology.* 1986;36: 264–267.
115. Lipkin PH, Roe CR, Goodman SI, Batshaw ML. A case of glutaric acidemia type I. Effect of riboflavin and carnitine. *J Pediatr.* 1988;112:62–65.
116. Travis S, Mathias MM, Dupont J. Effect of biotin deficiency on the catabolism of linoleate in the rat. *J Nutr.* 1972;102:767–772.
117. Roe CR, Hoppel CL, Stacey TE, Chalmers RA, Tracey BM, Millington DS. Metabolic response to carnitine in methylmalonic aciduria. *Arch Dis Child.* 1983;58:916–920.
118. Wolf B. Reassessment of biotin-responsiveness in "unresponsive" propionyl CoA carboxylase deficiency. *J Pediatr.* 1980;97:964–967.
119. Brusilow SW, Horwich AL. Urea cycle enzymes. In: Scriver CR, Beaudet AL, Sly WS, Valle D, eds. *The Metabolic and Molecular Bases of Inherited Disease.* 7th ed. New York: McGraw-Hill; 1995:1187–1232.
120. Ohtani Y, Ohyanagi K, Yamamoto Y, Matsuda I. Secondary carnitine deficiency in hyperammonemic attacks of ornithine transcarbamylase deficiency. *J Pediatr.* 1988;112:409–414.
121. Segal S, Berry GT. Disorders of galactose metabolism. In: Scriver CR, Beaudet AL, Sly WS, Valle D, eds. *The Metabolic and Molecular Bases of Inherited Disease.* 7th ed. New York: McGraw-Hill; 1995:967–1000.
122. Garibaldi LR, Canini S, Superti-Furga A, et al. Galactosemia caused by generalized uridine diphosphate ga-

lactose-4-epimerase deficiency. *J Pediatr*. 1983;103: 927–930.

123. Sardharwalla IB, Wraith JE, Bridge C, Fowler B, Roberts SA. A patient with severe type of epimerase deficiency galactosaemia. *J Inher Metab Dis*. 1988;11 (suppl 2):249–251.

124. Chen YT, Burchell A. Glycogen storage diseases. In: Scriver CR, Beaudet AL, Sly WS, Valle D, eds. *The Metabolic and Molecular Bases of Inherited Disease*. 7th ed. New York: McGraw-Hill; 1995:935–966.

125. Gitzelmann R, Steinmann B, van den Berghe G. Disorders of fructose metabolism. In: Scriver CR, Beaudet AL, Sly WS, Valle D, eds. *The Metabolic and Molecular Bases of Inherited Disease*. 7th ed. New York: McGraw-Hill; 1995:905–934.

126. Mock DM, Perman JA, Thaler MM, Morris RC. Chronic fructose intoxication after infancy in children with hereditary fructose intolerance. *N Engl J Med*. 1983;309:764–770.

127. Pineda O, Torun B, Viteri FE, Arroyave G. Protein quality in relation to estimates of essential amino acid requirements. In: Bodwell CE, Adkins JS, Hopkins DT, eds. *Protein Quality in Humans: Assessment and In Vitro Estimation*. Westport, CT: Avi Publication; 1981: 29–42.

128. Torun B, Pineda O, Viteri FE, Arroyave G. Use of amino acid composition data to predict nutritive value for children with specific reference to new estimates of their essential amino acid requirements. In: Bodwell CE, Adkins JS, Hopkins DT, eds. *Protein Quality in Humans: Assessment and In Vitro Estimation*. Westport, CT: Avi Publication; 1981:374–389.

129. Bower BD, Smallpiece V. Lactose-free diet in galactosaemia. *Lancet*. 1955;2:873.

130. Bell L, Sherwood WG, Chir B. Current practices and improved recommendations for treating hereditary fructose intolerance. *J Am Diet Assoc*. 1987;87:721–728.

131. Holman RT, Johnson SB, Hatch TF. A case of human linolenic acid deficiency involving neurological abnormalities. *Am J Clin Nutr*. 1982;35:617–623.

132. Pellock JM. Efficacy and adverse effects of antiepileptic drugs. *Pediatr Clin North Am*. 1989;36: 435–448.

133. Millington DS, Roe CR, Maltby DA, Inoue I. Endogenous catabolism is the major source of toxic metabolites in isovaleric acidemia. *J Pediatr*. 1987;110:56–60.

134. Petrowski S, Nyhan WL, Reznik V, et al. Pharmacologic amino acid acylation in the acute hyperammonemia of propionic acidemia. *J Neurogenet*. 1987;4: 87–96.

135. Bachmann C. Treatment of congenital hyperammonemias. *Enzyme*. 1984;32:56–64.

Chapter 14

Developmental Disabilities

Harriet H. Cloud

The nutritional needs of the child with developmental disabilities are as variable as they are for the child who is normal. They primarily involve energy, growth, regulation of the biochemical processes, and repair of cells and body tissue.

DEFINITION OF DEVELOPMENTAL DISABILITIES

A *developmental disability* was defined in Public Law 95-602, the Developmental Disabilities Assistance and Bill of Rights Act,[1] as a severe chronic disability that:

- is attributable to a mental or physical impairment or combination of mental and physical impairments;
- is manifested before the person attains age 22;
- is likely to continue indefinitely;
- results in substantial functional limitations in three or more areas of major life activity (self-care, receptive and expressive language, learning, mobility, capacity for independent living, and economic self-sufficiency);
- reflects the person's need for a combination of special interdisciplinary or generic care treatments, or other services that are lifelong or of extended duration and are individually planned and coordinated.

The etiology of developmental disabilities has been traced to chromosomal aberrations, such as Down syndrome (trisomy 21) and Prader-Willi syndrome; neurologic insults in the prenatal period; infectious diseases; trauma; congenital defects, such as cleft lip and palate; neural tube defects, such as spina bifida; inborn errors of metabolism; and other syndromes of lesser incidence.[2]

Nutritional considerations that involve the child with developmental disabilities include assessment of growth and the problems surrounding energy balance. This can lead to failure to thrive, obesity, or slow growth rate in height. The second major consideration includes feeding from the standpoint of oral motor problems, developmental delays of feeding skills, inability to self-feed, behavioral problems, and tube feedings. Other areas for nutritional consideration include drug–nutrient interaction, constipation, dental caries, urinary tract infections, and food or nutrition misinformation that the parent has related to hyperactivity and attention deficit disorders. Table 14–1 includes a list of developmental disorders and their nutritional considerations.

NUTRITIONAL NEEDS OF THE CHILD WITH DEVELOPMENTAL DISABILITIES

Energy needs for the child with developmental disabilities vary as they do for normal chil-

Table 14–1 Developmental Disabilities or Predisposing Conditions and Their Nutritional Considerations

Condition	*Nutrition Problems*	*Treatment Goal*
Down syndrome	Poor suck in infancy Constipation Failure to thrive Marked weight gain	Ability to suck vigorously Increased fiber and fluids Increased or decreased calories Increased activity
Prader-Willi syndrome	Failure to thrive in infancy Weak suck Obesity Hyperglycemia	Early identification Weight maintained for height Decreased calories Environmental control
Cornelia de Lange syndrome	Failure to thrive Feeding problems	Increased calories Early assessment and intervention
Cerebral palsy	Oral motor feeding problems	Assessment of problem Oral motor facilitation Texture progression Calorie progression
Spina bifida	Obesity Constipation Urinary tract infection Feeding problems	Weight loss or maintenance Kilocalories per centimeter of height Adequate fluid intake
Seizure disorders	Feeding problems Weight loss Drug–nutrient interaction Dental problems	Increased calories Vitamin D supplementation if Dilantin is given

dren; very little specific information is available for either. A decreased energy need is most apparent in chromosomal aberrations, such as Down syndrome; conditions accompanied by limited gross motor activity, such as in spina bifida; and syndromes characterized by low muscle tone, such as is found in Prader-Willi, Rubinstein-Tabyi, and Turner syndromes.

Energy needs of infants and children with developmental disabilities are highly individualized and vary widely.[2]

Lower Energy Needs

For the child with Down syndrome, Prader-Willi syndrome, or spina bifida, the growth rate has been found to be slower, basal energy needs lower, muscle tone lower leading to diminished motor activity, when compared with the child who is not developmentally disabled. Not to be forgotten is a familial predisposition to obesity. As a result, these children tend to become overweight and obese when fed according to normal standards. Determination of energy needs for children with these developmental disabilities—who tend to be short—led to the recommendation that energy needs be calculated per centimeter of height (see Table 14–2).[3] Recent studies have shown that the child with disorders such as Down Syndrome are frequently provided food intake greater than the Recommended Dietary Allowances (RDAs).[4]

Higher Energy Needs

Children with cerebral palsy often tend to be seriously underweight for height. Studies have been conducted to estimate the energy needs of the child with cerebral palsy, and have estimated energy needs utilizing indirect calorimetry and the doubly labelled water method. Recent studies have found that adults with cerebral palsy have higher resting metabolic rates than their controls.[5] A previous study by Bandini and colleagues[6] found that the resting energy expenditure of adolescents with cerebral palsy were lower than in adolescent controls. Stallings et al[7] completed a study of children ages 2–12 with spastic quadreplegia cerebral palsy compared with a normal control group. The conclusion was that growth failure and an abnormal pattern of resting REE are related to inadequate energy intake. Two other methods for determining energy needs of this population include using a nomogram for calculating body surface area and standards based on kcal/m^2/h.[8] This method can be used for males and females 6 years of age and above. Table 14–3 includes basal metabolic rates for infants and children from 1 week of age to 16 years and is based on weight.[8]

The information obtained in determining the basal energy need must be modified for growth and activity level. The RDAs are generally not appropriate to use in determining the energy needs of children with developmental disabilities. A more appropriate strategy would be to utilize basal energy needs with an individualized percentage added for growth rates and energy levels that encompasses slower growth rates and lowered motor activity. The dearth of research in this area makes it difficult to develop standards and requires that the dietitian and physician evaluate the child's nutritional needs carefully.

Protein, Carbohydrates, and Fats

Careful monitoring of protein intake is essential in the child with developmental disabilities. It is generally recommended that 15–20% of the total calories come from protein, which may be difficult for the child with an oral motor feeding problem, such as a child with cerebral palsy.

Table 14–2 Energy Needs of Selected Populations of Children with Developmental Disabilities*

Down syndrome	16.1 kcal/cm: male 1–3 years 14.3 kcal/cm: female 1–3 years
Prader-Willi syndrome	10–11 kcal/cm: maintenance 8–9 kcal/cm: weight loss
Spina bifida	7 kcal/cm: weight loss Maintenance: 50% of the kilocalorie level of normal children after 8 years of age
Cerebral palsy	13.9 kcal/cm: 5–11 years, mild to moderate activity 11.1 kcal/cm: 5–11 years, several restrictions on activity

*Values are kilocalories per centimeter of height.

Source: Reprinted from *Nutrition and Feeding for the Developmentally Disabled* by C Rokusek and E Heindicles with permission of the South Dakota University Affiliated Program, Interdisciplinary Center for Disabilities, © 1985.

Table 14–3 Basal Metabolic Rates: Infants and Children

Age 1 Week to 10 Months Metabolic Rate		*Age 11–36 Months Metabolic Rate*			*Age 3–16 Years Metabolic Rate*		
Weight (kg)	*(kcal/hr) M/F*	*Weight (kg)*	*(kcal/hr) M*	*F*	*Weight (kg)*	*(kcal/hr) M*	*F*
3.5	8.4	9.0	22.0	21.2	15	35.8	33.3
4.0	9.5	9.5	22.8	22.0	20	39.7	37.4
4.5	10.5	10.0	23.6	22.8	25	43.6	41.5
5.0	11.6	10.5	24.4	23.6	30	47.5	45.5
5.5	12.7	11.0	25.2	24.4	35	51.3	49.6
6.0	13.8	11.5	26.0	25.2	40	55.2	53.7
6.5	14.9	12.0	26.8	26.0	45	59.1	57.8
7.0	16.0	12.5	27.6	26.9	50	63.0	61.9
7.5	17.1	13.0	28.4	27.7	55	66.9	66.0
8.0	18.2	13.5	29.2	28.5	60	70.8	70.0
8.5	19.3	14.0	30.0	29.3	65	74.7	74.0
9.0	20.4	14.5	30.8	30.1	70	78.6	78.1
9.5	21.4	15.0	31.6	30.9	75	82.5	82.2
10.0	22.5	15.5	32.4	31.7			
10.5	23.6	16.0	33.3	32.6			
11.0	24.7	16.5	34.0	33.4			

Source: Reprinted from *Metabolism* by PL Altman and DS Dittmer (eds) with permission of the Federation of American Societies for Experimental Biology, © 1968.

These children often suffer from serious malnutrition, manifested by little or no weight gain and limited growth in height. One recent study of 75 gastrostomy fed children ages 2–6 years exhibited impressive growth in height and weight at 12 and 18 months after fundoplication surgery and initiation of the gastrostomy feeding.[9]

Carbohydrates are the primary source of energy for all individuals. According to the usual pediatric dietary recommendations, at least 50% of calories should come from carbohydrates, with no more than 10% coming from sucrose.

Children with developmental disabilities often have a high percentage of their carbohydrate calories coming from foods highly concentrated in sucrose, such as candy, carbonated beverages, cookies, etc. Dietary counseling related to better food choices of carbohydrate is frequently required, just as it is for normal children.

Fats should provide 30–35% of the total intake, increasing palatability and satiety, as well as providing a supply of the essential fatty acids. For the child who tends to be overweight and obese, fat intake should be carefully evaluated and controlled. For the underweight child, fat can provide an important source of supplemental calories.

Vitamins and Minerals

Research findings do not indicate that vitamin and mineral needs for the child with developmental disabilities are higher than normal. Studies have been completed for the vitamin needs of the child with Down syndrome, spina bifida, fragile X syndrome, and autism.[10–16]

Numerous studies have searched for nutritional deficiencies as causative factors in Down syndrome.[12] Traditionally, the studies have included numerous vitamins, minerals, fatty acids, digestive enzymes, lipotropic nutrients, and numerous drugs. Recent media coverage has promoted the use of antioxidants (Vitamins A, C, and E), minerals zinc, copper, manganese, and selenium, along with the amino acids glucosamine, tyrosine, and tryptophan. The expected outcome is improved growth; increased cognition, alertness, and attention span; and changed facial features. The key concept in the nutritional intervention is metabolic correction of genetic overexpression. It is reported that presence of the third chromosome 21 causes overproduction of superoxide dismutase and cystathionine beta synthase, which disrupts active methylation pathways. Vitamin supplements of antioxidants are considered key to the treatment. At this point nutritional supplements are considered an expensive, questionable approach. In addition, parents of children with attention deficit hyperactivity disorder (ADHD) report that omitting sugar from the diet decreases hyperactivity (see Chapter 5). Historically, this was reported, but is not found in the current literature.[14]

Blue green algae has also been promoted for children with Down syndrome and other developmental disabilities, purportedly to increase attention span and concentration. There is concern that little monitoring is part of initiation of these treatments. High dose supplementation of vitamin B_6 and magnesium has been proposed for autism to diminish tantrums, self-stimulation activities, and improve attention and speech.[16] Other proposed treatments include dimethyl glycine (GMG), gluten and casein free diets. Limited research is available to substantiate anything other than subjective reports that the child is helped.[16]

Studies involving children with spina bifida have involved ascorbic acid saturation and the impact of supplementation of ascorbic acid for producing an acidic urinary pH. Concern was shown in recent studies related to the effect of supplemental ascorbic acid on serum vitamin B_{12} levels. No evidence of B_{12} deficiency developed in one study of 40 children receiving long-term vitamin C supplementation.[13]

Since the 1980s, the literature has reflected a growing interest in vitamin supplementation in the prevention of spina bifida.[17] Nutritional deficiencies identified as possible etiologic factors include folic acid, vitamins, and zinc.[18] A British study[19] supplemented 234 mothers with a multivitamin/iron preparation 1 month prior to conception. Vitamins included were A, D, thiamine, riboflavin, pyridoxine, niacin, ascorbic acid, and folic acid. Supplemented mothers had a recurrence rate of 0.9%, compared with 5.1% of the 219 mothers without supplementation. Homocysteine-methionine metabolism appears to be altered in women with pregnancies affected by neural tube defects; however, the specific mechanisms of causation are not yet known.[20]

As a result of these studies it is the recommendation of the US Public Health Service (USPHS) that all women between the ages of 14 and 15 get an extra 400 mcg folate daily.[20] Fortification of flour with folic acid has been approved by the Food and Drug Administration although at a level that still requires folic acid supplementation as recommended by USPHS.[20] An additional concern related to children with spina bifida has been allergic reactions to latex brought about by repeated exposure to latex in multiple surgeries.[21] It has been recommended that children affected avoid bananas, water chestnuts, kiwi, and avocados. Mild reactions can occur from apples, carrots, celery, tomatoes, papaya, and melons.[22]

A special concern regarding adequacy of vitamin and mineral intake is the effect of certain medications commonly prescribed to developmentally disabled children on utilization of certain vitamins and minerals. Among these medications are antibiotics, anticonvulsants, antihypertensives, cathartics, corticosteroids, stimulants, sulfonamides, and tranquilizers (see Table 14–4).[23] Their nutritional effect can include nausea and vomiting, gastric distress, constipation, and interference with the absorption of vitamins and minerals. In some cases, vitamin and mineral supplements are recommended.[23]

NUTRITIONAL ASSESSMENT

Assessment of the child with developmental disabilities includes all components of nutritional assessment for normal children (as addressed in Chapter 2), as well as the inclusion of an evaluation of feeding skills and development. Guidelines for nutritional assessment of the child with developmental disabilities were developed by nutritionists from university-affiliated programs throughout the United States for persons with developmental disabilities. A copy of these guidelines is included in Table 14–5.[24]

Taking anthropometric measurements of children who are unable to stand and who have gross motor handicaps will require some ingenuity. Weights may be difficult to obtain on standing calibrated balance beam scales for the child with spina bifida or cerebral palsy. Chair and bucket scales are available for use in both clinics and schools, and bed scales are indicated for the severely affected. Recumbent boards can be constructed or commercially obtained. Alternate measures for height measurements include arm span, knee-to-ankle height, or sitting height.[24,25]

Standards for comparison of weight, height, and head circumference are found on the 1979 National Center for Health Studies (NCHS) growth charts.[26] Because these standards were developed on a normal population, the child with developmental disabilities may plot as short, especially when length or height for age is considered. This is particularly true for children with chromosomal aberrations, such as Down syndrome,[27] or for those with a neural tube defect, such as spina bifida. Growth curves have been developed for children with a number of disabilities (Table 14–6); however, for the most part, the NCHS charts are used. Proper interpretation is needed.

Weight for age, interpreted for the developmentally disabled, is also an important indicator of nutritional status and requires comparison with height for age. Again, it is the child with Down syndrome, spina bifida, cerebral palsy, Cornelia de Lange syndrome, and chromosomal aberrations in general whose height/weight relationship should be carefully monitored. Early identification of inappropriate relationships is critical so that early nutrition counseling related to energy balance can be given.

Growth velocity is an important anthropometric assessment parameter (see also Chapters 1 and 2). Growth velocity information assists the dietitian in evaluating changes in rate of growth over a specified period of time. Incremental growth curves are available for plotting growth velocity.[28] Skinfold thickness is a useful measurement for estimating body fat and is recommended, along with arm circumference measurement, in the nutrition assessment guidelines previously cited.

Biochemical measures for the child with developmental disabilities should include at least hemoglobin and hematocrit levels, complete blood count, urinalysis, and semiquantitative amino acid screening. The occurrence of these measures in an assessment would depend on biochemical testing that the child has received in the primary health care facility. Other tests may be indicated for children on anticonvulsant medication, who may have low serum levels of folic acid, ascorbic acid, calcium, vitamin D, alkaline phosphatase, phosphorus, and pyridoxine. A glucose tolerance test is recommended for the individual with Prader-Willi syndrome.[29]

The methods used to obtain dietary information about the child with developmental disabilities are identical to those used with the normal child; remember that the parent must be interviewed for the infant and young child, and often for the older child who has a degree of mental retardation, making it difficult to obtain the food intake. It is highly recommended that written dietary records be analyzed with computer software.

In addition to dietary information, an assessment of feeding skills and identification of feeding problems that influence the child's food intake is indicated. This part of the evaluation may include such members of the health care team as

Table 14–4 Drug–Nutrient Interactions of Medications Frequently Used for Children with Developmental Disabilities

Drug	*Indications for Use*	*Drug–Nutrient Interactions*	*Prevention of Nutritional Effect*
Anticonvulsants			
Diphenylhydantoin (Dilantin) Phenolbarbitol Carbamazepine (Tegretol) Valproic acid (Depakane)	Treatment of seizures	Altered metabolism and absorption of vitamins D, K, folate, B_{12}, B_6, calcium May produce gastrointestinal side effects such as nausea, vomiting, diarrhea, and lethargy	Vitamin D supplement recommended Emphasize high-folate food sources Folic acid supplement indicated only when drug levels and seizure frequency closely monitored Carnitine supplement for Depakane
Antibiotics			
Chloramphenicol Tetracycline	Treatment of infections	Both may alter intestinal function by decreasing flora and causing irritations Other side effects include nausea, vomiting	Decrease milk intake. Provide a multivitamin supplement. *Do not give* with iron supplement within 2 hours. Encourage increased fluids.
Laxatives			
Mineral oil	Constipation	Decreased absorption of fat-soluble vitamins Indigestion, Flatulence Weight loss Anorexia	Vitamin supplementation and taking 2 hours away from food. Utilization of a high-fiber liquid beverage is an acceptable strategy.
Stimulants			
Dexedrine Methylphenidate (Ritalin)	Attention deficit disorders Hyperactivity	Decreased appetite Decreased intake Poor growth	Take 1/2 hour after meals.

Source: Data from D.A. Roe, *Handbook on Drug and Nutrient Interactions,* 4th ed, American Dietetic Association.

the physical therapist, occupational therapist, dentist, and the psychologist. Observation of an actual feeding session is critical and may utilize an evaluation tool such as the Developmental Feeding Tool from the Boling Center for Developmental Disabilities, University of Tennessee (Exhibit 14–1).[30]

The feeding evaluation should include assessment of the oral mechanism, neuromuscular development, head and trunk control, eye–hand

Table 14–5 Guides for Nutritional Assessment of People with Mental Retardation or Other Disabilities

I. Anthropometric
  A. Purpose: to collect data related to growth and body composition
  B. Levels of assessment
    1. Minimal
      a. Weight*
        (1) Conditions: no shoes, light clothing
        (2) Suggested standard: reference data assembled by National Center for Health Statistics
      b. Height*
        (1) Conditions: recumbent length†
        (2) Suggested standard: reference data assembled by National Center for Health Statistics
      c. Head circumference*
        (1) Conditions: up to age 6 years
        (2) Suggested standard: reference data assembled by National Center for Health Statistics
    2. In-depth
      a. Skinfold triceps and subscapular desirable*
        (1) Conditions: obtain duplicate readings
        (2) Suggested standard: reference data assembled by Fomon and National Center for Health Statistics
      b. Arm circumference*
        (1) Conditions: desirable, if possible
        (2) Suggested standard: Gurney and Jelliffe nomogram
  C. Equipment specification and maintenance
    1. Calibrated weight scale (balance-type)
    2. Measuring board (stadiometer) for measuring recumbent length or vertical surface with leveler for measuring standing height
    3. Narrow flexible steel or plastic-coated tape measure for measuring circumference of head and arm
    4. Calibrated calipers
II. Clinical
  A. Purpose: to observe clinical signs of chronic or subacute disease
  B. Levels of assessment
    1. Minimal: review of past and present records of medical and dental examinations for signs suggestive of poor nutritional status
    2. In-depth
      a. Collection of health history with special attention to areas of nutritional risk, eg,
        (1) Prenatal: pattern and total amount of maternal weight gain, complications of pregnancy, etc.
        (2) Postnatal: client or family history of diabetes, coronary heart disease, infections, anemia, constipation, diarrhea, hyperactivity, food intolerances, pica, inborn errors of metabolism, malabsorption syndromes, etc.

continues

Source: Reprinted with permission from M.A.H. Smith, Nutritional Assessment of the Mentally Retarded and Developmentally Disabled, *Proceedings of the Third National Workshop for Nutritionists from the University Affiliated Facilities,* p. 129, © 1976, Boling Center for Developmental Disabilities, University of Tennessee, Memphis.

Table 14–5 continued

- b. Observation
  - (1) General appearance
  - (2) Speech
  - (3) Oral hygiene
- C. Suggested standards
  1. Fomon
  2. Christakis
  3. Goldsmith

III. Biochemical
- A. Purpose: to obtain objective data related to present nutrition status or recent dietary intake
- B. Levels of assessment
  1. Minimal
     - a. Complete blood count
     - b. Routine urinalysis including microscopic
     - c. Semi-quantitative amino acid screening‡
  2. In-depth
     - a. Serum total protein and albumin
     - b. Fasting blood glucose
     - c. Serum urea nitrogen
     - d. Transferrin saturation
     - e. Organic acids as primary screening for metabolic disorders
     - f. Quantitative urinary and plasma amino acid screening
  3. Other tests to respond to special conditions or problems (examples only)

Condition/problem	*Tests§*
a. Anticonvulsants	Folic acid, ascorbic acid, calcium, vitamin D, alkaline phosphatase, phosphorus, vitamin B_6
b. Prader-Willi Syndrome	Glucose tolerance test
c. Pica	Lead, hemoglobin

- C. Suggested standards
  1. Fomon
  2. Christakis

IV. Dietary
- A. Purpose: to determine a usual dietary pattern and/or nutrient intake
- B. Criteria for dietary assessment
  1. Family income
  2. Mechanical feeding problems
  3. Growth deviations
  4. Age
  5. Specific nutritional disorders or inborn errors of metabolism
  6. Feeding behavior problems
  7. Response to parents' or other professionals' concerns
- C. Levels of assessment
  1. Minimal
     - a. Twenty-four hour recall using food models and/or measures and food frequency with verbal questioning

continues

Table 14–5 continued

- b. Feeding history questionnaire to include parents' concerns regarding nutrition status
- 2. In-depth
  - a. 3-day dietary intake kept by parent
    - (1) Verbal instruction in dietary record keeping
    - (2) Kept during 2 week days and weekend day
    - (3) Dietary supplements and/or medications included
    - (4) Occurrences affecting validity recorded, ie, illness or holidays
    - (5) Quantity, preparation, and brand names of food included
    - (6) Where, when, and with whom client eats included
  - b. Activity record (as needed)
  - c. Pertinent historical information related to feeding
  - d. Present influences on dietary intake
- 3. Other
  Certain conditions (ie, inborn errors of metabolism or syndromes) may require further dietary investigation necessitating more detailed data collection

D. Suggested standards
- 1. Recommended Dietary Allowances
- 2. Fomon
- 3. FAO

V. Behavioral and Feeding Skill Development

A. Purpose: to determine the influence of level of feeding development and behavior on nutritional status

B. Levels of assessment
- 1. Minimal
  - a. Parental perception of feeding skills and behavior
  - b. Professional perception of feeding skills and behavior
- 2. In-depth
  - a. Review of past history and interview to determine feeding skill development and present level of functioning
  - b. Observations‖
    - (1) Physical
      - (a) Oral structure and function including primitive reflexes, sucking, swallowing, biting, chewing, occlusion, and caries
      - (b) Neuromuscular development including gross and fine motor skills, head and trunk control, eye-hand coordination, and position for feeding
    - (2) Behavioral
      - (a) Parent (caregiver)–child interaction
      - (b) Reinforcement patterns (positive and negative)
      - (c) Environmental influences

C. Suggested standards
- 1. Gesell and Amatruda
- 2. Vineland Adaptive Behavior Scales

* Measurement to be made by well-trained, motivated personnel.

† Standards for recumbent length for normal children are available only up to 2 years of age; however, this method yields more accurate measurement of physically handicapped children over 2 years, especially when they are unable to stand without support.

‡ Screening with multiple Guthrie tests and/or thin layer chromatography or chomatography alone.

§ Professional judgment is warranted and a current search of literature should be done to determine appropriateness of tests before they are used.

‖ Observations both at home and outside home with and without primary caregiver and/or conjoint professional assessments are valuable.

Table 14–6 List of Some Special Growth Charts

Condition	*Reference(s)*	*Printed Copies Available*
Achondroplasia	Horton WA, et al. *J Pediatr.* 1978;93:435.	Cedars-Sinai Medical Center, Birth Defects Center, 444 S. San Vincente Blvd., Los Angeles, CA 90048. (213) 855-2211 Camera-ready copies
Brachman (Cornelia) de Lange syndrome	Kline AD, et al. *Am J Med Genet.* 1993;47:1042.	
Cerebral palsy (quadriplegia)	Krick J, et al. *J Am Diet Assoc.* 1966;96:680.	Kennedy Krieger Insitute, 707 North Broadway, Baltimore, MD 21205. www.kennedykrieger.org
Down syndrome	Cronk CE, et al. *Pediatrics.* 1978;61:564 and *Pediatrics.* 1988;81:102.	
Marfan syndrome	Pyeritz RE. In: Emery AH, Rimoirn LD (eds). *Principles and Practice of Medical Genetics.* New York: Churchill Livingstone; 1983. Pyeritz, RE. In: Papadatas CJ, Bartsocas CS (eds). *Endocrine Genetics and Genetics of Growth* (*Prog Clin Biol Res* vol. 200).	Camera-ready copies
Myelomeningocele	Appendix 2. Ekvall S, ed. *Pediatric Nutrition in Chronic Disease and Developmental Disorders: Prevention, Assessment, and Treatment.* New York: Oxford University Press; 1993.	
Noonan syndrome	Witt DR, et al: *Clin Genet.* 1986;30:150.	Camera-ready copies
Prader Willii syndrome	Holm VA. Appendix A. In: Greenway LR, Alexander PC, eds. *Management of Prader-Willi Syndrome.* Springer-Verlag, 1995. Butler, et al. Pediatrics. 1991;88(4):853.	Camera-ready copies
Sickle cell disease	Phebus CK, et al: *J Pediatr.* 1984;105:28. Tanner JM, et al: *J Pediatr.* 1985;107.	

continues

Source: Reprinted from B.J. Scott et al., Monitoring Growth in Children with Special Health Care Needs. *Topics in Clinical Nutrition,* Vol. 13, No. 1, pp. 3–52, © 1997, Aspen Publishers, Inc.

Table 14–6 continued

Condition	*Reference(s)*	*Printed Copies Available*
Silver-Russell syndrome	Tanner JM, et al: *Pediatr Res.* 1975;9:611.	
Turner syndrome	Lyon AJ, et al: *Arch Dis Child.*	Genetech, Inc., 460 Point San Bruno Blvd., South San Francisco, CA 94080. Camera-ready copies
Williams syndrome	Morris CA, et al: *J Pediatr.* 1988;113:318.	Camera-ready copies

coordination, position for feeding, and social-behavioral components, which include the interaction between child and caregiver. Children with developmental disabilities frequently have oral motor feeding problems and positioning problems, and tend to be very easily distracted.[25]

MANAGEMENT OF NUTRITION CONCERNS

Once the nutritional problems have been identified for the child with developmental disabilities, various types of intervention programs may be implemented. First, however, the motivation level and degree of understanding of the parents and the family must be taken into consideration. Indeed, the new guidelines for intervention of the Surgeon General's report[31] on case management for children with developmental disabilities specify that all approaches should be family based. They should also be community centered and comprehensive in scope. The point is to take into account all aspects of a child's treatment program to avoid issuing an isolated set of instructions relevant to the treatment goals of only one discipline among the many involved in a child's care. This is an important philosophical consideration for the dietitian who would be working with this particular population.[32] The parent or another designated family member may be an individual's case manager, or another health care professional may be the case manager. Nutrition intervention would then become a part of the total intervention package, rather than something standing alone; indeed, it will work better if it is a part of that package.

Another important consideration is whether or not the family gives a high priority to a particular intervention procedure; this applies, again, to any discipline but, in this case, particularly to nutrition. For example, consider an obese spina bifida child who has frequent urinary tract infections and a major problem with constipation. The family of this child may give a lower priority to weight management until the other problems have been taken care of. If that is the case, suggestions should be withheld. When it is determined that suggestions related to any kind of nutritional problem should be given to the family, the coping and educational level of the family should be considered. Often, parents have difficulty coping with the fact that they have a developmentally disabled child, and may not be able to deal with too many suggestions at once. Cultural competence requires sensitivity to the cultural expectations and perspectives related to child care for successful intervention.[33] Increasing numbers of foreign populations are moving into this country and often are non-English speaking, requiring an interpreter to ensure that the family understands and accepts the intervention suggested.

It has been the author's experience that it is better to give one or two specific nutrition activi-

Exhibit 14–1 Developmental Feeding Tool (DFT)

Date ____________________
Staff member ______________
Child's name ____
Birth date ____________ Age __________ Sex ______ Race __________
Head circumference (cm) ________ (%ile NCHS) ______ Hand dominance __________
Height (cm) ______ (%ile NCHS) ______ Weight (kg) ______ (%ile NCHS) ________
Weight for height (%ile NCHS) ________ Hematocrit ________ Urine screen ________
Parent/Guardian ____
Address ____
City ____________________ State ____________ Zip __________
County ____________________ Telephone ____________________
Referrer ____________________

Yes	No	
		PHYSICAL
		Size
___	___	1. Weight (Avg. %ile NCHS)
___	___	2. Underweight
___	___	3. Overweight
___	___	4. Stature (Avg. %ile NCHS)
___	___	5. Short (below 5th %ile for ht. NCHS)
___	___	6. Tall (above 95th %ile for ht. NCHS)
___	___	7. Abnormal body proportions*
___	___	8. Head circumference (Avg. %ile NCHS)
___	___	9. Microcephalic
___	___	10. Macrocephalic
		Laboratory
___	___	11. Hematocrit (Normal)
___	___	12. Urine screen (Normal)*
		Health Status
___	___	13. Bowel problems*
___	___	14. Diabetes
___	___	15. Vomiting
___	___	16. Dental caries
___	___	17. Anemia
___	___	18. Food allergies/intolerance*
___	___	19. Medications*
___	___	20. Vitamin/mineral supplements*
___	___	21. Ingests nonfood items
___	___	22. Therapeutic diet*
___	___	23. General appearance (Normal)*
___	___	24. Head (Normal)*
___	___	25. Eyes (Normal)*
___	___	26. Ears (Normal)*
___	___	27. Nose (Normal)*
___	___	28. Teeth/gums (Normal)*
___	___	29. Palate (Normal)*
___	___	30. Skin (Normal)*
___	___	31. Muscles (Normal)*
___	___	32. Arms/hands (Normal)*
___	___	33. Legs/feet (Normal)*
		NEUROMOTOR/ MUSCULAR
		Tonicity
___	___	34. Body tone (Normal)*
		Head and Trunk Control
___	___	35. Head control (Normal)*
___	___	36. Lifts head in prone
___	___	37. Head lags when pulled to sitting
___	___	38. Head drops forward
___	___	39. Head drops backward
___	___	40. Trunk control (Normal)*
		Upper Extremity Control
___	___	41. Range of motion (Normal)*
___	___	42. Approach to object (Normal)*
___	___	43. Grasp of object (Normal)*
___	___	44. Release of object (Normal)*
___	___	45. Brings hand to mouth
___	___	46. Dominance established

continues

Source: M.A.H. Smith et al., Developmental Feeding Tool, in *Feeding Management for a Child with a Handicap*, M.A.H. Smith; ed., pp. 69–70, Boling Center for Developmental Disabilities, University of Tennessee, Memphis.

Exhibit 14–1 continued

Yes	No		
			Reflexes
___	___	47.	Grossly normal
___	___	48.	Asymmetrical tonic neck reflex*
___	___	49.	Symmetrical tonic neck reflex*
___	___	50.	Moro reflex*
___	___	51.	Grasp reflex*
			Body Alignment
___	___	52.	Scoliosis
___	___	53.	Kyphosis
___	___	54.	Lordosis
___	___	55.	Hip subluxation or dislocation suspected
			Position in Feeding
___	___	56.	Mother's lap
___	___	57.	Infant seat
___	___	58.	High chair
___	___	59.	Table and chair
___	___	60.	Wheelchair
___	___	61.	Other adaptive chair*
			ORAL/MOTOR
			Facial Expression
___	___	62.	Symmetrical structure/ function*
___	___	63.	Muscle tone lips/cheeks (Normal)
___	___	64.	Hypertonic muscle tone of lips
___	___	65.	Hypotonic muscle tone of lips
			Oral Reflexes
___	___	66.	Gag (Normal)*
___	___	67.	Bite (Normal)*
___	___	68.	Rooting (Normal)*
___	___	69.	Suck/swallow (Normal)*
			Respiration
___	___	70.	Mouth
___	___	71.	Nose
___	___	72.	Thoracic
___	___	73.	Abdominal
___	___	74.	Regular rhythm*
			Oral Sensitivity
___	___	75.	Inside mouth (Normal)*
___	___	76.	Outside mouth (Normal)*
___	___	77.	Hypersensitivity*
___	___	78.	Hyposensitivity*

Yes	No		
___	___	79.	Intolerance to brushing teeth
			FEEDING PATTERNS
			Bottle-Feeding
___	___	80.	Suckling tongue movements
___	___	81.	Sucking tongue movements
___	___	82.	Firm lip seal*
___	___	83.	Coordinated suck-swallow breathing
___	___	84.	Difficulty swallowing*
			Cup-Drinking
___	___	85.	Adequate lip closure*
___	___	86.	Loses less than 1/2 total amount*
___	___	87.	Wide up-and-down jaw movements
___	___	88.	Stabilizes jaw by biting edge of cup
___	___	89.	Stabilizes jaw through muscle control
___	___	90.	Drinks through a straw
			Feeding Patterns—Spoon Feeding
___	___	91.	Suckles as food approaches
___	___	92.	Cleans food off lower lip
___	___	93.	Cleans food off spoon with upper lip
			Feeding Patterns—Chewing
___	___	94.	Munching pattern
			Lateralizes Tongue:
___	___	95.	When food placed between molars
___	___	96.	When food placed center of tongue
___	___	97.	To move food from side to side
___	___	98.	Vertical jaw movements
___	___	99.	Rotary jaw movements
___	___	100.	Lip closure during chewing*
			Isolated, Voluntary Tongue Movements
___	___	101.	Protrudes/retracts tongue
___	___	102.	Elevates tongue outside mouth

continues

Exhibit 14–1 continued

Yes	No	
___	___	103. Elevates tongue inside mouth
___	___	104. Depresses tongue outside mouth
___	___	105. Depresses tongue inside mouth
___	___	106. Lateralizes tongue outside mouth
___	___	107. Lateralizes tongue inside mouth
		Special Oral Problems
___	___	108. Drools*
___	___	109. Thrusts tongue when utensil placed in mouth*
___	___	110. Thrusts tongue during chewing/swallowing*
___	___	111. Other oral-motor problem*
		NUTRITION HISTORY
		Past Status
___	___	112. Feeding problems birth to 1 year*
___	___	113. Breastfed
___	___	114. Bottle-fed
___	___	115. Weaned
		Current Status
___	___	116. Eats blended food
___	___	117. Eats limited texture
___	___	118. Eats chopped table foods
___	___	119. Eats table foods
___	___	120. Feeds unassisted
___	___	121. Feeds with partial guidance
___	___	122. Feeds with complete guidance
___	___	123. Drinks from a cup unassisted
___	___	124. Drinks from a cup assisted
___	___	125. Finger-feeds
___	___	126. Uses a spoon
___	___	127. Uses a fork

Yes	No	
___	___	128. Uses a knife
___	___	129. Average rate of eating
___	___	130. Fast rate of eating
___	___	131. Slow rate of eating
		Diet Review
___	___	132. Appetite normal
___	___	133. Eats 3 meals/day
___	___	134. Snacks daily
		Dietary Intake, Current
___	___	135. Milk/dairy products, 3–4/day
___	___	136. Vegetables, 2–3/day
___	___	137. Fruit, 2–3/day
___	___	138. Meat/meat substitute, 2–3/day
___	___	139. Bread/cereal, 3–4/day
___	___	140. Sweets/snacks, 1–2/day
___	___	141. Liquids, 2 cups/day
		SOCIAL/BEHAVIORAL
		Child–Caregiver Relationship
___	___	142. Child responds to caregiver
___	___	143. Caregiver affectionate to child
		Social Skills
___	___	144. Eye contact
___	___	145. Smiles
___	___	146. Gestures, ie, waves byebye
___	___	147. Clings to caregiver
___	___	148. Interacts with examiner
___	___	149. Responds to simple directions
___	___	150. Seeks approval
___	___	151. Toilet trained
___	___	152. Knows own sex
		Behavior Problems
___	___	153. Self-abusive
___	___	154. Hyperactive
___	___	155. Aggressive

COMMENTS ____

____

*List or specify on Comments section.

ties for a parent to work on at first; then to set up frequent follow-up visits for evaluation and providing of more suggestions. Also, be available to the parent by telephone for reinterpretation of what it was you might have said during the visit. This is particularly true when parents are distraught. Such parents may find it difficult to follow through on several suggestions given at one time, and, as a result, they may not attempt anything. Increasing numbers of parents have computer access to the internet which presents a new avenue for communication.

An important consideration for working on nutrition problems with this particular population is the cost of some of the intervention suggestions. The nutritionist should determine whether there is a community resource or insurance that can pay for the nutritional suggestions made. Variability in state coverage exists and requires research on the part of the nutritionist.

The general principle in the management of nutritional concerns is the importance of the interdisciplinary approach. Again, it has been the author's experience that most children with developmental disabilities have problems that require input from the physician, physical therapist, occupational therapist, social worker, psychologist, and nurse, in addition to the nutritionist. Pulling that team together in addressing these problems is important to have successful nutrition intervention. Some examples of the interdisciplinary approach include working with the occupational therapist in control of oral motor problems for the child with a feeding problem, with the physical therapist or occupational therapist on positioning, and with the psychologist on behavioral problems. All of these problems influence how the nutrition problem is addressed. Communication is a key element in the success of the interdisciplinary approach, which mandates group discussions, correspondence between groups, and good documentation. If one is fortunate, all the disciplines may be in the same facility. The success of an interdisciplinary effort can be phenomenal and can bring about very positive changes in the nutritional problems, so it is worth the effort to ensure that lines of communication are maintained.

MANAGEMENT OF NUTRITIONAL PROBLEMS

Obesity

Weight management of the child with developmental disabilities is indicated in any child who tends to plot in the > 75th percentile for weight/height relationship. Conditions that predispose a child to obesity are low muscle tone, limited physical activity, isolation, and slow growth in height, all of which are found in children with Down syndrome, Prader-Willi syndrome, spina bifida, Turner syndrome, Klinefelter syndrome, and mental retardation. The energy needs of such children are outlined in Table 14–2.

Prevention is the best nutrition intervention to avoid obesity. Counseling in appropriate feeding practices and frequent monitoring of height and weight are essential in a prevention program. Important topics to cover in counseling the parent for preventive weight management include:

- growth curves and growth rates
- learning to identify true hunger cues
- increasing activity
- selecting nutritious "lowered-calorie" foods
- food preparation practices
- the place of or emphasis on food in the family
- serving sizes

Successful programs for the obese individual should be individually planned and include a written diet. For the school-aged child, successful management will require contact with the child's school to determine food available through the school food service. Often, the family is unaware that school lunch programs may provide calorie restricted meals, low-fat milk, select menus, and salad bars, as well as the traditional school lunch by utilizing the meal prescription authorized under section 504 of the 1973 Rehabilitation Act and subsequent school lunch regulations. (Exhibit 14–2 shows a diet prescription.)

Childhood weight management must be carefully planned to avoid poor growth or nutritional deficiencies. Dietary records maintained by the parent and others caring for the child, such as teachers, day care workers, family, and friends, are useful for monitoring intake. The diet plan for the older developmentally disabled child who is also mentally retarded must be presented in a way that the child can understand. The interdisciplinary approach of working with a special education teacher to present written or pictorial information in an understandable format is necessary for success in this area.

Lack of exercise is often common in the child or adolescent with developmental disabilities. The availability of exercise programs for such children varies from school system to school system, as does the availability of general community-based programs of exercise. Exploring and coordinating community exercise resources is an important part of the dietitian's role in providing good nutritional care.[32]

Behavioral considerations are also an important consideration of weight management programs for the child with developmental disabilities. Important behavioral assessments to make include speed of eating, meal frequency, length of time spent eating, and where meals are taken. Three important behavior modifications to emphasize in the weight management plan include establishing a reward system for compliance with diet, increasing exercise, and targeting eating behaviors for change.

Intervention for obesity for the child with Prader-Willi syndrome requires special involvement of both the family and health care providers.[34] Total environmental control of food access, a low-calorie diet, consistent behavior management techniques, and physical exercise are necessary. Environmental control may include locking the refrigerator, cupboards, and the kitchen. Individuals with Prader-Willi syndrome often hide and hoard food, and exhibit emotional outbursts when food is withheld. Physical exercise is challenging due to the hypotonia, characteristic of the syndrome. The individual tires easily and often has limited gross motor skills.

It has been estimated that the caloric needs of the child with Prader-Willi syndrome are 37–77% of normal for weight maintenance, that weight loss occurs at 8–9 calories per centimeter of height, and that maintenance of appropriate weight can be accomplished at 10–11 calories per centimeter of height.[34]

Several hypocaloric regimens have been used in centers, with variable success. The use of a modified diabetic exchange list has been successful, along with a balanced low-calorie diet, a ketogenic diet, and a protein-sparing modified fast.[29]

Increasing physical activity and exercise is an important strategy, and daily exercise routines should be begun early to prevent problems secondary to hypotonia. Adaptive physical education programs in the school should be used with the school-aged child. Recent treatment has also included growth hormone therapy to increase stature.[35]

Failure to Thrive

Failure to thrive, which is defined as inadequate weight gain for height, is frequently found in the child with developmental disabilities. It may result from

1. impaired oral motor function and resultant feeding problems
2. excessive energy needs, such as occur in cerebral palsy and heart disease, and with gastrointestinal problems
3. infections and frequent illnesses
4. medications that may affect appetite
5. pica consumption leading to lead intoxication or parasites such as giardia
6. parental inadequacy related to feeding.

Nutrition intervention must begin with a careful assessment, including a feeding evaluation,

Exhibit 14–2 Diet Prescription for Meals at School

Name of student for whom special meals at school are requested:

____

Disability or medical condition that requires the student to have a special diet. Include a brief description of the major life activity affected by the student's disability.

____

Diet Prescription (check all that apply.)

☐ Diabetic ☐ Reduced Calorie

☐ Increased Calorie ☐ Modified Texture

☐ Other (Describe) ______________________

Foods Omitted and Substitutions (Please check food groups to be omitted. List specific foods to be omitted and suggest substitutions using the back of this form or attach information.)

☐ Meat and Meat Alternatives ☐ Milk and Milk Products

☐ Bread and Cereal Products ☐ Fruits and Vegetables

Textures Allowed (Check the allowed texture.)

☐ Regular ☐ Chopped ☐ Ground ☐ Pureed

Other Information Regarding Diet or Feeding (Please provide additional information on the back of this form or attach to this form.)

I certify that the above named student needs special school meals prepared as described above because of the student's disability or chronic medical condition.

______________________ ______________ ________

Physician/Recognized Medical Authority Signature Office Phone Number Date

Source: Reprinted with permission from CARE: Manual for School Food Service, © 1993, Alabama Department of Education.

with the opportunity for observation of parent/caregiver–child interaction. Management strategies will be individualized but will generally require increasing calories by increasing either formula concentration for the infant, use of supplemental formulas, or by providing energy-dense foods through carbohydrate or fat supplements (see Table 14–7).

Some children with developmental disabilities with failure to thrive require medical evaluation to determine the need for tube feeding or total parenteral nutrition on a temporary basis following a surgical procedure for a gastrointestinal disorder. Usually, this will be followed with a return to oral feeding.

Constipation

Constipation, defined as infrequent bowel movements of hard stools, often afflicts children with developmental disabilities, for various reasons, among them lack of activity, generalized hypotonia, and limited bowel muscle function. It can also result from insufficient fluid intake, lack of fiber in the diet, frequent vomiting, and medications. Parents frequently report using laxatives, mineral oil, and enemas on a regular basis to correct the problem. As a rule, laxatives and enemas are not recommended. They can lead to dependency, and mineral oil decreases the absorption of the fat-soluble vitamins A, D, E, and K.[23]

Treatment includes adjusting the diet to increase fiber and fluid content. Usual recommendations are as follows:

- Maintain adequate fluid intake, exceeding the daily requirement for age and including water and diluted fruit juice.
- Increase fiber content of the diet by replacing white bread and canned fruits with whole-grain breads and cereals, raw vegetables, fresh fruits, dried fruits, commercial fiber-rich beverages, and cereals fortified with 1–2 tablespoons unprocessed bran.
- Increase daily exercise.

Feeding Problems

Feeding problems are defined as the inability or refusal to eat certain foods because of neuromotor dysfunction, obstructive lesions, or psychosocial factors. Most feeding problems are the result of oral motor difficulties (see Table 14–8) caused by neuromotor dysfunction, developmental delays, positioning problems, a poor mother–child relationship, and sensory defensiveness.[25] All of these problems may contribute to such behavioral problems as refusal to eat, mealtime tantrums, resistance to texture changes, etc.

Intervention for feeding problems lends itself best to the team approach, utilizing occupational therapy, physical therapy, speech, nursing, psychology, nutrition, and social work.[25] A single written care plan developed by the team and prioritized with the parent's assistance according to the child's needs, should be provided.[30] Nutritional intervention may involve increasing calories, altering the texture of foods offered, and determining tube-feeding formulas. Additional nutrition education and counseling, oral motor therapy, and behavior management counseling are part of the feeding plan.

Dental Disease

Dental health care contributes to overall improved nutritional status but is often an unmet need in children and adolescents who are developmentally disabled. Dental caries and gum disease are prevalent in this population and are caused by plaque formation, tooth susceptibility, sugar consumption, and medication. Prevention and intervention include home care, professional treatment, and nutritional intervention.

Nutritional intervention involves decreasing the sucrose intake of the diet by eliminating candy, sugar-containing gum, sugar-containing carbonated beverages, cookies, cakes, and highly sweetened foods. Supplying adequate fluoride in the drinking water is helpful in the prevention of caries. In communities where the water supply is not fluoridated, toothpaste and

Table 14–7 Food that Can Be Added to Pureed Foods to Increase Calories

Food	*Calories*
Infant cereal	9/tbsp
Nonfat dry milk	25/tbsp
Cheese	120/oz
Margarine	101/tbsp
Evaporated milk	40/oz
Vegetable oils	110/tbsp
Strained infant meats	100–150/jar
Glucose polymers, powdered or liquid	30/tbsp

topical application of fluoride can be used. Bottled water is utilized by many families and may not contain flouride; however, some manufacturers are now adding fluoride and list it on the food label.

Gingival disease is often found where dental hygiene is poor. Children taking diphenylhydantoin (Dilantin) for seizures may suffer gingival hyperplasia, a side effect of the drug.[23] Nutrition counseling to decrease sucrose intake, increase intake of raw fruits and vegetables, and improve snacking practices, coupled with good dental hygiene instruction from the dentist and regular dental care are important components of dental intervention problems.

OTHER NUTRITIONAL CONSIDERATIONS

A ketogenic diet has been developed for children with intractable epileptic seizures that are nonresponsive to anticonvulsants.[36] Traditionally, the diet is recommended for children under age 2–5 with myoclonic, absence and atonic seizures. This diet is high in fat and very low in protein and carbohydrates. It is thought that the ketosis produced by the high fat to low carbohydrate ratio decreases the number and severity of the seizures. Generally, a 4:1 ratio of fat to carbohydrate is required. Fluids are limited, and protein is kept low. Historically, the diet was high in saturated fat content; however, in recent years, corn oil and medium-chain triglyceride (MCT) oil have been used, but protocols also contain whipping cream, bacon, butter, margarine, and mayonnaise.[36] One study of 58 children[36] showed excellent results in seizure control, utilizing an emulsion of MCT oil, to which a variety of flavorings were added. Daily vitamin and mineral supplements are required as the diet is low in calcium, iron, vitamin C, and other vitamins and minerals. The expense of the diet, compliance problems, and lack of palatability have made its use controversial. Like children on any metabolic diet, the child on a ketogenic diet requires close monitoring and frequent follow-up visits.

CONCLUSION

The nutritional needs of the child with developmental disabilities are important considerations in their treatment and program planning. The goal is to ensure a nutritional intake adequate for growth and to provide enough energy for participation in therapy. Research is needed to better define the nutritional requirements of this population. The RDAs for normal children are often inappropriate for this population.

Dietitians in programs serving this population are challenged to defend the cost-effectiveness of nutritional care and to develop nutrition education materials and programs specifically adapted for these children and adolescents, in collaboration with special education professionals.

Table 14–8 Feeding Problems Commonly Encountered

Problem	*Description*
Tonic bite reflex	Strong jaw closure when teeth and gums are stimulated
Tongue thrust	Forceful and often repetitive protrusion of an often bunched or thick tongue in response to oral stimulation
Jaw thrust	Forceful opening of the jaw to its maximal extent during eating, drinking, attempts to speak, or general excitement
Tongue retraction	Pulling back the tongue within the oral cavity at presentation of food, spoon, or cup
Lip retraction	Pulling back the lips in a very tight smile-like pattern at the approach of the spoon or cup toward the face
Sensory defensiveness	A strong adverse reaction to sensory input (touch, sound, light)

Source: Reprinted from S.J. Lane and H.H. Cloud, Feeding Problems and Intervention: An Interdisciplinary Approach, *Topics in Clinical Nutrition,* Vol. 3, No. 3, p. 26, © 1988, Aspen Publishers, Inc.

REFERENCES

1. Developmental Disabilities Assistance and Bill of Rights Act, Public Law 95-602. 1978;nos. 102,503.
2. Cloud H. Nutrition assessment of the individual with developmental disabilities. *Top Clin Nutr*. 1987;2:4.
3. Heinricks E, Rokusek C. *Nutrition and Feeding for the Developmentally Disabled*. Vermillion, SD: South Dakota Department of Education and Cultural Affairs; 1992.
4. Luke A, Sutton M, Raizen NJ, Schoeller DA. Nutrient intake and obesity in prepubescent children with Down syndrome. *J Am Diet Assoc*. 1996;96:1262–1263.
5. Johnson RK, Goran MI, Ferrara MS, Poehlman ET. Athetosis raises resting metabolic rate in adults with cerebral palsy. *J Am Diet Assoc*. 1996;96:145–148.
6. Bandini LG, Schneller DA, Fukagana NK, Wykes L, Dietz WH. Body composition and energy expenditure in adolescents with cerebral palsy or myelodysplasia. *Pediatr Res*. 1991;29:70–77.
7. Stallings VA, Cronk CE, Zemme BS, Charney EB. Body composition in children with spastic quadriplegic cerebral palsy. *J Pediatr*. 1995;126(5 pt 1):833–839.
8. Walker WA, Hendricks KM. Estimation of energy needs. In: *Manual of Pediatric Nutrition*. Philadelphia: WB Saunders Company; 1985.
9. Corwin DS, Isaacs JS, Georgeson KE, Bartolucci A, Cloud HH, Craig CB. Weight and length increases in children after gastrosomy placement. *J Am Diet Assoc*. 1996;96:874–879.
10. Bennett FC, McClelland S, Kriegsmann E, Andrus L, Sells C. Vitamin and mineral supplementation in Down syndrome. *Pediatrics*. 1983;72:707–713.
11. Bidder RT, Gray P, Newcombe RG, Evans BK, Hughes M. The effects of multivitamins and minerals on children with Down syndrome. *Dev Med Child Neurol*. 1989;31:532–537.
12. Pueschel SM. General health care and therapeutic approaches. In: Pueschel SM, Pueschel JK, eds. *Biomedical concerns in persons with Down Syndrome*. Baltimore: Paul H Brooks Publishing Co;1992:273–287.
13. Ekvall SM. Myelomeningocele. In: Ekvall SW, ed. *Pediatric nutrition in chronic diseases and developmental disorders*. New York: Oxford Press; 1993:111–113.
14. Patterson B. Ekvall SW, Mays SD. Autism. In: Ekvall SW, ed. *Pediatric nutrition in chronic diseases and developmental disorders*. New York: Oxford Press; 1993: 131–136.
15. Runyan D. Fragile X Syndrome. In: Ekvall SW, ed. *Pediatric nutrition in chronic diseases and developmental disorders*. New York: Oxford Press; 1993:399–402.
16. Quinn HP. Nutrition concerns for children with pervasive developmental disorder/autism. *Nutrition focus*. Center on Human Development and Disability, University of Washington, Seattle, WA. 1995;10(5):1–7.
17. Lawrence KM, James N, Campbell H. Blood folate levels and quality of the maternal diet. *Br Med J*. 1980; 285:216.
18. Bergman KE, Makoseh J, Tews KH. Abnormalities of hair zinc concentrations in mothers of newborn infants with spina bifida. *Am J Clin Nutr*. 1980;33:2145–2150.
19. Smithells RN, Nevin NC, Seller MJ, et al. Further experience of vitamin supplementation for prevention of neural tube defect recurrences. *Lancet*. 1983;1:1027.
20. Allen WP. Folic acid in the prevention of birth defects. *Curr Opin Pediatr*.1996;8(6):630–634.

21. Pittman T, Kiburz J, Gabriel K, Steinhardt G, Williams D, Slater J. Latex allergy in children with spina bifida. *Pediatr Neurosurg.* 1995;22(2):96–100.
22. Shapiro E, Kelly KJ, Setlock MA, Suwalski KL, Meyers P. Complications of latex allergy. *Dialogues in Pediatric Urology.* 1992;15(3):1–8.
23. Roe DA. *Handbook on Drug and Nutrient Interactions.* 4th ed. Chicago: American Dietetic Association; 1989.
24. Smith MAH. Nutritional assessment for persons with developmental disabilities. *Top Clin Nutr.* 1993;8(4):7–49.
25. Stevenson RD. Nutrition and feeding of children with developmental disabilities. *Ped Annals.* 1995;24(5): 255–260.
26. Hamill P, Drizd, TA, Johnson CL, et al. Physical growth: National Center for Health Statistics percentiles. *Am J Clin Nutr.* 1979;32:607–629.
27. Cronk C, Crocker AC, Pueschel SM, et al. Growth charts for children with Down syndrome: 1 month to 18 years of age. *Pediatrics.* 1988;81:102.
28. Roche AF, Hines JH. Incremental growth charts. *Am J Clin Nutr.* 1980;33:2041–2052.
29. Cassidy SB. Prader-Willi syndrome. *J Med Genetics.* 1997;34(11):917–923.
30. Smith MAH, Connolly B, McFadden S, et al. Developmental feeding tool. In: *Feeding Management for a Child with a Handicap.* Memphis, TN: The Boling Child Development Center, University of Tennessee Center for Health Sciences; 1982:69.
31. US Department of Health and Human Services, Public Health Service. *Surgeon General's Report: Children with Special Health Care Needs, Campaign '87. Commitment to Family-Centered, Community-Based, Coordinated Care.* DHHS publ no. (HRS) D/MC, 87-2.
32. American Dietetic Association. Nutrition services for children with special health care needs. *J Am Diet Assoc.* 1989;89:1133–1137.
33. Terry RD. Needed: a new appreciation of culture and food behavior. *J Am Diet Assoc.* 1994;95(5):501–503.
34. Hoffman CJ, Abeltman D, Pipes P. A nutrition survey of and recommendations for individuals with Prader- Willi who live in group home. *J Am Diet Assoc.* 1992; 92(7):823–830.
35. Hauffa BP. One-year results of growth hormone treatment of short stature in Prader-Willi syndrome. *Acta Paediatrica. Supplement.* 1997;423:63–65.
36. Kelly MT, Hays TL. Implementing the ketogenic diet. *Top Clin Nutr.* 1997;13(1):53–61.

NUTRITION RESOURCE LIST

1. Children with Special Health Care Needs. A Community Nutrition Pocket Guide. Isaacs JS, Cialone J, Horsley JW, Holland M, Murray P, Nardella M. Dietetics in Developmental and Psychiatric Disorders and the Pediatric Nutrition Practice Group of the American Dietetic Association, American Dietetic Association, Chicago, Ill. 1997, $15.00 Contact: Sparks Center, 1720 7th Ave. So, Birmingham, Ala. 35294-0017.
2. The Normal Acquisition of Oral Feeding Skills: Implication for Assessment and Treatment. S Evans Morris, JA, Preston 1982. Contact Therapeutic Media, Box 21056, Santa Barbara, CA 93121.
3. Nutrition Management of School Age Children with Special Needs. Second Edition. Horsley J, Allen E, and Daniel PW. Richmond: Virginia Dept of Health and Virginia Department of Education 1996. Contact: MCH Clearinghouse. (703) 821-8955.
4. Nutrition Focus for Children with Special Needs. (Newsletter) Contact: Sharon Feucht, Ed. Nutrition Focus CDMRC-WJ-10, University of Washington, Seattle, WA 98195. (6 issues/yr. $30.00)
5. Project SPOON (Specialized Program of Oral Nutrition for Children with Special Needs) Tluczek A and Sondel, S. eds, 1991. Available through University of Wisconsin Children's Hospital, 600 Highland Avenue, Madison, WI 53792, (608) 263-9059.
6. Feeding and Nutrition for the Child with Special Needs: Klein MD and Delaney TA, Tuscon, AZ: Therapy Skill Builders. 1994. Contact Therapy Skill Builders at 1-800-866-4446.
7. CARE: Special Nutrition for Kids. Alabama Department of Education, Child Nutrition Programs, Federal Administrative Services, 1995. (A video and workbook targeted for school food service managers.) Contact: National Food Service Management Institute, PO Drawer 188. University, MS 38677-0188, 1-899-321-3054.
8. Meeting Their Needs: Training Manual for Child Nutrition Program Personnel Serving Children with Special Needs, US Department of Agriculture, Food and Nutrition Services, Southeast Regional Office, Atlanta, GA and University of Alabama at Birmingham, Sparks Clinics, Birmingham, Ala. 1993.
9. Feeding for the Future: Exceptional Nutrition in the IEP. Wellman N, Sinofsky J, Crawford L, Frazee C, Rarback S, Murphy AB and Parham P. Florida International University, Florida NET Program and Florida Department of Education, Miami Fl, 1995. (Manual and video.)
10. Accommodating Children with Special Dietary Needs in School Nutrition Programs: Guidance for School Food Service Staff. US Department of Agriculture, Food and Consumer Services; Alexandria, VA, 1995. Contact: Regional USDA Office.

CHAPTER 15

Pulmonary Diseases

Nancy H. Wooldridge

Promoting optimal growth and development is an important outcome criterion for any child, but it is especially important for the child with chronic pulmonary disease. In this chapter, the nutritional management of cystic fibrosis, bronchopulmonary dysplasia, and asthma is discussed. Adequate nutrition in the care of the child with cystic fibrosis or bronchopulmonary dysplasia plays an important prognostic role in the outcome of these diseases. A discussion on asthma is included because it is the most common chronic disease of childhood.

CYSTIC FIBROSIS

Cystic fibrosis (CF), a genetic disorder of children, adolescents, and young adults, characterized by widespread dysfunction of the exocrine glands, is the most common lethal hereditary disease of the Caucasian race.[1] Characteristic of the disease is an abnormality in the cystic fibrosis transmembrane conductance regulator (CFTR) protein, causing an increased sodium resorption and a decreased chloride secretion. The result is the production of abnormally thick and viscous mucus, which affects various organs of the body. In the lungs, the thick mucus clogs the airways, causing obstruction and subsequent bacterial infections. The thick mucus prevents the release of pancreatic enzymes into the small intestine for the digestion of foods. Blockage of ducts eventually causes pancreatic fibrosis and cyst formation. About 85% of CF patients have pancreatic involvement, exhibited by such gastrointestinal symptoms as frequent, foul-smelling stools, increased flatus, and abdominal cramping. In a small percentage of patients, the ducts and tubules of the liver are obstructed by mucus, resulting in liver disease similar to cirrhosis. Another complication is CF-related diabetes (CFRD), seen particularly in the adolescent and young adult population. A unique characteristic of CF is an increased loss of sodium and chloride in the sweat. Sterility in males and decreased fertility in females is also seen.

The life expectancy of CF patients has greatly improved since the disease was first described as a distinct clinical entity by Andersen in 1938.[2] During the 1930s to 1950s, CF patients usually died at an early age, secondary to malabsorption and malnutrition. Pancreatic enzyme therapy, antibiotic therapy, and earlier diagnosis have been major contributory factors to the improvement. The Cystic Fibrosis Foundation currently reports the median age of survival to be 31.3 years.[3]

Genetics/Incidence

Cystic fibrosis is transmitted as an autosomal recessive trait. Both parents are carriers of the defective gene but exhibit no symptoms of the disease themselves. Each offspring of two carriers of the defective gene has a 25% chance of having the disease.

The CF gene was discovered in 1989 on the long arm of chromosome 7.[4] The CF gene product is called the *CF transmembrane conductance regulator* (CFTR), which is a cyclic adenosine monophosphate (cAMP)-regulated chloride channel and regulator of secondary chloride and sodium channels normally present in epithelial cells.[5–10] The most common mutation is called ΔF508 and accounts for about 67% of CF alleles among the Caucasian population worldwide.[11] However, more than 700 mutations of the *CFTR* gene have been identified. It is hoped that these genetic discoveries will lead to improved treatment of CF patients, including genetic therapy, and ultimately to a cure for the disease.

The incidence of CF in Caucasians is in the range of 1 in 2,500–3,200 live births, with a carrier rate of 1 in 20.[10,12] The incidence is 1 in 15,000 births among African Americans. The disease is rarely seen in the Asian or Native American populations.[12]

Manifestations/Diagnosis

Manifestations of the disease are numerous and are quite variable from patient to patient, due in part to the large numbers of mutations of the defective gene. A summary of common manifestations of CF is depicted in Table 15–1. Any child who repeatedly exhibits any of these symptoms should be tested for CF. In addition, CF should be ruled out when a child tastes salty when kissed or experiences heat prostration.

According to the consensus statement on the diagnosis of cystic fibrosis published by the CF Foundation,[13] the criteria for the diagnosis of CF are elevated levels of chloride found in the patient's sweat on two or more occasions, one or more of the characteristic features of the disease:

1. evidence of chronic sinopulmonary disease
2. evidence of gastrointestinal and nutritional abnormalities
3. evidence of salt loss syndromes
4. evidence of obstructive azospermia in males,

or a family history of the disease, or a positive newborn screening test result.

Sweat chloride is measured by a quantitative pilocarpine iontophoresis sweat test. A sweat chloride concentration greater than 60 mmol/L is indicative of the diagnosis of CF. With the advances in the genetic studies of CF, the diagnosis can also be made with the identification of two CF mutations.[13] The demonstration of abnormal nasal epithelial ion transport is also being investigated as a method of diagnosis but is presently limited to research centers.

Table 15–1 Manifestations of Cystic Fibrosis

Pulmonary	*Gastrointestinal*
Chronic cough	Failure to thrive
Repeated bronchial infections	Steatorrhea
Increased work of breathing	Hypoalbuminemia
Digital clubbing	Rectal prolapse
Bronchospasm	Frequent, foul-smelling stools
Cyanosis	Abdominal cramping
Chronic pneumonia	Voracious appetite
Nasal polyps	Anemia
	Vitamin deficiency

Health care practitioners in the community have become more familiar with CF and with the many ways that the disease may manifest itself. Several centers are investigating the use of newborn screening for CF and the impact of early diagnosis on the course of the disease. According to the 1996 CF Patient Registry, the median age at diagnosis was 6 months.[3] However, because of the variability of the disease, the diagnosis may not be recognized in some patients until adolescence or young adulthood.

Management

Rigorous daily management is required to control the symptoms of the disease. Daily chest percussion therapy and postural drainage, along with aerosolized medications, improve currently compromised lungs and retard future deterioration. Aerosolized, oral, or intravenous antibiotics are used to control pulmonary infections. Pancreatic enzyme replacement therapy is a crucial part of the management of the gastrointestinal symptoms. In patients with pancreatic insufficiency, enzymes are required with each meal and snack. Dosage is very individualized, depending on factors such as the extent of pancreatic involvement, the patient's dietary intake, and the patient's age. Vitamin and mineral supplementation is also recommended. Providing adequate nutrition for normal growth and development is one of the primary goals of disease management in CF. The complexity and multifaceted nature of the disease requires an interdisciplinary team approach with patient and family involvement in decision-making for proper management.

Effects on Nutritional Status

Chronic Energy Deficit

Many aspects of the disease of CF stress the nutritional status of the patient, directly or indirectly, by affecting the patient's appetite and subsequent intake. Aspects of pulmonary and gastrointestinal involvement affecting nutritional status are summarized in Table 15–2. Gastrointestinal losses occur in spite of pancreatic enzyme replacement therapy. Also, catch-up growth requires additional calories. All of these factors contribute to a chronic energy deficit and, if left untreated, can lead to a marasmic type of malnutrition. The primary goal of nutritional therapy is to overcome this energy deficit and to promote normal growth and development for CF patients.

Appetite

Many references have been made to the voracious appetites of CF patients. This may be true

Table 15–2 Aspects of Cystic Fibrosis That Affect Nutritional Status

Pulmonary	*Gastrointestinal*
Increased work of breathing	Malabsorption of fat
Chronic cough	Loss of fat-soluble vitamins
Cough–emesis cycle	Loss of essential fatty acids
Chronic antibiotic therapy	Malabsorption of protein
Fatigue, anxiety	Loss of nitrogen
Decreased tolerance for exercise	Anorexia
Repeated pulmonary infections	Gastroesophageal reflux
	Bile salts and bile acid loss
	Distal intestinal obstructive syndrome (DIOS)

of undiagnosed and untreated patients, particularly infants. In practice, however, dietetic professionals are often dealing with patients who have very poor appetites. Table 15–2 delineates some aspects of CF that contribute to this poor appetite and failure to thrive. Psychosocial issues that the patient may be dealing with will also impact appetite.

Nutritional Screening and Assessment

Because nutrition plays such an important role in the treatment of CF, routine nutritional screenings and thorough assessments are very important. In this section, anthropometric, dietary, biochemical, and clinical evaluations will be discussed. The CF Foundation has published a consensus report on the nutritional assessment and management in cystic fibrosis, as well as *Clinical Practice Guidelines for Cystic Fibrosis,* which includes nutrition management information.[14,15] Refer to Exhibit 15–1 for the CF Foundation's *recommendations for nutritional assessment status.*

Assessment

Anthropometric

Monitoring growth parameters is an important component of the screening, assessment, and follow-up of CF patients. As with any child, CF patients should be weighed and measured routinely, using appropriate techniques and equipment, such as those described by Fomon.[16] Weight for age, recumbent length or height for age, weight for height, and head circumference should be accurately measured and plotted on the National Center for Health Statistics (NCHS) growth curves at each clinic visit or hospitalization.[17] The detailed NCHS weight/height tables should be employed in determining weight/height percentiles for the preadolescent and adolescent patient.[18] (See Chapter 2 for additional information.) According to the *Clinical Practice Guidelines for Cystic Fibrosis*, anthropometric measurements, including midarm circumference and triceps skinfold thickness, should be obtained by a registered dietitian at least once a year on all patients younger than 18 years of age.[15] It is also recommended that the registered dietitian annually calculate weight as a percent of ideal weight for height.[15]

Growth charts are simple and readily accessible screening and assessment tools. Although they are intended for use with a healthy population of children, NCHS growth charts provide a way to monitor the growth of CF patients. Their use also seems appropriate when taking into consideration the fact that the CF patient will be comparing his or her own size to that of peers. General recommendations of cases needing further attention include the following:

1. weight for age less than the 5th percentile and greater than the 95th percentile
2. length or height for age less than the 5th percentile and greater than the 95th percentile
3. weight for height less than the 5th percentile or greater than the 95th percentile
4. a crossing of percentile levels in either an upward or downward direction

The CF Consensus Report[14] recommends calculating percentage of ideal weight for height, age, and gender, then expressing actual weight as a percentage of ideal weight for height. Nutrition intervention needs to be initiated for patients who are 85–89% of ideal weight for height. More aggressive nutrition therapy should be begun for those patients who are below 85% of ideal weight for height.[14] Refer to Exhibit 15–2 for the CF Foundation's recommendations for categories for nutritional management of patients with cystic fibrosis, which is based on the weight/height index.[15] The *Clinical Practice Guidelines for Cystic Fibrosis* also recommends calculating the patient's height as a percentage of the 50th percentile height for age to determine whether a patient's linear growth is stunted.[15] Based on the Gomez criteria,[19] if the patient's actual height divided by the 50th percentile height

Exhibit 15–1 Nutritional Status Assessment

Parameter	*Minimum Frequency*	*Indication*
Anthropometric Measurement		
Weight	every 3 months	routine care
Height (length < 2 yrs)	every 3 months	routine care
Head circumference	every 3 months until age 2 yrs	routine care
Midarm circumference	every 3 months	routine care
Triceps skinfold thickness	every 3 months	routine care
Nutritional Assessment		
Dietary intake—*This assessment will usually consist of a 24-hour recall with assessment of dietary pattern and should be performed by a dietitian.*	yearly	routine care diagnosis
3-Day fat balance—*Include both diet records to determine energy and fat intake, as well as a stool fat determination of energy*	as indicated	weight loss growth failure clinical deterioration diagnosis
Anticipatory dietary guidance	yearly	routine care diagnosis
Laboratory Studies		
CBC—*If there is any evidence of iron deficiency, iron status must be measured (ie, serum iron, iron binding capacity, and ferritin)*	yearly	routine care diagnosis
Serum or plasma retinol	yearly	routine care diagnosis
Serum or plasma α-tocopherol	yearly	rountine care diagnosis
Albumin	as indicated	*weight loss* *growth failure* *clinical deterioration* *diagnosis*
Electrolytes and acid base status	as indicated	*prolonged fever* *summer heat* *infancy* *breast feeding* *diagnosis*

Source: Reprinted with permission from *Clinical Practice Guidelines for Cystic Fibrosis,* Volume I, Section V, p. 11, Cystic Fibrosis Foundation.

for age times 100 is 85–89%, the patient is moderately stunted; if it is < 85%, the patient's height is severely stunted.

Other anthropometric measurements, such as triceps skinfold, midarm circumference, and midarm muscle circumference, should be obtained at least annually, according to standard procedures,[20] and compared with normative data.[21] These measurements are particularly beneficial when monitoring the effects of nutrition intervention over time.

Growth studies have found CF patients to be smaller and lighter than their age- and sex-matched peers. For example, Sproul and Huang[22] found the 50th percentile for CF patients from infancy to adolescence for height and weight to be between the 3rd and 10th percentiles on the growth charts for healthy children. These same investigators noted an absence of the adolescent growth spurt in the CF population. Growth deficiencies significantly correlated with the severity of respiratory disease but did not correlate with pancreatic insufficiency. A more recent study based on the 1993 National CF Patient Registry found that children with CF continue to have poorer growth at all ages, when compared with healthy peers.[23] In this study, the median height-for-age percentile and weight-for-age percentile for children with CF was at the 20th percentile of the NCHS growth charts. The largest differences were found in the infant and pre-adolescent populations. These investigators believe that this finding may be reflective of the high energy and nutrient requirements of infancy and adolescence.[23] This study did not correlate factors such as severity of respiratory disease or pancreatic insufficiency with growth.[23]

In contrast, the Toronto CF clinic reports that its patients conform to the normal distribution for height in both males and females and for weight in males.[24] This clinic has advocated a high-calorie diet, with 40% of total calories as fat, coupled with high doses of pancreatic enzymes, as part of its routine medical care since the early 1970s.

Dietary

As part of the nutritional assessment, dietary analysis provides important information about what and how much the CF patient is eating. Several methods of gathering the data can be utilized, including a 24-hour dietary recall, a 3- to 7-day food record, and a food frequency questionnaire. The health professional should analyze the diet's adequacy in terms of calories, protein, and other nutrients by looking for a variety of foods in adequate amounts. During this interview, information about the patient's appetite, eating patterns, and behavioral issues related to feeding should be noted.[15]

Biochemical

Undiagnosed infants, particularly those who are breastfed or who are on soy formula, often present with hypoalbuminemia and subsequent edema. The malabsorption of undiagnosed CF causes the inadequate absorption of protein. The low protein content of breast milk, as compared with modified cow's milk formulas, further compromises the infant's protein status. For reasons as yet unclear, the CF infant does not utilize soy protein effectively, although the use of soy formula coupled with enterically coated pancreatic enzyme therapy warrants further study.[25,26] Upon diagnosis of CF and the initiation of pancreatic enzyme therapy, the hypoalbuminemia is usually corrected because the infant is no longer malabsorbing protein. It is wise to check an albumin level in newly diagnosed infants.

Any time an inadequate protein intake is suspected, it may be beneficial to assess the albumin or prealbumin level. However, it is important to remember that other potential causes of an abnormal albumin value include infection and other physiologic stress, fluid overload, congestive heart failure, and severe hepatic insufficiency.[27] CF patients, who chronically have inadequate calorie intakes, usually have a marasmic type of malnutrition. Their visceral protein levels are usually in the normal range, whereas somatic protein stores are low.[27] Other laboratory measurements that should be obtained at diagnosis and when the patient's condi-

Exhibit 15–2 Categories for Nutritional Management of Patients with Cystic Fibrosis

Category	*Target Group*	*Goals*
I. Routine management	All CF patients	Nutritional education Dietary counseling Pancreatic enzyme replacement (patients with PI) Vitamin supplementation (patients with PI)
II. Anticipatory guidance	CF patients at risk to develop energy imbalance (ie, severe PI, frequent pulmonary infections, periods of rapid growth), but maintaining weight/height index ≥ 90% of ideal weight.	Further education to prepare patients for increased energy needs. Increased monitoring of dietary intake. Increased caloric density in diet as needed. Behavioral assessment and counseling.
III. Supportive intervention	Patients with decreased weight velocity and/or weight/height index 85–90% of ideal weight.	All of the above, plus Begin oral supplements as needed.
IV. Rehabilitative care	Patients with weight/height index consistently < 85% of ideal weight.	All of the above, plus Initiate enteral supplementation via NG tube or enterostomy as indicated.
V. Resuscitative/ palliative care	Patients with weight/height index < 75% of ideal weight or progressive "nutritional failure."	All of the above, plus continuous enteral feedings or TPN.

Source: Reprinted with permission from *Clinical Practice Guidelines for Cystic Fibrosis,* Volume I, Section V, p. 11, Cystic Fibrosis Foundation.

tion warrants include: electrolytes and acid-base status, complete blood count (CBC), plasma or serum retinol, and alpha-tocopherol (Exhibit 15–1). A CBC, plasma or serum retinol, alpha-tocopherol, and liver function tests are also recommended annually. If there is evidence of iron deficiency, further iron studies should be obtained, including serum iron, iron binding capacity, ferritin, and reticulocyte count.[14,15]

The long-term antibiotic therapy, common in the treatment of CF, alters the gut flora. Because an important source of vitamin K is microbiologic synthesis in the gut, vitamin K status is affected. For this reason, it is important to monitor prothrombin times routinely. Prothrombin time may also be a useful measure of hepatic synthetic function in patients with nutritional failure or biliary cirrhosis.[15]

In high-risk patients, including patients who have been on steroid therapy, routine measurement of vitamin D and bone mineralization status is recommended.[15] Such an evaluation may include serum calcium, phosphorus, and vitamin D levels, as well as dual emission xray absorptiometry (DEXA) study.[15]

With the increased life expectancy of CF patients, the frequency of glucose intolerance in this population has increased.[28] According to the CF Foundation statistics, 12% of CF patients are treated with insulin for diabetes, and as many as 50% may have abnormal glucose tolerance.[3,28] Because about one-third of CF centers do not routinely screen for CFRD, these numbers probably represent underreporting.[28] CFRD is a distinct clinical entity, because it has features of both type 1 and type 2 diabetes.[28,29]

The CF Foundation convened a consensus conference on CFRD in February 1998 and issued recommendations for monitoring glucose intolerance.[29] On an outpatient basis, it is recommended that a casual glucose level or a random blood glucose be obtained annually.[28,29] Based on the results, decisions should be made as follows:[28,29]

1. < 126 mg/dl—no further action is required.
2. ≥ 126 mg/dl (7.0 mM) measure fasting blood glucose (FBG).
3. FBG ≥ 126 mg/dl (7.0 mM) when confirmed by a second FBG or in conjunction with a casual glucose level of ≥ 200 mg/dl (11.1 mM) is diagnostic for CFRD.
4. An oral glucose tolerance test (OGTT) should be performed in all patients with symptoms of diabetes, including weight loss, delayed puberty, polyuria, and polydipsia, in spite of a normal FBG. A value ≥ 200 mg/dl (11.1 mM) is diagnostic of CFRD.

For inpatients, all CF patients with pancreatic insufficiency should have a casual glucose level measured on the first and third days of hospitalization.[28,29] Decisions should be made as follows:[28,29]

1. FBG ≥ 126 mg/dl (7.0 mM) in either measurement, a 2-hour postprandial glucose and a FBG the next morning should be performed.
2. FBG < 126 mg/dl (7.0 mM) and 2-hour postprandial glucose < 200 mg/dl (11.1 mM), no further action is required.
3. If repeated FBG ≥ 126 mg/dl (7.0 mM), it should be repeated the next morning. If fasting hyperglycemia persists for more than 48 hours, insulin treatment of diabetes should be begun.
4. FBG < 126 mg/dl (7.0 mM) but 2-hour postprandial glucose is > 200 mg/dl (11.0 mM), patients are not usually started on insulin.

CFRD should be identified as CFRD with fasting hyperglycemia (FBG > 126 mg/dl) or CFRD without fasting hyperglycemia.[28,29]

Any patient who exhibits weight loss, growth failure, and clinical deterioration would benefit from a 72-hour fecal fat study to include both diet records to determine energy and fat intake, as well as quantification of energy and fat losses in the stool.[15] Refer to Exhibit 15–1.

Clinical

An assessment of the patient's overall health status should be obtained. Questions about activity and energy levels should be asked. Any missed school or work days should be noted. It is recommended that a description of the patient's body habitus be noted.[15] A general review of systems should be performed by the physician and/or nurse. Questions about the patient's use of alternative and complementary medicine therapies should be asked (discussed later in this chapter).

Stool Pattern

Information about the patient's stool pattern should be monitored carefully at each clinic visit because this is a good indication of the adequacy of the enzyme therapy. Questions to be asked during a nutrition screening and assessment should include the following:

1. number of stools per day
2. consistency of stools
3. presence of oily discharge
4. rectal prolapse
5. foul-smelling, floating stools and/or flatus
6. abdominal cramping

Enzyme Therapy

Important aspects of enzyme replacement therapy that should be checked at every clinic visit and hospitalization are:

1. type
2. brand
3. amount taken
4. when taken
5. method of administration
6. timing with meals
7. calculation of units of lipase/kg body weight/meal

Refer to dosage section under Adequate Pancreatic Enzyme Replacement Therapy in this chapter and Table 15–3 for additional information.

Other Medications

It is important to note other medications that the patient may be taking at each clinic visit, including antibiotics, bronchodilators, H_2 blockers, antacids, prokinetic agents, steroids, diuretics, cardiac medications, vitamins, and minerals.

Pulmonary Status

The pulmonary status of the patient will directly influence the patient's nutritional status. The nutrition professional should note the presence of an acute pulmonary exacerbation and chronic disease. Older CF patients will be able to have pulmonary function tests to assess the extent of their pulmonary involvement. The Brasfield or X-ray score is also a quantitative measure of pulmonary status, designed as a simple, reproducible tool for scoring chest roentgenograms, with the perfect X-ray score being 25.[30]

Other Medical Complications

Evidence of other medical problems should be noted, including CF-related diabetes mellitus, liver disease, gastroesophageal reflux, and lactose intolerance. These conditions will also have a direct impact on the patient's nutritional status.

Nutritional Management

Adequate Diet for Normal Growth and Development

In the past, the gastrointestinal symptoms of the disease, such as increased number of bulky, foul-smelling stools, increased flatus, and abdominal cramping, were treated with a low-fat diet. Today, with the advent of better enzyme replacement therapy, fat restriction is no longer routinely imposed on all patients. Health professionals now appreciate the tremendous energy demands of the disease, although

Table 15–3 Examples of Pancreatic Enzymes

Product	*Form*	*Lipase USP units*	*Protease USP units*	*Amylase USP units*
Cotazym (Organon, Inc.)	Powder in a capsule	8,000	30,000	30,000
Cotazym-S	Enteric coated spheres	5,000	20,000	20,000
Creon 5 (Solvay Pharmaceuticals)	Delayed release mini microspheres	5,000	18,750	16,600
Creon 10	Delayed release mini microspheres	10,000	37,500	33,200
Creon 20	Delayed release mini microspheres	20,000	75,000	66,400
Pancrease (Ortho-McNeil)	Enteric coated microspheres	4,500	25,000	20,000
Pancrease MT4	Enteric coated microtablets	4,000	12,000	12,000
Pancrease MT10	Enteric coated microtablets	10,000	30,000	30,000
Pancrease MT16	Enteric coated microtablets	16,000	48,000	48,000
Pancrease MT20	Enteric coated microtablets	20,000	44,000	56,000
Pancrecarb MS-4 (Digestive Care, Inc.)	Enteric coated microspheres with bicarbonate buffer	4,000	25,000	25,000
Pancrecarb MS-8 (Digestive Care, Inc.)	Enteric coated microspheres with bicarbonate buffer	8,000	45,000	40,000
Ultrase (Scandipharm)	Enteric coated microspheres	4,500	25,000	20,000
Ultrase MT12	Enteric coated minitablets	12,000	39,000	39,000
Ultrase MT18	Enteric coated minitablets	18,000	58,500	58,500
Ultrase MT20	Enteric coated minitablets	20,000	65,000	65,000
Viokase Powder (A.H. Robins)	Powder (1/4 tsp)	16,800	70,000	70,000
Viokase Tablet	Tablet	8,000	30,000	30,000
Zymase (Organon, Inc.)	Enteric coated spheres	12,000	24,000	24,000

the specific energy, protein, and nutrient requirements of CF patients have not been determined quantitatively. It is difficult to meet the high energy needs within the confines of fat restriction. It is generally recommended that the diets of CF patients derive up to 40% of total calories from fat, based on the individual patient's tolerance.[31]

According to the CF Consensus Report on nutritional assessment and management in CF,[14] the CF patient may be able to grow normally on the RDA for age for energy.[32] The report also includes a method for determining estimated energy needs based on the World Health Organization (WHO) equation for basal metabolic rate,[33] an activity factor, and a pancreatic insufficiency factor for patients who do not thrive on the RDA for energy.[14] Several reports have advocated 120–150% of the RDA for age and sex for CF patients.[34–36] The energy metabolism of CF patients has been studied; generally, an increase in resting energy expenditure has been found, as compared with controls and/or predicted resting energy expenditure.[37–41]

Age-specific considerations in the nutritional management of CF are summarized in Table 15–4. Infants with CF may be successfully breastfed, as long as pancreatic enzymes are administered prior to each feeding. Standard iron-fortified infant formulas are alternatives to breast milk but also require the administration of pancreatic enzymes prior to each feeding. Some CF centers recommend the use of protein hydrolysate formulas. A recent study of newly diagnosed infants with cystic fibrosis compared nutrition and growth parameters of those infants fed standard infant formula with those fed a protein hydrolysate formula.[42] There was no significant difference in growth parameters between the two groups of infants. Therefore, these researchers concluded that their research failed to support the use of the more expensive protein hydrolysate formula for the routine care of newly diagnosed infants with CF.[42]

In practice, it is easy for a CF patient to achieve a high protein intake because the average American diet is so high in protein. It is much more difficult to achieve the calorie intake that is recommended. A recent 3-year longitudinal study of dietary intakes of CF patients reported that these patients did not meet the recommended 120% RDA for energy or a high-fat (40% of energy) diet.[43] In practice, this is a common observation.

To close the gap between caloric needs and the amount of calories the patient is able to consume, calorically dense foods can be added to the patient's diet. Margarine, cheese, sour cream, and cream cheese can be added easily to the patient's favorite foods, as tolerated by the patient. Exhibit 15–3 depicts one approach to increasing calories and protein.

A meta-analysis of the literature on treatment approaches to the nutrition management of CF patients, including oral supplementation, enteral nutrition, parenteral nutrition, and behavioral intervention and their effectiveness on weight gain was recently reported.[44] Weight gain was produced in CF patients with all interventions. The behavioral interventions were found to be as effective as were more invasive medical procedures.[44] The best choice of intervention for a CF patient must be made on an individual basis.

Pregnancy

With the increased life expectancy of patients with CF, more women with the disease are becoming pregnant. In addition to the usual nutrient recommendations of CF, the increased energy needs of pregnancy must be taken into consideration. Emphasis needs to be put on proper weight gain. In addition to the usual vitamin therapy, one prenatal vitamin per day is added to the regimen.[14] Mothers with CF have successfully breastfed their infants.[45] Breastfeeding further increases the energy demands on the CF patient and needs to be considered on an individual basis.[14]

Diabetes

As with any patient with CF, the treatment goals of CFRD are to provide a diet that promotes optimal growth and development in chil-

Table 15–4 Nutritional Management of CF Patients

1. Infants
   - Breast milk or standard iron-fortified infant formula should be recommended. Special formulas such as Alimentum* and Pregestimil† (protein hydrolysate formulas with medium-chain triglycerides) can be recommended for infants in special situations, such as gut resection or increased fat malabsorption.
   - Pancreatic enzymes should be given prior to feedings with any of the milks or formulas listed above.
   - Vitamin supplements and a source of fluoride should be given.
   - Introduction of solid foods should proceed as with a healthy infant. Some of the high-calorie, starchy vegetables and dessert baby foods can also be added to the diet to increase calorie intake. Salt supplementation may be needed.
2. Toddlers
   - Toddlers' diets should be based on a normal diet with a variety of foods.
   - Parents should be forewarned of the normal decrease in growth and appetite during this age.
   - Regular mealtimes and snack times should be encouraged.
   - Excessive snacking and drinking between meals should be discouraged.
   - Pancreatic enzymes and vitamins are continued.
3. Preschool and school age
   - A normal healthy diet with a variety of foods again should form the basis of the diet.
   - Parents lose control of what child eats away from home at preschool and school.
   - Arrangements need to be made for child to take enzymes during the school day.
   - Vitamins are continued.
   - Diet prescriptions for a high-calorie, high-protein diet can be sent to the school.
4. Adolescents
   - Patients begin exercising more independence in food choices.
   - Parents can provide appropriate food environment at home.
   - Patients can be taught to include quick-to-prepare high-calorie foods in daily diet.
   - Snack and fast foods can add a significant amount of calories to the diet and should not be discouraged.
   - Importance of high-calorie intake and enzyme and vitamin therapy should be emphasized by health professionals directly to patient and not via the parents.

* Ross Laboratories, Columbus, Ohio.
† Mead Johnson Nutritionals, Bristol-Myers Institutional Products, Evansville, Indiana.

dren and adolescents, achievement and maintenance of normal weight in adults, and optimal nutritional status.[28,29] Other treatment goals include controlling hyperglycemia to reduce diabetes complications, avoiding severe hypoglycemia, and assisting the patient in adapting to another chronic illness from a psychologic standpoint.[29] The patient with CFRD should be allowed as much flexibility as possible in the nutrition management of these two diseases.[29] The primary goal remains meeting the patient's caloric needs.[28] Because carbohydrates have the most effect on glycemic index, emphasis should be placed on total amount of carbohydrate eaten, rather than the carbohydrate source.[29] Simple sugars can be included in the diet plan. However, the patient needs to learn how to recognize the carbohydrate

Exhibit 15–3 Instructional Handout on Increasing Calories

Calorie-Protein BOOSTERS

—Some ways to hide extra calories and protein—

Powdered Milk **(33 cal/tbsp, 3 gm pro/tbsp)**
Add 2-4 tbsp to 1 cup milk. Mix into puddings, potatoes, soups, ground meats, vegetables, cooked cereal.

Eggs **(80 cal/egg, 7 gm pro/tbsp)**
Add to casseroles, meat loaf, mashed potato, cooked cereal, macaroni & cheese. Add extra to pancake batter and french toast. (Do not use raw eggs in uncooked items.)

Butter or margarine **(45 cal/tsp)**
Add to puddings, casseroles, sandwiches, vegetables, cooked cereal.

Cheeses **(100 cal/oz, 7 gm pro/oz)**
Give as snacks, or in sandwiches. Add melted to casseroles, potatoes, vegetables, soup.

Wheat germ **(25 cal/tbsp)**
Add a tablespoon or two to cereal. Mix into meat dishes, cookie batter, casseroles, etc.

Mayonnaise or Salad Dressings **(45 cal/tsp)**
Use liberally on sandwiches, on salads, as a dip for raw vegetables or sauce on cooked vegetables.

Evaporated milk **(25 cal/tbsp, 1 gm pro/tbsp)**
Use in place of whole milk, in desserts, baked goods, meat dishes and cooked cereals.

Sour Cream **(26 cal/tbsp)**
Add to potatoes, casseroles, dips; use in sauces, baked goods, etc.

Sweetened condensed milk **(60 cal/tbsp, 1 gm pro/tbsp)**
Add to pies, puddings, milkshakes. Mix 1-2 tbsp with peanut butter and spread on toast.

Peanut butter **(95 cal/tbsp, 4 gm pro/tbsp)**
Serve on toast, crackers, bananas, apples, celery.

Carnation Instant Breakfast **(130 cal/pckt, 7 gm pro/pckt)**
Add to milk, milkshakes.

Gravies **(40 cal/tbsp)**
Use liberally on mashed potatoes, meats.

High Protein Foods

- ★ MEATS—Beef, Chicken, Fish, Turkey, Lamb
- ★ MILK & CHEESE—Yogurt, Cottage Cheese, Cream Cheese
- ★ EGGS
- ★ PEANUT BUTTER (with Bread or Crackers)
- ★ DRIED BEANS & PEAS (with Bread, Cornbread, Rice)

Source: Courtesy of Pediatric Pulmonary Center, University of Alabama, Birmingham, Alabama.

content of foods, such as the "carbohydrate counting" method.[28,29] Patients should also be encouraged to spread their carbohydrate intake consistently throughout the day.[28] Fat should continue to contribute about 40% of total calories, and protein intake should provide about 20% of total calories.[28]

Patient and Family Education

Patient and family education on nutrition management and its importance in the patient's overall health care is an integral component of the individual patient's care plan. A qualified, registered dietitian should be available to the patient and family to assist them in meeting the nutritional needs of the patient in the least invasive way possible. Information about the nutrient content of foods and suggestions for increasing the patient's caloric intake should be available.

Luder and Gilbride[46] studied the effects of nutrition counseling that was provided quarterly for a 4-year period, based on self-management skills in a group of CF patients. These patients had significant increases in their energy intakes, as well as in their body mass index values, without decline in pulmonary function.[46] More and more emphasis is being placed on anticipatory guidance as an integral part of nutrition management (see Exhibit 15–2).[15]

Feeding issues are prominent in this patient population, and the health professional needs to provide anticipatory guidance to the parents or caretakers of these patients to avoid battles over eating.[47,48] The importance of behavioral programs in the nutritional care of CF patients is receiving more and more recognition.[49]

Supplemental Nutrition

Milkshakes and other high-calorie drinks can be used as supplemental feedings. Commercial oral feedings can also be used to boost calories, but they require additional expense and, in some instances, they may be difficult for the family to obtain.

Oftentimes, in spite of vigorous efforts by the patient, the patient's family, and dietetic professionals, it is very difficult to meet the patient's caloric needs by the oral route alone. At these times, alternate routes of supplemental feedings need to be considered.

CF centers have reported using various forms of tube feedings, including nasogastric, gastrostomy, and jejunostomy feedings. Tube feedings are sometimes administered on a continuous basis while the patient is asleep. Some centers use a partially predigested formula with or without enzymes; others use a nonelemental formula with enzymes. A recent study by Erskine et al[50] showed no difference in absorption between a predigested formula and a nonelemental formula with enzyme replacement. Predigested formulas are more costly than are nonelemental formulas.

Enzyme administration poses a problem with nocturnal tube feedings. Mixing enzymes directly into the feeding causes the product to begin to break down and may clog the feeding tube. Many centers instruct patients to take pancreatic enzymes prior to the initiation of the feeding and again if they wake up during the night. At the current time, there is no consensus on the type of tube feeding to use for CF patients or on the optimal enzyme administration. The CF Consensus Report on the nutritional assessment and management of CF suggests that the use of supplemental tube feedings be considered when optimization of feeding behaviors and addition of oral supplements have failed or when the patient's weight/height ratio falls below 85% of ideal.[14] The patient and family need to be given the facts about available therapies and should be involved in the decision making.[14]

Parenteral nutrition is used in special situations in CF care, such as after intestinal surgery. It is not a good choice of therapy for long-term calorie supplement because of its high cost and increased risks.[14]

Adequate Vitamin and Mineral Status

Vitamins

According to the CF Consensus Report on nutritional assessment and management of CF,[14] the following multivitamin regimen is recommended until further specific information is available on the vitamin needs of CF patients.

Multivitamins

1. Infants < 2 years of age: 1 mL liquid multivitamin preparation daily
2. Children 2–8 years of age: 1 tablet per day of standard multivitamin containing 400 IU vitamin D and 5,000 IU of vitamin A
3. Children > 8 years of age, adolescents, and adults: 1–2 tablets per day of a standard adult multivitamin

Vitamin E

1. 0–6 months of age: 25 IU per day
2. 6–12 months of age: 50 IU per day
3. 1–4 years of age: 100 IU per day
4. 4–10 years of age: 100–200 IU per day
5. >10 years of age: 200–400 IU per day

Vitamin K

1. 0–12 months of age: 2.5 mg per week (or 2.5 mg twice a week if on antibiotics)
2. > 1 year of age: 5.0 mg twice weekly when on antibiotics or with cholestatic liver disease

There are multivitamin preparations available on the market that contain water-miscible forms of vitamins A, D, E, and K: ADEK (Scandipharm, Birmingham, AL) and Vitamax (CF Pharmacy, Bethesda, MD). The use of these products may simplify the vitamin regimen and improve patient compliance.[15]

Minerals

Minerals such as zinc, iron, and selenium have been studied in the CF population.[51] Much more study is needed before specific supplementation recommendations can be made. CF patients who are on steroids, who have decreased dietary intake of calcium, and/or who are found to have decreased bone density may benefit from calcium supplementation. These minerals, as well as other macro- and micronutrients, are important in the overall nutriture of the CF patient; therefore, eating a variety of foods should be encouraged.

Additional salt should be added to the diet during times of increased perspiration, such as:

1. during hot weather
2. with fevers
3. during strenuous physical activity
4. with profuse diarrhea

The additional salt compensates for the increased losses of sodium and chloride from perspiration. In most instances, liberal use of the salt shaker and the inclusion of high-salt foods in the diet will supply the needed sodium and chloride. Salt supplements may be used in instances of very heavy perspiration. Breastfed infants may especially need supplementation with sodium chloride, particularly during hot weather.[14] According to the CF Consensus Report,[14] a safe dose is 2–4 mmol/kg body weight/day.

Adequate Pancreatic Enzyme Replacement Therapy

Types of Available Enzymes

There are many different brands and types of pancreatic enzymes available (see Table 15–3). They contain varying amounts of lipase, which breaks down fat; protease, which breaks down protein; and amylase, which breaks down carbohydrate.

The nonproprietary names of these products are *pancrelipase* or *pancreatin*. Most of the products feature an enteric coating, which protects the enzymes from inactivation in the acid environment of the stomach. The enzymes become activated in the alkaline pH of the duodenum. Pancreatic enzymes are also available in powder and capsule forms.

Dosage/Administration

There is a CF Consensus Statement on the use of pancreatic enzyme supplements.[52,53] Very high doses of pancreatic enzymes have been associated with fibrosing colonopathy in CF patients.[54,55] A recommended starting dose for infants is 2,000–4,000 units of lipase per 120 mL of formula or breastfeeding.[14,52,53] Another proposed weight-based enzyme dosing schedule is 1,000 units of lipase/kg body weight/meal for children younger than 4 years of age and 500 units of lipase/kg body weight/meal for those over age 4.[52,53] The usual enzyme dose for snacks is one-half of the mealtime dose. The recommendations are not to exceed a dose of 2,500 units of lipase/kg body weight/meal.[52–54] It is the amount of lipase presented to the gut at any one time that appears to be important in the context of fibrosing colonopathy. Calculating units of lipase/kg body weight/meal has become an integral component of routine care. For example, a 10-year-old child weighing 35.7 kg who takes a mealtime dose of 3 capsules of a pancreatic enzyme preparation containing 20,000 units of lipase per capsule will receive 1,681 units of lipase/kg body weight/meal (60,000 units of lipase divided by 35.7 kg = 1,681 units of lipase/kg body weight/meal). Careful monitoring of the patient's growth, stool pattern, and the absence or presence of gastrointestinal symptoms is necessary to determine the adequacy of therapy. Monitoring and adjusting the dosage as needed should be continued throughout the patient's treatment. If the CF patient is still exhibiting symptoms of malabsorption after reaching a maximum enzyme dose, it may be because the stomach contents are too acidic when reaching the small intestine and are inactivating the enzymes. In these cases, the addition of bicarbonate or drugs that inhibit gastric acid secretion may be helpful.[52,53]

Enzymes should be taken within an hour prior to meals and snacks to be most effective. The enterically coated enzymes should not be chewed or crushed.

Most of the enzymes are available in capsule form. For infants and small children who are unable to swallow a capsule, the capsule can be broken open and the contents mixed with a soft, acidic food such as applesauce. Enzymes mixed with food should be used within 30 minutes of mixing. When the enterically coated enzymes are mixed with a higher-pH food, such as pudding or milk, the enzymes will become activated and begin breaking down the food. Powdered enzymes are already in an activated form. Mixing enzymes directly into a tube feeding or infant formula causes enzymatic digestion to begin. This may cause the food to take on an unpleasant color, taste, or odor.

Patient Compliance

Administering enzymes to a very young infant can be a frustrating endeavor for the parent or caretaker, primarily because of the infant's natural extrusion reflex. After a few months of age, taking enzymes becomes part of a CF patient's daily routine. Parents of toddlers should be warned against allowing the child to "graze" throughout the day because this makes enzyme dosing difficult. In the preadolescent and adolescent age groups, patient compliance with enzyme administration can become a big issue. Sometimes, schools require the child to come to the school office for medications, and this may be a source of embarrassment and alienation from peers for the child with CF. The lack of compliance needs to be discussed with the child, and a solution must be found that is agreeable to the child, parents, and school authorities.

Pancreatic enzyme therapy is very expensive and contributes significantly to the overall cost of this disease. Enzymes are often covered by third-party payers and programs such as a state program for children with special health care needs.

Referral to Food/Nutrition and Other Resources

Referral to food and nutrition resources such as the U S Department of Agriculture's Special Supplemental Nutrition Programs for Women, Infants, and Children (WIC) and the Food Stamp Program should be made based on the individual's needs. In some states, referrals can be made to the state program for children with special health care needs for aid in obtaining supplemental feedings, enzymes, and vitamins. Children who participate in the Child Nutrition Program at their school will need diet prescriptions for high-calorie, high-protein diets sent to their schools.

CF has a tremendous impact on patients and their families—emotionally, physically, and financially. Most CF centers provide an interdisciplinary team approach to the care of these children and their families to better help them meet their many needs.

Drug Nutrient Interactions

Prolonged antibiotic therapy can alter the gut flora and subsequently influence vitamin K status. Some of the intravenous antibiotics can cause nausea in some patients. CF patients with an asthma component of their disease may be on bursts of steroids. As the CF patient's pulmonary disease progresses, cor pulmonale, or right-sided heart failure, develops. Diuretics may be prescribed at this point. Electrolyte and fluid status need to be carefully monitored.

Alternative and Complementary Medicine

As with other chronic diseases, the use of alternative and complementary medicine in CF care has sparked the interest of CF patients and health professionals. To date, little published science-based research exists in this area. More and more CF centers are surveying their patients to ascertain the extent of alternative medicine practices. Currently, CF patients are obtaining a lot of their information from the Internet, with many CF Internet sites having links to alternative medicine sites. CF centers will need to study alternative medicine practices further so that CF caregivers can advise patients and their families as to the safety and efficacy of various therapies.

The entire population of CF patients followed at Case Western Reserve University, Rainbow Babies, and Children's Hospital in Cleveland, Ohio participated in a survey of the use of nonmedical treatment.[56] The results indicated that nonmedical treatment was used by 66% of the population; 57% of the population used at least one religious treatment; 27% used at least one nonreligious treatment.[56] Group prayer (48%) was the most common nonmedical therapy, and 92% of those participating in group prayer perceived benefit. Chiropractors were consulted by 14%, with 69% of these patients perceiving benefit. Nutrition modalities other than those prescribed by the CF caregivers were employed by 11% of the population; 78% of these used these treatments frequently (>5 times); 87% perceived benefit. Meditation was used by 5%, with 94% reporting perceived benefit.

It is important for CF caregivers to include questions about alternative and complementary medicine practices when interviewing CF patients and their family members, especially in regard to ingested substances. This is especially important information to obtain from patients who may be participating in studies with experimental drugs because the possibility exists that substances such as unregulated botanical products may confound the study results.

Identification of Areas for Further Research

There are many unanswered questions about CF in general and, more specifically, in regard to nutrition. Much more research is needed to determine specific nutrient requirements of CF patients in regard to energy, protein, vitamins, and minerals. The most appropriate method for delivering these nutrients must be determined. The most appropriate time for nutrition intervention in the course of the disease must be determined. What are the psychosocial and emotional benefits and drawbacks with more invasive nutritional therapy? What effect does improved nutritional status have on the progression of the pulmonary disease, the ultimate killer of the vast majority of CF patients? What constitutes normal growth for a CF patient? With lung transplantation becoming more available to CF patients, appropriate nutrition management pre- and post-transplantation requires further study.

CF is a complicated disease, affecting many organs of the body. Proper nutritional care is an integral part of its therapy. The disease process is highly variable. Therefore, every patient and family deserve individualized treatment and support from an interdisciplinary team of health professionals, including qualified dietetic professionals.

BRONCHOPULMONARY DYSPLASIA

Bronchopulmonary dysplasia (BPD) was first described by Northway[57] in 1967 as a form of chronic lung disease seen in infants with severe hyaline membrane disease who required mechanical ventilation and high concentrations of oxygen for prolonged periods of time. Since that time, a commonly accepted definition of BPD has been a chronic lung disease with abnormal chest radiographic findings that requires the use of supplemental oxygen on the 28th day of life.[58] With more and more premature infants surviving at earlier gestational ages, the definition of BPD has been expanded to include the need for supplemental oxygen and an abnormal chest radiograph at or after the age of 36 weeks postconception.[58]

Today's definition of BPD usually includes infants who have had an acute lung injury with minimal clinical and radiographic findings, as well as those with major radiographic abnormalities. There is no standard nomenclature used in defining BPD, and it represents a continuum of lung disease.[59] This chronic disease is seen in young infants, the vast majority being premature infants, who require respiratory support during the first 2 weeks of life or longer for neonatal respiratory distress. The lungs are damaged by the barotrauma from the use of intermittent positive pressure ventilation (IPPV) and by oxygen toxicity from the high concentrations of oxygen required by these infants early in life.[58–60] Infection may play a role in the pathogenesis of BPD.[58,59] Other factors that may contribute to the development of the disease include increased fluids contributing to pulmonary edema[61] and inadequate early nutrition impeding lung reparative processes.[62,63]

Today, more and more preterm infants are surviving with the aid of mechanical ventilation. Consequently, BPD has become one of the most common sequelae of newborn intensive care unit stays. As BPD patients are followed over time, chronic lung disease remains a major clinical problem for many of these patients into late childhood and early adolescence.[59,64]

The disease is characterized by signs of respiratory distress, such as chest retractions, tachypnea, crackles, and wheezing. Supplemental oxygen therapy may be required, and there will be changes on the patient's chest radiograph. Pulmonary complications of BPD may include recurrent atelectasis, pulmonary infections, and respiratory failure requiring mechanical ventilation. Other complications of BPD include pulmonary edema, pulmonary hypertension, cor pulmonale, poor growth, neurodevelopmental delays, including delayed feeding skills, and cardiovascular problems.

The primary goal of BPD management is to provide the patient with the necessary pulmonary support during the acute and chronic phases of the disease to minimize lung damage and to maintain optimal oxygen saturation. This may include mechanical ventilation, supplemental oxygen, and diuretic therapy. Of equal importance is the provision of adequate nutrition, not only for growth and development, but also to compensate for the demands of the disease. Growth of new lung tissue can occur in humans until about 8 years of age. Theoretically, a BPD patient can "outgrow" the disease if proper pulmonary and nutritional support can be provided.

Effects on Nutritional Status

Increased Nutrient Requirements

Effects of Prematurity. Considering the fact that most babies who develop BPD are premature infants, it is easy to see that these infants have little fat, glycogen, or other nutrients in reserve, particularly iron, calcium, and phosphorus. Faced with the demands of prematurity and the stress of BPD, the infant can quickly develop a state of negative nutrient balance.

Effects of Bronchopulmonary Dysplasia. Several factors increase the caloric requirements of BPD patients, including:

1. increased basal metabolic rate
2. increased work of breathing
3. chronic illness/infections
4. respiratory distress/metabolic complications

Weinstein and Oh[65] reported that resting oxygen consumption was approximately 25% higher in eight infants with BPD, when compared with controls. Kurzner et al[66] found that infants with BPD and growth failure had increased resting oxygen consumption, as compared with control infants and infants with BPD and normal growth. Other investigators have also found an increase in resting energy expenditure in infants with BPD, as compared with controls.[67,68]

Treatment of the BPD patient usually includes a wide array of medications, including diuretics, bronchodilators, and steroids. The impact of these drugs on the patient's nutritional status is further discussed in the Drug–Nutrient Interaction section of this chapter.

Decreased Nutrient Consumption. Infants with BPD are very fluid sensitive because of the acute lung disease and the possible complication of cor pulmonale, or right-sided heart failure. Fluid restrictions are imposed, which places a limitation on the provision of calories and nutrients. Yeh[68] showed that infants with BPD had significantly lower energy intakes, as compared with controls.

These infants must be adequately oxygenated for growth and tissue repair to occur. Frequent intubations and mechanical ventilation interfere with the normal feeding sequence and feeding skill development. Therefore, these infants may be poor oral feeders and may develop adversive oral behavior.[58] Also, these patients may experience fatigue or decreased oxygen saturation during feeding because of their underlying pulmonary disease.[69,70]

Nutritional Screening and Assessment

Anthropometric

Obtaining daily weights in a BPD patient is essential during the early hospitalization(s) and critical stages of the disease. Weight data help to identify fluid overload in a patient, as well as growth.

Monitoring weight, length, and head circumference on a regular basis during the follow-up period will provide the necessary data to assess whether the patient is achieving expected growth. Measurements should be made using appropriate techniques and equipment (see Chapter 2) and be plotted on appropriate growth charts, using either the NCHS growth charts and correcting for gestational age or growth charts that allow assessment of infants of varying gestational age, such as those by Babson and Benda.[17,71] Other easily obtained and useful measurements are the midarm circumference and triceps skinfold.

It is unrealistic to expect true growth to occur when life-threatening events, such as respiratory failure, necrotizing enterocolitis, or other serious problems of prematurity, are taking place. The patient must be fairly stable for growth to occur. This is supported by a study by Shankaran et al,[72] who found a poor pattern of growth in BPD patients to be related to the severity of pulmonary disease. Similarly, Kurzner et al[66] found resting metabolic rate to be inversely correlated with body weight in infants with BPD.

Growth failure has been recognized as a complication of BPD. deRegnier et al[73] studied 16 very-low-birth-weight infants who developed BPD and compared them to birth-weight-matched control infants without BPD during the first 6 postnatal weeks. At the end of the study period, the infants with BPD had lower Z scores for weight and head circumference, as well as lower arm muscle area and arm fat area, as compared with controls. Length Z scores were not significantly different between the two groups. When the BPD infants achieved full enteral feedings, they gained at the same rate as the controls but did not achieve catch-up growth. These investigators speculate that early reductions in muscle and fat accretion and growth velocity may contribute to the long-term growth failure of BPD patients, and they emphasize the importance of delivering optimal nutrition early in the postnatal period.[73]

Johnson et al[74] studied 40 infants with BPD for 7 months after initial hospital discharge. During this study period, 73% of the infants experienced a decrease in weight-for-age Z score; 20% experienced a decrease in length-for-age Z score; and 65% experienced a decrease in weight-for-length Z score. Low socioeconomic status and postdischarge illness were associated with a significantly increased risk of growth failure.

In more long-term follow-up of BPD patients, Giacoia et al[64] studied 12 school-aged children with BPD and compared them with a preterm control group matched for birth weight, gestational age, and gender, as well as with an age-matched term control group. Both the BPD group and the preterm group were shorter than the healthy term control group. The BPD group had lower lean body mass, compared with the term control group, and had lower bone mineral content when compared with both control groups.[64] Another study of school-aged children with BPD was performed by Vrlenich et al,[75] who compared children who had been born prematurely with and without the development of BPD. The children with BPD were significantly smaller in weight and head circumference but not height. However, when possible confounders that are known to be correlates of poor growth were applied, the differences were no longer significant. These investigators suggest that the poor growth reported in children with BPD may be related to factors other than BPD.[75]

Adequate oxygenation must be maintained in the patient with BPD for growth to occur. Studies have shown that desaturation may occur during feeding and sleeping.[69,70,76] Moyer-Mileur et al[76] demonstrated positive growth trends in infants with BPD who maintained an oxygen saturation of greater than 92% while sleeping. These investigators also found that short-term pulse oxygen saturation studies were not always reliable predictors of oxygen saturation during prolonged periods of sleep. Groothuis and Rosenberg[77] found that BPD patients who were maintained on home oxygen therapy maintained their original weight percentiles, whereas those infants who discontinued oxygen therapy experienced significant decreases in weight gain.

Dietary

The BPD patient's dietary intake needs to be evaluated for calories, protein, fluid, and caloric distribution of fat, protein, and carbohydrate. The type of feeding—enteral versus parenteral—should be noted, as well as vitamin and mineral supplementation. This can then be compared with the patient's estimated nutrient and fluid requirements. Exhibit 15–4 contains an example of a clinical nutrition data collection form.

Of particular importance in the nutrition assessment of BPD patients is careful monitoring of the patient's ability to suck and swallow and of the patient's feeding skill development. The sucking reflex does not develop until about 34 weeks' gestation. Alternate methods of feeding are required until this reflex develops. Neurologic impairment may prevent the patient from being able to coordinate sucking and swallowing. Noxious stimuli to the patient's mouth, such as frequent intubations and suctioning, may seriously affect normal feeding skill development.

Maintaining adequate oxygenation during feedings is essential.[69,70] It is important to note whether the patient tires during feedings and whether he or she turns blue around the mouth or fingertips, indicating a drop in oxygen saturation. It is imperative that these problems be identified early and that appropriate intervention be instituted.

Biochemical

Biochemical monitoring of the BPD patient is summarized in Exhibit 15–5. Frequencies of measurement depend on the patient's clinical status, the type and amount of diuretic therapy, and the protocol of the individual institution.

Clinical

The patient's pulmonary status will have an impact on nutritional needs and intake. Noting the patient's pulmonary status is an important component of the nutrition assessment. If a BPD patient is ventilator-dependent, this is an indication of respiratory failure and of severe lung disease. Ventilator-dependent BPD patients require close follow-up because it may be difficult initially to determine their nutritional needs. A patient who has a low arterial partial pressure of oxygen is not properly oxygenating tissue, which may contribute to growth failure. These patients may require supplemental oxygen for tissue oxygenation and for growth. An increase in pulmonary symptoms, such as the presence of tachypnea, rales, rhonchi, and bronchiolitis/pneumonia, are indications of active pulmonary disease. The presence of chronic pulmonary disease and acute pulmonary exacerbations in BPD patients increases calorie needs and at the same time may increase their sensitivity to fluids.

Other medical conditions, such as cor pulmonale, gastroesophageal reflux with or without aspiration, esophagitis, repeated emesis, and the patient's medication regimen, should also be noted. The clinical nutrition data collection form found in Exhibit 15–4 lists the type of data needed to determine the patient's tolerance of the feedings, and Table 15–5 lists drug–nutrient interactions of medications commonly prescribed for BPD patients.

Nutrition Management

Determination of Caloric Requirements

As has already been discussed, the patient with BPD has high energy and nutrient needs. At the same time, numerous constraints are placed on the delivery of the calories and nutrients, such as fluid restrictions, gastrointestinal immaturity, and renal immaturity. Oh[78] describes three phases of nutritional management of infants with BPD, which are summarized below. The estimated caloric requirements of each phase and the components of the energy expenditure are depicted in Table 15–6.

Acute Phase

The BPD patient during this phase is critically ill and at risk for clinical morbidities, such as patent ductus arteriosus and necrotizing enterocolitis. No calories are needed for specific dynamic action or for growth. Efforts should be made to keep thermal losses to a minimum. Possible feeding complications during this phase include fluid overload and hyperglycemia. The BPD patient has decreased fluid tolerance because of pulmonary edema and reduced cardiac output. Caloric provision is often relegated to secondary importance, behind these two problems and electrolyte imbalance.

Intermediate Phase

This phase is characterized by a period of clinical improvements and a gradual introduction of oral feeding. Again, thermal losses should be kept to a minimum. Fluid overload continues to be a possible complication but, generally, the BPD patient is able to tolerate an increase in fluid during this phase.

Convalescent Phase

This is a period of recovery. Usually, but not always, the patient is exclusively feeding orally.

Exhibit 15–4 Clinical Nutrition Data Collection Form

Hx GA ____ Multi Ges ____ Apgars ____
BWt ____ BL ____ BHC ____

ID STAMP
Admit Date: ____
Address: ____
Phone: ____
Insurance: ____
WIC/County: ____

Maternal Hx ____
____
Initial Dx ____
____
Current Problems ____
____
____

DATE								
ANTHROPOMETRICS								
Weight								
Length								
HC								
FLUIDS/NUTRITION								
Goals								
kcal/kg/d								
pro/kg/d								
cc/kg/d								
Present Intake								
cc/kg/d								
kcal/kg/d								
pro/kg/d								
fat/kg/d								
% kcal enteral								
kcal distribution								
Enteral								
Formula								
Additives								
kcal/cc								
Route								
Rate								
IN cc								
Parenteral								
Days on TPN								
Route								
Glucose conc								
Fat conc								
Pro source								
mg glucose/kg/min								
NPC:N								
$Ca:PO_4$								

____ F/U day

Exhibit 15–4 continued

DATE								
IN PN								
IL								
IV								
BIOCHEMICAL								
FBP								
Glucose								
Ca/PO_4								
Mg								
Alk Phos								
Bili T/D								
TG								
Hct/Hgb								
T Pro/Alb								
Dexstix								
UGK								
TOLERANCE /OUTPUT								
Stools								
pH/Red sub								
Urine cc								
Emesis								
Residuals								
OG/NG								
GT								
Blood								
Drains								

MEDICATIONS: ______________________________

COMMENTS/PLANS: ______________________________

Source: Department of Clinical Nutrition, Children's Hospital, Birmingham, Alabama.

Exhibit 15–5 Biochemical Monitoring of the BPD Patient

Electrolytes: 1. Chloride								
2. Potassium								
3. Sodium								
Minerals: 1. Calcium								
2. Phosphorus								
3. Magnesium								
Other: 1. Albumin								
2. Alkaline phosphatase								
3. Hematocrit								
4. Hemoglobin								
5. $PaCO_2$								
6. pH								
Medications: Diuretics								
Steroids								
Bronchodilators								

Minimizing thermal losses continues to be important, as well as are monitoring activity, growth, and adequate oxygenation of tissues. Continued monitoring of intake, growth, and development is important. Nutritional recommendations must be individualized according to each patient's needs.

Determination of Protein Requirements

Adequate protein is necessary to achieve growth, but the immature kidney cannot handle high-protein loads. Protein should constitute about 8–12% of the total calories, with the remainder of the calories evenly divided between carbohydrate and fat.[79]

Provision of Adequate Calories and Protein. Translating these calorie and protein requirements into a feeding order can be very difficult in light of the restrictions previously described. This discussion will be divided into parenteral and enteral routes of feeding.

Parenteral Nutrition

During the acute phase of BPD, parenteral nutrition is often employed. Refer to Chapter 3 for specific guidelines in parenteral nutrition during the early postnatal period.

Studies have raised concern about the effect of intravenous fat in pulmonary-compromised patients.[80,81] Other studies have shown that the possible adverse effect of lipid infusion is related to the maturity of the infant and to the rate of the infusion.[82,83] The use of parenteral fat emulsions should be carefully monitored in patients with underlying infection, pulmonary disease, and/or hyperbilirubinemia.[84] The American Academy of Pediatrics recommends starting lipids in the low-birth-weight

Table 15–5 BPD Drug–Nutrient Interactions

Medication	*Nutrients Affected*	*Other Effects*
Diuretics (eg, furosemide)	↓ Na, ↓ K, ↓ Cl ↓ Mg, ↓ Ca ↓ Zn	Volume depletion Metabolic alkalosis Anorexia Diarrhea Hyperuricemia Gastrointestinal irritant
Bronchodilators (eg, theophylline)		Gastrointestinal distress Nausea Vomiting Diarrhea
Steroids (eg, prednisone)	↓ Ca, ↓ P	Growth suppression

Table 15–6 Calorie Requirements (kcal/kg/d) of Infants with Bronchopulmonary Dysplasia at Various Stages of Nutritional Management

Component	*Acute*	*Intermediate*	*Convalescent*
Basal metabolic rate	45	60	60
Stool losses	0–10	10	10
Thermal stress	0–10	0–10	10
Activity	5	5	10
Specific dynamic action	0	0–5	10
Growth allowance	0	20–30	20–30
Total	50–70	95–120	120–130

Acute = clinical illness, oral feeding difficult; intermediate = clinical improvement, gradual introduction of oral feeding; convalescent = recovery, oral feeding exclusively.

Source: Used with permission of Ross Products Division, Abbott Laboratories, Inc., Columbus, OH 43216. From *Bronchopulmonary Dysplasia and Related Chronic Respiratory Disorders,* © 1986, Ross Products Division, Abbott Laboratories, Inc.

infant at 0.5–1.0 g/kg/day and slowly increasing to a maximum of 2.0–3.0 g/kg/day.[85] Serum triglyceride levels should be kept below 150 mg/dL.[85]

For preterm infants, the American Academy of Pediatrics recommends starting glucose infusions at a rate less than 6 mg/kg/minute and steadily increasing to an infusion rate of 11–12 mg/kg/minute.[85] High-glucose loads in BPD patients have been shown to increase resting energy expenditure, increase basal oxygen consumption, and increase carbon dioxide production.[67] Infants with borderline respiratory function may not be able to excrete this additional carbon dioxide, and respiratory acidosis can result.

Enteral Nutrition

Enteral feedings must be begun at a slow rate and may initially be diluted to allow the immature intestine of the premature infant to adapt to the feedings (refer to Chapter 3). During this transitional phase, parenteral nutrition is often continued to meet the increased caloric needs of the patient. It is very important to maintain the delivery of adequate calories and protein while tolerance to enteral feedings is being established.

This transitional phase can become very complicated. An infant must be hungry before an oral feeding will be readily accepted. Continuous infusions of nutritional solutions may suppress natural hunger sensations. Hunger is particularly important when feeding skills are being developed. An appropriate schedule of parenteral feedings, enteral tube feedings, and oral feedings must be determined by members of the interdisciplinary health care team to best suit the individual patient's needs.

Fortified breast milk or premature infant formulas, which have higher concentrations of vitamins and minerals, may be used initially. The infant should continue with breast milk fortified with a human milk fortifier or with premature formula until reaching a weight of 2,000–2,500 g. At this point, the infant can most likely be transitioned to a premature follow-up formula or a standard infant formula concentrated to 22 or 24 kcal/oz. To meet some infants' very high energy needs, it may become necessary to further concentrate the formula to 26–30 kcal/oz. Currently, there is some controversy as to the best approach for further concentration of the formula. Some registered dietitians prefer to further concentrate the formula by adding less water. The proponents of this method argue that by concentrating formula in this manner, protein, vitamins, and mineral content per volume are not diluted. Another approach is using a 24-kcal/oz formula as a base and adding carbohydrate in the form of glucose polymers or rice cereal and/or lipids. When modulating formulas in this manner, it is important to maintain a proper balance of nutrients. Caloric distribution should continue to be approximately 8–12% protein, 40–50% carbohydrate, and 40–50% fat.[79] An example of a modulated formula is given in Table 15–7. When modulating formulas, care should be taken not to dilute the protein content to a level that is inadequate for growth.[86] Fat should not provide more than 60% of total calories because ketosis may be induced. Fat delays gastric emptying, and a high fat content may be contraindicated in patients who have gastroesophageal reflux.[86] Boehm et al[87] showed decreased fat absorption in patients with BPD, which may contribute to inadequate weight gain. Regardless of the approach taken, excessive osmolality and renal solute load should be avoided. It is important to maintain adequate vitamin and mineral intakes. Once an infant is on standard formula or breast milk, a supplement of a standard infant multivitamin preparation may be recommended until the infant is taking about 1L of formula.

Brunton et al[88] recently performed a prospective double-blind, randomized trial in which preterm infants with BPD received either a standard formula or an enriched formula. The enriched formula had the same caloric concentration as the standard formula (27 kcal/oz) but had higher concentrations of protein, calcium, phosphorus, and zinc. The study was conducted from 37 weeks postmenstrual age to 3 months chronologic age. The results included greater linear growth, greater radial bone mineral content, and greater lean mass in the infants who were fed the enriched formula. This study suggests that, in addition to calories, greater concentrations of protein and selected minerals may be necessary for catch-up growth in patients with BPD.[88]

When infants are receiving high-calorie formulas, careful monitoring is warranted. Increasing the caloric density may increase the potential renal solute load if fluid intake is limited. When the infant is growing and nitrogen is being utilized to form new tissue, the infant usually handles the solute load. However, if growth ceases or if there is increased fluid loss, such as with a febrile illness, renal solute load may become a problem for these infants, and

Table 15–7 Example of a Modulated Formula

	Carbohydrate (g)	*Protein (g)*	*Fat (g)*
30 mL Similac 24*	2.55	0.66	1.29
1 g Polycose* powder	0.94	—	—
1 mL Microlipid†	—	—	0.50
Total	3.49	0.66	1.79
Calories/g	× 4	× 4	× 9
	13.96	2.64	16.11
% Total calories	43	8	49

Total calories = 32.71/31 mL
1.06 cal/mL

*Ross Laboratories, Columbus, Ohio.
†Microlipid, Mead Johnson, Evansville, Indiana.

azotemia may result. Urine specific gravity should be monitored.[86]

The infant may be unable to consume an adequate amount of formula by mouth. It may be necessary to deliver the balance of the formula via tube feeding to achieve adequate intake. Oral gastric or nasogastric feedings are commonly used for short-term supplementary feedings, whereas gastrostomy feedings are used for long-term tube feeding.

Maintenance of Adequate Vitamin and Mineral Status

Calcium and Phosphorus. As previously stated, infants born prematurely are born without the benefit of the calcium and phosphorus accretion of the third trimester of gestation. In addition, the calcium and phosphorus status of premature infants with BPD is further compromised by diuretic therapy, steroid therapy, long-term use of parenteral nutrition, and feeding delays. Therefore, the adequacy of calcium and phosphorus intake requires special attention. Preterm human milk can be fortified with a commercial human milk fortifier. Premature formulas provide higher concentrations of these minerals. Adequate vitamin D (400 IU/day) intake is also important.[85]

Iron. Recommended iron intake is 2–4 mg of elemental iron/kg/day to a maximum of 15 mg/day.[85] Supplementation should begin no later than 2 months of age. Iron can be provided through a supplement or through the use of iron-fortified formulas. Proper iron nutriture is especially important in patients with BPD to maximize tissue oxygenation and minimize oxygen consumption.[60]

Trace Minerals. Particular attention should be given to the following trace minerals, which are components of an antioxidant enzyme system: copper, zinc, selenium, and manganese. No specific recommendations for these minerals have been established for the infant with BPD. Zinc can be decreased with diuretic therapy (refer to Table 15–5), and premature infants often are in negative zinc balance.[89] Monitoring serum zinc levels is important, especially with growth failure. Infants with BPD may be at risk for toxic accumulation of certain trace elements, such as copper and manganese, especially if the patient has cholestasis or other liver disease.[79]

Electrolytes. Electrolyte imbalance may result, especially when the infant is receiving diuretic therapy. The BPD infant can usually tolerate a sodium intake of 1.5–3.5 mEq/kg/day.[60] Potassium and chloride may need to be supplemented, depending on the diuretic therapy.[60,86] Careful monitoring is a must.

Vitamins A and E. Many studies have examined the role of vitamin A (retinol) in animals and premature infants who develop chronic lung disease.[90] Vitamin A is essential in the respiratory tract for maintenance of the integrity and differentiation of epithelial cells. Deficiency of vitamin A results in loss of cilia and other changes in the airways, which resemble the changes seen in BPD. Robbins et al[91] showed that vitamin A adequacy may decrease the incidence of BPD in infants with very low birth weight. With vitamin A supplementation, monitoring of plasma levels is essential.[91]

Adequate vitamin E status is particularly important in premature infants with BPD because vitamin E is a major antioxidant, protecting lipid-containing cell membranes from oxidation. Infants are most likely to receive adequate vitamin E when fed human milk or commercial formulas. Large doses of vitamin E appear to offer no additional protection against BPD. If, for medical reasons, the infant is not fed parenterally or enterally, the premature infant with BPD is at increased risk for developing vitamin E deficiency. Also at risk for vitamin E deficiency is the infant maintained by parenteral nutrition that includes large amounts of polyunsaturated fatty acids but little vitamin E.

Addressing Feeding Difficulties

The patient's ability to suck and swallow must be assessed. Feeding behavior should be assessed for age appropriateness, based on corrected age.

BPD patients are susceptible to developing feeding difficulties because of their usual prematurity and because of the nature of the life-sustaining respiratory therapy that they receive. Intubations and suctioning are noxious stimuli to the oral area and can interfere with normal feeding development. Supplemental oxygen is usually delivered by nasal cannula and does not interfere with oral feedings.

Occupational therapists and speech pathologists identify feeding problems and design treatment plans. Nonnutritive sucking can be instituted during a tube feeding so that the infant can begin to associate feelings of satiety with sucking. In some instances, feedings thickened with rice cereal may be easier for infants to handle. Overlooking problems in the development of feeding skills can result in serious aversions to eating or decreased and inadequate intake.

When critical steps in feeding skill development have been missed, it may be necessary to design a program that breaks eating down into small steps and to orient the child to each step. Instead of feeding according to chronological age, it is more important to feed the child according to his or her stage of feeding development. A behavioral program may be necessary to help the patient overcome fears related to eating or when food refusal is used manipulatively.

Singer et al[92] found that mothers of infants with BPD spent more time prompting the infant to feed, but these infants took in less formula and spent less time sucking than did the two control groups of premature infants without BPD and term infants. In the Johnson study, parents often expressed concern about getting their infant with BPD to take enough food and reported long feeding times.[74] Problematic feeding interactions between the caregiver and the infant may develop. It is important that the health care professional be aware of this potential problem and provide the family with anticipatory guidance in this area.

Family and Caretaker Education

The home care of the patient with BPD can be quite complex and may include supplemental oxygen, multiple medications and therapies, as well as nutrition management. Family and caretaker education by a registered dietitian is a very important component of the nutrition care plan, and adequate time must be devoted to education during the discharge planning process. Written instructions for mixing formulas in common household measures for volumes that will be used in 24 hours or less should be given to families. It is best to have the family member or caretaker demonstrate the proper mixing of formulas, especially formula that is being concentrated or contains additives. Reinforcement of these instructions needs to take place on an ongoing basis in outpatient follow-up.

Referral to Food/Nutrition Resources

Caring for a BPD patient can be very draining for the patient's family from an emotional, physical, and financial standpoint. It is important to assess the patient's and family's needs with regard to food and nutrition resources. Appropriate referrals must be made. Often, this can be done in cooperation with the nurse and/or social worker (see also Chapter 12).

Identification of Areas for Further Research

Effects of early onset of respiratory failure and vigorous ventilator support on nutrient and energy requirements for BPD patients should be assessed at various stages of the disease, particularly regarding energy, protein, vitamins A and E, and minerals such as calcium, phosphorus, and zinc. Assimilation and absorption of nutrients in BPD patients and whether a deficiency of one of these nutrients plays a role in the etiology of the disease also must be determined. General growth studies, including studies that establish appropriate growth for BPD patients at various stages of the disease, would provide guidance for health care practitioners. Nutritional requirements of BPD patients at various stages of the disease and appropriate methods and timing of nutrition intervention in BPD treatment require further study. The long-term sequelae of BPD and its current treatment modalities require ongoing investigation.

ASTHMA

Asthma is the most common chronic disease of childhood, affecting an estimated 4.8 million children.[93,94] Asthma is the most common cause of school absenteeism in the United States, with about 10.1 million lost school days per year.[95] It is reported that 17% of the visits to the Emergency Department by children is because of asthma.[96] The incidence and mortality of asthma are increasing worldwide.[97] There is increased incidence in childhood among males, children of lower socioeconomic groups, African Americans, and those with a family history of asthma or allergies.[97] Death rates from asthma are highest in African Americans aged 15–24 years.[98] Underdiagnosis and inappropriate treatment are major contributors to morbidity and mortality.[97]

Asthma is defined by the National Heart, Lung and Blood Institute (NHLBI) in its publication *Expert Panel Report 2: Guidelines for the Diagnosis and Management of Asthma* as a chronic inflammatory disorder of the airways.[99] Symptoms of this inflammation include recurrent episodes of wheezing, breathlessness, chest tightness, and cough, particularly at night and early in the morning.[99] These asthma episodes are associated with widespread but variable obstruction of airflow, which is often reversible, either spontaneously or with treatment.[99] Inflammation of the airways also causes an associated increase in airway responsiveness to a variety of stimuli.[99] Inflammation causes airway narrowing and increased airway secretions. Airway obstruction is caused by bronchoconstriction, airway edema, chronic mucus plug formation, and airway remodeling.[97]

According to the NHLBI guidelines,[99] asthma management consists of four components:

1. Assessment and monitoring
   a. Initial assessment and diagnosis of asthma
   b. Periodic assessment and monitoring
2. Control of factors affecting severity
3. Pharmacologic therapy

4. Education for a partnership in asthma care

The diagnosis of asthma can be made when the clinician determines that episodic symptoms of airflow obstruction are present, that airflow obstruction is at least partially reversible, and when alternative diagnoses have been excluded.[99] Diagnostic tools available to the clinician include obtaining a thorough history, spirometry, and chest radiograph. Other diagnostic tests available for the management of asthma include: allergy testing, nasal and sinus evaluation, gastroesophageal reflux assessment, and pulse oximetry to evaluate hypoxemia during an acute episode.[97] Differential diagnoses include: aspiration, cystic fibrosis, cardiac or anatomic defects, and lower respiratory tract infections.[97] The NHLBI guidelines include a classification system of asthma severity: mild intermittent, mild persistent, moderate persistent, and severe persistent. These classifications reflect the clinical manifestations of asthma.[99]

According to the NHLBI guidelines, the goals of asthma therapy are to:[99]

1. Prevent chronic symptoms
2. Maintain normal or near normal pulmonary functions
3. Maintain normal activity levels
4. Prevent recurrent exacerbations
5. Provide optimal pharmacotherapy with minimal or no side effects
6. Meet patient's and family's expectations and satisfaction with asthma care

A major goal of asthma treatment is to reduce inflammation. The first step toward this is for the patient to recognize and avoid the triggers of asthma. Triggers may include indoor allergens such as dust mites, mold, and animal dander, and outdoor allergens such as trees, grasses, weeds, and pollens.[97] Environmental tobacco smoke and air pollutants are major precipitants of asthma symptoms in children.[99] Other factors contributing to asthma severity include: rhinitis, sinusitis, gastroesophageal reflux, and viral respiratory infections.[99] In some children, weather or humidity changes, or exercise, especially in cold and dry air, may produce inflammation of the airways.[97] Food allergies may also cause asthma symptoms, although this is rare.[97]

In addition to reducing factors that increase the patient's asthma symptoms, pharmacologic therapy is an important component of asthma management.[99] Pharmacologic therapy is based on asthma severity and the classification of asthma. The goal is to reduce inflammation for persistent asthma, which includes long-term control medications. Long-term control medicines, taken daily, include inhaled corticosteroids, long-acting $beta_2$-agonists, cromolyn sodium, methylxanthine, leukotriene modifiers, and oral corticosteroids. Quick relief medications, inhaled short-acting $beta_2$-agonists, anticholinergics, and short course systemic corticosteroids are used to treat acute symptoms and exacerbations.[97,99]

Patient and family education in asthma care is an integral part of treatment. As the NHLBI guidelines[99] recommend, a partnership with the patient and family must be built by the health care professional. The patient and family need to be involved in problem solving for appropriate solutions for asthma trigger control and medication options. They should be able to recognize asthma symptoms and to treat appropriately and early. The patient and family members should demonstrate the proper use of inhalers and exhibit understanding of the proper use of other medications. Written instructions should be provided. Long-term follow-up is essential to adjust medication as needed and for education reinforcement. Because tobacco smoke is a common irritant and asthma trigger, smoking cessation information and counseling should be made available to family members.[97,99]

Food Allergies and Asthma

According to Sampson,[100] the confirmed incidence of adverse reactions to food is probably

1–2% in young children and 4–6% in infants[100] (see Chapter 8). The role of food allergies in asthma is controversial.[101] In a study by Adler et al,[102] 14.5% of children with asthma were reported by their parents to have food-provoked asthma symptoms. Several studies have been reported in the scientific literature investigating the true incidence of asthma symptoms caused by food allergies using double-blind, placebo-controlled food challenges.[103–105] The results of these investigations thus far include findings that IgE-mediated reactions to food can cause respiratory symptoms, including wheezing, but that it is uncommon, even in children with histories of other adverse reactions to food. Even when respiratory symptoms are exhibited after food ingestion, the changes in pulmonary function are not significant.[101] Further investigation in this area is needed before strong conclusions can be drawn but, based on currently available data, food allergies do not significantly contribute to asthma symptoms.

Effects of Nutrients on Asthma

Many studies have been performed investigating the role of various nutrients in protecting against asthma, as well as their effects on improving asthma symptoms. Nutrients that have been studied include vitamin C, fish oils, selenium, and electrolytes, including sodium and magnesium.[101]

Vitamin C

Antioxidants protect cell membranes from damage caused by free radicals and chemical oxidants. Of the antioxidant vitamins, vitamin C has received the most attention, with most of the studies involving adult subjects. According to the National Health and Examination Survey I, lower dietary vitamin C intakes were associated with lower forced expiratory volume at 1 second (FEV_1). However, the difference in this pulmonary function test between the highest and lowest levels of dietary vitamin C was not great, and the clinical significance of this finding was questioned.[106] Other studies of adult subjects showed that asthma patients had low blood levels of vitamin C and that low vitamin C intake was associated with weaker lung function.[101] In one pediatric study, children ages 8–11 who never ate fresh fruit had 4.3% weaker pulmonary function and had a 25.3% higher incidence of wheezing than did children who ate fruit more than once a day.[107] However, vitamin C intake was not specifically analyzed in this study. Other studies have suggested possible short-term protective effects of vitamin C on airway responsiveness.[101] There is no conclusive evidence linking vitamin C levels to asthma or identifying the role vitamin C may play in the treatment of asthma.[101] This area warrants further investigation before routine supplementation can be recommended for asthma patients.

Fish Oils

The ingestion of fish oils, which contain omega-3 fatty acids, causes arachidonic acid (AA) to be replaced by eicosapentaenoic acid (EPA) and docosahexaenoic acid (DHA) in cell membranes. This replacement leads to a decrease in the production of the inflammatory metabolites of AA. It is thought that this change in metabolites could have potential effects on airway inflammation, which is why fish oil ingestion and its relationship to asthma has been studied.[101]

As with the antioxidants, most of the studies have been with adult asthma patients.[101] A positive relationship between dietary fish intake and level of pulmonary function was found when the data from the NHANES I study was examined.[108] Two studies of Australian school children found an association between oily fish intake (tuna, salmon, herring) with a reduction in prevalence of increased airway responsiveness and a reduction in the incidence of asthma.[109,110] The majority of the studies do not show clinical improvement in asthma patients with the use of fish oils, despite some changes seen in inflammatory cell functions. The data are inconclusive at this point and do not support the use of fish oil in the treatment of asthma.[101]

Electrolytes

The relationship of increased sodium intake and asthma has been investigated by several groups of researchers.[101] These studies have been performed because it has been hypothesized that diets high in salt may increase bronchial reactivity. Although the data have shown small adverse effects of increased sodium intake on bronchial reactivity, no significant effects on the clinical symptoms of asthma have been shown.[101] Also, the data of many of the studies are confounded by other variables, such as other dietary constituents. Currently, there are little scientific data to support the use of low-salt diets in the treatment of asthma.[101]

Magnesium and its role in asthma have been studied in adult asthma patients. Clinical trials have been conducted on the effect of magnesium infusion during acute asthma exacerbations.[101] Small but transient changes in pulmonary functions were observed with the magnesium infusions but were not as effective as $beta_2$-agonist inhalation therapy.[101] One study in England by Britton et al[111] studied the relationship of magnesium intake, assessed from food frequency questionnaires, with pulmonary function (FEV_1), airway reactivity to methacholine, and self-reported wheezing. A magnesium intake of 100 mg/day or higher was associated with a 27.7-mL higher FEV_1, a reduction in relative odds of airway hyperresponsiveness of 0.82, and a reduction in wheeze symptoms.[111] These studies indicate that although intravenous magnesium supplementation may have a minimal role in the treatment of acute asthma, further study is needed of the role of magnesium supplementation in the treatment of chronic asthma.[101]

Selenium

The relationship of selenium to asthma has been studied because of selenium's role as an antioxidant. No current data demonstrate a positive effect of selenium supplementation on pulmonary function tests in asthma patients. Although some studies have indicated a possible correlation between low serum levels of selenium and asthma symptoms, there is not sufficient evidence to advocate the use of selenium supplementation in the treatment of asthma.[101]

The role that specific nutrients may play in asthma has sparked much interest in the scientific community. Much more research in this area is needed before specific recommendations can be made. The interest in this area will probably continue to grow, especially as the practice of alternative and complementary medicine receives more attention. The data gathered to date reinforces the importance to asthma patients of a diet consisting of a variety of food sources.

Effects of Asthma Treatment on Nutritional Status

Most of the effects of asthma treatment on the nutritional status of patients is related to the use of oral steroids and high-dose inhaled steroids. According to the NHLBI guidelines, medium to high-dose inhaled corticosteroids may be needed daily for long-term control in patients whose disease is classified as moderate persistent.[99] For patients whose disease is in the severe persistent classification, long-term control may require high-dose inhaled corticosteroids, as well as a long-acting bronchodilator and oral corticosteroids.[99] The primary goal is to treat the asthma with the smallest doses of medicines that will control the symptoms.

Linear Growth

According to the NHLBI guidelines, poorly controlled asthma may delay growth in children.[99] In general, children with asthma tend to have longer periods of reduced growth rates prior to puberty.[99] However, this delay in puberty does not appear to affect final adult height.[112] This delay in puberty is also not associated with the use of inhaled corticosteroids.[113] The potential for adverse effects on linear growth from inhaled corticosteroids appears to be dose-dependent. [99, 113–115] When inhaled corticosteroids are used as recommended, the majority of studies report no change in expected growth velocity.[114,115] In contrast, a few studies have demonstrated growth delay in children on inhaled corticosteroids.[99] High doses of inhaled corticosteroids have greater potential for growth suppression than do lower doses.[99] However, using high doses of inhaled corticosteroids with children having severe persistent asthma has less potential for decreasing linear growth than does using oral systemic corticosteroids.[99] The use of oral corticosteroids on a prolonged basis does stunt linear growth.[112]

Bone Density

Chronic corticosteroid use does induce osteoporosis.[116] That is why it is important that the smallest possible dose be used to control asthma symptoms. Many studies—again, mainly in adults—have been performed on the effect of inhaled corticosteroids on bone density, with varying results reported. Short-term effects on markers of bone turnover, such as osteocalcin, have been reported, but the long-term risk of osteoporosis is not clear.[117,118] Collagen turnover was found to be reduced in children receiving long-term (> 12 months) inhaled steroid treatment.[119] Martinati et al[120] found no adverse effect on bone mass in prepubertal children with mild moderate asthma when treated with beclomethasone dipropionate, as compared with children treated with cromolyn sodium, a nonsteroidal antiinflammatory drug. Much more research is needed before there is agreement as to the effect of the dose and duration of inhaled corticosteroids on bone density in patients, especially in children with asthma.

Investigators conclude that attention should be given to the maintenance of adequate calcium and vitamin D intake in patients on chronic steroid therapy.[116] Calcium supplementation may be necessary in some patients.[118] Calcium supplementation alone may be insufficient to block the progression of corticosteroid-dependent osteoporosis completely.[121] Other factors that may benefit the patient are weight-bearing exercise and the avoidance of other inhibitors of osteoblast production, such as alcohol excess.[116] In a study of adult asthmatic patients, Gagnon et al[122] did find a significant positive correlation between bone density and calcium intake in asthmatic patients.

Excessive Weight Gain

Common, well-known side effects of oral corticosteroid therapy include appetite stimulation, central distribution of fat, sodium and fluid retention, and steroid-induced glucose intolerance. For the asthma patient whose disease is in the persistent severe classification and who may require chronic oral steroid therapy to control asthma symptoms, anticipatory dietary guidance as to how to combat some of these side effects, such as limiting salt intake or limiting concentrated sweets, will be beneficial.

Luder et al[123] compared a group of inner city children with asthma to a group of their peers. The prevalence of overweight was significantly higher in children with moderate to severe asthma than in their peers. In the asthma group, a higher BMI was associated with significantly more severe asthma symptoms, such as lower pulmonary function measurements, more school absenteeism, and a greater number of prescribed asthma medications.[123]

Nutritional Management

The growth of children with asthma should be monitored on a regular basis (see Chapter 2). Any deviation in growth parameters should be investigated.

Based on the available data, a diet that provides a variety of foods, including fruits, vegetables, and dairy products, should be encouraged. Educational tools, such as the USDA/HHS *Food Guide Pyramid* or the USDA/HHS *Dietary Guidelines for Americans,* can be utilized. Patients and family members should be warned against eliminating whole food groups from the diet indiscriminately. Preadolescent and adolescent patients should receive information about healthy weight control practices. Chronically ill adolescents, including asthma patients, were found to have increased body dissatisfaction and to be at increased risk of engaging in unhealthy weight loss practices.[124]

Combating Steroid Side Effects

For those asthma patients who must take oral corticosteroids on a regular basis, additional factors should be more closely monitored. An adequate calcium intake is essential. These patients should be receiving at least the RDA for calcium and, in some instances, may require calcium supplementation.[32] Adequate vitamin D intake is also important.[116] The patient may need to modify energy intake to maintain weight control. The registered dietitian can assist the patient in identifying healthy ways to accomplish a healthy diet, especially if the patient develops steroid-induced hyperglycemia. Moderate exercise should be encouraged because this will help maintain bone density and will assist with weight control.

Alternative and Complementary Medicine

Many asthma patients and their families have turned to alternative and complementary medicine therapies. Relaxation techniques, such as biofeedback training and yoga, are commonly practiced. Herbs such as ma huang, echinacea, Asian mushrooms, and ginseng have been used by asthma patients. [125] These substances require scientific study before their effects on asthma are known. Asthma patients have also tried acupuncture and chiropractic spinal manipulation in attempts to control this chronic disease.[125]

Identification of Areas for Further Research

The areas that require further research have been indicated throughout this section. Much more scientific study of the role of specific nutrients in asthma must be done before recommendations for supplementation can be made. The effects of chronic steroid therapy and chronic inhaled steroid therapy on growth in children and on bone density requires continued study. It is exciting to realize that nutrition may play a major role in the treatment of this prevalent and chronic disease.

REFERENCES

1. Welsh MJ, Tsui L, Boat TF, Beaudet AL. Cystic fibrosis. In: Scriver CR, et al, eds. *The Metabolic Basis of Inherited Disease*. 6th ed. New York: McGraw-Hill; 1989:3799–3876.
2. Andersen DH. Cystic fibrosis of the pancreas and its relation to celiac disease: A clinical and pathologic study. *Am J Dis Child.* 1938;56:344–399.
3. Cystic Fibrosis Foundation Patient Registry 1996. *Annual Data Report*. Bethesda, MD: Cystic Fibrosis Foundation; August, 1997.
4. Riordan JR, Rommens JM, Kerem B, et al. Identification of the cystic fibrosis gene: Cloning and characterization of complementary DNA. *Science.* 1989;245:1066–1073.
5. Anderson MP, Gregory RJ, Thompson S, et al. Demonstration that CFTR is a chloride channel by alteration of its anion selectivity. *Science*. 1991;253:202–205.
6. Bear CE, Li CH, Kartner N, et al. Purification and functional reconstitution of the cystic fibrosis transmembrane conductance regulator (CFTR). *Cell.* 1992; 68:809–818.
7. Cheng SH, Rich DP, Marshall J, et al. Phosphorylation of the R domain by cAMP-dependent protein kinase regulates the CFTR chloride channel. *Cell.* 1991;66: 1027–1036.
8. Schwiebert EM, Egan ME, Hwang TH, et al. CFTR regulates outwardly rectifying chloride channels through an autocrine mechanism involving ATP. *Cell.* 1995;81:1063–1073.
9. Stutts MJ, Canessa CM, Olsen JC, et al. CFTR as a cAMP-dependent regulator of sodium channels. *Science*. 1995;269:847–850.
10. Welsh MJ, Smith AE. Molecular mechanisms of CFTR chloride channel dysfunction in cystic fibrosis. *Cell.* 1993;73:1251–1254.
11. Cystic Fibrosis Genetic Analysis Consortium. Population variation of common cystic fibrosis mutations. *Hum Mutat.* 1994;4:167–177.
12. Hamosh A, FitzSimmons SC, Macek M, et al. Comparison of the clinical manifestations of cystic fibrosis in black and white patients. *J Pediatr.* 1998;132:255–259.
13. Rosenstein BJ, Cutting GR, Cystic Fibrosis Foundation Consensus Panel. The diagnosis of cystic fibrosis: A consensus statement. *J Pediatr.* 1998;132:589–595.
14. Ramsey BW, Farrell PM, Pencharz P, Consensus Committee. Nutritional assessment and management in cystic fibrosis: A consensus report. *Am J Clin Nutr.* 1992;55:108–116.

15. Cystic Fibrosis Foundation. *Clinical Practice Guidelines for Cystic Fibrosis.* Bethesda, MD: Cystic Fibrosis Foundation; 1997.
16. Fomon SJ. *Nutrition of Normal Infants.* Philadelphia: Mosby; 1993.
17. National Center for Health Statistics. *NCHS Growth Curves for Children 0–18 Years* US Vital and Health Statistics, series 11, no. 165. Washington, DC: Health Resources Administration; 1977.
18. National Center for Health Statistics. *Height and Weight of Youths 12–17 Years.* US Vital and Health Statistics, series 11, no. 124. Washington, DC: Health Services and Mental Health Administration; 1973.
19. Gomez F, Calvan R, Frank S, et al. Mortality in second- and third-degree malnutrition. *J Trop Pediatr.* 1956;2:77–82.
20. Grant A, DeHoog S. *Nutritional Assessment and Support.* 5th ed. Seattle, WA: Anne Grant/Susan DeHoog; 1998.
21. Frisancho AR. New norms of upper limb fat and muscle areas for assessment of nutritional status. *Am J Clin Nutr.* 1981;34:2540–2545.
22. Sproul A, Huang N. Growth patterns in children with cystic fibrosis. *J Pediatr.* 1964;65:664–676.
23. Lai HC, Kosorok MR, Sondel SA, et al. Growth status in children with cystic fibrosis based on the National Cystic Fibrosis Patient Registry data: Evaluation of various criteria used to identify malnutrition. *J Pediatr.* 1998;132:478–485.
24. Corey M, McLaughlin FJ, Williams M, Levison H. A comparison of survival, growth, and pulmonary function in patients with cystic fibrosis in Boston and Toronto. *J Clin Epidemiol.* 1988;41:583–591.
25. Cannella PC, Bowser EK, Guyer LK, Borum PR. Feeding practices and nutrition recommendations for infants with cystic fibrosis. *J Am Diet Assoc.* 1993;93:297–300.
26. Michel S, Mueller D. Practical approaches to nutrition care of patients with cystic fibrosis. *Top Clin Nutr.* 1989;2:10–20.
27. Heimburger DC, Weinsier RL. *Handbook of Clinical Nutrition.* 3rd ed. St. Louis, MO: Mosby; 1997.
28. Hardin DS. The diagnosis and management of cystic fibrosis related diabetes. *Endocrinologist.* 1998;8:265–272.
29. Moran A. Highlights of the February 1998 consensus conference on CFRD. *Pediatr Pulmonol.* October 1998;suppl 17:104–105.
30. Brasfield D, Hicks G, Soong S, Tiller RE. The chest roentgenogram in cystic fibrosis: A new scoring system. *Pediatrics.* 1979;63:24–29.
31. Bell L, Durie P, Forstner GG. What do children with cystic fibrosis eat? *J Pediatr Gastroenterol Nutr.* 1984;3(suppl 1):S137–S146.
32. National Research Council. *Recommended Dietary Allowances.* Washington, DC: National Academy Press; 1989.
33. World Health Organization. Energy and protein requirements. *WHO Tech Report.* Series no. 724. 1985;924:000.
34. Daniels L, Davidson GP, Martin AJ. Comparison of the macronutrient intake of healthy controls and children with cystic fibrosis on low fat or nonrestricted fat diets. *J Pediatr Gastroenterol Nutr.* 1987;6:381–386.
35. Pencharz PB, Durie PR. Nutritional management of cystic fibrosis. *Annu Rev Nutr.* 1993;13:111–136.
36. Roy CC, Darling P, Weber AM. A rational approach to meeting macro- and micronutrient needs in cystic fibrosis. *J Pediatr Gastroenterol Nutr.* 1984;3(suppl 1):S154–S162.
37. Tomezsko JL, Stallings VA, Kawchak DA, et al. Energy expenditure and genotype of children with cystic fibrosis. *Pediatr Res.* 1994;35:451–460.
38. O'Rawe A, McIntosh I, Dodge JA, et al. Increased energy expenditure in cystic fibrosis is associated with specific mutations. *Clin Sci.* 1992;82:71–76.
39. Murphy M, Ireton-Jones CS, Hilman BC, et al. Resting energy expenditures measured by indirect calorimetry are higher in preadolescent children with cystic fibrosis than expenditures calculated from prediction equations. *J Am Diet Assoc.* 1995;95:30–33.
40. Shepherd RW, Vasques-Velasquez L, Prentice A, et al. Increased energy expenditure in young children with cystic fibrosis. *Lancet.* 1988;135:1300–1303.
41. Vaisman N, Pencharz PB, Corey M, et al. Energy expenditure of patients with cystic fibrosis. *J Pediatr.* 1987;111:137–141.
42. Ellis L, Kalnins D, Corey M, et al. Do infants with cystic fibrosis need a protein hydrolysate formula? A prospective, randomized, comparative study. *J Pediatr.* 1998;132:270–276.
43. Kawchak DA, Zhao H, Scanlin TF, et al. Longitudinal, prospective analysis of dietary intake in children with cystic fibrosis. *J Pediatr.* 1996;129:119–129.
44. Jelalian E, Stark LJ, Reynolds L, Seifer R. Nutrition intervention for weight gain in cystic fibrosis: A meta-analysis. *J Pediatr.* 1998;132:486–492.
45. Michel SH, Mueller DH. Impact of lactation on women with cystic fibrosis and their infants: A review of five cases. *J Am Diet Assoc.* 1994;94:159–165.
46. Luder E, Gilbride JA. Teaching self-management skills to cystic fibrosis patients and its effect on their caloric intake. *J Am Diet Assoc.* 1989;89:359–364.
47. Stark LJ, Jelalian E, Mulvihill MM, et al. Eating in preschool children with cystic fibrosis and healthy peers: Behavioral analysis. *Pediatrics.* 1995;95:210–215.

48. Stark LJ, Mulvihill MM, Jelalian E, et al. Descriptive analysis of eating behavior in school-age children with cystic fibrosis and healthy control children. *Pediatrics*. 1997;99:665–671.
49. Stark LJ, Mulvihill MM, Powers SE, et al. Behavioral intervention to improve calorie intake of children with cystic fibrosis: Treatment vs. waitlist control. *J Pediatr Gastroenterol Nutr*. 1996;22:240–253.
50. Erskine JM, Lingard CD, Sontag MK, Accurso FJ. Enteral nutrition for patients with cystic fibrosis: Comparison of a semi-elemental and nonelemental formula. *J Pediatr*. 1998;132:265–269.
51. Farrell PM, Hubbard VS. Nutrition in cystic fibrosis: Vitamins, fatty acids and minerals. In: Lloyd-Still JD, ed. *Textbook of Cystic Fibrosis*. Littleton, MA: John Wright; 1983.
52. Cystic Fibrosis Foundation. Cystic Fibrosis Foundation Consensus Conference. *Use of Pancreatic Enzyme Supplements for Patients with Cystic Fibrosis in the Context of Fibrosing Colonopathy*. March 23–24, 1995.
53. Borowitz DS, Grand RJ, Durie PR, Consensus Committee. Use of pancreatic enzyme supplements for patients with cystic fibrosis in the context of fibrosing colonopathy. *J Pediatr*. 1995;127:681–684.
54. FitzSimmons SC, Burkhart GA, Borowitz D, et al. High-dose pancreatic enzyme supplements and fibrosing colonopathy in children with cystic fibrosis. *N Engl J Med*. 1997;336:1283–1289.
55. Schwarzenberg SJ, Wielinski CL, Shamieh I, et al. Cystic fibrosis-associated colitis and fibrosing colonopathy. *J Pediatr*. 1995;127:565–570.
56. Stern RC, Canda ER, Doershuk CF. Use of nonmedical treatment by cystic fibrosis patients. *J Adolesc Health*. 1992;3:612–615.
57. Northway WH, Rosan RCC, Porter DY. Pulmonary disease following respiratory therapy of hyaline membrane disease. *N Engl J Med*. 1967;276:357–368.
58. Farrell PA, Fiascone JM. Bronchopulmonary dysplasia in the 1990s: A review for the pediatrician. *Curr Probl Pediatr*. 1997;27:129–163.
59. Abman SH, Groothius JR. Pathophysiology and treatment of bronchopulmonary dysplasia. Current issues. *Pediatr Clin*. 1994;41:277–315.
60. Cox JH. Bronchopulmonary dysplasia. In: Groh-Wargo S, Thompson M, Cox J, eds. *Nutritional Care for High-Risk Newborns*. Chicago: Precept Press; 1994:245–261.
61. Tammela OKT, Lanning FP, Koivisto ME. The relationship of fluid restriction during the first month of life to the occurrence and severity of bronchopulmonary dysplasia in low birth weight infants: A 1-year radiological follow-up. *Eur J Pediatr*. 1992;151:367–371.
62. Wilson DC, McClure G, Halliday HL, et al. Nutrition and bronchopulmonary dysplasia. *Arch Dis Child*. 1991;66:37–38.
63. Frank L, Sosenko IR. Undernutrition as a major contributing factor in the pathogenesis of bronchopulmonary dysplasia. *Am Rev Respir Dis*. 1988;138:725–729.
64. Giacoia GP, Venkataraman PS, West-Wilson KI, Faulkner MJ. Follow-up of school-age children with bronchopulmonary dysplasia. *J Pediatr*. 1997;130:400–408.
65. Weinstein MR, Oh W. Oxygen consumption in infants with bronchopulmonary dysplasia. *J Pediatr*. 1981;99:958–960.
66. Kurzner WI, Garg M, Bautista DB, et al. Growth failure in infants with bronchopulmonary dysplasia: nutrition and elevated resting metabolic expenditure. *Pediatr*. 1988;81:379–384.
67. Yunis KA, Oh W. Effects of intravenous glucose loading on oxygen consumption, carbon dioxide production, and resting energy expenditure in infants with bronchopulmonary dysplasia. *J Pediatr*. 1989;115:127–132.
68. Yeh TF, McClenan DA, Ajayi OA, Pildes RS. Metabolic rate and energy balance in infants with bronchopulmonary dysplasia. *J Pediatr*. 1989;114:448–451.
69. Singer L, Martin RJ, Hawkins SW, et al. Oxygen desaturation complicates feeding in infants with bronchopulmonary dysplasia after discharge. *Pediatrics*. 1992;90:380–384.
70. Garg M, Kurzner SI, Bautista DB, Keens TG. Clinically unsuspected hypoxia during sleep and feeding in infants with bronchopulmonary dysplasia. *Pediatrics*. 1988;81:635–642.
71. Babson SG, Benda GI. Growth graphs for the clinical assessment of infants of varying gestational age. *J Pediatr*. 1976;89:814–820.
72. Shankaran S, Szego E, Eizert D, Siegel P. Severe bronchopulmonary dysplasia: Predictors of survival and outcome. *Chest*. 1984;86:607–610.
73. deRegnier RA, Guilbert TW, Mills MM, Georgieff MK. Growth failure and altered body composition are established by one month of age in infants with bronchopulmonary dysplasia. *J Nutr*. 1996;126:168–175.
74. Johnson DB, Cheney C, Monsen ER. Nutrition and feeding in infants with bronchopulmonary dysplasia after initial hospital discharge: Risk factors for growth failure. *J Am Diet Assoc*. 1998;98:649–656.
75. Vrlenich LA, Bozynski ME, Shyr Y, et al. The effect of bronchopulmonary dysplasia on growth at school age. *Pediatrics*. 1995;95:855–859.

76. Moyer-Mileur LJ, Nielson DW, Pfeffer KD, et al. Eliminating sleep-associated hypoxemia improves growth in infants with bronchopulmonary dysplasia. *Pediatrics*. 1996;98:779–783.

77. Groothuis JF, Rosenberg AA. Home oxygen promotes weight gain in infants with bronchopulmonary dysplasia. *Am J Dis Child*. 1987;141:992–995.

78. Oh W. Nutritional management of infants with bronchopulmonary dysplasia. In: Farrell PM, Taussig LM, eds. *Bronchopulmonary Dysplasia and Related Chronic Respiratory Disorders*. Columbus, OH: Ross Laboratories; 1986:96–101.

79. Niermeyer S. Nutritional and metabolic problems in infants with bronchopulmonary dysplasia. In: Bancalari E, Stocker JT, eds. *Bronchopulmonary Dysplasia*. Washington, DC: Hemisphere Publishing Corp; 1988:313–336.

80. Green HL, Hazlett D, Demarec R. Relationship between intralipid-induced hyperlipemia and pulmonary function. *Am J Clin Nutr*. 1976;29:127–135.

81. Friedman Z, Marks KH, Maisels J, et al. Effect of parenteral fat emulsion on the pulmonary and reticuloendothelial systems in the newborn infant. *Pediatrics*. 1978;61:694–698.

82. Perira GR, Foxx WW, Stanely CA, et al. Decreased oxygenation and hyperlipemia during intravenous fat infusions in premature infants. *Pediatrics*. 1980;66:26–30.

83. Stahl GE, Spear MC, Egler JM, et al. The effect of lipid infusion rate on oxygenation in premature infants. *Pediatr Res*. 1984;18:406A.

84. American Academy of Pediatrics, Committee on Nutrition. Use of intravenous fat emulsions in pediatric patients. *Pediatrics*. 1981;68:738–743.

85. American Academy of Pediatrics, Committee on Nutrition. *Pediatric Nutrition Handbook*. Elk Grove Village, IL: American Academy of Pediatrics; 1998.

86. Reimers KJ, Carlson SJ, Lombard KA. Nutritional management of infants with bronchopulmonary dysplasia. *Nutr Clin Prac*. 1992;7:127–132.

87. Boehm G, Bierbach U, Moro G, Minoli I. Limited fat digestion in infants with bronchopulmonary dysplasia. *J Pediatr Gastroenterol Nutr*. 1996;22:161–166.

88. Brunton JA, Saigal S, Atkinson SA. Growth and body composition in infants with bronchopulmonary dysplasia up to 3 months corrected age: A randomized trial of a high-energy nutrient-enriched formula fed after hospital discharge. *J Pediatr*. 1998;133:340–345.

89. Higashi A, Ikeda T, Iribe K, Matsuda I. Zinc balance in premature infants given the minimal dietary zinc requirement. *J Pediatr*. 1988;112:262–266.

90. Zachman RD. Role of vitamin A in lung development. *J Nutr*. 1995;125:1634S–1638S.

91. Robbins ST, Fletcher AB. Early vs. delayed vitamin A supplementation in very-low-birth-weight infants. *J Parenter Enteral Nutr*. 1993;17:220–225.

92. Singer LT, Davillier M, Preuss L, et al. Feeding interactions in infants with very low birth weight and bronchopulmonary dysplasia. *J Dev Behav Pediatr*. 1996;17:69–76.

93. Adams PF, Marano MA. *Current estimates from the National Health Interview Survey, 1994. Vital Health Stat*. 1995;10:94.

94. Centers for Disease Control and Prevention. *Asthma—United States, 1989–1992. MMWR*. 1995;43:952–955.

95. National Heart, Lung, and Blood Institute and World Health Organization. *Global Initiative for Asthma*. NIH Publ no. 95–3659. Bethesda, MD, 1995.

96. Crain EF, Weiss KB, Fagan MJ. Pediatric asthma care in US emergency departments. *Arch Pediatr Adolesc Med*. 1995;149:893–901.

97. Johnston J. Lower respiratory disorders. In: Millonig VL, Baroni MA, eds. *Pediatric Nurse Practitioner Certification Review Guide*. 3rd ed. Potomac, MD: Health Leadership Associates; 1999.

98. Centers for Disease Control and Prevention: Asthma mortality and hospitalization among children and young adults—United States, 1990–1993. *MMWR*. 1996;45:350–353.

99. National Heart, Lung, and Blood Institute. *Highlights of the Expert Panel Report 2: Guidelines for the Diagnosis and Management of Asthma*. NIH Publication no. 97–4051A. Bethesda, MD: 1997.

100. Sampson HA. IgE-mediated food intolerance. *J Allergy Clin Immunol*. 1988;81:495–504.

101. Monteleone CA, Sherman AR. Nutrition and asthma. *Arch Intern Med*. 1997;157:23–34.

102. Adler BR, Assadullahi T, Warner JA, Warner JO. Evaluation of a multiple food specific IgE antibody test compared to parental perception, allergy skin tests and RAST. *Clin Exp Allergy*. 1991;21:683–688.

103. Bock SA. Respiratory reactions induced by food challenges in children with pulmonary disease. *Pediatr Allergy Immunol*. 1992;3:188–194.

104. James JM, Berhisel-Broadbent J, Sampson HA. Respiratory reactions provoked by double-blind food challenges in children. *Am J Respir Crit Care Med*. 1994;149:59–64.

105. Onorato J, Merland N, Terral C, et al. Placebo-controlled double-blind food challenge in asthma. *J Allergy Clin Immunol*. 1986;78:1139–1146.

106. Schwartz J, Weiss ST. Relationship between dietary vitamin C intake and pulmonary function in the first National Health and Nutrition Examination Survey (NHANES I). *Am J Clin Nutr*. 1994;59:110–114.

107. Cook DG, Carey IM, Whincup PH, et al. Effect of fresh fruit consumption on lung function and wheeze in children. *Thorax*. 1997;52:628–633.

108. Schwartz J, Weiss ST. The relationship of dietary fish intake to level of pulmonary function in the first National Health and Nutrition Examination Survey (NHANES I). *Eur Respir J*. 1994;7:1821–1824.

109. Peat JK, Salome CM, Woolcock AJ. Factors associated with bronchial hyperresponsiveness in Australian adults and children. *Eur Respir J*. 1992;5:921–929.

110. Hodge I, Salome CM, Peat JK, et al. Consumption of oily fish and childhood asthma risk. *Med J Austr* 1996;164:137–140.

111. Britton J, Pavord I, Wisniewski A, et al. Dietary magnesium, lung function, wheezing, and airway hyperreactivity in a random adult population. *Lancet*. 1994;344:357–363.

112. Price JF. Asthma, growth and inhaled corticosteroids. *Respir Med*. 1993;87:23–26.

113. Merkus PJFM, van Essen-Zandvliet EEM, Duiverman EJ, et al. Long-term effect of inhaled corticosteroids on growth rate in adolescents with asthma. *Pediatrics*. 1993;91:1121–1126.

114. Agertoft L, Pedersen S. Effects of long-term treatment with an inhaled corticosteroid on growth and pulmonary function in asthmatic children. *Respir Med*. 1994;88:373–381.

115. Allen DB, Bronshky EA, LaForce CF, et al. Growth in asthmatic children treated with fluticasone propionate. *J Pediatr*. 1998;132:472–477.

116. Hosking DJ. Effects of corticosteroids on bone turnover. *Respir Med*. 1993;87:15–21.

117. Barnes NC. Safety of high-dose inhaled corticosteroids. *Respir Med*. 1993;87:27–31.

118. Boner AL, Piacentini GL. Inhaled corticosteroids in children. Is there a "safe" dosage? *Drug Safety*. 1993;9:9–20.

119. Crowley S, Trivedi P, Risteli L, et al. Collagen metabolism and growth in prepubertal children with asthma treated with inhaled steroids. *J Pediatr*. 1998; 32:409–413.

120. Martinati LC, Bertoldo F, Gasperi E, et al. Effect on cortical and trabecular bone mass of different anti-inflammatory treatments in preadolescent children with chronic asthma. *Am J Respir Crit Care Med*. 1996;153:232–236.

121. Picado C, Luengo M. Corticosteroid-induced bone loss. *Drug Safety*. 1996;15:347–359.

122. Gagnon L, Boulet LP, Brown J, Desrosiers T. Influence of inhaled corticosteroids and dietary intake on bone density and metabolism in patients with moderate to severe asthma. *J Am Diet Assoc*. 1997;97:1401–1406.

123. Luder E, Melnik TA, DiMaio M. Association of being overweight with greater asthma symptoms in inner city black and Hispanic children. *J Pediatr*. 1998;132:699–703.

124. Neumark-Sztainer D, Story M, Resnick MD, et al. Body dissatisfaction and unhealthy weight-control practices among adolescents with and without chronic illness: A population-based study. *Arch Pediatr Adolesc Med*. 1995;149:1330–1335.

125. Dinsmoor R. Alternative therapies—Are they effective in treating asthma? *Asthma Magazine*. Sept/Oct, 1998.

RESOURCES

Booklets

Luder E. *Living with Cystic Fibrosis: Family Guide to Nutrition.* McNeil Pharmaceutical, 1993.

Power Packed Packet: Rocket Fueled Ideas for Your High Calorie High Protein Diet. Available from Pediatric Pulmonary Center, University of Alabama at Birmingham, 1600 7th Avenue South, ACC 620, Birmingham, AL 35233.

Managing Nutrition and Malabsorption in CF. Baylor College of Medicine, 1993. To order, contact your Genentech Representative.

Advance. Newsletter of the Asthma and Allergy Foundation of America, 1125 15th St. NW, Suite 502, Washington, DC 20005; (202) 466–7643; (800) 7-ASTHMA; http://www.aafa.org

Cookbooks

A Way of Life: Cystic Fibrosis Nutrition Handbook and Cookbook. 2nd ed. 1997. Available from Pediatric Pulmonary Center, Food and Nutrition Services, University of Wisconsin Hospital and Clinics, 600 Highland Avenue, Room F4/120, Madison, WI 53792–1510.

Fat and Loving It!!! A Book Written for the Individual with Cystic Fibrosis. Gail Farmer and Sherri Willcox, 1990. Available from Gail Farmer, P.O. Box 5127, Belmont, CA 94002.

Web Pages

Gaining and Growing: Assuring Nutritional Care of Very Low Birth Weight Infants in the Community. http://Weber.u.washington.edu/~growing. Donna Johnson, PhD, RD, Pediatric Pulmonary Center, University of Washington.

Pediatric Pulmonary Centers, Maternal and Child Health Bureau, Health Resources and Services Administration, Department of Health and Human Services. http://salud.unm.edu/asthma/ppc.htm

Chapter 16

Gastrointestinal Disorders

Jacqueline Jones Wessel

The gastrointestinal tract is the site of the assimilation of macro- and micronutrients, vitamins, and minerals. The function of the gastrointestinal tract may be disrupted by disease and result in alterations in nutritional requirements. The intent of this chapter is to provide information about the nutritional assessment and management of children with various gastrointestinal disorders or conditions.

The gastrointestinal tract may be thought of as a tube that processes and absorbs nutrients. Many nutrients are absorbed throughout the intestinal tract, whereas others are absorbed only from specific sites. Absorption of the latter class of nutrients is particularly vulnerable to disease or surgical resection. In Figure 16–1 the principal sites of absorption of macro- and micronutrients, vitamins, and minerals are presented.

Most symptoms of gastrointestinal disease can arise from disorders located in a specific region of the bowel, the entire bowel, or distant sites; eg, vomiting can occur due to pyloric stenosis, gastroenteritis, or brain tumor. In Figure 16–2, conditions that involve portions of the gastrointestinal tract rather than the entire tract are presented. Table 16–1 groups common symptoms according to their most common location of origin. The differential diagnosis of these symptoms and treatment of the etiology of symptoms are presented.

DIAGNOSTIC TESTS

A myriad of tests is available to evaluate gastrointestinal function. The tests most commonly performed are presented in Table 16–2. For each test, the procedure and potential diagnoses are listed.

ACUTE DIARRHEA

Acute diarrhea, namely diarrhea of less than 7 days' duration, is among the most common reasons for seeking the assistance of a pediatrician. Under most circumstances, a normal diet should be continued throughout the illness. When dehydration is imminent, the use of maintenance glucose-electrolyte solutions may prevent progression of the illness. When patients become dehydrated, oral rehydration solutions or intravenous fluids may be required. The composition of commonly used oral maintenance and rehydration solutions is presented in Table 16–3. The American Academy of Pediatrics recommends that children with mild to moderate dehydration be rehydrated within 4–6 hours, then offered age-appropriate foods, with resumption of breastfeeding for breastfed infants.[1] For bottle-fed infants, there is controversy regarding whether a lactose-free formula is necessary.[1–6] The most practical solution would seem to be if a child's diarrhea worsens on return to a lactose-containing formula, lactose-free feedings should be used until the illness has resolved.[7]

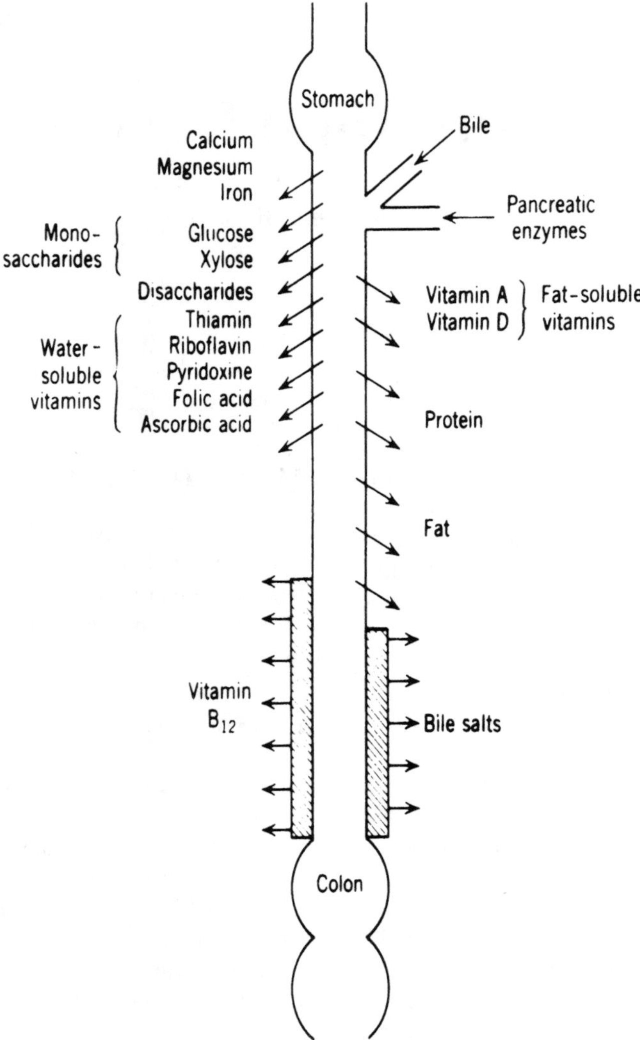

Figure 16–1 Principal sites of absorption of nutrients. *Source:* Reprinted from *Handbook of Physiology*, Vol 3, ed 6 by CC Booth with permission of the American Physiological Society, © 1968.

Full-strength formula should be used because dilution of formula has not improved outcome.[8] A soy protein, lactose-free formula with added soy polysaccharide fiber has been used in the treatment of acute diarrhea. The fiber-containing formula decreased the duration of diarrheal symptoms significantly in two studies on infants and toddlers.[9, 10]

CHRONIC DIARRHEA OF INFANCY

Chronic diarrhea of infancy, also called *protracted diarrhea of infancy,* is a reversible clinical condition.[11] It is considered to be a nutritional disorder.[12,13] As with all diarrheal illnesses in infants, chronic diarrhea is dangerous if not treated promptly and appropriately,

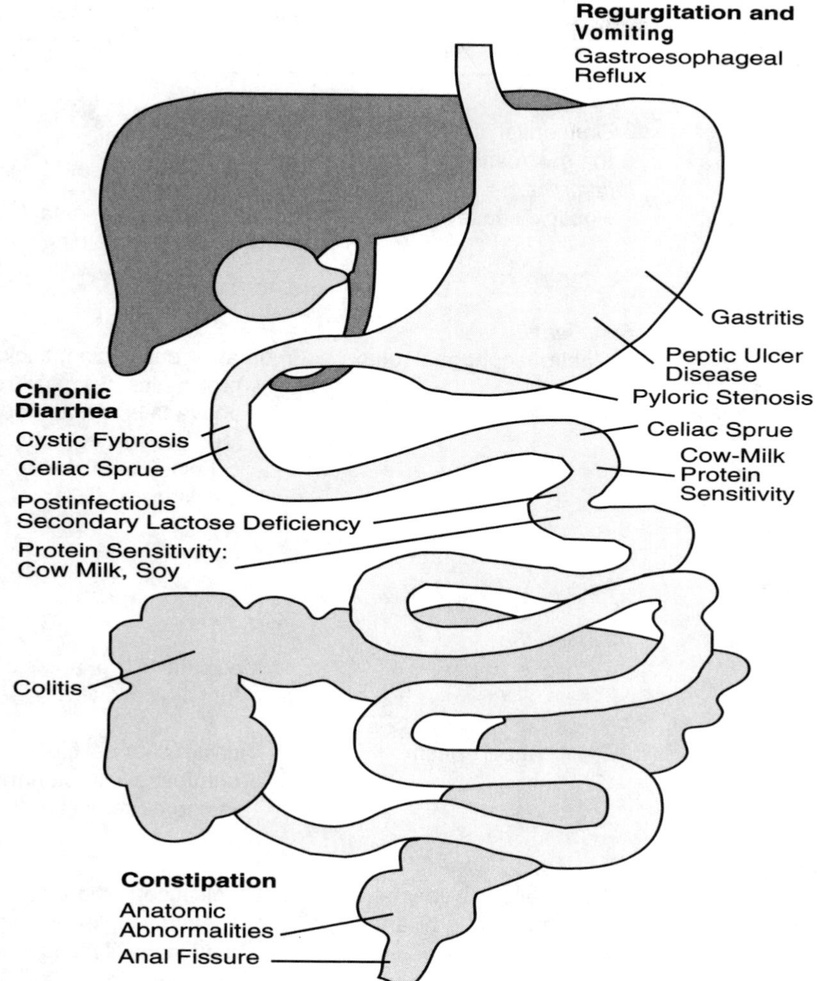

Figure 16–2 The site of pathology within the gastrointestinal tract varies with the disease process. *Source:* Used with permission of Ross Products Division, Abbott Laboratories, Inc., Columbus, OH 43216. From *Problems Relating to Feedings in First Two Years,* © 1977, Ross Products Division, Abbott Laboratories, Inc.

because it can result in dehydration and severe malnutrition.[14] Chronic diarrhea is mostly commonly seen in the first 6 months of life and occurs typically after an acute bout of diarrhea. The pathogenesis is largely unknown and is most likely multifactorial. Chronic diarrhea results in a malnourished infant with characteristic large-volume, acidic, often gassy diarrhea.[11]

In an effort to reduce stooling, diet is usually restricted, and malnutrition results.[14] As discussed earlier, the recommendations for diet therapy for diarrhea are to resume normal diet after 4–6 hours of rehydration.[1] The typical treatment, however, is bowel rest, then clear liquids, followed by a transitional diet, such as the BRAT diet (bananas, rice, apple juice,

Table 16–1 Common Pediatric Gastrointestinal Disorders

Presenting Symptom	*Differential Diagnosis*	*Treatment*
Stomach and Esophagus Vomiting/ regurgitation	*Structural:* Congenital anomaly of the gastrointestinal tract	Surgery
	Inflammatory: Peptic disease	Medications, eg, antacids; avoid caffeine-containing foods, alcohol, smoking
	Functional: Gastroesophageal reflux	Infants: positioning, thickened feeds, prokinetics. Surgical treatment if above fails, eg, fundoplication. Medications, eg, antacids; avoid caffeine-containing foods, alcohol, smoking
Dysphagia (choking after eating), odynophagia (pain with swallowing)	*Structural:* Congenital anomalies	Surgery
	Inflammatory: Peptic strictures	Medications, eg, antacids; dilatation, fundoplication
	Functional: Esophageal spasms	Calcium channel blockers and nitrates; avoid extreme temperatures in foods
Pancreas and Liver Jaundice	*Structural:* Extrahepatic biliary tract obstruction, eg, biliary atresia	Surgical correction; fat-soluble vitamin supplementation (fat source: MCT); choleretic agents, eg, phenobarbital, cholestyramine, ursodeoxycholate
Failure to tolerate feeds, persistent bilious vomiting, and distended upper abdomen	Annular pancreas	Surgery
Recurrent abdominal pain, jaundice	Gallstones	Surgery, lithotripsy, dissolution therapy
	Choledochal cyst	Surgery

Source: Reprinted from L.J. Boyne and L.A. Heitlinger, Gastrointestinal Disorders, in *Handbook of Pediatric Nutrition,* P.M. Queen and C.E. Lang, eds., © 1993, Aspen Publishers, Inc.

Table 16–1 continued

Presenting Symptom	*Differential Diagnosis*	*Treatment*
	Inflammatory:	
Anorexia, nausea, vomiting, jaundice	Hepatitis	Diet as tolerated; steroids for autoimmune hepatitis
Abdominal pain	Pancreatitis	NPO; nasogastric suctioning; TPN if prolonged course. Medications: pain control (eg, meperidine), H_2 antagonists (ie, cimetadine), pancreatic enzyme replacement. When improved, high-CHO, low-fat diet. Elemental diet may be beneficial.
	Functional:	
	Hereditary metabolic disorders	See Chapter 13
Meconium ileus, failure to thrive, chronic diarrhea	Pancreatic insufficiency, eg, cystic fibrosis, Shwachman/ Diamond syndrome	Enzyme replacement therapy; fat-soluble vitamin supplementation; high-calorie, high-fat diet
Small bowel and colon		
	Structural:	
Failure to thrive, diarrhea	Short bowel syndrome	TPN progressing to MCT-predominate hydrolysate formula; vitamin and mineral supplements
Abdominal distention, steatorrhea	Lymphangiectasia, protein-losing enteropathy	Surgical excision, if possible. Fat-soluble vitamin supplementation. High-calorie, high-protein, low-LCT diet; high-MCT diet or TPN may be necessary.
Anemia, gastrointestinal bleeding	Congenital malformations, eg, Meckel's diverticulum, duplication cysts	Surgery
	Inflammatory:	
Diarrhea, vomiting	Infectious enteropathies	Oral rehydration solutions, followed by lactose and/or sucrose restrictions*
Failure to thrive, abdominal distention, steatorrhea	Gluten-sensitive enteropathy (celiac disease)	Gluten-free diet
Failure to thrive, vomiting, diarrhea	Dietary protein intolerance	Hydrolysate formula, elimination diet
Postprandial abdominal pain	Inflammatory bowel disease, small bowel (Crohn's) disease	High-calorie diet; B_{12} supplementation if ileum affected

continues

Table 16–1 continued

Presenting Symptom	*Differential Diagnosis*	*Treatment*
Rectal bleeding, diarrhea, tenesmus	Ulcerative colitis or Crohn's disease of the colon	High-calorie diet; folate supplementation; low-residue diet,[†] if strictures or active colitis; other foods as tolerated
	Functional:	
Fermentive diarrhea after introduction of sucrose-containing foods	Congenital enzyme deficiency, eg, sucrase/isomaltase deficiency	Dietary restrictions of sucrose-containing foods
Severe, watery diarrhea from first day of life	Lactase deficiency	Dietary restrictions with calcium supplement or enzyme replacement, ie, Lactaid, Lactrase
Chronic diarrhea, normal growth pattern	Irritable bowel syndrome (chronic nonspecific diarrhea, toddler's diarrhea, or spastic colon)[‡]	Normal diet for age, increased fiber intake, decreased intake of sorbitol-containing beverages (apple and pear juice)
	Structural:	
Constipation	Hirschsprung's disease; post-NEC strictures	Surgery
	Functional:	
	Constipation	Complete bowel clean out using saltwater enemas, mineral oil; high-fiber diet, bowel habit training. In infants, increase CHO content of diet using sucrose, dextrimaltose

LCT, long-chain triglycerides; MCT, medium-chain triglycerides; NEC, necrotizing enterocolitis; TPN, total parenteral nutrition.

* The use of oral rehydration solutions should be closely monitored. Oral rehydration solutions should be used for 6–8 hours, then infant refeeding should begin to prevent further weight loss. To refeed, oral rehydration solutions may be alternated with a full-strength lactose-free formula for the first few feedings, or a concentrated formula may be reconstituted with the rehydration solution. Studies have shown that early refeeding does not exacerbate the diarrhea, and the child recovers more quickly. Frequently, the cow milk–based formula the child may have been consuming prior to the enteropathy may be used instead of a lactose-free formula. If a lactose-free formula is preferred, the previous formula may be reintroduced after a period of one or more weeks.

† The use of milk or a low-residue diet should be dictated by the individual tolerance of the patient.

‡ This disorder often follows a bout of infectious enteropathy or antibiotic therapy and is exacerbated by increased fluid intake or strict elimination diets. A good rule of thumb is to "feed the child, not the diarrhea."

Table 16–2 Common Diagnostic Tests for Pediatric Gastrointestinal Disorders

Test	*Procedure*	*Diagnosis*
Barium swallow	Swallow barium sulfate; upper gastrointestinal tract and small bowel visualized by fluoroscopy. NPO 4 hours.	Hiatal hernia, stricture, dysmotility disorders, varices
Esophageal pH monitoring	8 French tube with pH sensor on end, inserted for 24 hours. Infants fed 1/2 formula, 1/2 apple juice every 4 hours. Older child fed applesauce, and apple juice added to diet.	Gastroesophageal reflux
Esophago-gastro-duodenoscopy (EGD)	Fiberoptic tube into upper gastrointestinal tract; lining visualized and biopsies taken. NPO.	Esophagitis, gastritis, duodenitis, peptic ulcer disease, caustic substance ingestions
Upper GI with small bowel follow-through	Swallow barium sulfate; look for strictures and mucosal lesions by fluoroscopy. NPO.	Inflammatory and structural lesions
Breath hydrogen	Oral sugar load of 1 g/kg to a maximum of 25 g. End expiratory breath collection. NPO.	Lactose or other sugar intolerance. Peak after 90 minutes, rise of >20 ppm is positive.
D-xylose	D-xylose administered in AM after fast after midnight. Dose: 0.35 g/kg. Blood drawn 1 hour after administration.	Malabsorption syndrome. Normal if > 20 mg/dL.
Quantitative fecal fat	Diet with > 30% total calories as fat for 2 days prior to stool collection. Three-day stool collection after charcoal marker noted in stool. (Do not use diaper creams, eg, A&D ointment. Reverse disposable diaper for easier collection.)	Pancreatic insufficiency, eg, cystic fibrosis; mucosal atrophy, eg, celiac disease
Barium enema	Barium sulfate by enema. Lumen and mucosa of colon visualized by fluoroscopy.	Colitis, polyps, Hirschsprung's disease
Colonoscopy	Insertion of flexible fiberoptic tube via anus into large bowel. Visual examination of colonic lining, biopsies obtained (alternative to barium enema). NPO.	Colitis, polyps
Liver and pancreas tests		
Bilirubin	Blood (serum) test to determine excretory function of liver	Hepatitis, biliary tract disease
Biliary tract nuclear scan	Intravenous injection of a bile salt analogue; images obtained over liver and bowel for 24 hours	Obstructive lesions of biliary tree (eg, impacted gall stones, biliary atresia); poor uptake is indicative of hepatitis

Source: Reprinted from L.J. Boyne and L.A. Heitlinger, Gastrointestinal Disorders, in *Handbook of Pediatric Nutrition,* P.M. Queen and C.E. Lang, eds., © 1993, Aspen Publishers, Inc.

continues

Table 16–2 continued

Test	*Procedure*	*Diagnosis*
Plasma ammonia level	Blood (plasma) test to determine *detoxification* capabilities of liver	Hepatic encephalopathy, hepatic failure, Reye's syndrome
Prothrombin time	Blood (whole blood) test to determine *synthetic* function of liver; vitamin-K-dependent, clotting factors	If prothrombin time is prolonged and patient is not on antibiotics, hepatic protein synthesis diminishes.
Ultrasonography	Study to determine gross structure of liver, evaluate liver and biliary systems	Gallstones, pancreatic pseudocysts, biliary tract anomalies, biliary tract obstructions, hepatic tumors
Aminotransferase levels	Blood (serum) test to determine inflammation of liver due to virus, toxin	Infectious, toxic, or autoimmune hepatitis
Serum amylase and lipase levels	Blood (serum) test to determine pancreatic inflammation or obstruction	Acute or chronic pancreatitis. Amylase is elevated in mumps, pregnancy and lactation, pelvic inflammatory disease, and small bowel disease.
Liver-spleen nuclear scan	Intravenous injection of a marker of blood flow. Poor uptake by liver and uptake by spleen, lung, and bone marrow indicative of portal hypertension	Obstruction of extrahepatic blood vessels (eg, portal vein thrombosis), cirrhosis, hepatic failure
Computed tomography scan of abdomen	Multiple radiographs of abdomen with or without intraluminal and/or intravenous contrast. Computer reconstructs multiple images to generate "slices" through the abdomen. NPO.	Demonstration of organ size, consistency, blood flow, and function (kidney); identification of tumors and areas of inflammation (eg, abscess)

Table 16–3 Composition of Oral Electrolyte-Glucose Solutions (Concentration When Reconstituted)

Solution	*Na+ (mEq/l)*	*K+ (mEq/l)*	*Cl− (mEq/l)*	*Carbohydrate (g/l)*	*Osmolality (mOsM/l)*
Rehydration					
WHO-ORS*	90	20	80	20[1]	310
Rehydralyte†	75	20	65	25[1]	310
Maintenance					
Infalyte‡	50	25	45	0[1]	200
Ricelyte§	50	25	45	20[2]	290
Pedialyte†	45	20	35	25[1]	270
Resol‖	50	20	50	20[1]	269
Other clear liquids					
Cola¶	2	0.1		50–150[3]	550
Gingerale¶	3	1		50–150[3]	540
Apple juice¶	3	28		100–150[4]	700
Chicken broth	250	8		0	450
Tea	0	0		0	5

* Continued use of this product without the addition of free water could lead to hypernatremia.
† Ross Laboratories, Columbus, OH.
‡ Pennwalt, Rochester, NY.
§ Mead Johnson, Evansville, IN.
‖ Wyeth-Ayerst Laboratories, Philadelphia, PA.
¶ These products also contain fructose.
1 Containing glucose
2 Containing rice-syrup-solids
3 High fructose syrup
4 Sucrose

Source: Reproduced with permission from *AAP News* vol. 5, p. 5, 1989.

applesauce, and toast).[15] Restrictive diets, such as the BRAT diet, are nutritionally incomplete. Severe malnutrition can result if the restrictions are followed for an extended period of time.[14] Thus, transitional diets should be used only until the diet can be further advanced to a more appropriate nutrition regimen.

In chronic diarrhea, the enterocyte is damaged, and the absorptive ability of the intestine is compromised. There is a downward spiral as the infant or child becomes weak and compromised from malnutrition. Voluntary oral intake decreases, and the infant becomes more dehydrated and more malnourished, and the enterocyte cannot heal. In the acute phase, small intestinal mucosal biopsy reveals villous atrophy.[16] Mucosal disaccharidase activity is significantly decreased, with lactase most severely affected, then sucrase, and glucoamylase the least affected.[17] The intestinal absorptive capacity is decreased by approximately tenfold,[11] and there is a linear relationship with the ability to absorb glucose.[16]

The treatment for chronic diarrhea of infancy is providing nutrition.[11] The first step is appropriate fluid resuscitation. Next, cautious refeeding, through enteral feedings or enteral and parenteral nutrition, is started slowly, due to the possibility of metabolic alterations from refeeding syndrome.[18] Carbohydrate intake should be increased gradually; however, adequate normal levels of protein, lipid, and vitamins can be given.[19]

For the first week of treating chronic diarrhea, daily serum potassium, phosphorus, glucose, and magnesium levels should be monitored to determine whether the child has refeeding syndrome.[20] Supplementation of potassium and phosphorus may be needed. When a malnourished patient is rapidly refed by either the enteral or parenteral route, metabolic and clinical problems may occur as the result of the reversal of the adaptive mechanism to starvation.[21] Fluid and electrolyte shifts result; as the body becomes anabolic, minerals shift from extracellular to intracellular, and serum levels decrease. Hypophosphatemia, hypokalemia, and hypomagnesemia may develop if energy intake is advanced too rapidly. As a result, respiratory failure and circulatory collapse may occur.[22] Mezoff et al[23] looked at the incidence of hypophosphatemia in children during nutritional recovery and found that abnormal anthropometric measurements, arm circumference, and arm muscle circumference < fifth percentile may be predictive of patients at risk for refeeding syndrome.

Parenteral nutrition (PN) may be indicated if a child is very malnourished. Parenteral nutrition may be combined with enteral nutrition administered in the form of nasogastric feedings. In infants and young children with intestinal problems, absorption of many nutrients may be improved by using continuous enteral feedings. A crossover study in infants with protracted diarrhea showed greater absorption of zinc, calcium, copper, fat, and nitrogen during continuous feedings than with bolus feedings.[24] Small bolus oral feedings may be retained for oral motor stimulation.

The calories needed for catch-up growth in infants may be in the range of 140–200 kcal/kg/day.[25] Supplemental zinc may be needed, due to diarrheal losses. One recommendation is 8,000 mcg/L if administered through parenteral nutrition or 2–3 times the RDA if given orally.[26, 27] Supplemental vitamin A may also be needed in the nutritional therapy for chronic diarrhea.[28, 29] Cereal and other infant foods should be continued as tolerated; however, juices should be avoided, due to high osmolality (such as found in the BRAT diet). A lactose-free formula may be tolerated in some infants. Studies in the treatment of acute diarrhea show shorter duration of acute bouts of diarrhea with a lactose-free formula, compared with a lactose-containing formula.[30] Some infants may need a semi-elemental protein hydrolysate formula such as Alimentum (Ross Products) or Pregestimil (Mead Johnson). Also, because short peptides are absorbed better than an equimolar amount of amino acids,[31, 32] a semi-elemental formula may be superior to an elemental amino-acid-based formula such as Neocate (Scientific Hospital Supply).

As the infant improves with less diarrhea, PN or intravenous (IV) hydration should be decreased, with a concurrent increase in enteral feedings. Larger bolus oral feedings are then added gradually, as tolerated. Slow progression is often necessary. If this period is prolonged, the transition from continuous feeding to oral bolus feedings can often be accomplished in the home setting.

As the enterocytes heal, calorie needs gradually decrease as absorption improves. If the infant was breastfed, and the mother is willing to express milk for a continuous feeding regimen, breast milk can be used. As there is calorie loss from continuously infused breast milk through protein and lipid loss,[33,34] adjustments should be made in the calorie determinations. Alterations in the continuous infusion feeding method can be made to maximize nutrient delivery by using the shortest amount of tubing available and slanting the feeding syringe.[35] Another option is to use a formula in combination with breast milk in the continuous infusion for greater lipid delivery,[36] saving the expressed breast milk for oral feedings.

No studies to date have been found using a formula with fiber for the treatment of chronic diarrhea, as has been used in acute diarrhea in infants.[9, 10] Fiber has been used as part of a food-based regimen in several studies in underdeveloped countries. The World Health Organization has developed an algorithm for the treatment of persistent diarrhea, using locally available foods and simple clinical guidelines for use in underdeveloped countries.[37] Kolacek et al[38] compared a modular diet using food with a semi-elemental infant formula in the treatment of chronic diarrhea. The modular diet was found to decrease the duration of diarrhea and to decrease the time to nutritional recovery.[38] In another study, infant formula fermented with *Lactobacillus bulgaris* and *Streptococcus thermophilus* was compared with standard infant formula in the treatment of persistent diarrhea. Clinical treatment failure occurred in 45% of the formula group, as compared with 15% of the "yogurt" formula group.[39] These creative studies, based on the culture or available foods, illustrate that our traditional formula-based plan is not the only method of treatment.

Recent reports indicate that the incidence of chronic diarrhea has declined in the United States over the past two decades, presumable due to better treatment of acute diarrheal episodes.[11] Severe malnutrition is still seen as a result of management of diarrhea.[14] Education of parents and medical personnel as to the nutritional ramifications of the treatment of diarrhea may continue to improve patient outcomes.

CELIAC DISEASE

Celiac disease is also called *gluten-induced enteropathy* because it is an intolerance to gliadin, a constituent of the protein gluten. This disease is a form of malabsorption syndrome, primarily affecting the proximal portion of the small intestine, with destruction of the villi. The principal abnormality is the failure of the jejunal mucosa to adequately absorb digested substances, particularly nutrients. As a consequence, there is malabsorption of fat, carbohydrate, protein, vitamins, and minerals, resulting in general malnutrition. The classic symptoms of celiac disease are loss of weight, nausea and vomiting, abdominal pain, weakness, diarrhea consisting of pale, bulky, frothy, foul-smelling stools. Nutritional deficiency signs may develop from malabsorption such as anemia, cheilosis, glossitis, peripheral edema, tetany, rickets, and hypoprothrombinemia with a tendency to bleed. The condition is completely relieved if gluten, derived chiefly from wheat, barley, oats, and rye, is excluded from the diet.

Traditionally, the diagnosis of celiac disease was made in infants and toddlers several months after the introduction of solid foods to the diet. The classic symptoms of chronic diarrhea, abdominal distension, and poor growth would cause parents to seek medical attention, and an intestinal biopsy for definitive diagnosis would be conducted. Recently available serologic tests for antigliadin and antiendomysium antibodies are now being used as a screening tool, and school-aged children and adults are now being diagnosed after years of silent disease.[40] Celiac disease should be considered in children with unexplained short stature, poor weight gain, diarrhea, or abdominal pain. Nontraditional expressions of celiac disease involve the musculoskeletal, central nervous, reproductive, and hematologic systems, as well as skin and mucous membranes. Associated conditions include insulin-dependent diabetes mellitus (IDDM), thyroid disease, Sjogren's disease, rheumatoid arthritis, collagen vascular disease, and liver disease.[40] Celiac disease and IDDM have a common autoimmune pathogenesis and share the same genetic locus in chromosome 6.[40, 41]

The infant foods to use and avoid are presented in Table 16–4. There is recent debate concerning whether or not to exclude oats from the diet.[42] Strict adherence to a gluten-free diet is essential for the treatment of this disease. Growth may be adversely affected, and, thus, growth should be periodically assessed to ensure optimal results. In adults, osteoporosis is a common finding in patients with celiac disease. Recently, a study examined bone mineral density in children and adolescents at diagnosis. The celiac-diagnosed patients exhibited significantly lower density than did control children. However, after 1 year of a gluten-free diet, their studies had normalized.[43] At diagnosis, it is not uncommon for anthropometric, biochemical, and bone density data to be significantly abnormal. Another study has shown normalization of body mass composition after 1 year of a gluten-free diet.[44] These studies emphasize the need for early diagnosis and prompt treatment to restore optimal nutritional status.

INFLAMMATORY BOWEL DISEASE

The two major diseases of inflammatory bowel disease (IBD) are Crohn's disease (CD) and ulcerative colitis (UC). Crohn's disease may occur in any portion of the gastrointestinal tract. Ulcerative colitis is, by definition, confined to the colon, with minimal involvement of the terminal ileum.[45] Other diseases that do not fit into either category are termed *indeterminate colitis.*[46] The two diseases have many features in common: diarrhea, gastrointestinal blood and protein loss, abdominal pain, weight loss, anemia, and growth failure.[45]

Approximately 30% of children with IBD will have growth failure; children with Crohn's disease are three times as likely to have permanent

Table 16–4 Gluten-Free Diet for Infants with Celiac Disease

	Use	*Avoid*
Formula	Breast milk or iron-fortified infant formula	None
Dry cereal	Beech-Nut, Mead Johnson: Rice Cereal; Gerber: Rice Cereal with Bananas; Heinz: Instant Rice Cereal	All others
Jarred cereal	Beech-Nut, Gerber: Strained Rice with Applesauce and Bananas; Gerber: Junior Rice with Mixed Fruit; Heinz: Instant Rice Cereal with Bananas and Apple Juice, Rice Cereal with Pears and Apple Juice; Mead Johnson: Bananas 'n Rice	All others
Fruits, juices	All plain	None
Vegetables	All except those to avoid, plus Mead Johnson: Peas 'n Rice, Carrots 'n Rice	Gerber: Mixed Vegetables, Strained Creamed Spinach, Junior Creamed Green Beans
Meats	All plain meats, egg yolks	None
	Beech-Nut: Chicken Rice Dinner, Turkey Rice Dinner, Vegetable Chicken Dinner, Cottage Cheese with Pineapple	All other dinners and high-meat dinners
Teething, finger foods	Gluten-free rice wafers, rice cakes; Gerber: Turkey, Chicken, or Meat Sticks	

Note: Gluten or possible gluten-containing foods are those that have the following ingredients listed on a food label: wheat, rye, oats, barley; flour or cereal products; malt, malt flavor; hydrolyzed vegetable or plant protein; modified food starch; or gluten-containing flavorings, vegetable gums, emulsifiers, or stabilizers. Gluten may be present in foods, either as a basic ingredient or added during preparation/processing by the manufacturer. Reading food labels is very important in *strict* adherence to a gluten-free diet.

Source: Reprinted with permission from Merritt RJ and Hack S, Infant feeding and enteral nutrition, in *Nutrition in Clinical Practice* (1988;3:47–64), Copyright © 1988, American Society for Parenteral and Enteral Nutrition.

growth stunting than are patients with UC.[45] Children with IBD have growth failure, due to inadequate intake, malabsorption, excessive nutrient losses, and increased nutrient needs.[46] Inadequate intake may be due to abdominal discomfort, effort to decrease diarrhea, and lack of interest in a restricted diet. Altered taste perceptions can occur in children with zinc deficiency.[27] Medications such as metronidazole may also affect intake by changing taste perceptions. Children with Crohn's disease have dietary intakes of energy significantly less than nonaffected peers.[47]

Nutrient deficits have been noted in 30–40% of adolescents and children with IBD.[47] Malabsorption can occur as a result of inflammation of the mucosa. Protein-losing enteropathy may result. Malabsorption may also occur as a result of bacterial overgrowth, due to altered motility or strictures. Bile salt malabsorption can alter lipid absorption. Lactose intolerance is seen in approximately one-sixth of children with CD and UC.[27] Patients who have had bowel resections may also malabsorb fat and other nutrients, as a result of their shortened bowel length. Patients with resections or disease in the terminal ileum may not be able to absorb sufficient vitamin B_{12} and will need evaluation by Schilling test and intramuscular supplementation, 1 mg every 3 months, if results are abnormal. Other single nutrient deficiencies seen in IBD are those of folic acid and iron. Multiple deficiencies are more common and include those of protein, calcium, magnesium, zinc, vitamin D, and vitamin B_{12}.[49] Folic acid deficiency has been reported in 38% of patients with CD[50, 51] and 58% of those with UC.[52] Zinc deficiency may be a result of malabsorption and losses from diarrhea and/or fistula drainage; clinical signs of deficiency are sometimes seen.[49] Magnesium deficiency can also occur due to increased losses and may complicate active disease.[53–55]

Medications used in the treatment of IBD may affect nutrition. For example, sulfasalazine (Azulfidine) interferes with folate absorption.[27] Corticosteroid therapy interferes with mineral absorption of calcium, phosphate, and zinc; doses greater than 12 mg/m^2 of body surface area can induce catabolism and affect linear growth.[56]

Malnutrition appears to be the primary cause of growth failure in IBD.[45] Several nutritional rehabilitation studies have demonstrated the beneficial effect of supplemental nutrition therapy on growth. After supplementation, growth velocity equaled or exceeded normal controls. Some studies document the use of parenteral nutrition;[57–60] others have demonstrated successful results with enteral supplementation.[61–67] Although both methods increased the rate of growth, parenteral nutrition is associated with greater complications and cost. Thus, the gastrointestinal tract should be used whenever possible for nutritional rehabilitation in IBD.

Nutritional support appears to have both a primary and an adjunctive role in the treatment of IBD.[48] Primary nutrition therapy appears to be more effective in the treatment of Crohn's disease than in ulcerative colitis.[47,50] Uncontrolled studies in children have used elemental formulas (with either amino acids or peptides) administered via nasogastric tube with immunosuppressive drugs. Hypoallergenic foods were gradually introduced. Symptoms resolved, growth rates improved, and corticosteroid doses were considerably reduced. A 70% remission rate continued for 12–18 months after nutrition therapy was initiated.[45, 68–70] Controlled studies were conducted in children with Crohn's disease, comparing enteral formula against immunosuppressive drugs and sulfasalazine in the treatment of active disease.[71–73] The enteral formulas contained either amino acids, protein hydrolysate, or intact protein (casein) and were administered orally or by nasogastric tube for 1–2 months. Height velocity was superior in the enteral nutrition group, despite more sustained energy intake in the medications group.[45] Despite these positive studies in children and several others in adults, comparing altered diet with the use of medications,[74–76] the European Cooperative Crohn's Disease study found opposite results using a semi-elemental formula.[77] In another study with adult CD patients, elemental formula was more effective in inducing remissions than was semi-elemental formula.[78]

Marine oils, which are high in omega 3 long-chain fatty acids, appear to modulate the immune response of the large bowel and may be advantageous in patients with UC. In adult studies, a reduction in disease activity and a reduction in corticosteroids were noted in UC patients receiving omega 3 oils but not in CD patients.[79–81] Histologic samples showed a difference in the fatty acid composition of the colon and a reduction in the number of inflammatory cells and inflammatory mediators.[79,81,82] There was, however, no difference in the relapse rate between treatment and control groups.[82] Olestra, the fat-free fat substitute, has been studied in adult patients with IBD in remission; it did not affect the disease activity in this study.[83] Although there does not seem to be a role for a fat substitute in the day-to-day diet of a pediatric patient with IBD, it is helpful to know that it does not appear to be harmful if ingested occasionally.

Nutritional rehabilitation requires increased calories and protein, with 140–150% of RDA for age.[27] Multivitamin and minerals, folate, zinc, and iron supplementation should be considered, and vitamin B_{12} sufficiency should be assessed (Table 16–5). A high-calorie, high-protein well-balanced diet should be encouraged. Restrictions should be based on individual tolerance, rather than on the potential hazard of various foods. There is very little evidence that eating or avoiding specific foods affects the frequency of relapses or the severity of the disease.[45] Controlled studies have not supported the use of a low-residue, high-fiber or refined low-sugar diet to maintain remission of Crohn's disease.[84–86] Dairy products need not be restricted in all patients with IBD. However, lactose malabsorption is more common in patients with small bowel Crohn's disease than in patients with disease involving the colon or UC. Advice concerning intake of dairy products should be individualized to avoid unnecessary dietary restrictions.[87] During periods of illness or weight loss, oral nutritional supplementation can be useful. The choice of formula used depends on disease activity and tolerance. If voluntary intake is insufficient, nasogastric nocturnal continuous or intermittent enteral supplementation may be considered. If there is no evidence of gastric Crohn's disease, a gastrostomy may be useful and more acceptable than a nasogastric tube. Parenteral nutrition should be reserved for patients who have bowel obstructions, short bowel syndrome, or who are unable to tolerate sufficient quantity of enteral nutrition because of active disease.

Nutritional issues are often neglected in the management of IBD.[88] The pediatric nutritionist must play an integral role in the treatment

Table 16–5 Vitamin and Mineral Supplementation Suggestions for Use in Children and Adolescents with Inflammatory Bowel Disease

Nutrient	*Dose*
Multivitamin with minerals	1 tablet daily
Iron	4 to 6 mg/kg in 3 divided doses
Folate (for sulfasalazine therapy)	1 mg/day
Vitamin B_{12} (evaluate need with Schilling test)	1 mg IM q 3 months
Calcium	1200 mg
Magnesium	200–400 mg
Zinc	50–100 mg elemental zinc divided into 3 doses

Source: Data from A.M. Davis, et al., Pediatric Gastrointestinal Disorders, in *The ASPEN Nutrition Support Practice Manual,* R. Merritt, ed., pp. 27:12–13; © 1988, American Society for Parenteral and Enteral Nutrition.

plan for both ulcerative colitis and Crohn's disease. Further research is needed to better define the benefits of nutrition therapy as adjunctive therapy and to investigate the role of specific nutrients in the primary treatment of IBD.

LACTOSE INTOLERANCE

Lactose intolerance (LI) is the most common of all of the syndromes of carbohydratre malabsorption. It is characterized by bloating, flatulence, and diarrhea after ingestion of lactose-containing foods. The breath hydrogen test is the diagnostic test to determine LI (see Table 16–2). Carbohydrate that is malabsorbed in the small intestine is fermented by colonic bacteria, and hydrogen gas is released. Intermittent breath samples are taken and analyzed.[90]

Lactose intolerance may be primary or secondary. Secondary disorders are most common in infancy. There are three major disorders of primary lactose intolerance: developmental, congenital, and late-onset.[89]

Developmental Lactose Intolerance

Lactase activity develops late in the third trimester of pregnancy,[91] so premature infants typically have lower levels of lactase activity.[92] There is no evidence to suggest that lactase can be induced—that by giving infants lactose, there is a more rapid development of lactase activity.[91] Premature infant formulas contain a combination of lactose and glucose polymers as the carbohydrate composition.[93] Premature infants were studied with breath hydrogen tests to assess the degree of lactose intolerance. Although the infants had positive breath tests, they did not have clinical symptoms of LI, such as diarrhea. The infants gained weight appropriately and had low mean stool output.[94] In practice, most infants do quite well.[93] Malabsorption may be normal for premature infants, and salvage of carbohydrate by the colon is operational in premature infants. This process may, in fact, be beneficial; associated with the development of fecal flora, which prevents the colonization of the colon with enteropathogens.[89]

Congenital Lactose Intolerance

Congenital lactase deficiency is very rare. Lactase activity remains abnormal throughout life in this disorder.[89] As a result, individuals with this condition must severely restrict and omit lactose in their diets.

Late-Onset Lactose Intolerance

The other primary disorder, late-onset LI, is also known as *adult-onset lactose intolerance.* Lactose intolerance is common among individuals with different racial and ethnic backgrounds such as adult Eskimos, Native Americans, Asians, some Africans, and Semitics.[95] It is uncommon in Northern Europeans, in several tribes in Africa, and in India.[96] In the United States, it is seen in up to 70% of African Americans[97] beginning between age 6 and the teenage years.[98] In the Caucasian population, LI is less common, with less than 20% affected.[97] If LI is found in an African American child under 3 years of age or a Caucasian child under 5 years, the possibility of damage to the intestinal mucosa should be considered.[99]

Most cases of secondary lactose intolerance are caused by an acute diarrheal disease,[100–102] and the deficiency is temporary.[96–97] Lactose can generally by reintroduced into the diet after several weeks. Rotavirus, the leading cause of diarrhea in older infants and toddlers, is very likely to be associated with temporary lactose intolerance.[101] Secondary LI is also seen with chronic diarrhea of infancy, food protein intolerance, parasitic infections, and gluten-sensitive enteropathy.[90]

Lactose-free infant formulas include Lactofree (Mead Johnson) and Similac Lactose Free (Ross), or soy formulas such as Isomil (Ross Products) and Prosobee (Mead Johnson), which can be used for infants with LI. For older children, milk and dairy products may need to be eliminated from the diet temporarily. Because these foods are an excellent source of calcium, protein, and other vitamins and minerals, it is best not to eliminate these foods altogether. Not all milk substitutes or "imitation" milk products are equal; some do not contain the nutrients normally found in milk, such as rice milk or soy milk products not containing calcium supplementation. In an extreme case, pellagra, beri-beri, iron deficiency anemia, and zinc and essential fatty acid deficiency were found in an infant consuming an "imitation" milk product that contained less than 2% of the RDA for B complex, zinc, iron, and essential fatty acids.[103] Milk-free diets often require calcium and other mineral/vitamin supplementation. Calcium supplements are available in carbonate, gluconate, lactate, and citrate, and some with Vitamin D added. Dolomite and bone meal calcium supplements should be avoided because they have been linked with lead poisoning.[104] Stoker and Castle[104] describe a method for testing the physical ability of a calcium supplement to be absorbed by placing a tablet in a glass of vinegar for 30 minutes. If it has not dissolved in 30 minutes, they do not classify it as an easily absorbed source of calcium.

Many children and adolescents with LI can better tolerate a low-lactose diet than they can a lactose-restricted diet. Some foods with lactose are better tolerated than others, and factors, such as the fat content of the food or beverage, amount consumed, and timing (whether it is ingested by itself, or with a meal) are important. Ingesting small amounts at a time and taking the lactose-containing food with a larger meal reduces the chance of side effects and malabsorption. Higher-fat lactose-containing foods sometimes are tolerated better than low- or fat-free products. When reintroducing new foods to the diet, a recommendation is to wait 48 hours before each new food or change in amount of food already tolerated.[104]

Many products are now commercially available as lactose-reduced or lactose-free products, such as Lactaid milk. Lactase enzyme tablets, which can be swallowed or chewed, are available and can be taken with a meal containing lactose. Lactaid drops can be added to milk to break down lactose. The package insert directions should be followed for the needed (70% or 90%) lactose reduction. Some products, such as naturally aged cheese (blue, brie, cheddar, and swiss), seem to be tolerated; increased aging improves tolerance.[104]

CONSTIPATION

Constipation is common in childhood. Encouraging fluids is the first line of therapy. In children over age 2 years, high-fiber diets are often recommended. When fiber alone fails, lubricants and laxatives may be required. The fiber content of common foods is presented in Table 16–6. Medications such as phenytoin may slow peristalsis, and diuretics that alter fluid balance may cause constipation as well.[105]

When stooling is chronically difficult or painful, children may withhold stool, aggravating the existing problem. Encopresis may result due to the stretched rectal wall, allowing softer stool to leak out involuntarily.[105] A bowel program after a thorough clean-out may include a high-fiber diet, adequate fluid, and increased physical activity.

Iron contained in infant formula may be perceived by mothers to cause constipation. They may make this association because of their experience with iron supplementation in pregnancy.[105] Iron in formula has not been associated with an adverse side effect of constipation.[106–109] If parents choose low-iron formula, an iron supplement is necessary by 4–6 months, when iron stores become depleted.[110] (see also Chapter 4 for further details).

PANCREATIC INSUFFICIENCY AND CHOLESTATIC LIVER DISEASE

The pancreas has numerous endocrine and exocrine functions. The exocrine functions enable the body to digest and absorb complex carbohydrates, protein, and fat. Remarkably, only when 90% of the pancreatic function is lost do alterations in digestion and absorption occur.[111]

Table 16–6 Good Sources of Dietary Fiber

Food	*Grams of Fiber*
Apple, 1 med. w/ skin	2.2
Apple, 1 med. w/o skin	2.0
Apricot, dried, 3 oz	7.8
Blueberries, 1 cup raw	4.4
Dates, dried, 10	4.2
Kiwi, 3 oz	3.4
Pear, 1 med. raw	4.1
Prunes, dried, 3 oz	7.2
Prunes, stewed, 3 oz	6.6
Raisins, 3 oz	5.3
Raspberries, 1 cup	5.8
Strawberries, raw, 1 cup	2.8
Avocado, California, raw, 1 med.	3.0
Beans, black, boiled, 1 cup	7.2
Beans, great northern, boiled, 1 cup	6.0
Beans, kidney, boiled, 1 cup	6.4
Beans, lima, boiled, 1 cup	6.2
Beans, baby lima, boiled, 1 cup	7.8
Beans, navy, boiled 1 cup	6.6
Beans, green, canned 1/2 cup	6.8
Broccoli, boiled, 1/2 cup	2.2
Chickpeas (garbanzo beans), 1 cup	5.7
Cowpeas (blackeye peas), 1 cup	4.4
Lentils, boiled, 1 cup	7.9

Ready to Eat Cereal	*Fiber Grams*	*Serving*
Fiber One	13	1/2 c
All Bran	10	1/2 c
Shredded Wheat and Bran	8	1 1/4 c
100% Bran	8	1/3 c
Raisin Bran	8	1 c
Multi Bran Chex	7	1 c
Cracklin' Oat Bran	6	1 3/4 c
Mini Wheats	6	1 c
Mini Wheats with raisins	5	3/4 c
Mini Wheats with strawberries	5	3/4 c
Shredded Wheat	5	1 c
Grape Nuts	5	1/2 c
Fruit n Fiber	5	1 c
Wheat Chex	5	1 c
Complete Wheat	5	3/4 c
Bran Flakes	5	3/4 c

continues

Table 16–6 continued

Ready to Eat Cereal	*Fiber Grams*	*Serving*
Great Grains	4	2/3 c
Banana Nut Crunch	4	1 c
Raisin Bran Crunch	4	1 c
Cranberry Almond Crunch	3	1 c
Healthy Choice Low Fat Granola	3	1/2 c
Grape Nut Flakes	3	3/4 c

Source: Data for sections on fruits and vegetables from references 163 and 164; data for section on ready-to-eat cereals from a supermarket survey of manufacturer's labels as of April 1999.

Diseases that may cause pancreatic insufficiency include: cystic fibrosis, Shwachman syndrome, Jeune's thoracic dystrophy, Johanson-Blizzard syndrome, Alagille syndrome, and severe protein calorie malnutrition.[111] Pancreatic insufficiency has also been reported after graft-versus-host disease following stem cell transplantation.[112] Diagnosis of insufficiency typically is based on an abnormal fecal fat or nitrogen test and evidence that the malabsorption is related to the pancreas, as it may occur with intestinal and liver diseases.[111] The fecal fat or nitrogen test is conducted using a 72-hour pooled stool collection taken while the individual is consuming an age-appropriate normal diet. The nitrogen or fat intake is evaluated and compared with excretion, and the percent of absorption is calculated. Normal individuals absorb approximately 93% of ingested protein and fat.[111] The "gold standard" for evaluating pancreatic dysfunction is direct collection of pancreatic output during stimulation.[111]

Cystic fibrosis is the most common etiology of pancreatic insufficiency. Nutritional treatment includes oral pancreatic supplements, fat-soluble vitamin supplementaion, and close follow-up of nutrition intake and growth parameters. In 1995, a consensus conference from the Cystic Fibrosis Foundation determined guidelines for pancreatic enzyme replacements.[113] Pancreatic enzyme replacements are made in a fixed-dose ratio of lipase, protease, and amylase, and are typically dosed in units of lipase because it is the most important determinant of effectiveness of therapy for steatorrhea.[114] The enzymes should be taken at the start of each meal that contains fat or protein.[115] The panel reviewed weight-based and fat-based dosing of enzymes. For weight-based dosing, the panel recommended that initial doses of supplemental lipase should begin at 1,000 IU of lipase/kg/meal for children younger than 4 years and 500 IU lipase/kg/meal for children older than 4 years. The dose may be increased gradually to a maximum of 2,500 IU lipase/kg/meal if weight gain is inadequate or abdominal symptoms persist.[113] The dose should rarely exceed 2,500 IU lipase/kg/meal. Excess lipase is suspected as the etiology of fibrosing colonopathy.[113] In other disorders of pancreatic insufficiency, there are no guidelines for pancreatic enzymes. However, most clinicians use the dosing guidelines for cystic fibrosis.[111]

Cholestasis may present in the newborn period with symptoms of elevated conjugated bilirubin (> 20% of the total), jaundice, light or acholic stools, and hepatomegaly.[116] Further testing can determine whether the problem is intrahepatic (medical) or extrahepatic (surgical). Intrahepatic liver disease may result from viral and metabolic disease such as galactosemia, as

Table 16–7 Vitamin Supplementation in Cystic Fibrosis and Hepatic Disorders

Vitamin Needed	*Dose*
Cystic fibrosis	
Vitamin A	1–2 × RDA
Vitamin D	1–2 × RDA
Hepatic disorders	
Vitamin A (Aquasol A)	5000 IU/d
Vitamin D	2,000–10,000 IU/d
or	
25-Hydroxycholecalciferol	50 μg/d
Vitamin E	50–400 IU/d
Vitamin K	2.5–5 mg/d

Source: Adapted with permission from Merritt RJ and Hack S, Infant feeding and enteral nutrition, in *Nutrition in Clinical Practice* (1988;3:47–64), Copyright © 1988, American Society for Parenteral and Enteral Nutrition.

well as "idiopathic" neonatal hepatitis. Extrahepatic causes of injury include biliary atresia and intrahepatic duct hypoplasia or paucity.[116] Other causes of cholestasis include bacterial endotoxin from sepsis and TPN-associated cholestasis.[117] Unfortunately, parenteral nutrition-associated cholestasis is common in pediatrics.[118,119] Infants or children with cholestasis who are receiving parenteral nutrition often need to reduce their intake of copper[120] and manganese because these nutrients are excreted through the biliary system (see also Chapter 25).

Fat-soluble vitamin malabsorption is a problem that occurs with pancreatic insufficiency and cholestatic liver disease. Supplementation at levels exceeding the Recommended Dietary Allowances (RDAs) for normal healthy children is recommended for children with these disorders. The recommended dosage for supplementation of fat-soluble vitamins is presented in Table 16–7.

For infants receiving enteral formulas, those containing 50–60% medium-chain triglycerides (MCT) and 40–50% long chain triglycerides (LCT) are typically recommended for patients with cholestasis. For premature infants, premature formulas, such as Similac Special Care (Ross Products) or Enfamil Premature (Mead Johnson), have this lipid profile. For term infants, Alimentum (Ross Products) or Pregestimil (Mead Johnson) contain MCT/LCT in this mix. In cholestasis, there is insufficient bile for micelle formation for optimal LCT absorption; MCT do not require bile for absorption. MCT oil does not contain essential fatty acids or aid in the absorption of fat soluble vitamins,[121] so a source of linoleic acid is essential. Infants typically require 2.7% of calorie intake as essential fatty acids.[122] Essential fatty acid deficiency has been reported with the use of a high-MCT formula, such as Portagen (Mead Johnson), in an infant with hepatobiliary disease and presumed LCT malabsorption.[123,124]

SHORT BOWEL SYNDROME

Short Bowel Syndrome (SBS) is a condition in which the patient has an anatomic or functional loss of more than 50% of expected small intestine.[125] These patients have difficulty sustaining appropriate growth and development with normal age-appropriate enteral nutrition. Although most patients have had a significant bowel resection, SBS cannot be solely described by an arbitrary amount of remaining small intestine. Some patients may have had a rather small amount of bowel resected, but the entire bowel was damaged, causing difficulty with enteral nutrition.[114] The injury may be a result of necrotizing enterocolitis (NEC), volvulus, intestinal atresias, gastroschisis, ruptured omphalocele, or vascular infarct.[125] The result of the injury and/or resection is decreased small intestine surface area, which leads to malabsorption and large volume watery diarrhea. The degree of malabsorption varies with the area and extent of missing or injured bowel. Recovery depends on the degree of functional intestinal adaptation.

Absorption of fluids and nutrients occurs throughout the small intestine, but half of the mucosal surface is contained within the proximal quarter of the small intestine.[126] The duodenum and jejunum are the primary sites of digestion and absorption of proteins, carbohydrates, lipids, and most vitamins and minerals. Vitamin B_{12} is an exception; it is absorbed only in the ileum. Bile salts are also absorbed in the ileum; this is necessary for enterohepatic circulation. If the bile acid pool becomes depleted, there is decreased fat and fat soluble vitamin absorption.[127] Many gut hormones are produced in the ileum, including enteroglucagon and peptide YY that affect gastrointestinal motility. Resection of the ileum can impair nutrient-regulated gut motility.[128] The ileum can adapt to take the place of the jejunum. However, due to some of these specific roles of the ileum, the jejunum cannot adapt to the role of the ileum.[127]

The presence of the ileocecal valve is very important. It slows transit time and acts as a barrier to bacteria moving into the small bowel from the colon. Bacterial overgrowth in the small bowel can be a major problem and lead to increased diarrhea and malabsorption.[125] The colon absorbs water, can salvage malabsorbed carbohydrate, and can absorb sodium. Patients with a jejunostomy or ileostomy will have watery stomal output high in sodium, zinc, and other minerals. There are different schools of thought in the surgical community as to whether to perform a primary anastomosis—putting the bowel back together and creating continuity—at the time of a bowel resection. Sometimes, patients are also too labile, and a temporary ostomy is created. Whereas having all the bowel in continuity maximizes the gastrointestinal surface area for absorption of nutrients, there are advantages of an ostomy. Fluid management is easier to monitor because it is easy to measure ostomy output and analyze it as needed for electrolytes, carbohydrate, etc. Measuring urine output is easily done by weighing the urine-only diapers in infants. After an anastomosis, output is difficult to gauge because it is reported as mixed stool and urine. When a patient is stooling heavily and fluid intake is inadequate, stool and urine can look very similar, further complicating assessment. The use of urine specific gravity, obtained by putting cotton balls in the urine area of the diaper, becomes a useful tool to assess hydration status in infants and young children.

Parenteral Nutrition

The first phase in the treatment of a new patient with SBS is the provision of parenteral nutrition (TPN), which should be started as soon as possible. Due to the possible long-term aspect of this form of nutrition, consideration should be given to central vein access. Initially gastric contents are drained. Gastric drainage may consist of 140 mEq/L of sodium, 15 mEq/L of potassium, and 155 mEq/L of chloride.[129] Replacement fluids should be used to replace GI losses for easier fluid and electrolyte management. Initial TPN needs vary, depending on age and nutritional status, but for infants, it is usually between 100 and 105 kcal/kg/day, 3–3.5 g protein/kg/day, and 3.0 g lipid/kg/day. As soon as stooling begins, additional sodium and zinc may be needed to compensate for stool or ostomy losses. Ileostomy output may contain 80–140 mEq/L of sodium, 15 mEq/L of potassium, 40 mEq/L of bicarbonate, 115 mEq/L of chloride[129] and 12 mg of zinc/L.[130] Adjustments should be made in the TPN solution accordingly. Laboratory data and other parameters should be monitored carefully to minimize complications associated with PN therapy. TPN-associated cholestasis is a major cause of death in patients with SBS[119] (see also Chapter 25).

Gastric acid hypersecretion can occur after a large bowel resection. It is seen most often after a large resection when enteral feedings are initiated.[131] IV ranitidine can be effective in inhibiting acid secretion[132] and can be put in the TPN as an additive. Normal dosage should be used at first, gastric pH checked, and dosage titrated for effective therapy with the assistance of a pharmacist. Hypersecretion is usually transitory, so the periodic review of medications and dosages should include gastric pH testing. Ranitidine may decrease intrinsic factor secretion, which can affect vitamin B_{12} absorption. The potential for bacterial contamination of the bowel may be increased with the long-term use of H_2 blockers.[128]

Enteral Nutrition

Enteral nutrition should be started as soon as the patient is stable and gastrointestinal motility has returned.[133] Enteral nutrition is necessary to promote intestinal adaptation. Adaptation, with cellular hyperplasia, villous hypertrophy, intestinal lengthening, and motility improvement may take a year or more.[134] There is great controversy as to the ideal formula for infants and toddlers with SBS. Breast milk is tolerated well (if available), and animal studies suggest it stimulates mucosal growth.[135] Premature infants with smaller resections may do well with premature infant formulas, depending on their tolerance to lactose. Premature infant formulas, such as Similac Special Care (Ross Products) or Enfamil Premature (Mead Johnson) with a carbohydrate source of approximately 50% lactose and 50% glucose polymers and lipid mix of MCT and LCT,[92] have been used successfully in SBS.[136] However, protein hydrolysate formulas, such as Alimentum (Ross Products) and Pregestimil (Mead Johnson), are often used to feed infants and toddlers with SBS (see Table 4–7 and Table 8–2). Although most protein is absorbed as di- or tripeptides, such as are found in protein hydrolysates,[138] sometimes there appears to be an allergic component, as well as SBS. An amino-acid-based formula, such as Neocate (Scientific Hospital Supply), is tolerated well.[137] For older infants and toddlers, fiber-containing complex formulas,[128] such as Pediasure with Fiber (Ross Products), is tolerated well. In transitioning from TPN to enteral nutrition, enteral feedings should be started at a low rate and gradually increased. Patients during this phase of treatment must be closely monitored for GI tolerance, electrolyte imbalance, and growth.

Continuous gastric feeding is usually the preferred feeding method for infants and toddlers with SBS, due to the studies showing greater absorption of nutrients and clinical experience.[24,139] Orogastric tubes may be used in premature infants because they are obligate nose breathers.[140] Nasogastric tubes are used in older infants. For long-term use, a gastrostomy tube should be considered.

Until the infant is able to eat by mouth, an oral motor stimulation program should be in place. Specially trained occupational therapists or speech pathologists can work with the nursing staff and parents on a feeding plan. As soon as the team feels that the infant is developmentally ready and can tolerate small amounts of bolus feedings, feeding should begin. Continuous feedings should continue to be the preferred enteral route of nutrition, but oral stimulation is very important for development of feeding skills. Feeding aversion in patients with SBS is very difficult to treat.[141] Preventing aversive feeding behavior is very important.

If at all possible, solid foods should be introduced when the infant is 4–6 months of age. Cereals such as rice cereal are usually well tolerated. Fruit juices should be avoided because they may cause increased diarrhea. Most fruits, vegetables, and meats are tolerated, but there is considerable individual variation on specific food intolerances. Only one new food should be tried at a time, waiting 3 days before adding a new food. Some centers report a greater number of food allergies in their patients with SBS and use greater caution with the introduction of hyperallergenic foods. Lactose need not be banned from the diet forever; a study has shown tolerance to a diet with 20 g/day later in the course of therapy.[142]

The transition from parenteral nutrition to all enteral nutrition may be slow. Malabsorption is common with enteral feedings, and calorie needs per kg increase as the percentage of enteral nutrition increases. At least 20–30% of the enteral formula may be malabsorbed.[138] Calorie needs are difficult to estimate, but may be higher than normal for age. Several articles have been written documenting poor growth and abnormal laboratory tests from sodium loss from ileostomy drainage.[143–145] Similar losses could occur in a patient with a subtotal proximal colon resection and a primary anastomosis. Urine sodium values can be used to titrate the amount of additional sodium needed in combination with stool volume; supplementation can be initiated using the average stool output and the midrange estimate of 110 mEq/L of sodium contained in ileostomy fluid. Usually, sodium chloride is used, but if the patient has bicarbonate loss and is acidotic, a combination of sodium chloride and sodium citrate can be used.

Small bowel bacterial overgrowth can develop when the ileocecal valve is absent, when there is slow motility, or when there is a partial small bowel obstruction.[138] Symptoms of overgrowth are diarrhea and/or air within the bowel wall.[138] Antibiotic treatment is available, and some centers routinely administer antibiotics, such as metronidazole (Flagyl), to their patients for 1–2 weeks every month for overgrowth treatment. Metabolic acidosis can occur from the absorption of d-lactic acid produced by bacteria from malabsorbed carbohydrate, which may cause drowsiness and mental confusion. This has been seen in young children who are eating a mixed diet.[146, 147]

For patients who have successfully been weaned from parenteral nutrition, vitamin supplementation may be necessary. Vitamin B_{12} may need to be supplemented with an intramuscular administration of 1 mg every 3 months. Iron, folate, and magnesium may also need to be supplied.[27] An assessment should be made for each child to determine individual needs.

Infants and children may need supplemental continuous enteral infusion for a long time. Very small enteral pumps using a backpack or fanny pack are now available. The taste and acceptability of formula often becomes an issue during the transition to oral feedings. Some patients may take one formula by mouth and use another for gastric feeds. Some patients who are off of parenteral nutrition still need IV hydration daily. Portable IV pumps can contribute to making their lifestyle more normal.

For patients who do not seem to be making progress weaning from parenteral nutrition, there are other options. Medications that delay gastric emptying or reduce gastrointestinal transit time may be beneficial to an improved outcome. In adults, growth hormone, glutamine, and a modified diet have been used in a supervised treatment plan to enhance nutrient absorption and to decrease dependence on parenteral therapy.[148]

Cholestasis occurs in 30–60% of children with SBS; liver failure develops in 3–19% of children who acquired SBS in the neonatal period.[149–151] Although it has always been assumed that parenteral nutrition was the leading culprit in the etiology, a recent study points out the close association between cholestasis and bacterial or fungal infections.[152] Alternative surgical procedures, such as bowel lengthening or tapering enteroplasty, may be considered for those patients who are not making progress.[118,153–155] Bowel transplantation is now clinically feasible and may offer hope for patients who have no other options. Combined liver and bowel transplantation is reserved for those patients with life-threatening progressive liver disease.[156] Although there has been much progress made in bowel transplantation over the past 5 years, better immunosuppressive drugs and more donors are needed to improve outcomes.[156]

LIVER TRANSPLANTATION

The most common disease requiring liver transplantation in childhood is biliary atresia (over 50% of cases); other less prominent causes are inherited metabolic disorders (alpha-1-antitrypsin deficiency, glycogen storage disease, Wilson's disease, tyrosinemia), intrahepatic holestasis syndromes (ie, Alagille, Byler), chronic hepatitis with cirrhosis, and fulminant viral or toxic hepatitis. Indications for transplantation include hepatic failure, intractable ascites, recurrent variceal hemorrhage, and hypersplenism.

The patient with end-stage liver disease awaiting transplantation presents a formidable challenge to the medical team. The particular liver disease involved, the magnitude of liver dysfunction, the presence of complications, and the transplantation procedure itself combine to present a complex treatment process, including meeting nutritional needs for healing and growth.[157] Pretransplant nutritional care involves both assessment of current status and development of a therapeutic diet tailored to the liver disease and degree of debilitation. Assessment parameters the dietitian should follow include:

1. anthropometrics: height/length, weight, triceps skinfolds, midarm circumference, abdominal girth
2. laboratory studies: complete blood count with differential; platelet count; prothrombin and partial thromboplastin times; serum levels of total and direct bilirubin, alanine aminotransferase, aspartate aminotransferase, alkaline phosphatase, total protein, prealbumin, albumin, ammonia, electrolytes, calcium, inorganic phosphorous, blood urea nitrogen, creatinine, serum bile salts, and vitamins A, D, and E; serologic testing for titers of hepatitis A and B, Epstein-Barr virus, cytomegalovirus, herpes virus, human immunodeficiency virus
3. radiology: ultrasound (to check for patency of vascular structures)

The pretransplant diet should be planned. Calories should be provided at 140% of the RDA for age. The use of glucose polymers or medium-chain triglyceride oil added to food or feedings can help to boost energy intake to these levels. Enteral drip feedings (intermittent or continuous) may be necessary to ensure intake. For infants, protein should be provided at 2.0 to 2.5 g/kg of dry weight if parenteral nutrition is being employed or at 2.5 to 3.0 g/kg of dry weight if enteral feeding is used. The parenteral nutrition solution used should contain a balanced amino acid mixture. If the patient is encephalopathic, the protein intake should be reduced to 1.0–1.5 g/kg of dry weight. Branched-chain amino acid solutions may also be considered and improvement in status evaluated. Water-miscible fat-soluble vitamins are often indicated. Zinc and iron are provided as needed, and sodium may need to be restricted to help control ascites.[146, 147]

Immediately after transplantation, TPN may be initiated, using a balanced amino acid solution with dextrose and an appropriate intravenous lipid source. For infants, the TPN solution should provide nutrients at the following specified levels: 2.0–2.5 g protein/kg of dry weight; 2–3 g lipid/kg of dry weight; and 80–100 kcal/kg of dry weight.[159] Sodium, potassium, calcium, and phosphorous amounts are based on serum levels.

Routine posttransplant care includes monitoring fluid balance closely, which requires strict intake and output measurements and daily weights. The following laboratory tests should be monitored daily: complete blood count and differential and levels of blood and urine glucose, triglycerides, electrolytes, calcium, phosphorous, magnesium, albumin, and liver enzymes. When bowel movements resume, stools should be checked for pH, reducing substances, and occult blood.[160,161]

Enteral feedings may begin when the postoperative ileus has resolved (exhibited by stooling). Enteral feedings are increased with concurrent decrease in TPN. For the infant and younger child, continuous nasogastric feeding using a MCT-oil-containing formula is often the feeding of choice. Feedings should be advanced as tolerated to oral regular formula as the stooling pattern normalizes. For the older child, continuous nasogastric feedings, intermittent feedings, or an oral defined diet may be used. The diet should be advanced as tolerated to a soft low-residue diet, then to a regular diet. Multivitamin supplements should be used, but each child's need for supplemental zinc, iron, and vitamin E should be assessed. A mild sodium restriction may be indicated to prevent fluid retention caused by steroid use.[161,162]

Possible problems in the resumption of oral feeding include oral defensiveness due to prolonged use of TPN and developmental delay in sucking and chewing skills in infants. Appropriately trained occupational therapists or speech pathologists should be consulted to devise an interdisciplinary treatment plan for these problems.

The postdischarge follow-up of liver transplant recipients includes assessment of anthropometric values and the patient's diet log at each clinic visit. Long term, the transplant patient should receive the dietary supplements only if indicated. Problems that the dietitian should be alert for in this population include fat malabsorption, metabolic bone disease, dental caries, hypertension, and anemia.[162] Referrals can then be made to the appropriate care teams.

REFERENCES

1. American Academy of Pediatrics, Committee on Nutrition. Use of oral fluid therapy and posttreatment feeding following enteritis in children in a developed country. *Pediatrics.* 1985;75:358–361.
2. Wall CR, Webster J, Quirk P, et al. The nutritional management of acute diarrhea in young infants: Effect of carbohydrate ingested. *J Pediatr Gastroenterol Nutr.* 1994;19:170–174.
3. Liftshitz F, Maggioni A. The nutritional management of acute diarrhea in young infants. *J Pediatr Gastroenterol Nutr.* 1994;19:148–150.
4. Brown KH. Dietary management of acute childhood diarrhea: Optimal timing of feeding and appropriate use of milks and mixed diets. *J Pediatr.* 1991;118: S92–98.
5. Santosham M, Foster S, Reid R, et al. Role of soy-based, lactose-free formula during treatment of acute diarrhea. *Pediatrics.* 1985;76:292–298.
6. Santosham M, Goepp J, Burns B, et al. Role of soy-based lactose-free formula in the outpatient management of diarrhea. *Pediatrics.* 1991;87:619–622.
7. Goepp JG. Acute diarrhea. In: Walker WA, Watkins, JB, eds. *Nutrition in Pediatrics: Basic Science and Clinical Applications.* Hamilton, Ontario: BC Decker; 1997:594.
8. Chew F, Penna FJ, Peret Filho LA, et al. Is dilution of cow's milk formula necessary for dietary management of acute diarrhoea in infants aged less than 6 months? *Lancet.* 1993;341:194–197.
9. Brown KH, Perez F, Peerson JM, et al. Effect of dietary fiber (soy polysaccharide) on the severity, duration, and nutritional outcome of acute, watery diarrhea in children. *Pediatrics.* 1993;92:241–247.
10. Vanderhoof JA, Murray ND, Paule CL, et al. Use of soy fiber in acute diarrhea in infants and toddlers. *Clin Pediatr.* 1997;36:135–139.
11. Klish WJ. Chronic diarrhea. In: Walker WA and Watkins JB, eds. *Nutrition in Pediatrics: Basic Science and Clinical Applications.* Hamilton, Ontario: BC Decker; 1997:603.
12. Lo CW, Walker WA. Chronic protracted diarrhea of infancy: A nutritional disorder. *Pediatrics.* 1983;72: 786.
13. Chronic diarrhoea in children: A nutritional disease. [editorial]. *Lancet* 1987;1:143.
14. Baker SS, Davis AM. Hypocaloric oral therapy during an episode of diarrhea and vomiting can lead to severe malnutrition. *J Pediatr Gastroenterol Nutr.* 1998;27: 1–5.
15. Bezerra JA, Stathos TH, Duncan B, et al. Treatment of infants with acute diarrhea: What's recommended and what's practiced. *Pediatrics.* 1994;80:1–4.
16. Klish WJ, Udall JN, Rodriguez JT, et al. Intestinal surface area of infants with acquired monosaccharide intolerance. *J Pediatr.* 1978;92:566–571.
17. Calvin RT, Klish WJ, Nichols BL. Disaccharidase activities, jejunal morphology and carbohydrate tolerance in children with chronic diarrhea. *J Pediatr Gastroenterol Nutr.* 1985;4:949–953.
18. Solomon SM, Kirby KF. The refeeding syndrome: A review. *J Parenteral Enteral Nutr.* 1985;85:28–36
19. Lee PC, Werlin SL. Carbohydrates. In: Baker RD Jr, Baker SS, and Davis AM, eds. *Pediatric*

Parenteral Nutrition. New York: Chapman & Hall, 1997:103.

20. Blackman JA, Nelson CLA. Reinstituting oral feedings in children fed by gastrostomy tube. *Clin Pediatr*. 1985;24:434.
21. Heymsfield S. Metabolic changes associated with refeeding. *ASPEN Update*. 1982;4:1–2
22. Weisner RL, Krumdieck CL. Death resulting from overzealous total parenteral nutrition: The refeeding syndrome revisited. *Am J Clin Nutr,* 1981;34:393–399.
23. Mezoff AG, Gremse DA, Farrell MK. Hypophosphatemia in the nutritional recovery syndrome. *Am J Dis Child*. 1989;143:1111.
24. Parker P, Stroop S, Greene H. A controlled comparison of continuous versus intermittent feeding in the treatment of infants with intestinal disease. *J Pediatr*. 1987;99:360.
25. Thobani S, Molla AM, Synder JD. Nutritional therapy for persistent diarrhea. In: Baker SS, Baker RD Jr, Davis AM, eds. *Pediatric Enteral Nutrition*. New York: Chapman & Hall;1994:291.
26. Sachdev HPS, Mittal NK, Mittal SK, et al. A controlled trial on utility of oral zinc supplementation in acute dehydrating diarrhea in infants. *J Pediatr Gastroenterol Nutr*. 1988;7:877.
27. Davis AM, Baker SS, Baker RD Jr, et al. Pediatric gastrointestinal disorders. In: Meritt RM, ed. *The ASPEN Nutrition Support Practice Manual*. Silver Spring, MD: ASPEN;1998:27–33.
28. Rahmathullah L, Underwood BA, Thulasiraj RD, et al. Reduced mortality among children in southern India receiving a small weekly dose of vitamin A. *N Engl J Med*. 1990;323:929.
29. Brown KH. Appropriate diets for the rehabilitation of malnourished children in the community setting. *Acta Paediatr Scand*. 1991;374(suppl):151.
30. Wall CR, Webster J, Quirk P, et al. The nutritional management of acute diarrhea in young infants: effect of carbohydrate ingested. *J Pediatr Gastroenterol Nutr*. 1994;19:170–174.
31. Keohane PP, Grimble CK, Brown B, et al. Influence of protein composition and hydrolysis method on intestinal absorption of protein in man. *Gut*. 1985; 26:907.
32. Hegarty JE, Fairclough PD, Moriarity KJ, et al. Comparison of plasma and intraluminal amino acid profiles in man after meals containing a protein hydrolysate and equivalent amino acid mixture. *Gut*. 1982;23: 670.
33. Stocks RJ, Davies DP, Allen F. Loss of breast milk nutrients during tube feeding. *Arch Dis Child*. 1985;60:164.
34. Greer FR, McCormick A, Loker J. Changes in fat concentration of human milk during the delivery by intermittent bolus and continuous mechanical pump infusion. *J Pediatr*. 1984;105:745.
35. Narayan I, Singh B, Harvey D. Fat loss during feeding of human milk. *Arch Dis*. 1984;59:475.
36. Lavin, M, Clark RM. The effect of short-term refrigeration of milk and the addition of breast milk fortifier on the delivery of lipids during tube feeding. *J Pediatr Gastroenterol Nutr*. 1989;8:496.
37. Evaluation of an algorithm for the treatment of persistent diarrhea: A multicenter study. International Working Group on Persistent Diarrhoea. *Bull WHO*. 1996;74:479–489.
38. Kolacek S, Grguric J, Perci M, et al. Home-made modular diet versus semi-elemental formula in the treatment of chronic diarrhoea of infancy: A prospective randomized trial. *Eur J Pediatr*. 1996;155:997–1001.
39. Touhami M, Boudraa G, Mary JY, et al. Clinical consequences of replacing milk with yogurt in persistent infantile diarrhea. [French] *Ann Padiatrie*. 1992;39: 79–86.
40. Fasano A. Where have all the American celiacs gone? *Acta Paediatr Suppl*. 1996;412:20–24.
41. Visakorpi JK. Silent coeliac disease: The risk groups to be screened. In: Auricchio S, Visakorpi JK, eds. Common food intolerances. I: Epidemiology of coeliac disease. *Dyn Nutr Res Basel: Karger*. 1992; 2:84–92.
42. Thompson T. Do oats belong in a gluten-free diet? *J Am Diet Assoc*. 1997;97:1413–1416.
43. Mora S, Barera G, Ricotta A, et al. Reversal of low bone density with a gluten-free diet in children and adolescents with celiac disease. *Am J Clin Nutr*. 1998; 477–481.
44. Rea F, Polito C, Marotta A, et al. Restoration of body composition in celiac children after one year of gluten-free diet. *J Pediatr Gastroenterol Nutr*. 1996; 23:408–412.
45. Motil KJ, Grand RJ. Inflammatory bowel disease. In: Walker WA, Watkins JB, eds. *Nutrition in Pediatrics: Basic Science and Clinical Applications*. Hamilton, Ontario: BC Decker;1997:516.
46. Bern EM, Calenda KA, Grand R. Inflammatory bowel disease. In: Baker SS, Baker RD Jr, Davis AM, eds. *Pediatric Enteral Nutrition*. New York: Chapman & Hall;1994:305.
47. Motil KJ, Grand RJ. Nutritional management of inflammatory bowel disease. *Pediatr Clin North Am*. 1985;32:447.
48. O'Morain CA. Does nutritional therapy in inflammatory bowel disease have a primary or an adjunctive role? *Scan J Gastroenteral*. 1990;S172:29–34.

49. Goldschmid S, Graham M. Trace element deficiencies in inflammatory bowel disease. *Gastroenterol Clin North Am.* 1989;18:579.

50. Seidman EG, Lelieko N, Ament M, et al. Nutritional issues in pediatric inflammatory bowel disease. *J Pediatr Gastroenterol Nutr.* 1991;12:424.

51. Harries AD, Heatlry RV. Nutritional disturbances in Crohn's disease. *Postgrad Med J.* 1983;59:690.

52. Elsborg L, Larsen L. Folate deficiency in chronic inflammatory bowel diseases. *Scand J Gastroenterol.* 1979;14:1019.

53. Gerlach K, Morowitz DA, Kirsner JB. Symptomatic hypomagnesemia complicating regional enteritis. *Gastroenterology.* 1970;59:567–574.

54. Hessov I, Haselblad C, Fadth S, et al. Magnesium deficiency after ilieal resection for Crohn's disease. *Scand J Gastroenterol.* 1983;18:643.

55. LaSala MA, Lifshitz F, Silverberg M, et al. Magnesium metabolism studies in children with chronic inflammatory disease of the bowel. *J Pediatr Gastroenterol Nutr.* 1985;4:75.

56. Hyams JS. Crohn's disease. In: Hyams WS, Hyams JS, eds. *Pediatric Gastrointestinal Disease: Pathophysiology, Diagnosis, Management.* Philadelphia: WB Saunders Co; 1993;750–764.

57. Kelts DG, Grand RJ, Shen G, et al. Nutritional basis for growth failure in children and adolescents with Crohn's disease. *Gastroenterology.* 1979;76:720–727.

58. Layden T, Rosenberg J, Nemchausky B, et al. Reversal of growth arrest in adolescents with Crohn's disease after parenteral nutrition. *Gastroenterology.* 1976;70:1017–1022.

59. Fleming CR, McGill DB, Berkber S. Home parenteral nutrition as a primary therapy in patients with extensive Crohn's disease of the small bowel and malnutrition. *Gastroenterology.* 1977;73:1077–1081.

60. Strobel CT, Byrne WJ, Ament ME. Home parenteral nutrition in children with Crohn's disease: Effective management alternative. *Gastroenterology.* 1979;77:272–279.

61. Kirschner BS, Klich JR, Kalman SS, et al. Reversal of growth retardation in Crohn's disease with therapy emphasizing oral nutritional restitution. *Gastroenterology.* 1981;80:10–15.

62. Morin CL, Roulet M, Roy CC, et al. Continuous elemental enteral alimentation in children with Crohn's disease and growth failure. *Gastroenterology.* 1980;79:1205–1210.

63. Motil KJ, Grand RJ, Maletskos CJ, et al. The effect of disease, drug, and diet on whole body protein metabolism in adolescents with Crohn's disease and growth failure. *J Pediatr.* 1982;101:125–140.

64. Motil KJ, Grand RJ, Matthews DE, et al. Whole body leucine metabolism in adolescents with Crohn's disease and growth failure during nutritional supplementation. *Gastroenterology.* 1982;82:1359–1368.

65. Aiges H, Markowitz J, Rosa V, et al. Home nocturnal supplemental nasogastric feedings in growth retarded adolescents with Crohn's disease. *Gastroenterology.* 1988;97:905–910.

66. Belli DC, Seldman E, Bouthillier L, et al. Chronic intermittent elemental diet improves growth failure in children with Crohn's disease. *Gastroenterology.* 1988;94:603–610.

67. Polk DB, Hattner JAT, Kerner JA. Improved growth and disease activity after intermittent administration of a defined formula diet in children with Crohn's disease. *J Parenter Enter Nutr.* 1992;16:499–504.

68. Morin CL, Roulet M, Roy CC, et al. Continuous elemental and enteral alimentation in the treatment of children and adolescents with Crohn's disease. *J Parenter Enter Nutr.* 1982;6:194–199.

69. O'Morain C, Segal AM, Levi AJ, et al. Elemental diet in acute Crohn's disease. *Arch Dis Child.* 1983;53:44–47.

70. Navarro J, Vargas J, Cezard JP, et al. Prolonged constant rate elemental enteral nutrition in small bowel Crohn's disease. *J Pediatr Gastroenterol Nutr.*1982;1:541–546.

71. Sanderson IR, Udeen S, Davies PSW, et al. Remission induced by an elemental diet in small bowel Crohn's disease. *Arch Dis Child.* 1987;62:123–127.

72. Thomas AG, Taylor F, Miller V. Dietary intake and nutritional treatment in childhood Crohn's disease. *J Pediatr Gastroenterol Nutr.* 1983;17:75–81.

73. Ruuska T, Avilahti E, Maki M, et al. Exclusive whole protein enteral diet versus prednisolone in the treatment of acute Crohn's disease in children. *J Pediatr Gastroenterol Nutr.* 1993;19:175–180.

74. O'Morain C, Segal AW, Levi AJ. Elemental diet as primary treatment of acute Crohn's disease: A controlled trial. *Br Med J.* 1984;288:1859–1862.

75. Saverymuttu S, Hodgson HJF, Chadwick VS. Controlled trial comparing prednisolone with an elemental diet plus nonabsorbable antibiotics in active Crohn's disease. *Gut.* 1985;26:994–998.

76. Okada M, Yao T, Yamamoto T, et al. Controlled trial comparing an elemental diet with prednisolone in the treatment of active Crohn's disease. *Hepatogastroenterology.* 1990;37:72–80.

77. Lochs H, Steinhardt HJ, Klaus-Wentz B, et al. Comparison of enteral nutrition and drug treatment in active Crohn's disease. Results of the European Cooperative Crohn's Disease Study IV. *Gastroenterology.* 1991;11:881–888.

78. Giaffer MH, North G, Holdsworth CD. Controlled trial of polymeric versus elemental diet in treatment of active Crohn's disease. *Lancet.* 1991;355:816.
79. Lorenz R, Weber PC, Szimnau P, et al. Supplementation of ulcerative colitis in chronic inflammatory bowel disease—a randomized, placebo-controlled, double-blind cross-over trial. *J Intern Med.* 1989; 225(suppl):225–232.
80. Aslan A, Triadafilopoulos G. Fish oil fatty acid supplementation in active ulcerative colitis: A double blind, placebo-controlled, crossover study. *Am J Gastroenterol.* 1992;87:432–437.
81. Stenson WF, Cort D, Rogers J, et al. Dietary supplementation with fish oil in ulcerative colitis. *Ann Intern Med.* 1992;116:609–614.
82. Hawthorne AB, Daneshmend TK, Hawkey CJ, et al. Treatment of ulcerative colitis with fish oil supplementation: A prospective 12-month randomized trial. *Gut.* 1992;33:922–928.
83. Zorich NL, Jones NB, Kesler JM, et al. A randomized double-blind study on disease activity in patients with quiescent inflammatory bowel disease. Olestra in IBD Study Group. *Am J Med.* 1997;103:389–399.
84. Seidman EG. Nutritional management of inflammatory bowel disease. *Gastroenterol Clin North Am.* 1989;17:129.
85. Levenstein S, Prantera C, Luzi C, et al. A low residue or normal diet in Crohn's disease: A prospective controlled trial of Italian patients. *Gut.* 1985;26:989.
86. Levi AJ. Diet in the management of Crohn's disease. *Gut.* 1985;26:985.
87. Mishkin S. Dairy sensitivity, lactose malabsorption, and elimination diets in inflammatory bowel disease. *Am J Clin Nutr.* 1997;65:564–567.
88. Husain A, Korzenik JR. Nutritional issues and therapy in inflammatory bowel disease. *Semin Gastroenterol Dis.* 1998;9:21–30.
89. Ulshen MH. Carbohydrate absorption and malabsorption. In: Walker WA, Watkins, JB, eds. *Nutrition in Pediatrics: Basic Science and Clinical Applications.* Hamilton, Ontario: BC Decker; 1997:649.
90. Lifshitz CH. Breath hydrogen testing in infants with diarrhea. In: Lifshitz F, ed. *Carbohydrate intolerance in infancy.* New York: Marcel Dekker; 1982:31–42.
91. Antonowicz C, Chang SK, Grand RJ. Development and distribution of lysosomal enzymes and disaccharidases in human fetal intestine. *Gastroenterology.* 1974;67:51.
92. MacLean WC, Fink BB. Lactose malabsorption by premature infants: Magnitude and clinical significance. *J Pediatr.* 1980;97:383.
93. Sapsford A. Enteral nutrition products. In: Groh Wargo S, Thompson M, Cox JH, eds. *Nutritional Care for High Risk Newborns.* Chicago: Precept Press; 1994:178.
94. MacLean WC, Fink BB. Lactose malabsorption by premature infants: Magnitude and clinical significance. *J Pediatr.* 1980;97:383.
95. Simons FJ, Johnson JD, Kretchmer N. Perspective on milk drinking and malabsorption of lactose. *Pediatrics.* 1977;59:98.
96. Sahi T. Genetics and epidemiology of adult type hypolactasia. *Scand J Gastroenterol.* 1994;29:(suppl 202):7–20.
97. Bayless TM, Rothfeld TM, Massa C, et al. Lactose and milk intolerance: Clinical implications. *New Eng J Med.* 1975;292(22):1156–1159.
98. Huang S, Bayless TM. Lactose intolerance in healthy children. *N Eng J Med.* 1967;276:1283.
99. Hyams JS, Stafford RJ, Grand RJ, Watkins JB, et al. Correlation of lactose breath hydrogen test, intestinal morphology, and lactase activity in children. *J Pediatr.* 1980;97:609–612.
100. Saavedra JM, Perman JA. Current concepts in lactose malabsorption and intolerance. *Annu Rev Nutr.* 1989;9:475–502.
101. Hyams JS, Krause PJ, Gleason PA. Lactose malabsorption following rotavirus infection in young children. *J Pediatr.* 1981;99:916–918.
102. Davidson GP, Goodwin D, Robb TA. Incidence of lactose malabsorption in children hospitalized with acute enteritis: Study in a well nourished urban population. *J Pediatr.* 1984;105:587–590.
103. Yelton L, Cox JH. Pediatric human immunodeficiency virus infection. In: Cox JH, ed. *Nutrition Manual for At-Risk Toddlers and Infants*, Chicago: Precept Press; 1997:174.
104. Stoker TW, Castle JL. Special diets. In: Walker WA, Watkins JB, eds. *Nutrition in Pediatrics: Basic Science and Clinical Applications.* Hamilton, Ontario: BC Decker; 1997:771.
105. Goldberg D. Clinical assessment. In: Cox JH, ed. *Nutrition Manual for At-Risk Toddlers and Infants*, Chicago: Precept Press; 1997:59.
106. Reeves JD, Yip R. Lack of adverse side effects of oral ferrous sulfate therapy in 1 year old infants. *Pediatrics.* 1985;75:352–355.
107. Nelson SE, Ziegler EE, Copeland AM, et al. Lack of adverse reactions to iron fortified formula. *Pediatrics.* 1988;81:360–364.
108. Oski FA. Iron fortified formulas and gastrointestinal symptoms in infants: A controlled study. *Pediatrics.* 1980;66:168–170.
109. Committee on Nutrition, American Academy of Pediatrics. Iron fortified formulas. *Pediatrics.* 1989;84: 1114–1115.

110. Oski FA. Iron deficiency in infancy and childhood. *New Eng J Med.* 1993;329:190–193.

111. Rothbaum R. Pancreatic disease. In: Walker WA, Watkins JB, eds. *Nutrition in Pediatrics: Basic Science and Clinical Applications.* Hamilton, Ontario: BC Decker; 1997:632.

112. Maringhini A, Gertz MA, DiMagno EP. Exocrine pancreatic insufficiency after allogenic bone marrow transplantation. *Int J Pancreatol.* 1995;17:243–247.

113. Borowitz DS, Grand RJ, Durie PR, Consensus Committee. Use of pancreatic enzyme supplements for patients with cystic fibrosis in the context of fibrosing colonopathy. *J Pediatr.* 1995;127:681–684.

114. Durie PR, Pencharz PB. A rational approach to the nutritional care of patients with cystic fibrosis. *J Roy Soc Med.* 1989;82:11–20.

115. Nutrition management of pulmonary disease. In: Williams CP, ed. *Pediatric Manual of Clinical Dietetics.* Chicago: American Dietetic Association; 1998: 322.

116. Balistreri WF. Liver disease associated with alpha1-antitrypsin deficiency. In: Balistreri WF, Stocker JT, eds. *Pediatric Hepatology.* New York: Hemisphere Publishing; 1990:159.

117. Sokol RJ. Medical management of neonatal cholestasis. In: Balistreri WF, Stocker JT. *Pediatric Hepatology.* New York: Hemisphere Publishing; 1990:41.

118. Benjamin SR. Hepatobiliary dysfunction in infants and children associated with long-term parenteral nutrition: A clinico-pathologic study. *Am J Clin Pathol.* 1981;76:276.

119. Farrell MK. Physiologic effects of parenteral nutrition. In: Baker RD, Jr, Baker SS, Davis AM, eds. *Pediatric Parenteral Nutrition.* New York: Chapman & Hall; 1997:36.

120. Suchy FJ, Mullick F. Total parenteral nutrition-associated cholestasis. In: Balistreri WF, Stocker JT, eds. *Pediatric Hepatology.* New York: Hemisphere Publishing; 1990:29.

121. Committee on Nutrition, American Academy of Pediatrics. Commentary on breastfeeding and infant formulas including proposed standards for formulas. *Pediatrics.* 1976;57:278.

122. Kleiman R, Warman KY. Nutrition in liver disease. In: Baker SS, Baker RD Jr, Davis AM, eds. *Pediatric Enteral Nutrition.* New York: Chapman & Hall; 1994:261.

123. Pettei MJ, et al. Essential fatty acid deficiency associated with the use of a medium chain triglyceride formula in pediatric hepatobiliary disease. *Am J Clin Nutr.* 1991;53:1217–1221.

124. Gourley GR, Fasrrel PM, Odell GB. Essential fatty acid deficiency after hepatic portoenterostomy for biliary atresia. *Am J Clin Nutr.* 1982;36:1194.

125. Ziegler MM. Short bowel syndrome in infancy: Etiology and management. *Clin Perinatol.* 1986;13: 167.

126. Taylor SF, Sokol RJ. Infants with short bowel syndrome. In: Hay WW, ed. *Neonatal Nutrition and Metabolism.* St. Louis, MO: Mosby Year Book; 1991:437.

127. Klish WJ. The short gut. In: Walker WA, Watkins JB, eds. *Nutrition in Pediatrics.* Boston: Little Brown; 1985;561.

128. Vanderhoof JA. Short bowel syndrome. In: Walker WA, Watkins JB, eds. *Nutrition in Pediatrics: Basic Science and Clinical Applications.* Hamilton, Ontario: BC Decker; 1997:610.

129. Heird WC, Winters RW. Fluid therapy for the pediatric surgical patient. In: Winters RW, ed. *Principles of Pediatric Fluid Therapy.* Boston: Little Brown; 1985:595.

130. Collier S, Forchielli ML, Lo CW. Parenteral nutrition requirements. In: Baker RD Jr, Baker SS, Davis AM, eds. *Pediatric Parenteral Nutrition.* New York: Chapman & Hall; 1997:78.

131. Hyman PE, Everett SL, Harada T. Gastric acid hypersecretion in short bowel syndrome in infants: Association with extent of resection and enteral feeding. *J Pediatr Gastroenterol Nutr.* 1987;5:191

132. Hyman PE, Garvey TQ Abrams CE. Tolerance to intravenous ranitidine. *J Pediatr.* 1987;110:794.

133. Purdum PP, Kirby DF. Short bowel syndrome: A review of the role of nutrition support. *J Parenter Enter Nutr.* 1990;15:93.

134. Vanderhoof JA, Langnas AN, Pinch IW, et al. Short bowel syndrome. *J Pediatr Gastroenterol Nutr.* 1992; 14:359.

135. Heird WC, Schwartz SM, Hansen IH. Colostrum induced enteric mucosal growth in beagle puppies. *Pediatr Res.* 1984;18:512A.

136. Puangco MA, Schanler RJ. Comparing preterm and elemental formulas in infants with gastrointestinal (GI) resection. 22nd Clinical Congress Abstracts. American Society for Parenteral and Enteral Nutrition, #26, 1997.

137. Lifschitz CH. Enteral feeding in short small bowel. In: Baker SS, Baker RD Jr, Davis AM, eds. *Pediatric Enteral Nutrition.* New York: Chapman & Hall; 1994:280.

138. Bines J, Francis D, Hale D. Reducing parenteral nutrition requirements in children with short bowel syndrome: Impact of a amino acid based complete infant formula. *J Pediatr Gastroenterol Nutr.* 1998;26:123–128.

139. Christie DL, Ament, ME. Dilute elemental diet and continuous infusion technique for management of short bowel syndrome. *J Pediatr.* 1975;87:705.

140. Miller MJ, Carlo WJ, Strohl KP, et al. Determination of oral breathing in premature infants. *Pediatr Res.* 1985;19:354A.
141. Linsheid TR, Tarnowski KJ, Rasnake LK, et al. Behavioral treatment of food refusal in a child with short gut syndrome. *J Pediatr Psychol.* 1987;12: 451.
142. Marteau P, Messing B, Arrigoni E, et al. Do patients with short bowel syndrome need a lactose free diet? *Nutrition.* 1997;13:13–16.
143. Mews CF. Topics in neonatal nutrition. Early ileostomy closure to prevent salt and water losses in infants. *J Perinatol.* 1992;12:297–299.
144. Bower TR. Sodium deficit causing decreased weight gain and metabolic acidosis in infants with ileostomy. *J Pediatr Surg.* 1988;23:567–572.
145. Schwarz KB, Ternberg JL, Bell MJ, Keating JP, et al. Sodium needs of infants and children with an ileostomy. *J Pediatr.* 1983;102:509–513.
146. Perimutter DH, Boyle JT, Campos JM, et al. D-lactic acidosis in children: An unusual metabolic complication of small bowel resection. *J Pediatr.* 1983;102: 234.
147. Gurevitch J, Sela B, Jonas A, et al. D-lactic acidosis: A treatable encephalopathy in pediatric patients. *Acta Paediatrica.* 1993;82:11.
148. Bryne TA, Morrissey TB, Nattakom TV, et al. Growth hormone, glutamine, and a modified diet enhance nutrient absorption in patients with severe short bowel syndrome. *J Parenter Enter Nutr.* 1995;19: 296–302.
149. Caniano DA, Starr J, Ginn-Pease ME. Extensive short bowel syndrome in neonates: Outcomes in the 1980s. *Surgery.* 1998;105:119–124.
150. Galea MH, Holliday H, Carachi R, et al. Short bowel syndrome: A collective review. *J Pediatr Surg.* 1992;27:592–596.
151. Cooper A, Floyd TF, Ross AJ. Morbidity and mortality of short bowel syndrome acquired in infancy: An update. *J Pediatr Surg.* 1984;19:711–717
152. Sondheimer JM, Asturias E. *Cadnapaphornichai.* Infection and cholestasis in neonates with intestinal resection and long term parenteral nutrition. *J Pediatr Gastroenterol Nutr.* 1998;27:131–137.
153. Chaet MS, Warner BW, Farrell MF. Intensive nutritional support and remedial surgical intervention for extreme short bowel syndrome. *J Pediatr Gastroenterol Nutr.* 1994;19:295–298.
154. Thompson JS. Surgical management of short bowel syndrome. *Surgery.* 1993;113:4–7.
155. Warner BW, Chaet MS. Nontransplant surgical options for management of the short bowel syndrome. *J Pediatr Gastroenterol Nutr.* 1997;17:1–12.
156. Goulet O, Jan D, Brousse N. Intestinal transplantation. *J Pediatr Gastroenterol Nutr.* 1997;25: 1–11.
157. Hendricks K. Nutrition aspects of chronic liver disease. *Pediatr GI Nutr News.* Massachusetts General Hospital; 1988;2.
158. Goulet OJ, deGoyet JDV, Ricour C. Preoperative nutritional evaluation and support for liver transplantation in children. *Transplant Proc.* 1987;14:3249–3255.
159. Weisdorf S, Lysne J, Cerra F. Total parenteral nutrition in hepatic failure and transplantation. In: Lebenthal E, ed. *Total Parenteral Nutrition: Indications, Utilization, Complications, and Pathophysiological Considerations.* New York, NY: Raven Press; 1986.
160. Sutton M. Nutritional support in pediatric liver transplantation. *Diet Nutr Support.* 1989; March/April: 1–9.
161. Khazal P, Freese D, Sharp H. A pediatric perspective on liver transplantation. *Pediatr Clin North Am.* 1988; 35:409–433.
162. Byers S, Wood RP, Kaufman S, Williams L, Antonson D, Vanderhoof J. Liver transplantation therapy for children: Part I. *J Pediatr Gastroenterol Nutr.* 1988;7:157–166.
163. Pennington JAT. *Bowes and Church's Food Values of Portions Commonly Used.* 15th ed. Philadelphia, PA: JB Lippincott; 1989.
164. United States Department of Agriculture. *USDA Provisional Table on the Dietary Fiber Content of Selected Foods*, HNIS/PT-106; 1988.

SUGGESTED READING

Baker SS, Baker RD Jr, Davis AM. *Pediatric Enteral Nutrition.* New York: Chapman & Hall; 1994.

Baker RD Jr, Baker SS, Davis AM. *Pediatric Parenteral Nutrition.* New York: Chapman & Hall; 1997.

Cox JH, ed. *Nutrition Manual for At-Risk Toddlers and Infants*, Chicago: Precept Press; 1997.

Groh Wargo S, Thompson M, Cox JH, eds. *Nutritional Care for High Risk Newborns.* Chicago: Precept Press; 1994.

Lebenthal E. *Textbook of Gastroenterology and Nutrition in Infancy.* 2nd ed. New York, NY: Raven Press; 1990.

Meritt, RM, ed. The ASPEN Nutrition Support Practice Manual. Silver Spring, MD: American Society for Parenteral and Enteral Nutrition; 1998.

Walker WA, Watkins JB. *Nutrition in Pediatrics: Basic Science and Clinical Applications.* Hamilton, Ontario: BC Decker; 1997.

Williams CP. *Pediatric Manual of Clinical Dietetics.* Chicago: American Dietetic Association; 1998.

PARENT ASSISTANCE

American Pseudo Obstruction and Hirschsprung's Disease Society (800) 394-2747

Center for Children with Chronic Illness and Disability, Box 721, University of Minnesota, 420 Delaware St SE, Minneapolis, MN 55455

Children's Motility Disorder Foundation (800) 809-9492

Crohn's and Colitis Foundation of America (800) 343-3637

Intestinal Disease Foundation (412) 216-5888

National Foundation for Ileitis and Colitis, Inc., 444 Park Avenue South, New York, NY 10016. (212) 685-3440. Support group

Pediatric Crohn's and Colitis Association (617) 290-0902

OLEY Foundation (for families of parenteral and enteral nutrition customers) (518) 262-5079

United Ostomy Association (800) 826-0826

CHAPTER 17

Chronic Renal Disease

Nancy S. Spinozzi

Infants and children with chronic renal disease, regardless of etiology, face multiple and frequent dietary manipulations throughout their course of treatment. This occurs at a time when growth and development are at their most dynamic stages and behavioral adaptations to eating and making food choices are greatly influenced. Dietary modifications, along with the physical and emotional effects of chronic illness, can result in outcomes counterproductive to these activities, which are so vital to the normal maturation of the child. However, with better understanding of the particular disease and its medical and nutritional management (including the timely initiation of recombinant human growth hormone), it is possible to overcome what not too long ago were negative, though tolerated, outcomes—growth retardation and metabolic bone disease.

Chronic renal failure (CRF) in infants and children is almost equally represented by acquired and congenital etiologies.[1] Table 17–1 lists the predominant diagnoses in children less than 16 years of age with CRF. Fortunately, acquired diseases such as chronic glomerulonephritis have less impact on growth, due to their more insidious onset. Congenital diseases, however, can result in early and severe growth retardation. Therefore, infants and toddlers (ages 0–4 years) presenting with chronic renal insufficiency (CRI) must be aggressively nourished to promote at least a normal growth rate, preferably greater than the 5th percentile of length for age.[2,3] The earlier the age of onset of renal failure (GFR < 30% of normal), the more potentially severe its impact on growth will be.[4–6]

The consequences of chronic renal failure and its treatments for children all potentially influ-

Table 17–1 Common Etiologies of Chronic Renal Failure in Children Younger than 16 Years

Etiology	*Predominant Diagnosis*
Congenital/hereditary	Hypoplasia/dysplasia Obstructive uropathy
Acquired	Chronic glomerulonephritis (GN) Membranoproliferative GN Focal segmental sclerosing GN

Table 17–2 Consequences of Chronic Renal Failure

Water/electrolyte imbalance
Accumulation of endogenous/exogenous toxins
Hypertension
Acidosis
Anemia
Renal osteodystrophy
Anorexia/undernutrition
Need for steroid therapy

ence growth (see Table 17–2). If any of these conditions are left inadequately managed (and each of them is successfully manageable), linear growth of the child will be delayed.[7,8] If properly treated, growth retardation can be arrested; however, catch-up growth is difficult to achieve.

The characteristic symptoms of CRF in children signaling increasing uremia are noted in Table 17–3. Several of those listed, including nausea, growth retardation, swelling, and shortness of breath may respond favorably to dietary modifications.

Despite aggressive attempts at optimizing nutritional intake and preventing renal osteodystrophy, normal growth velocity in children with CRI and end-stage renal disease (ESRD) is unattainable in most cases. However, in 1994, the results of a multicenter study on the use of recombinant human growth hormone (rhGH) demonstrated that improved growth velocity was possible in children receiving 0.05 mg/kg/day of rhGH.[9] Of note is that adequate nutrition and control of renal bone disease continue to be significant therapies in the management of children with CRF.[10]

A recently published series of clinical practice guidelines,[11] sponsored by The National Kidney Foundation, Inc., has provided practitioners invaluable information on ESRD care (hemodialysis, peritoneal dialysis, vascular access, and anemia). The guidelines reflect the insufficient quantity of pediatric research and experience currently available; however, an increasing collection of data by the North American Pediatric Renal Transplant Cooperative Study (NAPRTCS) and several ongoing multicenter studies promise to provide continued expertise for the pediatric practitioner.

Table 17–3 Symptoms of Uremia in Children

Nausea
Weakness
Fatigue
Decreased school performance
Loss of attention span
Growth retardation
Changes in urine output
Shortness of breath
Swelling of face/extremities/abdomen
Amenorrhea in adolescent girls

To summarize, the impact of CRF on growth in children depends on the severity and duration of the renal insufficiency, the diagnosis, and the age of onset. The treatments for CRF, dialysis, and transplantation will affect growth as well.

CONSERVATIVE MANAGEMENT

Treating children with CRF without dialysis requires judicious and frequent monitoring of diet intake, biochemical parameters, and growth.[12] It has long been recognized that renal osteodystrophy contributes significantly to growth retardation in children with renal insufficiency.[13]

Calcium and Phosphorus

Early in the course of renal disease, synthesis of 1,25-dihydroxycholecalciferol (1.25 (OH)2D3) and the excretion of excessive dietary phosphate decrease, leading to the development of renal osteodystrophy and secondary hyperparathyroidism if left untreated. Hyperphosphatemia is considered a late indicator of bone deformities. Current therapy may include any or all of the following: dietary restriction of high-phosphorus foods and fluids (primarily dairy products, chocolate, nuts, and colas), supplementation of vitamin D (1.25 (OH)2D3) and calcium, and the prescription of non–aluminum, non–magnesium-containing phosphate binders (calcium carbonate and/or acetate), to be taken with meals.[14–18]

In infants, PM 60/40 (Ross Products) is the formula of choice, given its preferred calcium/phosphorus ratio of 2:1.[3] However, this formula does contain lactose and may not be tolerated by all infants. A soy-based formula would be indicated for the lactose-intolerant infant. PM 60/40 contains less phosphorus than do the more common infant formulas, and it may be inadequate in providing sufficient phosphorus for the anabolic, growing infant. An inspection of the nutrient content of alternative infant formulas (Carnation Good Start, Similac by Ross Products, and Enfamil by Mead Johnson) should be considered and selection made on a case-by-case basis.[2]

Sodium, Potassium, and Fluid

Sodium and fluid restriction might be necessary to prevent or control the incidence of hypertension and edema not uncommonly associated with CRI. Usually, a no-added-salt diet for height age is sufficient. Limitation of fluid should be based on the child's urine output and insensible losses. Hyperkalemia is rarely a problem, as long as kidney function is greater than 5% of normal. However, should potassium restriction become necessary, limiting high-potassium foods in the diet is generally adequate.

For infants requiring sodium and/or potassium restriction, formulas such as PM 60/40 or Carnation Good Start are appropriate. Furthermore, if the volume of formula must be restricted, it is unlikely that any significant contribution of sodium or potassium will come from formula. To the contrary, infants with increased urine losses of sodium will need some sodium supplementation.

Protein/Energy

Energy needs are at least 80% of the Recommended Dietary Allowance (RDA) for height age[19] and may be greater than 100%. It is generally accepted that protein restriction much below the RDA for height age is contraindicated in growing children. With dietary phosphate restriction alone, a considerable limitation of protein intake could occur without restriction of protein per se. Routine nutritional assessment, including anthropometric measurements and dietary intake, will indicate whether the prescribed protein and calorie levels are adequate.[20]

Infants with CRI without dialysis intervention have been studied at Children's Hospital in Boston, where it was found that the most efficient nitrogen retention occurs when calorie intake ranges between 8 and 11.9 kcal/cm of height and protein intake is maintained at or below 0.15 g/cm of height. This protein intake represented 5–7% of the total calories ingested.[2]

Accomplishing these nutritional goals, particularly in the presence of limited fluid intake (voluntary or involuntary), is possible only by caloric supplementation of the formula to as much as 60 kcal/oz. Increasing caloric density by three times normal dilution requires a methodical approach (Figure 17–1).[21] Attempts should be made to maintain caloric distribution as follows, with the lower intakes of fat calories recommended for children over the age of 2 years:

- Carbohydrate, 35–65%
- Protein, 5–16%
- Fat, 30–55%

Carbohydrate sources such as Polycose (Ross Laboratories, Columbus, Ohio) and Moducal (Mead Johnson) are coupled with an oil (canola, corn oil, or medium-chain triglyceride [MCT] oil for premature infants), as illustrated in Figure 17–2. Concentration of the formula, with or without the addition of a protein supplement such as Promod (Ross Laboratories), increases protein content. Caloric density can be advanced 2–4 kcal/oz, as tolerated.[2]

Ensuring the consistent daily intake of a sufficient volume of formula to meet an infant's nutritional goals for growth most often can be achieved only after the initiation of enteral tube feedings.[20–23] The presence of gastroesophageal reflux in infants with CRI is considered a major factor contributing to feeding problems in this

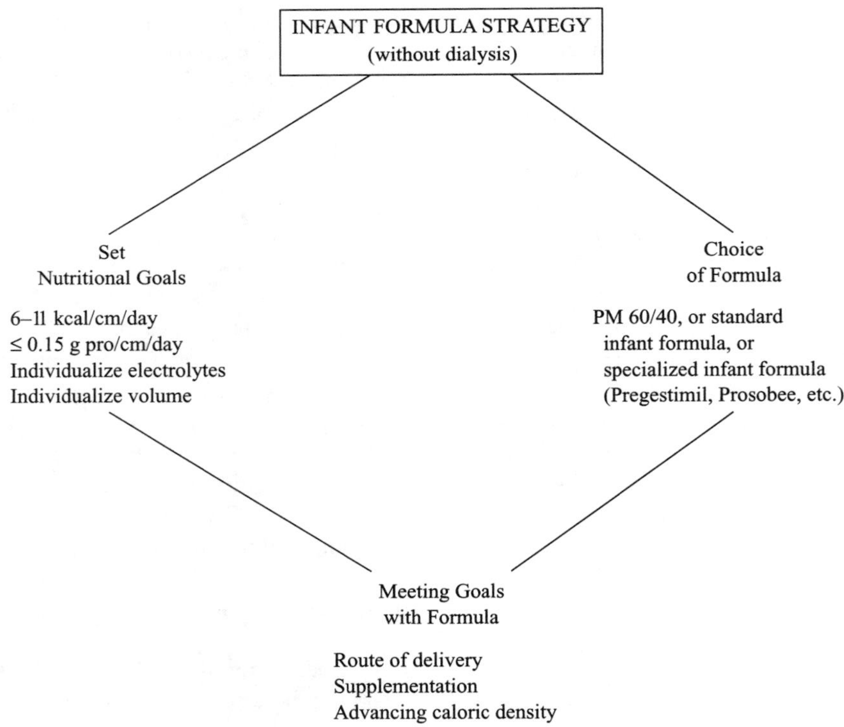

Figure 17–1 Infant Formula Strategy

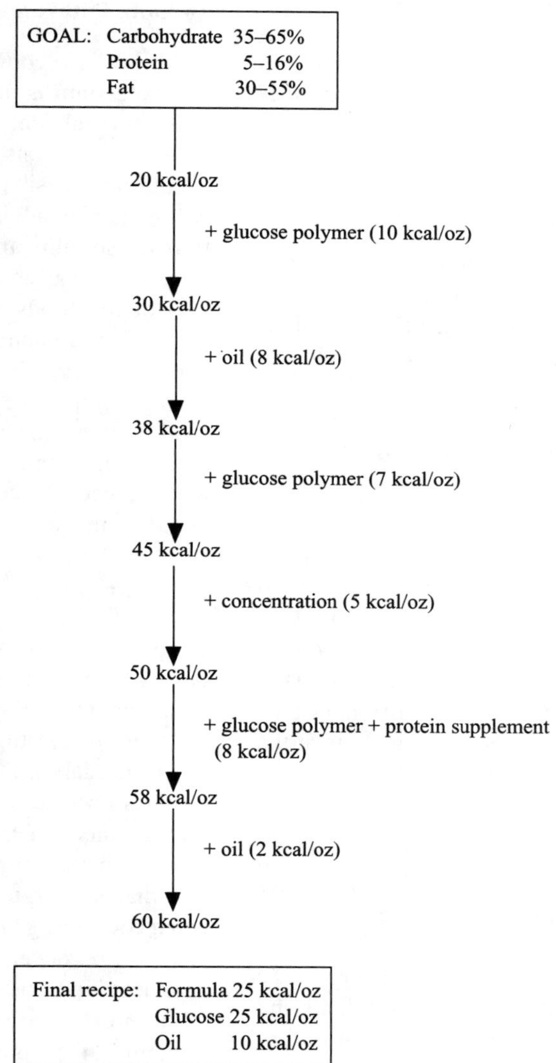

Figure 17–2 Increasing Caloric Density of Formula: An Example. (*Editors' note:* Very low fat intake in children less than 2 years of age may compromise development of the brain and central nervous system.)

age group.[24] However, continuous nighttime infusions of formula via feeding pump allows maximum tolerance of formula.

Once nutritional goals are realized and a feeding regimen established, additional oral stimulation through nonnutritive sucking can begin.[25] In the author's experience, once children are successfully transplanted, they eventually return to normal feeding practices.

Vitamins and Minerals

Because few children with CRI have consistently adequate diets, it is suggested that a multivitamin be routinely recommended. Additionally, 0.5–1.0 mg folic acid should be included. Iron supplementation may be indicated as well, especially if the child is receiving erythropoietin and ferritin, and/or transferrin saturation levels are depressed.[26,27]

Lipids

Hypertriglyceridemia secondary to decreased hepatic lipase activity is common in CRI. Management with carbohydrate restriction is controversial, given the limited caloric intake of many infants and children. Most practitioners currently choose not to restrict carbohydrate at the expense of compromised growth.[28,29]

DIALYSIS

Dialysis is indicated once a child experiences symptoms that significantly interfere with activities of daily living. Peritoneal dialysis (continuous cycling or continuous ambulatory) is the preferred choice of dialytic care for infants and small children. Both hemodialysis and peritoneal dialysis are options for larger children. Nutritional management is dictated by the type of dialytic therapy chosen; however, the principles are similar to those described for conservative management.

Calcium and Phosphorus

Management of calcium and phosphorus balance continues to be necessary even while on dialysis and is the same as that stated previously.

Sodium, Potassium, and Fluid

A child's recommended intake for sodium and potassium is directly related to the child's residual renal function and the type and effectiveness of dialysis. Likewise, the degree of ultrafiltration possible and the child's urine output will dictate an advisable fluid intake. If restriction of sodium and potassium is necessary (which it usually is), the elimination or limitation of the foods containing especially large amounts of sodium and potassium is generally sufficient. Severely restricted diets often encourage noncompliance and dull a child's interest in food. Individualization of diet, taking into consideration the child's food preferences, is essential to successful control of sodium, potassium, and fluid intake.[30,31]

Protein/Energy

The nutritional requirements for protein and energy for patients undergoing peritoneal dialysis are not clear. It is known that some protein is lost to the dialysate, whereas glucose is absorbed from the dialysate. The degree to which these changes occur can be determined only through measurement of individual patients. Periodic calculations of urinary and dialysate urea nitrogen, dialysate protein and amino acids, and miscellaneous nitrogen losses are necessary.[32] Diets can then be developed and altered when measurements indicate the need, promoting growth while preventing obesity.[33] During periods of peritonitis, there is an increased loss of protein to the dialysate, and the child usually feels ill. Careful attention to dietary intake is important to prevent a potentially significant loss of lean body weight during this time of infection.

Protein and energy requirements for children on hemodialysis have been studied using urea kinetic modeling as well as actual nitrogen balance techniques.[34,35] It was concluded that a protein intake of 0.3 g/cm/day and an energy intake of 10 kcal/cm/day produced positive nitrogen balance. The protein catabolic and urea generation rates of the children in positive balance were uniformly lower; therefore, there was no increase necessary in dialysis requirements with these levels of intake.

The routine use of urea kinetic modeling is especially helpful in determining dialysis and nutritional adequacy in children.[36,37] Monthly monitoring of protein catabolic rates and urea generation provide insight into subtle changes in dialysis treatment and/or diet intake that otherwise might go unnoticed. Kinetic modeling, usually conducted by the dietitian, allows the dietitian access to the fundamental parameters and concepts of dialysis prescription, ensuring maximum confidence in the nutrition counseling of patients.

Lipids

Hyperlipidemia remains a problem in children on dialysis.[38] Treatment with carbohydrate restriction or carnitine supplementation remains controversial.

Vitamins

It is advisable that children on either hemodialysis and peritoneal dialysis be provided water-soluble vitamins and folate, which are lost to dialysate.[39] Although studies have not been conducted in children, it is current practice to provide 1 mg folate, 5–10 mg vitamin B_6, and up to 100 mg ascorbic acid per day. Additional water-soluble vitamins should be given according to the RDAs for height age.[12] There are specially formulated dialysis vitamin preparations on the market (Nephro-Vite Rx by R&D Laboratories, Marina del Rey, California, and Nephrocaps by Fleming & Co., Fenton, Missouri) that fulfill most patients' needs. Infants can be given a standard liquid multivitamin, such as Polyvisol by Mead Johnson, and young children can take a flavored chewable multivitamin; however, both should be accompanied by folate.

TRANSPLANTATION

The ultimate goal of all pediatric ESRD programs is transplantation. This is the only treatment option thus far that provides children with the opportunity for normal growth and development, and potentially for catch-up growth.[40] Clinicians must be constantly vigilant for signs of rejection and infection, especially in the first postoperative year. Immunosuppression and antibiotic therapy result in side effects related to inefficient digestion and metabolism of nutrients, as well as to growth retardation.[41] Alternate-day steroid therapy has been shown to promote normal and, at times, catch-up growth. The medical course of the patient and the individual transplant program's protocol for immunosuppression will dictate just how quickly a patient can begin alternate-day dosing. The usual immunosuppressive medications prescribed today include azathiaprine, prednisone, cyclosporine, and FK506; OKT3 and antilymphocyte globulin are used as short-term therapies.

For small children receiving adult kidneys, it is advisable that parenteral nutrition be considered immediately postoperatively, due to the likelihood of ileus developing from the manipulation of bowel necessary to accommodate an adult kidney into a small body cavity.

Once feedings are resumed, the dietary recommendations are once again individualized. If kidney function is not normal, attention to sodium, potassium, phosphorus, and fluid will be necessary. A rise in blood urea nitrogen (BUN) level and a slow recovery to normal is usual, even with normal kidney function, due to the catabolic stress of surgery. If it is possible, aggressive nutritional support of the patient should resume soon after transplant.[42]

With the attainment of normal kidney function, a no-added-salt diet is still advisable.[43] Hypertension, now a potential result of high-dose steroid therapy, is frequently seen after transplantation, and sodium restriction, at least during the acute phase (first 6–8 months after transplant), is helpful. Also, tubular loss of phosphate is often present, requiring phosphorus supplementation. Dietary phosphorus intake usually is not adequate to maintain blood levels above 3.0 mg/dL.

Finally, children may develop steroid-induced hypoglycemia, requiring a no-concentrated-sweets diet. Occasionally, insulin is indicated. However, because hyperglycemia in the transplanted patient is due to insulin resistance and is usually a temporary situation while steroids are at their highest dosage, it is current practice not to attempt tight control of blood sugar. Rather, fasting sugars within the 200–300 range are acceptable. At this point, a diabetic diet (eg, one with a designated caloric level using commercially recognized exchanges of food groups and portion size) should begin (see Chapter 20).

Perhaps the most important aspect of the diet at this time is instruction in appropriate portion sizes. Most children have never learned to eat

Table 17–4 Major Nutritional Considerations

Nutrient	*Indication for Treatment*	*Modification*
Phosphorus	CRI, elevated parathormone level, elevated alkaline phosphatase level, with or without hyperphosphatemia	Phosphate binders; low-phosphate diet; calcium and vitamin D supplement
	Posttransplant tubular loss; hypophosphatemia	Add supplement
Sodium	Hypertension; fluid retention	↓
	Daily steroid therapy	↓
	Increased urine losses	↑
	Increased peritoneal dialysate losses	↑
Potassium	< 5% GFR; hyperkalemia	↓
	Diuretic therapy; hypokalemia (peritoneal dialysis or posttransplant losses; diarrhea)	↑
Protein	Infants with CRI (no dialysis)	≤ 0.15 g/cm/d
	Children with CRI (no dialysis)	Limit to RDA for height age
	Children on hemodialysis	≤ 0.30 g/cm/d
	Infants/children on peritoneal dialysis	Usually ↑
	Posttransplant	RDA for height age
Energy	Undernutrition/anorexia	80% RDA for height age
	Infants with CRI (no dialysis)	6–11.9 kcal/cm/d
	Children on hemodialysis	10 kcal/cm/d
	Dextrose absorption from peritoneal dialysate	Varies depending on absorption
	Posttransplant steroid therapy	Varies depending on dose
	Steroid-induced hyperglycemia	No concentrated sweets

nutritionally balanced meals. Additionally, the increased appetite accompanying prednisone therapy should be manipulated in a positive, healthy fashion before a taste develops for high-carbohydrate, high-fat foods. It is common to hear parents describe the mealtimes of their newly transplanted children as lasting all day, with one meal overlapping another.

Once steroids are tapered to levels where hypertension and hyperglycemia are no longer problematic, a diet appropriate for height age is indicated. Continued assessment of nutritional adequacy of the diet is necessary, even with normal kidney function.

CONCLUSION

The nutritional intake of the child is especially important to ensure optimal growth and development during all stages of renal disease. The diet must be adequate and consistent. This is no easy task, in light of the symptomatology accompanying the disease. Anorexia and taste changes commonly associated with CRF[44,45] constantly challenge attempts to promote optimal nutritional care. Additionally, dietary modification (see Table 17–4) and implementation must be individualized for all age groups, taking into account developmental levels, growth potentials, and renal functional limitations. Input from the entire renal team at all times is critical to ensuring successful nutritional management of this population. Frequent evaluation of food intake, growth, kidney function, and developmental stages is essential to adequate care.

REFERENCES

1. Fine RN. Growth in children with renal insufficiency. In: Nissenson A, Fine RN, Gentile D, eds. *Clinical Dialysis.* Norwalk, CT: Appleton-Century Crofts; 1984: 661.
2. Spinozzi NS, Nelson P. Nutrition support in the newborn intensive care unit. *J Renal Nutr*. 1996;6:188–197.
3. Wassner SJ, Abitol C, Alexander S, et al. Nutritional requirements for infants with renal failure. *Am J Kidney Dis.* 1986;7:300–305.
4. Betts PR, White RHR. Growth potential and skeletal maturity in children with chronic renal insufficiency. *Nephron*. 1976;16:325–332.
5. Broyer M. Growth in children with renal insufficiency. *Pediatr Clin North Am*. 1982;29:991–1003.
6. Rizzoni G, Broyer M, Guest G, et al. Growth retardation in children with chronic renal disease: scope of the problem. *Am J Kidney Dis*. 1986;7:256–261.
7. Rizzoni G, Basso T, Setari M. Growth in children with chronic renal failure on conservative treatment. *Kidney Int*. 1984;26:52–58.
8. Kleinknecht C, Broyer M, Hout D, et al. Growth and development of nondialyzed children with chronic renal failure. *Kidney Int*. 1983;24(S15):40–47.
9. Fine RN, Kohout EC, Brown D, Perlman AJ. Growth after recombinant human growth hormone treatment in children with chronic renal failure: Report of a multicenter randomized double-blind placebo-controlled study. *J Pediatr*. 1994;124:374–382.
10. Berard E, Crosnier H, Six-Beneton A, et al. Recombinant human growth hormone treatment of children on hemodialysis. *Pediatr Nephrol*. 1998;12:304–310.
11. Dialysis Outcomes Quality Initiative: *Clinical Practice Guidelines*. New York: National Kidney Foundation; 1997.
12. Hellerstein S, Holliday MA, Grupe WE, et al. Nutritional management of children with chronic renal failure. *Pediatr Nephrol*. 1987;1:195–211.
13. Salusky IB, Goodman WG. The management of renal osteodystrophy. *Pediatr Nephrol*. 1996;10:651–653.
14. Brookhyser J, Pahre SN. Dietary and pharmacotherapeutic considerations in the management of renal osteodystrophy. *Adv Renal Replacement Ther*. 1995;2:5–13.
15. Tamanah K, Mak RH, Rigden SP, et al. Long-term suppression of hyperparathyroidism by phosphate binders in uremic children. *Pediatr Nephrol*. 1987;1:145–149.
16. Schiller LR, Santa Ana CA, Sheikh MS, et al. Effect of the time of administration of calcium acetate on phosphorus binding. *N Engl J Med*. 1989; 320: 1110–1113.
17. Schmitt, J. Selecting an appropriate phosphate binder. *J Renal Nutr*. 1990;1:38–40.
18. Salusky IB, Goodman WG. The management of renal osteodystrophy. *Pediatr Nephrol*. 1996;10:651–653.
19. Betts PR, Macgrath G. Growth pattern and dietary intake of children with chronic renal insufficiency. *Br Med J*. 1974;2:189.
20. Stover J, Nelson P. Nutritional recommendations for infants, children and adolescents with ESRD. In: Gillit D, Stover J, Spinozzi NS, eds. *A Clinical Guide to Nutritional Care in ESRD*. Chicago: American Dietetic Association; 1987:71–94.

21. Yiu VWY, Harmon WE, Spinozzi NS, et al. High-calorie nutrition for infants with chronic renal disease. *J Renal Nutr.* 1996;6:203–206.
22. Brewer ED. Supplemental enteral tube feeding in infants undergoing dialysis: Indications and outcome. *Semin Dial.* 1994;7:429–434.
23. Reed EE, Roy LP, Gaskin KJ, Knight JF. Nutritional intervention and growth in children with chronic renal failure. *J Renal Nutr.* 1998;8:122–126.
24. Ruley EJ, Boch GH, Kerzner B, Abbott AW. Feeding disorders and gastroesophageal reflux in infants with chronic renal failure. *Pediatr Nephrol.* 1989;3:424–429.
25. Bebaum JC, Pererra GR, Watkins JB, et al. Non-nutritive sucking during gavage feeding enhances growth and maturation in premature infants. *Pediatrics.* 1983;71:41–45.
26. Eschbach MD, Egrie JC, Downing MR, et al. Correction of the anemia of end-stage renal disease with recombinant human erythropoietin. *N Engl J Med.* 1987;310:73–78.
27. Van Wyck DB, Stivelman JC, Ruiz J. Iron status in patients receiving erythropoietin for dialysis-associated anemia. *Kidney Int.* 1989;35:712–716.
28. Arnold WC, Danford D, Holliday MC. Effects of calorie supplementation on growth in children with uremia. *Kidney Int.* 1983;24:205.
29. Betts PR, Magrath G, White RHR. Role of dietary energy supplementation in growth of children with chronic renal insufficiency. *Br Med J.* 1977;1:416.
30. Wolfson M. Nutritional management of the continuous ambulatory peritoneal patient. *Am J Kidney Dis.* 1996;27:744–749.
31. Salusky IB. The nutritional approach for pediatric patients undergoing CAPD/CCPD. *Adv Perit Dialysis.* 1990;6:249–251.
32. Schleifer CR, Teehan BP, Brown JM, Raimondo J. The application of urea kinetic modeling to peritoneal dialysis: A review of methodology and outcome. *J Renal Nutr.* 1993;3:2–9.
33. Harvey E, Secker D, Braj B, Picone G, Balfe JW. The team approach to the management of children on chronic peritoneal dialysis. *Adv Renal Replacement Ther.* 1996;3:3–13.
34. Spinozzi NS, Grupe WE. Nutritional implications of renal disease. *J Am Diet Assoc.* 1977;70:493–497.
35. Grupe WE, Harmon WE, Spinozzi NS. Protein and energy requirements in children receiving chronic hemodialysis. *Kidney Int.* 1983;24:S6–S10.
36. Harmon WE, Spinozzi NS, Meyer A, Grupe WE. The use of protein catabolic rate to monitor pediatric hemodialysis. *Dial Transplant.* 1981;10:324.
37. Grupe WE, Spinozzi NS, Harmon WE. Nutritional assessment of hemodialysis in children using urea kinetics. In: Brodehl J, Ehrich JHH, eds. *Pediatric Nephrology: Proceedings of the Sixth International Symposium of Paediatric Nephrology.* Berlin, Germany: Springer-Verlag; 1984:86–91.
38. Querfeld U, Salusky IB, Nelson P, et al. Hyperlipidemia in pediatric patients undergoing peritoneal dialysis. *Pediatr Nephrol.* 1988;2:447–452.
39. Warady BA, Kriley M, Alon U, Hellerstein S. Vitamin status of infants receiving long-term peritoneal dialysis. *Pediatr Nephrol.* 1994;8:354–356.
40. Inglefinger JR, Grupe WE, Harmon WE, et al. Growth acceleration following renal transplantation in children less than 7 years of age. *Pediatrics.* 1981;68:255–259.
41. Neu AM, Warady BA. Dialysis and renal transplantation in infants with irreversible renal failure. *Adv Renal Replacement Ther.* 1996;3:48–59.
42. Seagraves A, Moore EE, Moore FA, et al. Net protein catabolic rate after kidney transplantation: impact of corticosteroid immunosuppression. *J Parenter Enteral Nutr.* 1986;10:453–455.
43. Gammarino M. Renal transplant diet: recommendations for the acute phase. *Dial Transplant.* 1987;16:497.
44. Spinozzi NS, Murray CL, Grupe WE. Altered taste acuity in children with ESRD. *Pediatr Res* (abstract). 1978;12:442.
45. Shapera MR, Moel DI, Kamath SK, et al. Taste perception of children with chronic renal failure. *J Am Diet Assoc.* 1986;86:1359–1365.

CHAPTER 18

Failure to Thrive

Kattia M. Corrales and Sherri L. Utter

INTRODUCTION

Failure to thrive (FTT) is a serious condition of undernutrition and poor growth usually identified in the first 3 years of life. Inadequate nutrient intake is central to the pathogenesis of FTT because growth deficiency in a child is essentially the result of not taking, not being offered, or not retaining adequate calories.[1] The etiology of FTT has historically been classified as either organic (OFTT) or nonorganic (NOFTT). OFTT indicates malnutrition due to an underlying medical condition causing inadequate intake, absorption, or utilization of nutrients. NOFTT suggests a social or behavioral dysfunction leading to inadequate oral intake (Exhibit 18–1). However, a dichotomous classification is often inappropriate, because many children with FTT will present with both physiologic and psychosocial conditions that inhibit their growth. The development and progression of FTT involves a complex and multifactorial process influenced by several factors, including the infant's medical status and temperament, as well as familial, economic, and psychosocial conditions. A multidisciplinary team, including a pediatrician, child psychologist or behaviorist, dietitian, nurse clinician, and social worker is often most effective in the treatment of FTT.[2-4]

DIAGNOSTIC CRITERIA AND EVALUATION OF GROWTH

Despite the common use of the term, an exact and consistent method for identifying FTT has not been established.[5] FTT is defined by both anthropometry and by diagnostic criteria related to the etiology of undernutrition. The important issue, however, is not the terminology used to define it, but the choice of growth indices.[5] FTT is typically defined as growth that deviates from the norms established by the National Center for Health Statistics (NCHS) growth charts. (These charts are recommended for use, regardless of race or ethnic origin.)[6] Weight, height, and head circumference are plotted to obtain percentiles for weight for age, height for age, head circumference for age, and weight for height. The following methods are commonly used as cut-off points to identify growth failure:

1. Growth below a specified percentile on the growth chart:
   - Weight for age plotting less than the fifth percentile in the absence of constitutional delay
   - Weight for height plotting less than the fifth percentile
2. Poor growth velocity:
   - Decreased growth velocity where weight drops more than two major percentiles over 3–6 months.

Exhibit 18–1 Risk Factors for Failure to Thrive

Organic Factors

Inability to take in adequate calories

- Difficulty with sucking, mastication, swallowing
- Neurologic disease
- Systemic disease resulting in anorexia/food refusal

Inability to retain/utilize adequate calories

- Persistent vomiting
- Gastroesophageal reflux
- Rumination syndrome
- Malabsorprtion/maldigestion
  - Inflammatory bowel disease, celiac disease, short gut syndrome, cystic fibrosis, HIV
- Poor nutrient utilization
  - Renal tubular acidosis, inborn errors of metabolism

Increased calorie requirements

- Congenital heart disease
- Brochopulmonary dysplasia
- Fevers
- Hyperthyroidism

Altered growth potential

- Perinatal complications
  - Prematurity, intrauterine growth retardation, exposure to drugs/toxins
- Congenital anomalies
- Chromosomal abnormalities
- Endocrinopathies
  - Growth hormone deficiency, hypothyroidism, hypercortisolism

Nonorganic Factors

Inability to provide adequate calories

- Poverty
- Inadequate breast milk production

Psychosocial issues

- Disordered feeding environment
- Dysfunctional parent–child interaction
  - Behavioral feeding problem, neglect, abuse, sickly/difficult child, isolated/overwhelmed mother, emotionally/physically unavailable father
- Stress and loss in the social environment
  - Marital stress, family history of death and loss, chronic illness, poverty

Lack of knowledge/misinformation regarding feeding practices

- Errors in formula preparation
- Excessive juice consumption
- Misperceptions about diet and feeding practices
- Unusual health and nutrition beliefs

Source: Data from references: 16, 21, 22, 32, 70, and 74.

- Decrease of more than 2 standard deviations over a 3- to 6-month period

Evaluation of growth

It is best to assess the progression of growth longitudinally when evaluating for FTT. A single point on the growth chart does not provide information about a child's growth pattern or deviation from previously established growth channels. Although normal shifting of percentiles for linear growth may occur during the first 2 years of life,[7] a weight decrease of more than two major percentiles from a previously established growth channel should be considered evidence of growth failure.[8,9] Edwards et al[10] found that the maximum weight percentile achieved by a child between 4 and 8 weeks of age is a better predictor of the percentile at 12 months than is the birth weight percentile. They propose that FTT be defined as a weight deviation of two or more major percentiles below the maximum weight percentile achieved by 4–8 weeks for a period of a month or more.[10]

Weight for age should not be used as the single measure for identifying FTT because some children are both underweight and short, relative to reference standards (weight for age and height for age less than the 5th percentile), but have weight for height ratios within the normal range. These children may be genetically small, be demonstrating constitutional growth delay, or they have suffered a nutritional insult earlier in life, yet not be acutely malnourished or showing a weight for height deficit.[11–13] Genetic short stature can be evaluated by determining the midparental height (average height of both parents at any time between 25 and 45 years of age) using the Tanner-Whitehouse charts,[14] assuming, of course, that the parents grew normally and realized their true growth potential. Bone age can be determined to help differentiate stunting from genetic short stature.[15,16] If bone age lags behind chronologic age and equals height age, this suggests the child has room to make additional gains in height. In genetic short stature bone age typically equals chronologic age.

Premature and small-for-gestational-age (SGA) infants are generally small at birth, relative to reference standards, but exhibit different patterns of growth in infancy and early childhood.[12,17] Potential for catch-up growth in high-risk infants varies with birth weight, degree of prematurity, severity of perinatal medical illness, and ponderal index classification, which reflects timing and duration of intrauterine growth retardation.[12,18] Premature infants without serious medical problems and asymmetric SGA infants (where birth weight is disproportionately more depressed than length or head circumference) are capable of significant catch-up growth in the first 6–9 months of life.[18–20] Nutritional therapy should support maximal growth rates during this period. Symmetrical SGA infants (where weight, height, and head circumference are equally depressed) have a poorer prognosis for catch-up growth, despite treatment. All growth parameters are affected in these infants, suggesting chronic growth retardation early in gestation.[19,21,22] With adequate nutrition, their growth rates should parallel reference curves.[16] Guidelines for the assessment and nutritional management of premature and SGA infants appear in Chapter 3.

When plotting the measurements of premature infants on growth charts, the age at measurement should be corrected. Corrected age is chronologic age less the number of weeks the child was premature (ie, the difference between 40 weeks and gestational age). Severity of growth deficit in premature infants will be overestimated if uncorrected ages are used to analyze anthropometric data. Measurements should be corrected for prematurity until the age of 18 months for head circumference, 24 months for weight, and 3.5 years for height.[1]

Breastfed infants gain weight in a different pattern than the mostly formula-fed infants used to establish the NCHS growth charts.[12] Breastfed infants gain weight more slowly after the first 3 months of life and may be leaner between 4 to 18 months.[23] Therefore, due to their normally slower growth velocity, breastfed infants may appear to be faltering after 2–3 months when their measurements are plotted on the NCHS growth charts.

CLASSIFICATION OF SEVERITY OF UNDERNUTRITION

Gomez and Waterlow Criteria

Determining that a child is at or below the fifth percentile on the growth chart can help to identify a growth problem but does not relate the severity of undernutrition. Degree of undernutrition can be determined using criteria established by Gomez and Waterlow[24,25] that compare actual weight and/or height with the expected standard (at the 50th percentile on the NCHS growth chart) (Table 18–1). These criteria are divided into four levels of degree of undernutrition: normal, mild, moderate, and severe. The Gomez[24] criteria evaluate weight for age but do not account for stature; thus, a child who is short in stature but at an appropriate weight for height may appear underweight. The Waterlow[25] criteria take into account both weight and height. Weight for height is evaluated as an index of wasting due to acute undernutrition. Height for age is evaluated as an index of stunting due to chronic undernutrition.

Standard Deviation

The standard deviation (SD) score, also called the *Z score*, is useful in expressing how far a child's weight and height fall from the median, or 50th percentile, on the reference growth charts for children of the same age and sex.[26]

$$Z = \frac{\text{measurement value} - \text{median for age value of reference population}}{\text{standard deviation for age of reference population}}$$

Categorizing growth according to progressive decrements in SD scores (–2.0, –3.0, –4.0) can be used to describe the relative severity of undernutrition. Percentiles and equivalent SD scores for weight for age, height for age, and weight for height can be easily calculated using computer software developed by the Centers for Disease Control (CDC) and the World Health Organization (WHO).[27] A SD of zero is equivalent to the 50th percentile; –1.65 SD corresponds to the 5th percentile cut-off used in the National Nutrition Surveillance System. The WHO recommends that a cut-off point of –2.0 SD below the NCHS reference median weight for age, height for age, and weight for height be used to discriminate between well-nourished and poorly nourished children.[28] When compared over time,

Table 18–1 Classification of Severity of Undernutrition

	Gomez Criteria	*Waterlow Criteria*	
Grade of Malnutrition	*Percent of Median Weight for Age (Underweight)*	*Percent of Median Weight for Height (Wasting)*	*Percent of Median Height for Age (Stunting)*
Normal	90–110	90–110	≥ 95
I. Mild	75–89	80–89	90–94
II. Moderate	60–74	70–79	85–89
III. Severe	<60	< 70	< 85

Source: Data from references 24 and 25.

a positive change in SD indicates growth, whereas a negative change indicates a slowing of the growth rate. Categorizing growth in this manner is the most accurate technique for classifying growth deficits in children and is the preferred method by the WHO but proves more difficult in the clinical setting without the necessary software.[19]

Anthropometry

Essentially, growth is the desired final outcome in FTT. Consistent and accurate technique in measuring growth parameters is imperative. Routine use of upper arm measurements may not be indicated but may be useful, especially in the malnourished child with edema. Triceps skinfolds and midarm muscle circumference may provide a better index of nutritional status than does the weight for height measurement because the arm is relatively free of edema.[29] Techniques for obtaining accurate anthropometric data are covered in Chapter 2.

MEDICAL EVALUATION

A complete medical history and physical examination are necessary to assess possible organic causes leading to FTT. Exhibit 18–2 provides guidelines for obtaining information to assess the FTT patient. A variety of medical conditions, especially those chronic in nature, can result in poor weight gain. A child should be evaluated for possible gastrointestinal symptoms, such as vomiting and diarrhea; recurrent infections; medication use; and previous hospitalizations. Because perinatal factors exert a powerful influence on patterns of postnatal growth, the perinatal history should be investigated. A family history should also be obtained to evaluate for chronic illnesses, mental illness, parental height, and growth pattern of siblings. The physical examination should evaluate for dysmorphic features to identify syndromes that may be associated with poor growth, gross motor skills and tone, as well as signs of neglect or abuse.

Because poor nutrition and psychosocial factors are the most frequent causes of FTT, laboratory testing is rarely warranted unless findings on the history and physical examination indicate a need.[30,31] A few screening tests may be useful. Screening for lead toxicity and anemia should be considered because approximately 50% of children with FTT present with iron deficiency, and lead intoxication can result in poor growth.[15,32,33] Nutritional status can be further evaluated with serum protein tests, such as those for albumin and prealbumin. Alkaline phosphatase can be checked to evaluate for rickets (elevated) or zinc deficiency (depressed). Zinc deficiency has been implicated in poor growth.[19,34] Urinalysis, serum electrolytes, blood urea nitrogen, and creatinine levels can help evaluate for infection or renal dysfunction. If stool patterns are abnormal, the stool can be checked for pH, reducing substances, ova, parasites, or occult blood to evaluate for possible infection, malabsorption, or allergy.

PSYCHOSOCIAL EVALUATION

Poverty and Familial Stress

Although FTT can occur in any socioeconomic group,[35] incidence is especially high in urban and rural families living in poverty.[19,36,37] Rates of poverty have not decreased significantly since the 1970s and appear to be more prevalent in African American and Latino children and in children of single-parent families. It is estimated that one-third of all children living in the United States live in poverty for at least 1 year.[38] Poverty has been and continues to be a significant contributor to FTT as it not only limits resources, such as food, shelter, and access to medical care, but also can compound already existing familial stress.

Parental stress and marital discord have been significantly correlated with FTT.[39] Parental depression or intellectual impairment, drug abuse, and social isolation, especially in regard to a mother with poor support from extended family or from the child's father,[40] have also been asso-

Exhibit 18–2 Guidelines for the Assessment of Failure to Thrive

Health History	*Clinical Exam*	*Biochemical Data* *
Individual:	Nausea, vomiting	Hematocrit (Hct)
Gestational age	Diarrhea, steatorrhea, or constipation	Hemaglobin (Hgb)
Birth weight	Stool size, frequency, consistency, color, odor	Urinalysis (SG, pH)
Type of delivery/APGAR scores/complications	Clinical manifestations of malnutrition	Erythrocyte sedimentation rate
Prenatal history	Rumination	Electrolytes
Growth history/pattern	Signs of abuse or neglect	Albumin
Activity level/energy	Poor oral health, diaper rash, general hygiene	Prealbumin
Developmental milestones	Accurate anthropometrics	Blood urea nitrogen/creatinine
Illness (including acute/recurring/chronic)	Dysmorphic features	Lead (Pb)
Hospitalizations (accidents/injuries/surgeries)	Gross motor skills and tone	Alkaline phosphatase
Medications	Developmental assessment	Urine culture
		Stool for pH, reducing substances, ova, parasites, occult blood
Family:		Sweat test
Mental illness		TB test
Alcohol/drug abuse		
Genetic disorder		* Laboratory testing should be limited to screening tests or those indicated by findings on the history and physical.
Chronic or metabolic disorder		
Eating disorder		
Parental height		
Growth and development of siblings		
Maternal age		

Social History	Nutrition History	Caregiver–Child Interaction
Multiple caregivers	24-hour recall/3–5 day food record	Evidence of bonding (richness of interaction, eye and physical contact, sense of mutual pleasure, warmth and affection, consistency of response)
Support systems available to caregiver	Formula/Breastfeeding history	Caregiver's attentiveness to child's cues
Maturity of caregiver	Formula preparation	Appropriateness of caregiver's expectations
Social environment (marital dissatisfaction, financial stress, disorganized lifestyle)	History of food allergies/intolerances	Clarity of child's cues to caregiver
History of abuse or neglect of child, sibling, or caregivers	Food restrictions/special diets	Caregiver's tolerance level
Socioeconomic status	Age at introduction of solids/acceptance	Appropriateness of caregiver's expectations
Perception of problem by caregivers	Amount of juice, soda, water and/or milk consumed	
Involvement in public programs (EIP, WIC, Food Stamps)	Meal time/snacks (who feeds, where, duration)	
History of loss	Self-feeding skill	
	Difficulty chewing/swallowing/sucking	
	Cues for hunger/satiety	
	Rewards/punishments	
	Feeding behavior/environment	

Source: Data from references 21, 22, 32, and 70.

ciated with growth failure[19,36,41–44] Familial stress is a risk factor in FTT because it can impair a parent's ability to perceive and provide for a child's emotional and physiologic needs. A parent who is in ill health, depressed, experiencing economic problems, or abusing drugs may not be able to respond to a child's hunger cues or to provide a stable home environment.[19] A history of neglect and abuse in the parent's own childhood, as well as signs of present abuse in the FTT child, should always be explored in the evaluation of these cases. Whereas child abuse may not make up a significant number of FTT cases,[45,46] one study found that a surprising 80% of mothers of children with FTT had experienced child abuse in their own childhood. Withholding of food[47] and death by suspicious circumstances[44] have been reported in the FTT literature.

PARENT–CHILD INTERACTIONS

Children with growth failure have been described as temperamental, lethargic, passive, and developmentally and physically immature.[1,42] They may be apathetic and hypervigilant, and may demonstrate delays in cognitive and motor development.[48] They may have sleeping and elimination difficulties; be overly sensitive to stimulation; and exhibit oppositional behavior, defiance, and clingingness.[22,40] Feeding difficulties, which are prevalent in this population, may present in the form of abnormal duration of feeding time, poor appetite, delayed tolerance to different food textures, and deviant food behavior.[49,50] The child, as a result, may be viewed as difficult and sickly, and the caretaker may feel incompetent in parenting. The end result is a breakdown in the parent–child relationship.

Whether aberrant behavior is inherent in the child or is the child's reaction to familial stress is not entirely clear. Ramsay et al[49] found that many feeding skill disorders in FTT children were present at birth. They argued that these could be the result of a neurophysiologic process manifested by oral sensorimotor impairment of varying degrees, ranging from mild, in the case of the healthy-looking child with NOFTT, to severe, in the case of the child with cerebral palsy.[49] However, the role of parent–infant interactions in the development of feeding disorders has also been extensively explored.[40,47,51,52] Chatoor et al[52] describe a developmental model that can help explain the complex interrelationship between parent and child resulting in feeding disorders.[52] They describe three stages of child development at which adaptive and maladaptive feeding behaviors can occur:

1. Disorders of homeostasis are thought to develop during the first 2 months of life when the child attempts to reach a balance between internal and external states and to form the basic rhythms of sleep, wakefulness, feeding, and elimination. For example, a child with congenital abnormalities, who may have delayed introduction and advancement of feedings or limited interaction with caregivers, may not achieve a balance between internal state and environmental limits. A parent who is unable to offer a stable environment for the child or to attend to the infant's cues on hunger, satiety, and emotional needs can contribute to disorders of homeostasis.
2. During the attachment phase, which begins between 2 and 6 months of age, the infant begins to interact with his or her environment in a more complex manner. At this stage of mutual interaction, a variety of factors can contribute to attachment disorders, including poor parenting skills, social isolation, and economic hardship, as well as a temperamental or overly sensitive infant who has difficulties in establishing normal patterns of sleep and eating. Because most interactions between infant and caregiver at this stage revolve around feeding, it is not surprising that a history of vomiting, diarrhea, and poor weight gain are common presenting features in poorly

attached children. Fleisher et al[53] go on to argue that vomiting and rumination disorders in children may often be directly related to psychosocial issues. If these issues are missed, invasive and unnecessary medical intervention may occur.[53]

3. During the separation and individuation stage, which typically occurs between 6 months and 3 years of age, the child begins to deal with issues of autonomy and independence.[48] The child also begins to differentiate between somatophysiologic states, such as hunger, satiety, anger, frustration, and the need for affection. Separation disorders are thought to be related to the child's need for autonomy and the parent's inability to "let go." As the parent becomes more anxious about the child's eating, the child becomes more willful about gaining independence. Specific problems include a child who refuses to sit for meals, displays excessive aversion to different food textures or mixed foods, or is actively resistant to being fed.[48,51] A parent who force-feeds, coaxes with toys or other distractions to get the child to eat, or does not accept messes at meals contributes to the poor feeding situation.

NUTRITION EVALUATION

Diet History

A complete diet history should be obtained to identify both nutritional and behavioral problems in feeding. Information about amounts and types of food eaten, food textures, portion sizes, and timing of feedings should be obtained. A 24-hour-diet recall or, if possible, a 3- to 7-day food record can be used to gather this information. Questions during the diet history should also address the child's feeding capacities, including the preferred duration and pace of feeding, the child's ability to remain focused on feeding, and the child's readiness or ability to self-feed. Guidelines for general nutrition assessment are described in Chapter 2. Exhibit 18–2 provides guidelines for the assessment of failure to thrive.

The most common mistake in formula preparation is improper dilution of formula, usually either secondary to a poor understanding of proper preparation or a parent's attempt to preserve formula due to financial concerns.[1] Polydipsia, polyuria, and a voracious appetite have been described as indications of an overly diluted formula.[45] Overly concentrated formula, on the other hand, can lead to early satiety, vomiting, or diarrhea and a subsequent net loss in nutrients.[21] Another commonly identified problem in formula preparation is the addition of large quantities of cereal or baby food to the bottle, which displaces nutrients such as protein and fat.

In the breastfed child, poor weight gain may result from an inadequate milk supply, poor maternal diet, inadequate let-down reflex, infrequent or short feedings, milk-suppressing medications, a sick baby, or a baby with a poor suck.[45] Exclusive breast feeding beyond 6 months of age without the introduction of solids can limit nutrient intake and inhibit the development of feeding milestones.[54,55]

Large amounts of juice, as well as other sugary beverages or water, can displace consumption of more nutrient-dense foods and be detrimental to growth.[56,57] Excessive juice consumption (>12–16 oz per day) has also been associated with malabsorption and diarrhea in children.[58] A reduction or complete removal of juice from the child's diet may result in weight gain.

Finally, parental health beliefs and misconceptions about what constitutes a healthy diet for infants and children should be explored in the diet history. For example, a history of heart disease or obesity in the family, or simply the pursuit of a "healthy diet" may induce parents to limit sweets, fats, and food portions in their children's diets, even when children are not growing properly.[54,59] Vegetarian diets may not provide adequate amounts of several nutrients required for growth, such as protein, calcium, iron, vitamin B_{12}, riboflavin, and zinc.[60,61]

Caregivers should be instructed on ways to make these diets more appropriate. Chapter 7 provides more information regarding vegetarian diets in children.

ASSESSMENT OF THE DIET

The caloric content of the diet must be compared with the child's specific needs for growth to evaluate whether the usual intake is inadequate. Protein, calcium, zinc, and iron intake should also be evaluated. The Recommended Dietary Allowances (RDAs) and the Recommended Daily Intakes (RDIs) can be used for this assessment (see Chapter 2 and Appendix K). Children with increased metabolic needs from chronic illness or increased losses from vomiting, diarrhea, or malabsorption may have nutritional needs different from the RDAs or RDIs.

Feeding Observation

Particular attention should be paid to behavioral factors that may lead to inadequate caloric intake. A feeding observation can be extremely helpful in identifying parent–infant interactions, as well as particular problems with feeding. Feeding observations can be done in the clinic or hospital setting but are more informative if done in the home. Particular points to note during a feeding observation are detailed in Exhibit 18–3. Several practical checklists have been developed specifically to assist in the observation of feeding interactions in NOFTT.[62,63]

Nutritional Therapy

Nutritional therapy of the child with FTT has three principal goals:

1. Achievement of appropriate weight for height
2. Provision of macro- and micronutrient needs necessary for growth
3. Concrete and individualized nutrition instruction to caregivers.

Catch-up growth is a period of accelerated growth achieved by providing calories in excess of the RDAs. Approximately 20–30% more energy may be needed for a child to achieve catch-up growth. Protein requirements will also increase.[64] Guidelines for estimating catch-up growth requirements are detailed in Exhibit 18–4. It is important to note that malnourished children in developing countries have shown catch-up growth at levels as high as 150–240 kcal/kg and 3.1–4.4 g protein/kg.[64–66] However, calculation of catch-up needs is simply an estimate. Weight gain at or above an expected rate for age is a better determinant of whether the child is receiving sufficient calories and protein (Table 18–2). When looking at growth patterns of children hospitalized with NOFTT, Ellerstein et al[67] found that most infants younger than 6 months of age began to gain weight in as little as 2–3 days (2–9 days lag time). Older infants showed the greatest variability, with weight gain in 2–17 days. All of the children 2 years of age or greater gained weight between the third and seventh days.

Aggressiveness of refeeding should be determined by the degree of malnutrition. Refeeding the severely malnourished child too quickly can result in vomiting, diarrhea, circulatory decompensation, and metabolic alterations (Exhibit 18–5). In these instances the diet may require restriction to normal calories for age for the first 7–10 days, then gradually be increased toward catch-up growth requirements.[19] A multivitamin with minerals, including zinc and iron, is recommended to ensure that micronutrient needs are met.[13,15,19] Efforts to promote catch-up growth should continue until the child regains previous growth percentiles.[13] Intake and rate of growth will spontaneously decelerate toward the normal level for age as deficits in weight for height are repleted.[13] Catch-up growth in length may lag several months behind that in weight.[19]

It is often difficult to meet catch-up growth needs without increasing the caloric density of the diet via high-calorie foods or additives (Exhibit 18–6). Because nutritional intervention is often more effective if accompanied by

Exhibit 18–3 Feeding Observation

General observations

- Does the child eat alone? Who feeds the child or sits with the child during meals? How many people are involved in the feeding?
- Note the location of feeding (kitchen, living room, day care, car), mealtime atmosphere, size and preparation of meals.
- Is food offered on schedule or is the child allowed to "graze" all day?

Child behaviors

- Does the child have a poor suck, tire easily, and fall asleep after short feeding?
- Throws food, cries, vomits or ruminates, spits up, gags, turns head, arches, holds food in mouth, plays with food?
- Is the child interested in eating (reaches for bottle or spoon, opens mouth eagerly) or easily distracted (plays with food/toys, talks instead of eating) or uninvolved (looks around, opens mouth only when food touches lips)?
- Make eye contact with the caregiver?
- Take greater than 30 minutes to eat?
- Refuse to stay seated?
- Express hunger or satiety? Request or refuse particular foods? How does the child communicate his/her likes/dislikes?

Caregiver behaviors

- Does the caregiver position or sit the child so that eye contact is possible, or is there little interaction between caregiver and child during feeding?
- Feeds mechanically or props bottle?
- Fails to establish a consistent feeding pattern?
- Ignores or seems unaware of the child's feeding cues?
- Is bothered by messiness? Cleans child excessively during feeding?
- What is the caregiver's reaction when the child does not eat? Does the caregiver become frustrated and angry? Force feeds?
- Appears anxious, depressed, overwhelmed, easily distressed, uninterested, hostile?
- Does not facilitate or encourage self-feeding? Distracts child with toys? Offers rewards for eating?
- Terminates or interrupts feeding inappropriately, causing distress in the infant?

Source: Adapted with permission from M. MacPhee and J. Schneider, A Clinical Tool for Nonorganic Failure-to-Thrive Feeding Interactions, *Journal of Pediatric Nursing,* Vol. 11, No. 1, pp. 29–39, © 1996, W.B. Saunders Company and E. Satter, The feeding relationship: problems and interventions, *Journal of Pediatrics*, Vol. 117, pp. 182–183, © Mosby-Yearbook.

techniques for behavioral change, it is important that any problematic behaviors identified during the feeding observation or diet history be addressed early. Concrete nutritional and behavioral guidelines should be developed. All individuals involved in caring for the child, including day care workers, babysitters, and grandparents, need to be included in the treatment plan.

Community-based management of FTT must be coordinated, interdisciplinary, and family-focused. Periodic home visits by public health

Exhibit 18–4 Estimating Catch-Up Growth Requirements

1. Plot the child's height and weight on the NCHS growth chart
2. Determine the child's recommended calories for age (RDA or RDI)
3. Determine the IDEAL WEIGHT (50th percentile) for the child's HEIGHT
4. Multiply the RDA calories by IDEAL BODY WEIGHT FOR HEIGHT (kg)*
5. Divide this value by the child's actual weight

Catch-up growth requirement

$$\frac{\text{RDA calories for age}^{\dagger} \times \text{ideal weight for height (kg)}}{\text{Actual weight}}$$

Protein requirements

$$\frac{\text{RDA for protein for age} \times \text{ideal weight for height}}{\text{Actual weight}}$$

* Ideal weight for age can be used in this part of the equation.

† Catch-up growth equations for children with developmental delay may utilize RDA for height age. (Determine at what age present height would be at 50th %ile. Use RDA for that age.)

Table 18–2 Average Gains in Weight and Height for Age

Age	*Weight (grams/d)*	*Height (mm/d)*
Premie	15–30	0.17
0–3 months	20–30	1.03
3–6 months	15–21	0.68
6–12 months	10–13	0.47
1–6 years	5–8	0.23
7–10 years	5–11	0.15

Source: Data from S.J. Fomon et al., Body Composition of Reference Children from Birth to Age 10 Years, *American Journal of Clinical Nutrition,* Vol. 35, p. 1169, © 1982, American Society for Clinical Nutrition.

nurses (or dietitians, if available in the community) can be incorporated as part of the treatment plan. Visiting nurses can reinforce care plans in the home environment and also get a first-hand view of specific family dynamics that may be contributing to the child's poor growth. Intervention by a social worker can be instrumental in helping a family to find resources for food and shelter and to apply to such programs as the Supplemental Nutrition Program for Women, Infants and Children (WIC), Food Stamps, Medical Assistance, and Aid to Families with Dependent Children (AFDC).

When nutritional and behavioral approaches fail to promote weight gain, additional therapies may include appetite stimulation, tube feedings,

Exhibit 18–5 Metabolic Alterations Associated with Refeeding Syndrome

Severe hypophosphatemia
Hypokalemia
Hypomagnesemia
Glucose intolerance
Fluid intolerance

Source: Reprinted with permission from S.M. Solomon and D.F. Kirby, The Refeeding Syndrome: A Review, *Journal of Parenteral and Enteral Nutrition*, Vol. 14, pp. 90–96, © 1990, American Society for Parenteral and Enteral Nutrition.

and hospitalization. Cyproheptadine hydrochloride (Periactin), typically used as an antihistamine, has been prescribed in persistent FTT due to its appetite-stimulating activity.[68] However, both the American Academy of Pediatrics and the Food and Drug Administration believe that the potential side effects (central nervous system effects) of this drug outweigh any perceived benefits.[68] Tube feedings are rarely indicated but may prove helpful as a temporary measure to allow for focus on behavioral modification.[13,69] Parenteral nutrition is seldom indicated. Considerations for hospitalization include failed outpatient management, evidence of physical abuse and severe neglect, poor parental functioning, severe malnutrition, and medical instability.[32,70] Interventions such as physical therapy, speech therapy, or day care can benefit both the child and parent. These can offer stimulation and supervision to the child and can alleviate stress in the parent, allowing the parent to return to work or focus on his or her own psychosocial treatment.[71]

PROGNOSIS

Outcomes are variable due to the many possible factors that can contribute to FTT. Deficiencies in growth during infancy and childhood do harbor potential risk for subsequent lasting deficits in growth, development, and social and emotional functioning.[21,72,73] Therefore, FTT should be identified as early as possible and treated by a multidisciplinary team. Focus should be on the achievement of appropriate weight for height and on maintaining growth velocity. In many situations, the prognosis can be excellent if medical, nutritional, and psychosocial needs of these children and families are met.[1,13]

Exhibit 18–6 Caloric Supplementation and Feeding Suggestions

Method		*Considerations*
Infants		
• Formula: Increase caloric density by 2 kcal/oz every 2–3 days.		• Caloric density should not be increased over 24 kcal/oz by concentration. High formula osmolality and renal solute load can result in vomiting and dehydration in the child.
20 kcal/oz	Normal dilution	
24 kcal/oz	Increased concentration example: 13 oz liquid concentrate to 8 oz of water	
26–30 kcal/oz	Add fortifiers to 24 kcal/oz formula: carbohydrate additive (8 kcal/tsp), vegetable oil (45 kcal/tsp), protein additive, MCT oil (only if medically indicated)	• Monitor for weight gain and signs of intolerance (vomiting, diarrhea, stool reducing substances). • If not tolerating caloric increase, return to previous step for 2 to 3 more days.
• Breastmilk: Increase caloric density by 2 kcal/oz every 2–3 days.		• Consult lactation specialist for additional suggestions on breastfeeding.
24 kcal/oz:	1 tsp formula to 3 oz of breast milk	
26–30 kcal/oz:	Add fortifiers to 24 kcal/oz breast milk to increase caloric density.	
• Food:	- Use high calorie baby foods. Read labels to determine caloric content. example: plain meats, high meat dinners; bananas, peaches, apricots; mixed vegetables, sweet potatoes, custards/puddings; cereals prepared with concentrated formula. - Baby foods can be fortified with moderate amounts of infant cereal, dry milk powder, carbohydrate additive, oil/margarine.	
• Juices:	Avoid	
Toddlers		Feeding Suggestions
• Beverages: 25–30 kcal/oz Milk drinks	Add dry milk powder (15 kcal/tbsp), cream (30–50 kcal/tbsp), instant breakfast powder (30 kcal/oz); nutritional supplements, frappes, milkshakes.	• Establish a regular feeding schedule. (example: three meals, three snacks) • Restrict food or liquids, except water, to meals/snacks only. • Offer solids first, then liquids.

Source: Adapted with permission from J.M. Rathbun and K.E. Peterson, Nutrition in Failure-to-Thrive, in *Pediatric Nutrition: Theory and Practice,* F.J. Grand, J.L. Suthpen and W.H. Dietz, eds., pp. 627–643, Butterworth-Heinemann Publishers, Newton, Massachusetts; and *Feeding Your Toddler,* Combined Program in Pediatrics GI/ Nutrition, Children's Hospital, Boston, Massachusetts.

- <u>Solid foods</u>: Increase caloric density of foods preferred by child.
  - Semi-solids: Add carbohydrate additives, vegetable oil/butter/margarine (45 calories/tsp).
  - Entrees: Add gravies, sauces, cheese (100 kcal/oz), mayonnaise (100 kcal/tbsp), cooked meats (50–75 kcal/oz).
  - Finger foods: String cheese, luncheon meats, chicken nuggets, eggs, small sandwiches, French fries, muffins, waffles, fried vegetables, buttered pasta.
    Use cream cheese (50 kcal/tbsp), peanut butter (100 kcal/tbsp) on crackers/bread.
- <u>Juice</u>: Limit to 4 oz/day or remove from diet completely.

- Offer small portions and allow the child to ask for seconds.
- Reinforce positive behaviors. Ignore the negative.
- Limit meals and snacks to 20–30 minutes.
- Decrease distractions during feeding.
- No force feeding.

REFERENCES

1. Bithoney WG, Dubowitz H, Egan H. Failure to thrive/growth deficiency. *Pediatr Rev.* 1992;13:453–459.
2. Bithoney WG, McJunkin J, Michalek J, Egan H, Snyder J, Munier A. Prospective evaluation of weight gain in both nonorganic and organic failure to thrive children: an outpatient trial of a multidisciplinary team intervention strategy. *Dev Behav Pediatr.* 1989;10:27–31.
3. Bithoney WG, McJunkin J, Michalek J, Snyder J, Egan H, Epstein D. The effect of a multidisciplinary team approach on weight gain in nonorganic failure to thrive children. *Dev Behav Pediatr.* 1991;12:254–258.
4. Hobbs C, Hanks HGI. A multidisciplinary approach for the treatment of children with failure to thrive. *Child Care Health Dev.* 1996;22:273–284.
5. Wilcox WD, Nieburg P, Miller DS. Failure to thrive: A continuing problem of definition. *Clin Pediatr.* 1989;28:391–394.
6. World Health Organization. *A Growth Chart for Use in Maternal and Child Health Care.* Geneva: World Health Organization; 1978.
7. Smith DW, Truog W, Rogers FE, et al. Shifting linear growth during infancy: Illustration of genetic factors in growth from fetal life through infancy. *J Pediatr.* 1976;89:225–230.
8. Fomon SJ. Normal growth, failure to thrive and obesity. In: *Infant Nutrition.* Philadelphia: WB Saunders Co; 1974.
9. Karlberg P, Angstrom I, Karlberg J, Kristiansson B. Evaluation of growth during the first two years of life. In: Kristiansson B, ed. *Low Rate of Weight Gain in Infancy and Early Childhood.* Goteborg, Sweden: Department of Paediatrics, University of Goteborg; 1980.
10. Edwards AGK, Halse PC, Waterston AJR. Recognizing failure to thrive in early childhood. *Arch Dis Child.* 1990;65:1263–1265.
11. Horner JM, Thorsson AV, Hintz RL. Growth deceleration patterns in children with constitutional short stature: An aid to diagnosis. *Pediatrics.* 1978;62:529–534.
12. Lifshitz F, Tarim O. Worrisome growth patterns in children. *Int Pediatr.* 1994; 9:181–188.
13. Maggioni A, Lifshitz F. Nutritional management of failure to thrive. *Pediatr Clin North Am.* 1995;42:791–810.
14. Tanner JM, Goldstein H, Whitehouse RH. Standards for children's height at ages 2–9 years allowing for height of parents. *Arch Dis Child.* 1970;45:755–762.
15. Frank DA, Silva M, Needlman R. Failure to thrive: Mystery, myth, and method. *Contemp Pediatr.* 1993;10: 114–133.
16. Avery ME, First LR, eds. *Pediatric Medicine.* Baltimore: Williams & Wilkins; 1989.
17. Binkin, NJ, Yip R, Fleshood L, Trowbridge FL. Birth weight and childhood growth. *Pediatrics.* 1988;82:828–834.
18. Fitzhardinge PM, Inwood S. Long-term growth in small-for-date children. *Acta Paediatr Scand.* 1989(suppl);349:27–33.
19. Frank DA, Zeisel SH. Failure to thrive. *Pediatr Clin North Am.* 1988;35:1187–1206.
20. Altigani M, Murphy JF, Newcombe RG, Gray OP. Catch-up growth in preterm infants. *Acta Paediatr Scand.* 1989(suppl);357:3–19.
21. Gahagan S, Holmes R. A stepwise approach to evaluation of undernutrition and failure to thrive. *Pediatr Clin North Am.* 1998;45:169–187.
22. Rathbun JM, Peterson KE. Nutrition in failure to thrive. In: Grand RJ, Sutphen JL, Dietz WH, eds. *Pediatric Nutrition: Theory and Practice.* Boston: Butterworth; 1987:627–643.
23. Dewey KG, Heinig MJ, Nommsen LA, Peerson JM, Lonnerdal B. Growth of breast-fed and formula-fed infants from 0 to 18 Months: The DARLING study. *Pediatrics.* 1992;89:1035–1041.
24. Gomez F, Galvan R, Frenk S, Munoz JC, Chavez R, Vasquez J. Mortality in second and third degree malnutrition. *J Trop Pediatr.* 1956;2:77.
25. Waterlow, JC. Classification and definition of protein-calorie malnutrition. *BMJ.* 1972;3:566–569.
26. Waterlow JC, Buzina R, Keller W, Lane JM, Nichaman MZ, Tanner JM. The presentation and use of height and weight data for comparing the nutritional status of groups of children under the age of ten years. *Bull WHO.* 1977;55:486–498.
27. Dean AG, Dean JA, Burton AH, Dicker RC. *Epi Info V.5.* A word processing, database, and statistics program for epidemiology on microcomputers. Stone Mountain, GA: USD, Inc; 1990.
28. WHO Working Group. Use and interpretation of anthropometric indicators of nutritional status. *Bull WHO.* 1986;64:929–941.
29. Blackburn GL, Thornton PA. Nutritional assessment of the hospitalized patient. *Med Clin North Am.* 1979;63: 1103–1115.
30. Homer C, Ludwig S. Categorization of etiology of failure to thrive. *Am J Dis Child.* 1981;135:848–851.
31. Sills, RH. Failure to thrive. *Am J Dis Child.* 1978;132: 967–969.
32. Duggan C. Failure to thrive: Malnutrition in the pediatric outpatient setting. In: Walker WA, Watkins JB, eds. *Nutrition in Pediatrics: Basic Science and Clinical Applications.* Boston: Decker Publishers; 1996:705–714.
33. Bithoney WG. Elevated lead levels in children with nonorganic failure to thrive. *Pediatrics.* 1986;78:5.
34. Walravens PA, Hambidge KM, Koepfer DM. Zinc supplementation in infants with a nutritional pattern of

failure to thrive: A double-blind, controlled study. *Pediatrics*. 1989;83:532–538.

35. Wright CM, Waterston A, Aynsley-Green A. The effect of deprivation on weight gain in infancy. *Acta Paediatr Scand.* 1994(a);83:357–359.

36. Hufton IW, Oates RK. Nonorganic failure to thrive: A long-term follow-up. *Pediatrics.* 1977;59:73–77.

37. Raynor P, Rudolf MC. What do we know about children who fail to thrive? *Child Care Health Dev.* 1996;22: 241–250.

38. Corcoran ME, Chaudry A. The dynamics of childhood poverty. *Future Child.* 1997;7:40–54.

39. Altemeier, WA, O'Connor SM, Sherrod KB, Vietze PM. Prospective study of antecedents for nonorganic failure to thrive. *J Pediatr.* 1985;106:360–365.

40. Dahl M. Early feeding problems in an affluent society. *Acta Paediatr Scand.* 1987;76:872–880.

41. Lobo ML, Barnard KE, Coombs JB. Failure to thrive: a parent–infant interaction perspective. *J Pediatr Nurs.* 1992;7:251–260.

42. Bithoney WG, Newberger EH. Child and family attributes of failure-to-thrive. *Dev Behav Pediatr.* 1987;8: 32–38.

43. Pollitt E, Eichler AW, Chon C. Psychosocial development and behavior of mothers of failure to thrive children. *Am J Orthopsychiatr.* 1975;45:525–537.

44. Weston JA, Colloton M. A legacy of violence in nonorganic failure to thrive. *Child Abuse Negl.* 1993;17: 709–714.

45. Schmitt BD, Mauro RD. Nonorganic failure to thrive: An outpatient approach. *Child Abuse Negl.* 1989;13: 235–248.

46. Wright CM, Talbot E. Screening for failure to thrive: What are we looking for? *Child Care Health Dev.* 1996; 22:223–234.

47. Krieger I. Food restriction as a form of child abuse in ten cases of psychological deprivation dwarfism. *Clin Pediatr.* 1974;13:127–133.

48. Chatoor I, Egan J. Nonorganic failure to thrive and dwarfism due to food refusal: A separation disorder. *J Am Acad Child Psychiatr.* 1983;22:294–301.

49. Ramsay M, Gisel EG, Boutry M. Non-organic failure to thrive: Growth failure secondary to feeding skill disorder. *Dev Med Child Neurol.* 1993;35:285–297.

50. Glaser HH, Heagarty MC, Bullard DM, Pivchik EC. Physical and psychological development in children with early failure to thrive. *J Pediatr.* 1968;73:690–698.

51. Satter E. The feeding relationship: Problems and interventions. *J Pediatr.* 1990;117:S181–S189.

52. Chatoor I, Schaeffer S, Dickson L, Egan J. Non-organic failure to thrive: A developmental perspective. *Pediatr Ann.* 1984:123:832–843.

53. Fleisher DR. Functional vomiting disorders in infancy: Innocent vomiting, nervous vomiting, and infant rumination syndrome. *J Pediatr.* 1994;125:S84–S94.

54. Pugliese MT, Weyman-Daum M, Moses N, Lifshitz F. Parental health beliefs as a cause of nonorganic failure to thrive. *Pediatrics.* 1987;80:175–182.

55. Weston JA, Stage JA, Hathaway P, et al. Prolonged breast-feeding and nonorganic failure to thrive. *Am J Dis Child.* 1987;141:242–243.

56. Dennison BA, Rockwell HL, Baker SL. Excess fruit juice consumption by preschool-aged children is associated with short stature and obesity. *Pediatrics.* 1997;99:15–22.

57. Smith MM, Lifshitz F. Excess fruit juice consumption as a contributing factor in nonorganic failure to thrive. *Pediatrics.* 1994;93:438–443.

58. Hyams JS, Etienne NL, Leichtner AM, Theuer RC. Carbohydrate malabsorption following fruit juice ingestion in young children. *Pediatrics.* 1988;82:64–68.

59. McCann JB, Stein A, Fairburn CG, Dunger DB. Eating habits and attitudes of mothers of children with non-organic failure to thrive. *Arch Dis Child.* 1994;70:234–236.

60. Truesdell DD, Acosta PB. Feeding the vegan infant and child. *J Am Diet Assoc.* 1985;85:837–840.

61. Zmora E, Corodicher R, Bar-Ziv J. Multiple nutritional deficiencies in infants from a strict vegetarian community. *Am J Dis Child.* 1979;133:141.

62. MacPhee M, Schneider J. A clinical tool for nonorganic failure-to-thrive feeding interactions. *J Pediatr Nurs.* 1996;11:29–39.

63. Chatoor I, Schaeffer S, Dickson L, Egan J, Conners K, Leong N. Pediatric assessment of non-organic failure to thrive. *Pediatr Ann.* 1984;123:844–850.

64. Whitehead RG. Protein and energy requirements of young children living in developing countries to allow catch-up growth after infections. *Am J Clin Nutr.* 1977; 30:1545.

65. Ashworth A, Feacham RG. Interventions for the control of diarrheal disease among young children: Prevention of low birth weight. *Bull WHO.* 1985;63:165–184.

66. Kerr D, Ashworth A, Picou D, et al. Accelerated recovery from infant malnutrition with high calorie feeding. In: Gardner LI, Amacher P, eds. *Endocrine Aspects of Malnutrition*. Santa Ynez, CA: Krock Foundation; 1973.

67. Ellerstein NS, Ostrov BE. Growth patterns in children hospitalized because of caloric-deprivation failure to thrive. *Am J Dis Child.* 1985;139:164–166.

68. Lemons PK, Dodge NN. Persistent failure-to-thrive: A case study. *J Pediatr Health Care.* 1998;12:27–32.

69. Tolia V. Very early onset nonorganic failure to thrive in infants. *J Pediatr Gastroenterol Nutr.* 1995;20:73–80.

70. Yetman RJ, Coody DK. Failure to Thrive: A clinical guideline. *J Pediatric Health Care*. 1997;11:134–137.
71. Hathaway P. Failure to thrive: knowledge for social workers. *Health Social Work*. 1989;14:122–126.
72. Corbett SS, Drewett RF, Wright CM. Does a fall down a centile chart matter? The growth and developmental sequelae of mild failure to thrive. *Acta Paediatr*. 1996; 85:1278–1283.
73. Grantham-McGregor SM, Powell CA, Walker SP, Himes JA. Nutritional supplementation, psychosocial stimulation and mental development of stunted children: The Jamaican study. *Lancet*. 1991; 338:1–5.
74. Berhrman RE, Kliegman RM. Failure to thrive. In: *Nelson Essential of Pediatrics*. Philadelphia: WB Saunders Co; 1998:37–39.

SUGGESTED READING

Satter E. *How To Get Your Kid to Eat...But Not Too Much*. Palo Alto, CA: Bull Publishing Company; 1987.

Scott BJ, Artman H, St. Jeor ST. Growth assessment in children: A review. *Top Clin Nutr*. 1992;8:5–31.

CHAPTER 19

Cardiology

Jacqueline Jones Wessel

Nutrition issues for pediatric cardiology range from specific medical nutrition therapy for infants and children with congenital heart disease (CHD) to population screening guidelines for cholesterol education. Both issues will be discussed in this chapter.

CONGENITAL HEART DISEASE

Nutrition support for infants and children with CHD covers a wide range of topics from acute care in infancy to chronic care in childhood. The magnitude of the effect of the cardiac defect on growth, development, and nutritional status depends on the particular lesion and its severity.[1] Malnutrition and growth retardation are common in infants and children with CHD.[2–4] A recent study evaluated the nutritional status of 48 children admitted for surgical repair of CHD. All of the children were markedly malnourished; 83% had at least five biochemical or hematologic indices of malnutrition; and 52% had weights below the third percentile.[4] Controversy exists concerning the etiology of growth failure and the role of inadequate energy intake, hypermetabolism, malabsorption, and cardiac anomaly (see Table 19–1).

Inadequate energy intake has been cited as a component of the growth failure in infants and children with CHD.[5–9] Energy intake of children with CHD was 76% of the intake of unaffected children of the same age;[8] infants with CHD had

Table 19–1 Types of Cardiac Lesions

Acyanotic		*Cyanotic*
Obstructive Malformations	*Left-To-Right Shunt Malformations*	
Pulmonary stenosis	Patent ductos arteriosis (PDA)	Transportation of great arteries (TGA)
Aortic stenosis	Ventricular septal defect (VSD)	Tetralogy of Fallot
	Atrial septal defect (ASD)	

Source: Data from references 1 and 16.

an intake of 82% of the estimated average requirements in a study by Barton et al.[9]

Hypermetabolism has been described in CHD.[9] Total daily energy expenditure (TDEE) was measured in infants with CHD by the doubly labeled water method. TDEE includes basal metabolism, as well as the energy of activity, sweating, and the mechanical labor of the heart and lungs.[10] A significantly higher TDEE was found for infants with CHD (101 +/ – 3 kcal/kg/day), as compared with the TDEE for healthy infants (67 +/ – 14 kcal/kg/day).[9] The calculated increase in total daily energy expenditure was 36% above that of healthy infants, except for one infant who had a very high TDEE.[10] Another study did not find significantly higher resting energy expenditure, measured by respiratory gas exchange method, in infants with CHD, except for a subgroup of infants with pulmonary hypertension and cardiac failure.[11] Leitch et al[12] found increased TDEE but not increased REE as a primary factor in reduced growth of infants with CHD as compared to age-matched controls.

Malabsorption has been suggested as a cause for growth failure. Mild protein malabsorption and more significant fat malabsorption were found in infants with congestive heart failure (CHF) and cyanosis.[13] Fat malabsorption with steatorrhea, bile salt loss, and delayed gastric emptying was found by Yahav et al[7] but malabsorption was not felt to be sufficient to cause growth failure. Vaisman et al[14] noted increased fat malabsorption in sicker infants, with total body water 120% of predicted, but infants regularly receiving diuretics did not significantly malabsorb.[14]

Delayed gastric emptying has been found in infants with CHD.[15] This may predispose an infant to gastroesophageal reflux and increase the potential for aspiration.[16] Premature satiety may be a result of delayed emptying,[1] as well as further compromising energy and nutrient intake.

The type of cardiac lesion affects the pattern of growth failure. Cardiac lesions are designated as *cyanotic* and *acyanotic*, depending on the hemodynamic effect. Patients with cyanotic heart lesions (Table 19–1) usually exhibit reduced height and weight.[16] Acyanotic lesions with a large degree of left-to-right shunting typically affect weight rather than height in the early stages.[2,16,17] The greater occurrence of pulmonary hypertension in children with left-to-right shunts may affect their growth; these children tend to weigh less than do children with cyanotic heart lesions.[16,18] Obstructive malformations, such as pulmonary stenosis and coarctation of the aorta, typically result in impaired linear growth, with linear growth more affected than weight[2,19] (Table 19–2). Strategies to nourish these challenging infants and children in the acute and chronic aspects of care will be discussed.

ACUTE CARE

In infancy, nutrition support is essential during the diagnosis, corrective surgeries, and postoperative rehabilitation period. Parenteral nutrition is often used in the acute phase, then enteral nutrition through tube feedings, and a transition to breast or bottle feedings.

Some infants with cardiac problems are admitted to the Newborn Intensive Care Unit in an acutely ill state within the first days of life. Some can be stabilized and surgery deferred for weeks; others may need immediate surgery. Depending on the type of cardiac defect, multiple surgeries may be planned for a staged repair. As in any surgery, the best outcome is achieved in the patient who is in good nutritional status and positive nitrogen balance. The immediate goal for nutrition support in infants is to achieve the best nutritional status possible in preparation for surgery. Other, less immediate nutrition support goals are to encourage normal growth and support normal feeding skill development. Optimal nutrition support may be impossible, due to the many complicating factors in these patients. Also, providing for normal growth and development may not be possible or realistic in the short-term future of the acute care setting.

The nutrition support plan may be viewed as having four phases. The immediate goals of the acute phase are to minimize catabolism, pre-

Table 19–2 Factors Affecting Growth Failure in Infants and Children with Congenital Heart Disease

Factor	*Effect*
1. Type of cardiac lesion	
Cyanotic	Reduced height and weight
Acyanotic	
Obstructive	Linear growth affected more than weight
Left-to-right shunt	Reduced weight more than height in early stages Weigh less than cyanotic children Large shunts affect body fluid compartments
2. Inadequate energy intake	Energy intake may average only 80–90% of an infant/child without CHD
Decreased energy for feeding	May approach feeding eagerly but tires quickly and cannot finish the feeding
Anorexia, early satiety seen in children[12]	Poor intake
3. Increased metabolic rate	
Increased energy cost for infants and children with CHD	36% increase in metabolic rate observed in children[10]
4. Dysmotility and malabsorption	
Delayed gastric emptying	Premature satiety; increased potential for gastroesophageal reflux
CHF may cause compressive hepatomegaly, reducing gastric capacity	Increased potential for gastroesophageal reflux and aspiration
Mild abnormalities in absorption of nutrients; tendency toward fat malabsorption with increased total body water	Mild steatorrhea, bile salt loss[7] Sicker infants with elevated body water may have lower intake and mild fat malabsorption[13]
5. Prenatal factors	
Trisomy 21 (Down syndrome)	Postnatal growth delay may be characteristic of syndrome[19]

Source: Data from references 16, 17, 18, and 19.

serve lean body mass, and correct abnormal laboratory values as possible. It is usually not possible for calories to be provided for growth at this time and may well be inappropriate. This phase typically involves the use of parenteral nutrition and intravenous (IV) fluids. The second phase goal is to begin enteral nutrition. Parenteral and enteral nutrition are used simultaneously in the gradual transition to full enteral feedings. The third phase is to provide for optimal growth. Calories are increased gradually, as tolerated, to provide sufficient calories for growth. Because of higher calorie needs, higher-calorie formulas are often used. The fourth phase is to provide for feeding skill development. After calorie needs are determined, ways of providing this intake are investigated. Whereas feedings by mouth may be used, they may not be relied upon totally to provide sufficient consistent intake for appropriate growth in many circumstances. Strategies for encouraging age-appropriate feeding skills are used.

Nutrition support in the acutely ill infant, however, requires careful attention. The infant may be fluid restricted; there may be arterial lines needing at least 1 cc/hour/line to keep patent; and medications may use significant amounts of fluid for dilution and administration. It is not uncommon to have only 60–80 cc/kg of fluid allotted for nutrition in the first phase of nutrition support.

Laboratory values may not be normal. The use of diuretics may deplete total body potassium; calcium, phosphorus, and magnesium levels may also be abnormal.[20] Due to the need for fluid restriction, the renal lab values may reflect some degree of dehydration, with elevated sodium and blood urea nitrogen (BUN). Acid base status may also be altered, further complicating potassium management.

Some infants may develop other problems. Renal problems may develop, such as acute tubular necrosis. Some infants may temporarily need peritoneal dialysis, further complicating nutrition support (see Chapter 17). For infants and children needing support prior to surgery or those unable to be weaned from the bypass pump after surgery, extracorporeal life support (ECLS), also known as *extracorporeal membrane oxygenation* (ECMO) may be used.[21,22]

EXTRACORPOREAL LIFE SUPPORT

Extracorporeal life support offers its own unique nutrition problems.[23] Some strategies are to fluid restrict while on bypass, with as little as 60 cc/kg allotted for nutrition. Total parenteral nutrition (TPN) can be infused as part of the ECLS circuitry, and hyperosmolar central line-type solutions can be used as tolerated for calories. Due to the fluid restriction, glucose infusion rate (GIR) should be calculated with each fluid change. A low-volume amount of D25% (25% dextrose) may yield a modest GIR; care should be taken if fluids are liberalized with altering dextrose percent. Although there has been concern about the effect of IV lipid on the membrane,[24] many centers have found that the use of IV lipid has not been associated with increased problems. Some centers infuse IV lipid through a peripheral line. Research is being conducted to provide clarification on this issue.[24]

Problems have been noted with calcium and direct bilirubin for patients using ECLS. Ionized hypocalcemia can be a problem in infants and children after ECMO initiation[25]; and later in the course of the ECLS run, hypercalcemia can be a concern.[26] The elevation of direct bilirubin has been noted in neonates treated with ECLS.[27–30] A study reviewing outcomes found 39% of ECLS neonates to have direct hyperbilirubinemia; 46% of these infants had severe elevations. However, 9 weeks after ECLS treatment, all cases were resolved.[29] Cholestasis has been associated with a plasticizer, di-(2 ethylhexyl) phthlate (DEHP) used in the ECLS circuitry tubing and hemolysis that occurs during ECLS.[28–30] Another study did not find plasma DEHP levels to correlate with short-term toxicity.[30] Heparin bonding of the tubing used in the circuit resulted in very little leaching of DEHP, as compared with standard tubing.[30]

The use of enteral feeding while patients are on ECLS has been controversial. Continuation of transpyloric feedings after the initiation of ECLS has been successful in pediatric burn patients[31]; others have used enteral nutrition successfully in other pediatric ECLS patients.[32] A small study has shown that minimal enteral or trophic feedings for neonates during the third to ninth days of ECLS can be successful. Assessment of intestinal integrity, however, showed intestinal integrity of ECLS patients to be compromised.[33] Although minimal enteral feeding did not result in further deterioration, this finding should suggest caution with enteral feedings. The risk/benefit ratio of initiating feedings on ECLS should be assessed on an individual basis. Neonates are at a greater risk of feeding hazards on ECLS, due to the possibility of acquiring necrotizing enterocolitis. Many ECLS runs are short, and the risks of feeding a neonate may not be worth the benefit of enteral nutrition. For the longer ECLS neonatal run, such as a bridge to cardiac transplantation, the benefits of enteral nutrition may outweigh the risks.

PARENTERAL NUTRITION SUPPORT

To plan the nutrition support for an acutely ill infant, the multidisciplinary team should review all fluids objectively. Laboratory tests, including renal panel, and levels of glucose, calcium, phosphorus, and magnesium should be monitored daily. A bed scale can be helpful for the nursing staff to obtain daily weights used to evaluate fluid status. The pharmacist can determine whether the medications are appropriate and are concentrated appropriately. Any dextrose used in fluid administration should be counted toward the overall glucose infusion rate and carbohydrate and calorie intake. Sodium used in these fluids also should be calculated because it can represent a significant and unexpected intake. Line patency fluids should be counted toward electrolyte, carbohydrate, calorie (if dextrose is a component), and fluid intake. Parenteral nutrition fluids should be written last, accounting for the content of the other fluids. Because fluid is such an issue and may require altering in the course of the day, it may be helpful if total nutrient admixtures are not used and lipids run separately. Parenteral nutrition is usually very concentrated in the cardiac infant, due to fluid restrictions. Central lines are generally used because peripheral parenteral nutrition lines should not contain more than 12.5% dextrose. With increasing dextrose concentrations, the osmolality of solutions increases dramatically. Typically, the maximum dextrose concentration used in central lines is 25%. Higher dextrose percentages increase the risk of thrombosis. The risks and benefits of providing higher calories through a higher percentage of glucose should be considered carefully. Glucose infusion rates should be calculated daily or with every dextrose-containing fluid change. Postoperative infants may tolerate only a GIR of 10–12 mg glucose/kg/minute.

Intravenous lipids are a concentrated source of calories and a source of essential fatty acids. Twenty-percent lipids are typically used (see Chapter 25). A 30% lipid solution is available but pediatric applications for this product have not been seen in the literature. Lipids should be used over the greatest amount of time possible—24-hour infusion, if not contraindicated by a lipid incompatible medication. Triglyceride levels may be monitored to assess tolerance to this therapy.

Protein needs are important to consider in this stressed population. Chaloupecky et al[34] found that the provision of a small amount of IV protein, 0.8 g/kg/day, blunted the muscle proteolysis hypercatabolic response in infants after cardiac surgery, in contrast to an isocaloric maintenance dextrose solution. Starting parenteral nutrition with protein immediately postoperatively would seem to be warranted, even if only half of maintenance fluids can be used for this endeavor, due to electrolyte fluctuations.

It may not be possible for mineral needs for bone development to be met in the short term, due to the use of IV nutrition and fluid restriction. Diuretic use may alter calcium status. Premature and term infant calcium and phosphorus requirements for bone mineralization often cannot be realized until later. The use of premature infant or premature follow-up formulas may be considered as a component of the nutrition support for a fluid-restricted infant with higher mineral needs.

ENTERAL NUTRITION SUPPORT

Gut perfusion may not be optimal in some infants with cardiac anomalies. They also may have had a period of asphyxia, further complicating the question of gut integrity. Because the risk of necrotizing enterocolitis is higher in infants with compromised intestine,[35,36] a slow, cautious approach to enteral feeding, such as the protocol used for feeding premature infants, would seem reasonable.[37] Parenteral nutrition can be the backup nutrition source until full-volume enteral feedings have been established. Trophic feedings, a method of using 10 cc/kg or less of breast milk or formula and keeping feedings at this level for 5–7 days,[38] may also be indicated for premature cardiac infants or term infants felt to have compromised gut. Breast milk use would be preferable for these infants, if possible, due to the lower association with necrotizing enterocolitis (NEC)[39] and other positive benefits—ease of digestion and absorption, immunochemical and cellular component protection,[40] and promotion of mother–infant interaction.[41]

In the transition from parenteral to enteral nutrition, caution should be used with the addition of hyperosmolar medications. NEC has also been associated with hyperosmolar formula, and the addition of medications can make an isotonic feeding hypertonic.[41,42] Hyperosmolar medications have also been known to cause osmotic diarrhea.[43] Many infants with CHD will need additional calories.[44] Increased calorie density of infant formulas from 20 kcal/oz to 30 kcal/oz may be necessary. Once at or close to full allowed volume, density can be gradually increased. The volume of enteral fluid tolerated by each patient should be determined by the multidisciplinary team; different styles of management exist, and the fluid used is often related to the extent of diuretic therapy employed by a team. Diuretics may be used to lessen the effects of high-volume feedings but side effects of potassium wasting, acid-base problems,[15] and potential for calcium and magnesium problems exist. Usually if the calorie increase is done slowly, increasing by 1–2 kcal/oz at a time, infants tolerate this change.[41] To increase the caloric density of formulas, they can be made using less water with powdered or concentrated formula, which keeps the original proportion of carbohydrate, protein, and fat the same. Although this change does increase the osmolality of the formula, in practice, the medications added to formulas alter the osmolality to a much greater extent than the formula alone.[41] Osmolality of products commonly used in intensive care nurseries is discussed elsewhere.[43,45,46] In practice, some clinicians use an IV preparation of a medicine, such as IV potassium chloride instead of the oral form, which has a greater osmolality due to the syrup suspension of the medication.[41]

The enteral formulas used for infants and children with CHD are the same as for other children. Although a moderate sodium restriction (2.2–3.0 mEq/day) for children has been suggested,[15] there is not a great deal of difference (0.1 mEq/dL) between standard term infant formulas such as Similac (Ross Products Division, Abbott Laboratories, Columbus, Ohio) and Enfamil (Mead Johnson, Evansville, Indiana), and the electrolyte- and mineral-restricted formula Similac PM 60/40 (Ross Products Division, Abbott Laboratories, Columbus, Ohio) used for infants with renal disease.[47] Mineral and potassium restriction is not needed in CHD, and the lower potassium in the special formula, 0.31–0.39 mEq/dL less than standard,[47] may increase the amount of supplementation needed. However, when the caloric density of formulas is increased, the amount of electrolytes and minerals is also increased and should be calculated as well.

Calorie needs of infants and children with CHD are greater than those without cardiac problems. Studies using nutrition intervention in either the in- or outpatient setting have shown that normal growth can be achieved using higher calorie intakes. Continuous intragastric infusion of an average of 137 kcal/kg/day in 146 mL/kg/day of formula was used with a small group of 2- to 24-week-old infants with normal growth in weight and length.[48] Partial (12-hour) and total (24-hour) continuous nasogastric tube feedings of 31.8-kcal/oz formula were compared with oral feedings in a group of young infants over a 5-month period. The formulas were made using a cow's milk- or soy protein-based formula with added rice cereal and glucose polysaccharides. Approximately 147 kcal/kg and 167 mL/kg were given in the 24-hour infusion group and 70 kcal/kg from tube feeding plus oral intake, for a total of 122 kcal/kg in the 12-hour infusion group; the oral feeding control group averaged 95 kcal/kg. Comparing Z scores, only the 24-hour infusion group had improvement in length and weight.[49] Another study using 24-hour continuous infusion with infants at ages from 1 week to 9 months who had previously displayed poor growth showed a growth improvement of 198%. The calorie range used was 120–150 kcal/kg with a 24- to 30-kcal/oz range in calorie densities of the formulas.[50] Infants with mild CHD were given higher-calorie formula recipes to increase calorie intake by 20% in oral feedings. Favorable growth was seen in 60% of the group with the higher calorie intake.[51] Higher-calorie formulas were used in a study with oral feedings and infants with CHD. Calories were increased by 32%, and weight gain improved significantly. The author's recommendation is to begin supplementation from the time of diagnosis to optimize growth.[52] A study using nutritional counseling in underweight infants and children with CHD showed increased oral calorie intake and improved anthropometric studies over a 6-month period of counseling.[53] Interestingly, a small study reviewing feeding and growth of breastfed versus bottle-fed infants with CHD showed better growth in the breastfed infants.[54] A naturalistic study reviewing the behavioral and physiologic response of infants during feeding did not show a pattern in infants with CHD, as compared with healthy controls, but there was a wide range of individual differences among the 20 infants studied.[55]

The exact energy intake amount is difficult to estimate, but many infants will need 135–155 kcal/kg in enteral nutrition. Toddlers and children may need 20–33% more than normal estimated needs. Postrepair, the calorie needs will usually decrease but may still stay 10–15 kcal/kg above the average. Calorie needs may be estimated using indirect calorimetry while in the hospital; many nurseries, however, do not have the equipment to accurately assess infants under 5.0 kg. The best method is to set an estimated goal, assess growth parameters, and make adjustments as needed until appropriate growth is achieved.

CHRONIC CARE

Feeding methodology often becomes an issue in the follow-up care of infants and children with cardiac problems. In infancy, when caloric needs are very high, a typical infant will eat eagerly for a set time, then quit. Parents and caregivers may assume the infant is full, but it may be that the infant has just used the energy it has available for eating and cannot be cajoled or stimulated into taking more. Other infants and children may refuse to eat or eat very poorly. Thommessen et al[56] found 65% of parents of infants and children with CHD document feeding problems. The reported feeding problems were a good predictor for low voluntary food intake and low growth outcome.[56]

Some options are to use higher-calorie formulas or supplements to decrease the volume needed for optimal caloric intake. Other options include using an indwelling nasogastric tube and finishing the feed by a bolus tube feeding. If an infant is close to the goal, the infant may be able to feed by mouth all day and get tube feedings overnight to make up the daytime deficit. This is usually calculated daily by parents or caregivers and given either by bolus feedings or continuous infusion at night. In situations where caregivers are unable to make these calculations, estimations can be used, with frequent checks to make sure that the estimates are still appropriate. For some infants, 24-hour infusions may be needed. Attempts can be made to compress feedings into a shorter infusion time, giving a few hours off of infusion for social and developmental needs. For infants and children not able to take feedings by mouth, an oral stimulation program should be initiated, and oral motor follow-up care can be instituted by an experienced occupational therapist or speech pathologist.

For infants and children who are thought to need tube feeding assistance for greater than 3 months, a gastric tube (G-tube) is a positive step toward simplifying the care. G-tubes can be inserted in surgery or by endoscopy (percutaneous endoscopic gastrostomy). G-tubes and tube feedings should be viewed as tools to improve the quality of life. Without the pressure of forced or unpleasant mealtimes or around-the-clock marathons, feedings can be pleasurable, with the best possible behavioral and developmental outcome. Feedings should typically not exceed 30 minutes in length and should be a pleasant time for both caregiver and the infant or child.

Growth must be monitored carefully. Preventive measures and early nutritional intervention is the best approach to correcting growth problems in childhood. Multidisciplinary teamwork is again important; growth or appetite problems can be caused by a change in clinical course or by a change in medications. Celiac disease has been found in children with CHD and poor growth.[57] It is necessary to consider all possibilities for failure to thrive when cardiac status is stable and calorie intake appears sufficient for good growth. Reevaluation of all parameters on an ongoing basis provides the best outcome.

NUTRITION MANAGEMENT OF PEDIATRIC HYPERLIPIDEMIA

The aim of nutrition support in pediatric hyperlipidemia is to provide nutrition for normal growth and development, as well as to normalize lipid levels as much as possible to decrease the risk of cardiovascular disease.[58] The guidelines for diet modification are for children over 2 years of age. Before that, age restriction of fat intake may result in altered growth.[59] The National Cholesterol Education Program (NCEP) and the American Heart Association (AHA) advocate dietary changes for all healthy children over 2 years of age and for adolescents.[59,60] The dietary changes suggested for all are actually very similar to the Step I guidelines and can be incorporated into the use of the food pyramid (see Appendix L) with low-fat dairy products. The American Academy of Pediatrics recommends that total fat intake should not fall below 20% of total calories for children and adolescents.[59]

The NCEP has guidelines for cholesterol and lipoprotein screening in children and adolescents with positive family histories of cardiovascular disease or hypercholesterolemia (> 240 mg/dL)[59] (see Table 19–3).

The Step I diet is used for children and adolescents with elevated total or low-density (LDL) cholesterol and is used initially for 3 months. If the serum levels do not decrease to acceptable levels after 3 months, the Step II diet is used for 6–12 months. There is further reduction in cholesterol intake and saturated fatty acid percentage in the diet. Step I and II diets have been shown to decrease total and LDL cholesterol by

Table 19–3 Steps I and II Dietary Modifications

Nutrient	*Step I Diet*	*Step II Diet*
Total Fat	No more than 30% on average of total calories	Same
Saturated fatty acids	Less than 10% of total calories	Less than 7% of total calories
Polyunsaturated fatty acids	Up to 10% of total calories	Same
Monounsaturated fatty acids	Remaining fat calories	Same
Cholesterol	Less than 300 mg/day	Less than 200 mg/day
Protein	About 15–20% of total calories	Same
Calories	To achieve normal weight and promote normal growth and development	Same

Source: Reproduced with permission from *Pediatrics*, Vol. 89, pages 525–527, 1992.

10–15% within 3 weeks, with children with higher lipid levels having the greater response.[61,62] If serum levels are still not down to acceptable levels, medication may be considered for children over 10 years of age.[59] Details on the foods that constitute the Step I and II diet are described elsewhere.[63]

Increasing the fiber intake of the diet to the patient's age plus 5 g of dietary fiber is advocated for all children.[64] Fiber may be helpful in reducing cholesterol. However, studies on the effect of the lipid-lowering effect of fiber in children are inconclusive.[65]

Activity is important in reducing the likelihood of childhood obesity, and it is also an important facet of promoting cardiovascular health.[63] The activity level of the family influences the activity of the children. A family commitment to a healthy lifestyle, including diet and activity level, is essential.

REFERENCES

1. Greecher CP. Congenital heart disease. In: Groh-Wargo S, Thompson M, Cox J, eds. *Nutritional Care for High-Risk Newborns.* Revised ed. Chicago: Precept Press; 1994;266.
2. Mehrizi A, Drash A. Growth disturbance in congenital heart disease. *J Pediatr.* 1962;61:418–429.
3. Glassman MS, Woolf PK, Schwarz SM. Nutritional considerations in children with congenital heart disease. In: Baker SB, Baker, RD Jr, Davis A, eds. *Pediatric Enteral Nutrition.* New York: Chapman & Hall; 1994;340.
4. Mitchell IM, Logan RW, Pollock JCS, et al. Nutritional status of children with congenital heart disease. *Br Heart J.* 1995;73:277.
5. Krieger I. Growth failure and congenital heart disease. Energy and nitrogen balance in infants. *Am J Dis Child.* 1970;120:497–502.
6. Huse DM, Feldt RH, Nelson RA, et al. Infants with congenital heart disease. *Am J Dis Child.* 1975;129:65–69.
7. Yahav J, Avigad S, Frand M, et al. Assessment of intestinal and cardiorespiratory function in children with congenital heart disease on high calorie formulas. *J Pediatr Gastroenterol Nutr.* 1985;4:778–785.
8. Hansen SR, Dorup I. Energy and nutrient intakes in congenital heart disease. *Acta Paediatr.* 1993;82:166–172.
9. Barton JS, Hindmarsh PC, Scrimgeour CM, et al. Energy expenditure in congenital heart disease. *Arch Dis Child.* 1994;70:5–9.
10. Broekhoff C, Houwen RHJ, de Meer K. Energy expenditure in congenital heart disease. (Commentary) *J Pediatr Gastroenterol Nutr.* 1995;21:322–323.
11. Menon G, Poskitt EME. Why does congenital heart disease cause failure to thrive? *Arch Dis Child.* 1985;60:1134–1139.
12. Leitch CA, Karn CA, Peppard RJ, et al. Increased energy expenditure in infants with cyanotic congenital heart disease. *J Pediatr.* 1998;133:755–760.
13. Sondheimer JM, Hamilton JR. Intestinal function in infants with severe congenital heart disease. *J Pediatr.* 92;572–578.
14. Vaisman N, Leigh T, Voet H, et al. Malabsorption in infants with congenital heart disease with diuretic treatment. *Pediatr Res.* 1994;36:545–549.
15. Cavell B. Gastric emptying in infants with congenital heart disease. *Acta Paediatr Scand.* 1981;70:517–520.
16. Forchielli ML, McColl R, Walker WA, et al. Children with congenital heart disease: A nutrition challenge. *Nutr Rev.* 1994;52:348–353.
17. Umansky R, Hauck AJ. Factors in the growth of children with patent ductus arteriosis. *Pediatrics.* 1992;146:1078–1084.
18. Salzer JR, Haschke M, Wimmer M, et al. Growth and nutritional intake of infants with congenital heart disease. *Pediatr Cardiol.* 1989;10:17–23.
19. Stranway A, Fowler R, Cunningkam K, et al. Diet and growth in congenital heart disease. *Pediatrics.* 1976;57:75–86.
20. Pronsky ZM, Solomon E, Crowe JP, Young V, Smith C. *Food-medication interactions*, 10th ed. Pottstown, PA: Food Medication Interactions; 1997.
21. Walters HL III, Hakimi M, Rice MD, et al. Pediatric cardiac surgical ECMO: Multivariate analysis of risk factors for hospital death. *Am Thorac Surg.* 1995;60:329–336.
22. Ishino K, Wong Y, Alexi-Meskishvili V, et al. Extracorporeal membrane oxygenation as a bridge to cardiac transplantation. *Artif Organs.* 1996;30:728–732.
23. Brown RL, Wessel J, Warner BW. Nutritional considerations in the extracorporeal life support patient. *Nutr Clin Prac.* 1994;9:22–27.
24. Buck ML, Ksenich RA, Wooldridge P. Effect of infusing fat emulsion into extracorporeal membrane oxygenation circuits. *Pharmacotherapy.* 1997;17:1292–1295.
25. Meliones JN, Moler FW, Custer JR, et al. Hemodynamic instability after the initiation of extracorporeal membrane oxygenation: Role of ionized calcium. *Crit Care Med.* 1991;19:1247–1251.

26. Fridricksson J, Wessel JJ, Warner BW, et al. Hypercalcemia associated with extracorporeal life support ECLS. (Abstract) *ECMO*. Conference, 1997.

27. Walsh-Sukys MC, Cornell DJ, Stork EK. The natural history of direct hyperbilirubinemia associated with extracorporeal membrane oxygenation. *Am J Dis Child.* 1992;146:1176–1180.

28. Shneider B, Maller E, VanMarter L, et al. Cholestasis in infants supported with extracorporeal membrane oxygenation. *J Pediatr.* 1989;115:462–465.

29. Shneider B, Cronin J, VanMarter L, et al. A prospective analysis of cholestasis in infants supported with extracorporeal membrane oxygenation. *J Pediatr Gastroenterol Nutr.* 1991;13:285–289.

30. Karle VA, Short BL, Martin GR, et al. Extracorporeal membrane oxygenation exposes infants to the plasticizer di(ethylhexyl) phthalate. *Crit Care Med.* 1997;25:606–703.

31. Wessel JJ, Wieman RW, Gottschlich MM. Enteral feeding during pediatric extracorporeal membrane oxygenation (ECMO) patients. (Abstract) ASPEN 20th Clinical Congress; 1996:389.

32. Pettigano B, Heard M, Davis B, et al. Total enteral nutrition versus total parenteral nutrition during pediatric extracorporeal membrane oxygenation. *Crit Care Med.* 1998;26:358–363.

33. Piena M, Albers MJIJ, Gischler SJ, et al. Safety of enteral feeding in neonates during extracorporeal membrane oxygenation treatment after evaluation of intestinal permeability changes. (Abstract) *Crit Care Med.* 1998;26:A91.

34. Chaloupecky V, Hucin B, Tlaskal T, et al. Nitrogen balance, 3-methylhistidine excretion, and plasma amino acid profile in infants after cardiac operations for congenital heart defects: The effect of early nutritional support. *J Thorac Cardiovasc Surg.* 1997;14:1053.

35. Anderson DM, Kliegman RM. The relationship of neonatal alimentation practices to the occurrence of endemic necrotizing enterocolitis. *Am J Perinatol.* 1991;8:62.

36. Kliegman RM, Walsh MC. Necrotizing enterocolitis: Pathogenesis, classification, and spectrum of illness. *Curr Probl Pediatr.* 1987;17:213.

37. Book LS, Herbst JJ, Jung AL. Comparison of fast- and slow-feeding rate schedules to the development of necrotizing enterocolitis. *J Pediatr.* 1976;89:463.

38. Meetze, W, Valentine C, McGuigan, JE, et al. Gastrointestinal priming prior to full enteral nutrition in very low birth weight infants. *J Pediatr Gastroenterol Nutr.* 1992;15:163.

39. Lucas A, Cole TJ. Breast milk and neonatal necrotizing enterocolitis. *Lancet.* 1990;336:1519.

40. American Academy of Pediatrics. *Pediatric Nutrition Handbook.* Elk Grove Village: American Academy of Pediatrics; 1985:9.

41. Sapsford A. Enteral nutrition products. In: Groh-Wargo S, Thompson M, Cox J, eds. *Nutritional Care for High-Risk Newborns.* Revised ed. Chicago: Precept Press, 1994:176.

42. White KC, Harkavy KL. Hypertonic formula resulting from added oral medications. *Am J Dis Child.* 1982;136: 931.

43. Zenk L, Hutzable R. Osmolality of infant formulas, tube feedings, and total parenteral solutions. *Hosp Form. 577,* 8/1978.

44. Salzer HR, Haschke F, Wimmer M, et al. Growth and nutritional intake of infants with congenital heart disease. *Pediatr Cardiol.* 1989;10:17.

45. Ernst JA, Williams JM, Glick MR, et al. Osmolality of substances used in the intensive care nursery. *Pediatrics.* 1983;72:347.

46. Jew R, Osmolality of medications and formulas used in the newborn intensive care nursery. *Nutr Clin Prac.* 1997;12:158–163.

47. Sapsford A. Composition of human milk, selected infant formulas, and modular supplements. In: Groh-Wargo S, Thompson M, Cox J, eds. *Nutritional Care for High-Risk Newborns.* Revised ed. Chicago: Precept Press; 1994:421–429.

48. Bougle D, Iselin M, Kahyat A, et al. Nutritional treatment of congenital heart disease. *Arch Dis Child.* 1986; 61:799–801.

49. Schwarz, SM, Gewitz MH, See CC, et al. Enteral nutrition in infants with congenital heart disease and growth failure. *Pediatrics.* 1990;86:368–373.

50. Vanderhoof JA, Hofshire PJ, Baluff MA, et al. Continuous enteral feedings. An important adjunct in the management of complex congenital heart disease. *Am J Dis Child.* 1982;136:825–827.

51. Khajuria R, Grover A, Bidwai PS. Effect of nutritional supplementation on growth of infants with congenital heart diseases. *Indian Pediatr.* 1989;26:76–79.

52. Jackson M, Poskitt, EM. The effects of high energy feeding on energy balance and growth in infants with congenital heart disease and failure to thrive. *Br J Nutr.* 1991;65:131–143.

53. Unger R, et al. Calories count. Improved weight gain with dietary intervention after cardiac surgery in children. *Am J Dis Child.* 1992;146:1078–1084.

54. Combs VL, et al. A comparison of growth patterns in breast and bottle-fed infants with congenital heart disease. *Pediatr Nurs.* 1993;19:175–179.

55. Lobo ML, Michel Y. Behavioral and physiological response during feeding in infants with congenital heart

disease: a naturalistic study. *Prog Cardiovasc Nurs*. 1995;10:26–34.

56. Thommessen M, Heiberg A, Kase BF. Feeding problems with children with congenital heart disease: The impact on energy intake and growth outcomes. *Eur J Clin Nutr*. 1992;46:457–464.

57. Congdon PJ, Fiddler GI, Littlewood JM, et al. Coeliac disease associated with congenital heart disease. *Arch Dis Child*. 1982;57:78–79.

58. American Academy of Pediatrics Committee on Nutrition. Statement on cholesterol. *Pediatrics*. 1992;90: 469–473.

59. NCEP Expert Panel on Blood Cholesterol Levels in Children and Adolescents. National Cholesterol Education Program (NCEP). Highlights of the report of the expert panel on blood cholesterol levels in children and adolescents. *Pediatrics*. 1992;89:525–527.

60. American Heart Association Nutrition Committee. Nutrition and children: A statement for healthcare professionals from the nutrition committee. *Circulation*. 1997; 95:2332–2333.

61. Kris-Etherton PM, Krammel D, Russell ME, et al. The effect of diet on plasma lipids, lipoproteins, and coronary heart disease. *J Am Diet Assoc*. 1988;88:1373–1400.

62. DISC Collaborative Research Group: Efficacy and safety of lowering dietary intake of fat and cholesterol among school children in The Woodlands, Texas. *Pediatrics*. 1990;86:520–526.

63. Nutrition management of hyperlipidemia. In: Williams CP, ed. *Pediatric Manual of Clinical Dietetics*. Chicago: American Dietetic Association; 1998:265–283.

64. Williams CL, Bolella M, Wynder EL. A new recommendation for dietary fiber in childhood. *Pediatrics*. 1995; 96:985–988.

65. Kwiterovitch PO. The role of fiber in the treatment of hypercholesterolemia in children and adolescents. *J Pediatr*. 1995;S1005–S1009.

CHAPTER 20

Diabetes

Karen Hanson Chalmers

MEDICAL NUTRITION THERAPY FOR THE CHILD WITH DIABETES

Empowering parents to care for their children with type 1—insulin-dependent diabetes—is the ultimate challenge for many health professionals dealing with pediatric patients. Families already faced with altering their lifestyles to include insulin injections, blood monitoring, and scheduled meals must face these challenges in combination with feelings of anger, fear, denial, and guilt.

During the last two decades our knowledge base for childhood diabetes has been expanded through research and new technologies, giving health care managers new tools to help this population in balancing and improving their diabetes management, as depicted in Figure 20–1. These tools include intensive insulin therapy, new medications, self–blood glucose monitoring devices, psychologic intervention, inclusion and education for family and support persons, insulin/food adjustment for exercise, and state-of-the-art medical nutrition therapy. The challenge to the dietitian on the diabetes team is to support the family's efforts, help promote healthy eating habits by using information gained from current research, and gain insight into family dynamics.

Meal planning is one of the most important tools of diabetes self-management. However, studies have shown that "diet" is overwhelmingly the number one problem in diabetes care.[1] To date, many factors associated with poor adherence to meal planning principles are psychosocial (ie, anger, denial, frustration, poor understanding, social pressures, and restriction of favorite foods).[2] With the revised *American Diabetes Association Principles and Nutrition Recommendations: 1994*,[3] it is now possible to provide a positive approach to this potentially negative topic. Health educators on the diabetes team must not lose sight of the ability of food to provide more than nutrients, especially for children. Changes in eating should not be viewed as restrictions and losses, but rather as a healthful way for the entire family to eat.

To be successful, the meal plan must not only meet nutritional requirements but must be realistic and workable, without making major routine changes to those involved. Every attempt should be made to establish a meal plan that reflects the child's food preferences and the family's social and cultural attitudes. Flexibility and graduated goal setting are important keys to success, increasing the chances of the child's achieving optimal management and decreasing the development of complications. The goals for medical nutrition therapy are listed in Exhibit 20–1.

THE DIABETES TEAM

Diabetes requires teamwork. This was clearly demonstrated in the 1993 published results of the landmark Diabetes Control and Complications Trial (DCCT).[4] The DCCT supported the importance of a coordinated team approach

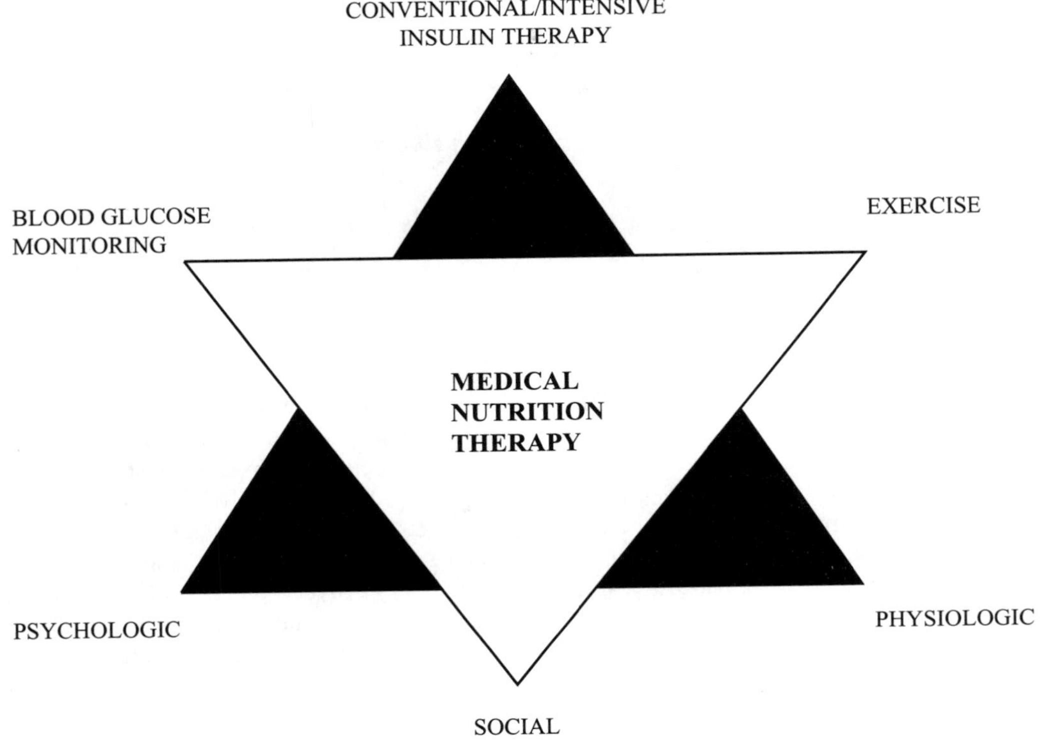

Figure 20–1 Tools for diabetes management.

Exhibit 20–1 Goals for Medical Nutrition Therapy for Children and Adolescents

1. To provide adequate nutrition to maintain normal growth and development based on the child's appetite, food preferences, and family lifestyle
2. To maintain near-normal blood glucose levels and reduce/prevent risks of short- and long-term diabetes
3. To achieve optimal serum lipid levels
4. To preserve social and psychologic well-being
5. To improve overall health through optimal nutrition
6. To provide level of information that meets interest and ability of family
7. To provide information on current research to help the family make appropriate nutrition decisions

to achieve nutrition goals. The ultimate therapeutic diabetes team utilized in the DCCT consisted of the patient and family as the primary players, along with the diabetes nurse educator, dietitian, behaviorist, and the diabetologist.[5] The DCCT also provided important information specific to successful nutrition intervention strategies, based firmly on scientific evidence. Shortly after the DCCT clinical findings were published, the American Diabetes Association published a revised set of nutrition guidelines in 1994, refocusing on an "individualized approach to nutrition self-management that is appropriate for the personal lifestyle and diabetes management goals of the individual with diabetes."[3(p.490)]

NUTRITION PRINCIPLES FOR THE MANAGEMENT OF DIABETES AND RELATED COMPLICATIONS

A positive approach to meal planning is to encourage family members and other support persons to follow the same lifestyle recommendations as the child with diabetes. In our attempt to maintain the "pleasures of the table," it is essential that the nutrition recommendations promote "normal," healthy eating and prevent isolating and dividing the child and family in their food choices. Today, there is no one "diabetic" diet, and the recommended *USDA/DHHS Dietary Guidelines for Americans: 1995*[6] applies to all healthy individuals, including those with diabetes. The current nutrition recommendations can be defined as simply a nutrition prescription based on assessment and treatment goals and outcomes.[7]

The 1994 American Diabetic Association nutrition recommendations redistributed the calories from macronutrients. The current recommended goals are shown in Table 20–1. Protein should provide 10–20% of daily calories, and the recommendations are no different for a child without diabetes. Carbohydrate distribution is based on nutritional assessment and on blood glucose and lipid goals. Fat distribution is also based on nutritional assessment and on weight and lipid goals, with less than 10% of calories from saturated fat.

Calories

Including enough calories (kcal) in the meal plan to maintain a consistent growth curve and to achieve and/or maintain a desirable body

Table 20–1 Historical Perspective of Nutrition Recommendations

	Distribution of Calories (%)		
Year	*Carbohydrate*	*Protein*	*Fat*
Before 1921	—	Starvation diets	—
1921	20	10	70
1950	40	20	40
1971	45	20	35
1986	<60	12–20	<30
1994	*	10–20	*†

* Based on nutritional assessment and treatment goals.
† Less than 10% of calories from saturated fats.

Source: Reprinted with permission from Nutrition Recommendations and Principles for People with Diabetes Mellitus, *Diabetes Care*, Vol. 21, pp. 532–535, © 1998, American Diabetes Association.

weight is of major importance. In growing children, caloric intake should not be restricted and should be the same as for children without diabetes. Because energy needs vary during periods of growth, comparing and validating calorie needs based on age, height, ideal body weight (IBW), activity, and average energy allowance per day (see Exhibit 20–2 and Appendix K) will provide the best method to estimate energy needs for an individual child.[8]

Mahan and Rosebrough[9] recommend adapting the Recommended Dietary Allowances (RDA) figures and basing the estimate of calorie and protein need on height for adolescents. From ages 11 to 22 years, the estimate ranges from 16 to 17 kcal/cm for boys and from 13 to 14 kcal/cm for girls. Other guidelines for determining calorie needs of children are found in Chapters 2 and 5.

Carbohydrate and Sweeteners

The percentage of calories from carbohydrate will vary and is individualized, based on nutritional assessment and treatment goals. One of the most common misconceptions about carbohydrate is the belief that sugars are more rapidly digested and absorbed than are starches and, thus, sugar contributes significantly to hyperglycemia. However, research published in the past 10–15 years found little or no scientific evidence that supports this theory. The basis for this belief likely originated from the glycemic index, which categorizes foods according to their effect on blood glucose level.[10] The glycemic index is not a precise tool because the exact effect of foods on blood glucose differs significantly among individuals and is affected by

Exhibit 20–2 Estimating Needs for Calories in Youth

1. Base calories on nutrition assessment
2. Validate calorie needs

Method 1	National Academy of Sciences *Recommended Dietary Allowances*[8] (see Appendix K)
Method 2	1,000 calories for first year
	Add 100 kcal per year up to age 11 years
	Girls 11–15 years, add 100 kcal or less per year after age 10 years
	Girls >15 years, calculate as an adult
	Boys 11–15 years, add 200 kcal per year after age 10 years
	Boys >15 years, add
	23 kcal/lb if very active
	18 kcal/lb if usual activity level
	16 kcal/lb if sedentary
Method 3	1,000 kcal for first year, add
	125 kcal × age for boys
	100 kcal × age for girls
	Up to 20% more kcal for activity
	For toddlers 1–3 years old, add 40 kcal per inch of length

Source: Reprinted with permission from *Maximizing the Role of Nutrition in Diabetes Management,* © 1994, American Diabetes Association.

many factors, such as processing, preparation, and digestion.[3] The American Diabetic Association recommends that the first priority should be given to the total amount of carbohydrate consumed, rather than the source of the carbohydrate, within the context of healthy eating.

Sucrose

Flexibility in allowing some sucrose into the diet may lead to better adherence to the meal plan. Sucrose may be incorporated into the diet of a child or adolescent on a regular basis, assuming adequate, consistent intake from all of the essential food groups. To moderate the impact of many new food choices on the blood glucose level, it is advisable to substitute sucrose and sucrose-containing foods for other carbohydrates in the diet, and not simply to add these foods to the meal plan.[11] Because most sources of sugar for children under 10 years are from milk and milk products, fruit drinks, and carbonated soft drinks, it is important to promote overall healthy eating and optimal dental status by limiting empty-calorie foods. Added sucrose-containing foods should be related to extra activity and special occasions, and these foods should be promoted as special "treat" foods.

Nutritive Sweeteners

Sweeteners other than sucrose also contain large amounts of carbohydrate and calories, and can impact glycemic control. Common sweeteners, such as corn syrup, honey, molasses, carob, dextrose, lactose, and maltose, do not decrease calories or carbohydrate and offer no significant advantage over foods sweetened with sucrose.[7] Although fructose has been shown to produce a somewhat smaller rise in blood glucose, compared with the other sweeteners listed above, research evidence suggests potential negative effects of large amounts of fructose (double the amount usually consumed or 20% of daily calories) on cholesterol and LDL cholesterol.[12]

Commonly used sugar alcohols, such as sorbitol, mannitol, xylitol, and hydrogenated starch hydrolysate, may produce less of a glycemic response and average about 2.4–3.5 kcal/g, compared with 4 kcal/g from other carbohydrates.[13] However, research indicates that sugar alcohols do not significantly reduce calories or the total carbohydrate content of the daily diet and have no significant advantage over other nutritive sweeteners. In addition, gastrointestinal side effects, such as stomach distress or diarrhea, are noted when sugar alcohols are ingested in large amounts (50 g/day for sorbitol, 20 g/day for mannitol).[3]

Nonnutritive Sweeteners

Acesulfame K, aspartame, and saccharin are the most common noncaloric sweeteners used in the United States today and approved by the US Food and Drug Administration (FDA). The FDA also determines an acceptable daily intake (ADI) for these intense sweeteners, as it does for all food additives. ADI is defined as the amount of a food additive that can be safely consumed on a daily basis over a person's lifetime without any adverse effects and includes a 100-fold safety factor.

Acesulfame K's ADI for children is 15 mg/kg/day (eg, one packet contains about 0.4 g).[9] It has no caloric value and is 200 times sweeter than sucrose. Also, it is not metabolized by the body and is eliminated unchanged in the urine. Acesulfame K is heat stable and blends well with other sweeteners. The amount of potassium (K) in this sweetener is minimal, with only 10 mg of potassium in one packet. No safety concerns have been raised about acesulfame K, and it has been reported safe for all individuals.[3,13]

Aspartame's ADI for children is 50 mg/kg/day (eg, 37 mg in one packet, about 200 mg in a 12-oz diet soda, 80 mg in an 8-oz yogurt or a 4-oz diet gelatin, and 47 mg in a 1/2-cup frozen dessert). Aspartame contains 4 kcal/g but is 160–220 times sweeter than sucrose; therefore, aspartame provides negligible calories. Aspartame is rapidly metabolized in the gastrointestinal tract and does not accumulate in the system at recommended intakes. Aspartame is not heat stable and may decompose on long exposure to high temperatures. The FDA has addressed many concerns related to ingestion of aspartame, leading the Centers for Disease Control and Prevention (CDC) to evaluate and report that data "do not provide for the existence of serious widespread, adverse health consequences."[14(p.400)] However, because aspartame is composed of phenylalanine and aspartic acid, medical nutrition therapy controls aspartame products in persons with phenylketonuria, a homozygous recessive inborn error of metabolism, where persons are unable to metabolize the amino acid phenylalanine.

Saccharin's ADI for children is 5 mg/kg/day. It is 200–700 times sweeter than sucrose. Saccharin is heat stable, is not metabolized by the body, and is excreted unchanged in the urine. Parents often question their child's safety, based on highly publicized research results in the 1970s, suggesting a possible causal relationship between saccharin and bladder tumors in laboratory rats. It has been documented that the saccharin samples used in the studies were impure, and the results were incorrectly interpreted. The American Diabetic Association has stated that saccharin poses no health hazard.[15,16]

Sucralose is the most recent noncaloric sweetener to be approved by the FDA and confirmed by many regulatory agencies throughout the world. The ADI for children is up to 15 mg/kg/day. Although sucralose is the only low-calorie sweetener made from sugar and is 600 times sweeter than sugar, it can be safely consumed by people with diabetes. Sucralose is not recognized by the body as either sugar or carbohydrate because it is not broken down or metabolized by the body. Furthermore, it does not affect blood glucose levels. Sucralose is heat stable and may be used during the cooking and baking process. The FDA states that no adverse or carcinogenic effects are associated with sucralose consumption.

Fiber

Total dietary fiber is defined as the sum of insoluble and soluble plant polysaccharides and lignin.[17] Soluble fiber is made up of pectins, gums, mucilages, and some hemicelluloses. Insoluble fiber is made up of noncarbohydrate components that include cellulose, lignin, and many hemicelluloses. Current estimates of fiber intake in both adults and children over the age of 2 years, with or without diabetes, are lower than the recommended 20–35 g per day. Data published in 1994 from a national nutrition survey reported that the average fiber intake of all children was 9–12 g/day and somewhat higher than figures previously reported.[18] This may indicate that education and intervention have begun to encourage increased intake from fiber-containing carbohydrate sources in children.

The 1986 Nutrition Recommendations and Principles for Individuals with Diabetes Mellitus suggested that soluble dietary fiber improved carbohydrate metabolism and stressed that "careful attention must be paid to insulin dose, because hypoglycemia can result if there is a radical change in fiber intake."[19(p.503)] This statement implied that large increases in dietary fiber resulted in a profound decrease in blood glucose and an increase in insulin sensitivity. Although increased soluble fiber intake has been positively linked to improved glycemic control in the past, interpretation of recent data collected in carefully controlled studies now indicates that the clinical significance of the effect of soluble fiber on blood glucose absorption, in the amounts consumed from foods, is probably insignificant. Therefore, recommendations for children with diabetes eating solid foods are the same as for children without diabetes—increase both types of fiber from a wide variety of food sources.

Dietary fiber may be useful in the treatment or prevention of constipation and gastrointestinal disorders (see Chapter 16). Furthermore, large amounts of soluble fiber (20 g/day) have been shown to have a beneficial effect on fasting total and LDL cholesterol levels, with maintenance of fasting HDL cholesterol concentration.[3]

However, a high-fiber diet for some children may result in an insufficient caloric intake of foods necessary for growth, due to the satiety value provided by fiber, as well as possible impairment of mineral absorption. Therefore, the amount of dietary fiber recommended for children should be based on the child's usual eating habits and lipid goals.[20]

Protein

Current nutrition recommendations for children with diabetes encourage protein from both animal and vegetable sources, comprising 10–20% of calories per day. Protein intake should be sufficient to ensure adequate growth and development, and maintenance of body protein stores in children and adolescents. At this time, there are no data to support a higher or lower protein intake than the RDAs for all children, 0.9–2.2 g protein/kg of body weight/day, as shown in Appendix K. Protein recommendations are higher for infants with 1.6–2.2 g protein/kg of body weight/day and lower for individuals with evidence of nephropathy, 0.8 g protein/kg of body weight/day or about 10% of daily calories from protein.

It is estimated that the average protein intake in the United States for all ages is about 14–18% of the total daily calories, with about 65% of this protein intake from animal products.[8] In a study assessing usual dietary intake of macro- and micronutrients of children with type 1 diabetes, it was noted that protein intake was within recommended levels. It is of concern, however, that the majority of the children are consuming levels at the upper limit of what is recommended.[20] Studies have demonstrated that one-third of patients with type 1 diabetes will develop nephropathy within 15–20 years after diagnosis.[21] Therefore, protein intake should be carefully assessed, with a focus on the family's overall protein intake.

Consistent competitive exercise may increase the need for some additional protein. This need should be met by increasing consumption of a nutritionally balanced diet, rather than by intake of liquid or powdered protein supplements.

Total Fat

Guidelines for fat intake were developed for children > 2 years of age by the National Cholesterol Education Program (NCEP) in 1991 to decrease risk of cardiovascular disease.[22] Type 1 diabetes has been associated with an increased risk of cardiovascular disease, but evidence suggests that blood glucose control may directly influence the levels of several plasma lipid components.[3] The NCEP recommends the Step 1 diet for children and adolescents with borderline or high LDL cholesterol levels. This diet includes the reduction of high dietary intakes of cholesterol to < 300 mg daily and no more than 30% of total calories from fat. Of the total fat, < 10% of calories should come from saturated fat, about 10% or fewer calories from polyunsaturated fat, and > 10% of calories from monounsaturated fat. If improvement in LDL cholesterol levels is not seen in 3 months, the NCEP recommends the Step 2 diet, which decreases saturated fat to less than 7% of calories and cholesterol to 200 mg per day. Studies have shown intake levels for cholesterol, fat, and saturated fat in children with type 1 diabetes are close to the recommendations.[20] This is likely supported by the fact that the national trend has been leaning toward decreasing overall fat intake.[18] Unfortunately, many children and adolescents do consume fat levels well above what is recommended, and these individuals may be at an even greater risk than children without diabetes.[20] Annual monitoring of lipid status is necessary to assess the effectiveness of any dietary fat modifications.[7] Careful consideration should be given to avoid strict fat restriction for children younger than 2 years of age, because the development of the brain and central nervous system are dependent in part on adequate intake of fats.

Vitamins and Minerals

There is often no need for additional vitamin and mineral supplements for the majority of people with diabetes, as long as the dietary intake is balanced and adequate. However, some children's normal eating habits exclude or severely limit foods or food groups throughout the growth cycle. Therefore, micronutrient adequacy should be evaluated periodically as children's food preferences change.

Vitamins and minerals often suggested as treatments for diabetes and other health issues include chromium, magnesium, zinc, and antioxidants.

Chromium

Chromium deficiency in both animal and human studies is associated with elevated blood glucose, cholesterol, and triglyceride levels; and reduction in body growth and longevity. Populations at risk for chromium deficiency include the elderly and those on long-term total parenteral alimentation. Fortunately, most people with diabetes are not chromium deficient, and the American Diabetes Association does not recommend chromium supplementation unless a deficiency is clearly documented.

Magnesium

Magnesium deficiency has been associated with insulin resistance, carbohydrate intolerance, and hypertension, among other disorders. Only those patients at high risk should be evaluated routinely, such as those in poor glycemic control (diabetic ketoacidosis and prolonged glycosuria), those on diuretics, or those with intestinal malabsorption.

Sodium

Sodium intakes for children and adolescents with diabetes are the same as those for the general population (see Chapters 4 and 5). Sensitivity to sodium varies greatly in its effect on people and blood pressure; however, it has not been demonstrated that those with diabetes are at a greater risk of developing hypertension associated with a high sodium intake. Routine monitoring of blood pressure is important and will help identify children and adolescents who may benefit from a reduction in sodium intake. Because sodium intake recommendations are the same as those for the general population, guidelines should be directed toward the entire family.

Zinc

Although insulin is stored as inactive zinc crystals in the beta cells and zinc is involved with insulin action, supplementation is suggested to benefit only those children with a zinc deficiency. When the dietary intake of children with type 1 diabetes was investigated, low intakes of zinc were noted in many of the children who were 4–6 years old; however, a nationwide sample of all children was reported to be inadequate in zinc intake, as well.[18] Low zinc intake may be attributed to limited animal products consumed by this young population, particularly meat. Poor growth has also been attributed to zinc deficiency in children with type 1 diabetes. Zinc supplementation in those children with low zinc levels increased their rate of linear growth.[23]

Antioxidants

Most vitamin and mineral intakes in a sample of 66 children with type 1 diabetes who were younger than 10 years of age exceeded the RDA; however, it was reported that exceptions to this in many of the children included such antioxidants as vitamins E and C.[18]

Recommendations

Vitamin and mineral supplements should not be used in place of a varied, balanced diet to ensure that children and adolescents receive adequate nutrients. Those who may be at risk and benefit from a multivitamin supplement with antioxidants would include those who are not consuming a variety of foods within the food groups, are strict vegetarians, are taking medications known to alter certain micronutrients, or those consistently in poor glycemic control, which can result in excess excretion of water-soluble vitamins.

Alcohol

Alcohol use and abuse should be discussed with the teenager in an objective manner.

Although the use of alcohol is not legal and is always discouraged for teens, facts about how alcohol affects the blood glucose level should be available to teens who express an interest in drinking. It should be made clear that alcohol lowers the blood glucose level and blocks gluconeogenesis, possibly leading to erratic behavior, loss of consciousness, or seizures, particularly if food is not consumed with the alcohol.[24] In addition, glucagon is not effective in the treatment of alcohol-induced hypoglycemia because alcohol depletes glycogen stores.

Alcohol should be used only when diabetes is under good control and in moderate amounts, defined as no more than one drink per day for most females and no more than two drinks a day for most males. One drink or portion is defined as 12 oz of beer, 5 oz of wine, or 1.5 oz of 80-proof distilled spirits. Each of these portions provides about 0.5 oz of alcohol, and it takes about 2 hours for the average 150-pound male to metabolize 1 oz of alcohol.[3]

Pointing out that alcohol alters the ability to think clearly may help the teen to use alcohol with caution or to avoid its use entirely. Wearing identification is especially important for individuals who choose to drink, because intoxication and symptoms of hypoglycemia can often be confused. Drinking alone should always be discouraged.

DESIGNING THE MEAL PLAN

The ultimate goals when designing a meal plan for a child who has been recently diagnosed with type 1 diabetes are to:

- promote positive behavioral changes
- provide healthy meals and snacks
- focus on healthy eating habits of the entire family

The amount of time required by the family to learn meal planning depends on multiple factors, such as family dynamics, emotional status, extended support system, preconceived ideas about the "diabetic diet," and the family's social and cultural attitudes. The child should participate in the initial visit and be reassured that he or she will not be put on a "diet" and have many of his or her favorite foods taken away. Rather, healthy guidelines (a meal plan) will be provided, based on the usual eating pattern, to help make healthy food choices. To avoid isolating the child and dividing the family, it should be emphasized to children that meal planning is simply a healthy eating plan for them, as well as for their entire family. Eating the same foods provides a sense of unity within the family.

Nutrition Counseling

At the time of diagnosis, the parent and/or child may be asked to keep a record of what is eaten at each meal and snack. This helps to establish the amount of food that is currently needed to satisfy the child's appetite. A newly diagnosed child is more likely to experience increased hunger due to glycosuria, therefore it is important to respond to their stimulated appetite so that hunger and restriction are not associated with having diabetes. The appetites of most children will usually stabilize by the third to fifth day of insulin management. An accurate measurement of weight and height (or length), information on recent weight loss, and calculation of IBW are needed to estimate the child's current nutrient needs. Determining the percentile of the height (length), weight, weight for height, and the range for IBW will identify the child's initial nutrition status and help guide the development of the meal plan.

Nutrition intervention in the hospital setting should be based on the family's ability, interest, and readiness to learn. Attempts to present all concepts upon initial diagnosis may result in confusion and family members' loss of confidence in their ability as caretakers. Only general guidelines should be provided, such as consistency with timing, amount and types of foods, and the relationship between food, insulin, and exercise, and their effect on blood glucose. Routine follow-up by phone is beneficial because many questions arise when the child returns home and normal activity resumes. Above all, it should be stressed that:

- Parents should not promote distorted eating to maintain blood glucose control.
- Any changes associated with food choices should be made slowly.
- Ranges should be used with young children for food choices (ie, 1–2 oz protein, 1/2–1 fruit), offering smaller amounts first and using the larger end of the range if more food is requested.
- The length of time required to achieve *initial* nutrition management survival skills while hospitalized varies considerably and may require 2–4 hours, with additional time for menu writing and selection by the caretakers, using the meal plan.
- After leaving the hospital, actual teaching may require from two to four outpatient visits to achieve *ultimate* nutrition education goals.

The initial visit as an outpatient should lay the groundwork in nutrition basics and serve to develop a sound and trusting relationship with the child and family. The Children's Checklist (Exhibit 20–3) is a detailed analysis of the child's and family's eating habits and behaviors, food preferences, and family lifestyle, and it will assist the registered dietitian in producing a realistic and workable meal plan for this very important population.

General guidelines to help develop a positive working relationship with the child and caretakers are as follows:

- Include children in the interview to allow them to be part of the decision-making process.
- Do not refer to or label a child as a "diabetic"—these are children who happen to have diabetes.
- Interview prepubertal children separately and together with family to stimulate self-management.
- Provide reassurance that many of the child's usual foods can be included in the meal plan.
- Describe the meal plan as a "road map" for healthy eating, rather than a rigid diet.
- Stress healthy eating practices for the entire family, rather than focusing on just the child with diabetes to avoid isolating and dividing the child and family in their food choices.
- Avoid negative words when explaining meal planning, such as *cannot, do not, never, should not, bad, restrict*, and especially the word *diet*. In a child's mind, *diet* connotes deprivation, as well as a short-term process, rather than an ongoing one.
- Ask about favorite foods and avoid eliminating these foods. Instead, stress balance, moderation, and variety.
- Review the reality of special treats for birthday parties, holidays, special occasions, and relate "treat" foods with extra exercise and active days.
- Encourage caregivers to include children in shopping and meal preparation.
- Revise or draft a realistic and workable meal plan with input from the parent and/or child.
- Advise caregivers that omitting foods from the meal plan because of a single high blood glucose reading is not advisable. An elevated blood glucose level caused by stress may decrease rapidly when the stress is reduced, and hypoglycemia may occur if food is omitted.[25]

Continued nutritional follow-up and education are required every 6 months to 1 year as the child grows and develops, and as the family works to gain expertise in the nutritional management of diabetes.

Meal Planning Approaches

One of the primary reasons that patients with diabetes have such a difficult time understanding "food issues" is a lack of nutrition education

Exhibit 20–3 Children's Checklist: Assessing the Child Newly Diagnosed with Diabetes

Growth (Anthropometrics):
- Height
- Weight
- Weight for height
- History of growth pattern
- Recent weight changes

Biochemical Indices:
- Blood glucose
- Glycosylated hemoglobin
- Lipid profile
- Microalbumin
- Ketones

Psychosocial Information:
- Identify the family unit at home (two parents, single, divorced, separated parents, siblings, other family or friends)
- Evaluate emotional state of parents, child, siblings (anger, fear, guilt, denial, anxiety)
- Assess child's interactions with parents and siblings
- Identify person(s) responsible for shopping/cooking
- Evaluate knowledge/comprehension levels
- Identify cultural/religious systems that influence attitudes
- Identify family members or friends with diabetes
- Assess parent and family beliefs about the "diabetic diet"

Child's Usual Food Intake Prior to Symptoms of Diabetes

Home:
- Eats scheduled meals/snacks
- Includes staple foods, such as milk, cheese, yogurt, bread
- Eats meats, fruits, and vegetables on a regular basis
- Consumes beverages at meals/snacks other than milk
- Drinks soda/juice/water for thirst
- Includes dessert foods with most meals/snacks

School:
- Brings lunch from home
- Scheduled snacks are part of regular class activities
- Obtains snack at school or snack sent from home
- Scheduled gym class
- Participates in school sports or activities after school

Weekends:
- Evaluate meals prepared or eaten with others on weekends
- Identify meal schedule if different from weekdays
- Determine restaurant eating habits on weekends
- Assess sports/activities scheduled on weekends

continues

Exhibit 20–3 continued

Eating Behaviors

Child:

- Overeats or undereats
- Relies on convenience and fast foods
- Experiences food jags often
- Refuses many family foods offered
- Sits at the table for all meals and snacks
- Finishes meals in a reasonable amount of time
- Respects limits set for acceptable eating behavior at the table
- Food allergies

Family:

- Evaluate parents as role models
  - healthy eaters, structured meals, planned meals, limit junk food in home
  - unhealthy eaters, overweight, chronic dieters
- Identify supervision at meals/snacks
- Evaluate limit-setting around food choices
- Assess cultural/religious eating behaviors
- Identify whether food is used as a reward

and counseling by a registered dietitian. Instead, patients may simply be told to restrict sugar or may be given a basic sample menu to follow without an adequate educational foundation. The DCCT provided important insight into the role of nutrition intervention in intensive diabetes treatment and stated that registered dietitians are best qualified to match appropriate meal planning approaches to the needs of the patient.[26]

A *meal planning approach* simply means the "educational resource" used by the dietitian/diabetes educator to teach the client how to plan meals.[26] Today, there are several effective methods of teaching patients about food. All methods can be equally effective when "geared to the patient's intellectual level, repeated frequently, and evaluated."[27(655)]

The two most common approaches used with children are exchange lists for meal planning and carbohydrate counting. These methods give structure to meal planning, providing the right balance between food, insulin, and exercise.

The Exchange System

The lists of food choices (exchange lists) are based on three main food groups—the carbohydrate group (starch, fruit, milk, vegetables, and other carbohydrates), the meat and meat substitute group (protein), and the fat group (see Exhibit 20–4).[28] Examples of the specific amounts of carbohydrate, protein, fat, or combination of these nutrients in each food group are found in Table 20–2. Foods with similar nutrient values are listed together and may be exchanged or traded for any other food on the same list. Portion sizes for each food are listed and are measured after cooking. Exchange lists are used to achieve a consistent timing and intake of carbohydrate, protein, and fat, and provide needed variety when planning meals. Exchange lists and a meal plan can be a starting point for those patients on intensive insulin management and can help them to understand and learn the carbohydrate content of foods.

Exhibit 20–4 Exchange Lists for Meal Planning*

Carbohydrate Group

Starch/Bread

Cooked cereal	1/2 cup
Bran cereal, flaked	1/2 cup
Frankfurter or hamburger bun	1/2 (1 oz)
Bread (white or whole-wheat)	1 slice (1 oz)
Peas, green	1/2 cup
Potato, mashed	1/2 cup
Popcorn, popped (no fat added)	3 cups

Vegetable

1/2 cup cooked or 1 cup raw vegetable:
Beans (green)
Broccoli
Carrots
Cauliflower
Peppers (green)
Spinach (cooked)
Summer squash
Tomato (1 large)

Fruit

Apple (raw, 2" across)	1
Applesauce (unsweetened)	1/2 cup
Banana (9" long)	1/2
Orange (2 1/2" across)	1
Strawberries (raw, whole)	1 1/4 cups
Apple juice/cider	1/2 cup
Grape juice	1/3 cup
Orange juice	1/2 cup

Milk

Skim/low-fat/reduced-fat/whole	8 oz

Other Carbohydrates

Sandwich cookies	2 small
Potato chips	12–18
Frozen yogurt, low-fat	1/3 cup
Jam, sugar or syrup	1 tbsp

Meat/Meat Substitute Group

Lean	
Lean beef (round, flank)	1 oz
Chicken (without skin)	1 oz
Cottage cheese	1/4 cup
Medium-Fat	
Ground beef	1 oz
Pork chop	1 oz
86% fat-free luncheon meat	1 oz
High-Fat	
Frankfurter (turkey or chicken) (10/lb)	1 frank
Cheese (American, Cheddar, or Swiss)	1 oz

Fat Group

Margarine	1 tsp
Mayonnaise	1 tsp
Mayonnaise (reduced-calorie)	1 tbsp
Salad dressing	1 tbsp
Salad dressing (reduced-calorie)	2 tbsp

Free Food

Carbonated drinks (sugar free)	
Cocoa powder (unsweetened)	1 tbsp
Raw vegetables	1 cup
Gelatin (sugar free)	
Catsup	1 tbsp
Taco Sauce	1 tbsp
Pickle, dill	

*Partial listing; shows amounts to equal one exchange.

Source: Reprinted from *Exchange Lists for Meal Planning,* with permission of American Diabetes Association, Inc. and the American Dietetic Association, © 1995.

Table 20–2 Nutrient Content of Exchanges

Groups/Lists	*Carbohydrate (g)*	*Protein (g)*	*Fat (g)*	*Calories*
Carbohydrate Group				
Starch	15	3	1 or less	80
Fruit	15	—	—	60
Milk				
Skim	12	8	0–3	90
Reduced-fat	12	8	5	120
Whole	12	8	8	150
Other Carbohydrates	15	varies	varies	varies
Vegetables	5	2	—	25
Meat and Meat Substitute Group				
Very lean	—	7	0–1	35
Lean	—	7	3	55
Medium-fat	—	7	5	75
High-fat	—	7	8	100
Fat Group	—	—	5	45

Source: Reprinted from *Exchange Lists for Meal Planning,* with permission of American Diabetes Association, Inc. and the American Dietetic Association, © 1995.

Carbohydrate Counting

A growing number of older children is maintaining glucose levels on multiple daily injections (MDI) or continuous subcutaneous insulin infusion (CSII) using pump therapy. The carbohydrate counting system allows the users greater flexibility in the timing of meals, the amount of food eaten at each meal, and the selection of specific foods. The meal planning objective is to coordinate food intake (carbohydrate) by matching the peak activity of insulin with the peak levels of glucose resulting from the digestion and absorption of food.[26] With this system, only the carbohydrate value of the food is counted, which allows more precise adjustment of premeal, short-acting insulin (regular or humalog) using an insulin/carbohydrate ratio. The insulin/carbohydrate ratio is based on the assumption that carbohydrate intake is the main consideration in determining meal-related insulin requirements, together with self-monitored blood glucose (SMBG) and targeted blood glucose values set by the physician and the patient. The general rule is that approximately 1 unit of short-acting insulin will be needed for every 10–15 g carbohydrate.[25] Care must be taken not to overeat because increased availability of insulin and food may promote unwanted weight gain. A good understanding of how carbohydrate affects blood glucose, what food groups contain carbohydrate, which reference books provide carbohydrate content of specific foods, and of portion control is necessary for carbohydrate counting to be effective. Continuous reinforcement of healthy eating habits is advisable because many young people tend to omit food groups, as well as meals, to accommodate busy schedules or to control weight.

Insulin Therapy

Insulin regimens for children may range from one to two daily injections of intermediate-acting insulin (NPH or Lente) or long-acting insulin

(Ultralente), possibly combined with a small amount of short-acting insulin (regular or humalog), called *conventional insulin therapy,* to four or more daily injections using a short-acting insulin with either an intermediate or long-acting insulin, or CSII/pump therapy, called *intensive insulin therapy*. A MDI regimen allows more freedom in the scheduling of meals and may eliminate the need for many snacks; however, intensive insulin therapy does increase the risk of hypoglycemia. The onset, peak, and duration of the common types of insulin are listed in Table 20–3.

Many circumstances require that permanent or temporary insulin adjustments be made. As a child grows and food intake increases, the insulin dose also increases. During brief periods of illness or times of stress or decreased activity, insulin needs also may increase. A change in the child's level of activity, which may be especially dramatic at the beginning and end of the school year, usually requires a decrease in the insulin dosage. When a problem or behavior that affects insulin dosage resolves or changes, the child's insulin dose will require readjustment. Otherwise, a larger intake in response to the higher insulin level may result in inappropriate weight gain or hypoglycemia, whereas too little insulin may result in hyperglycemia.

Snacks

Because insulin is continuously released after injection, it is necessary to prevent hypoglycemia between meals by encouraging snacks between meals and at bedtime. Typically, a snack of 15–20 g carbohydrate is recommended for young children, and a snack of 20–30 g carbohydrate or higher is recommended for adolescents. The times of recess and physical education (PE) classes and the type and length of after-school activities will influence the kind and amount of food needed for snacks. If PE is offered only on Mondays and Wednesdays at 10:00 AM, for example, the child may need a larger snack on those days, preferably a snack with 20–30 g carbohydrate and 1–2 oz protein. A long-lasting snack (2–3 hours) for very active days and extended appetite control must have carbohydrate, protein, and fat in it. For inactive children whose main activity is not likely to increase beyond watching television and studying, snacks may require only 15–20 g carbohydrate.

AGE-SPECIFIC DEVELOPMENTAL CONSIDERATIONS

The most important psychosocial issues facing families with children with diabetes are:[29]

Table 20–3 Summary of the Activity of Insulin Types

	Rapid-Acting (Humalog)	*Short-Acting (Regular)*	*Intermediate-Acting (NPH, Lente)*	*Long-Acting (Ultralente, Human)*
Onset	within 15 min	approx 1/2 hr	1–3 hrs	approx 4–8 hrs
Peak	30–90 min	2–4 hrs	6–12 hrs	approx 12–18 hrs
Duration	3–5 hrs	6–8 hrs	18–26 hrs	approx 24–28 hrs

Source: From *The Joslin Guide to Diabetes,* page 116, by Richard S. Beaser and Joan V.C. Hill, 1995, Simon & Schuster (Fireside). Copyright © 1995 by The Joslin Diabetes Center. Adapted with permission.

- how responsibilities for diabetes management are defined and supported within the family
- how these treatment responsibilities are shared among family members
- how and when these responsibilities are transferred from parent to child as the child develops

As the child progresses through the different stages of development, it is important to address the changes facing parents and/or children with diabetes and to focus on the normal developmental issues at each stage. Exhibit 20–5 outlines the psychosocial and developmental adjustments that children, adolescents, and families must face and consider in managing diabetes.

Age-Specific Food Considerations

Birth to 12 Months

Initially, infants consume 100% of their calories as breast milk or formula, and most eat every 3–4 hours. The American Academy of Pediatrics recommends that all babies be breastfed for the first 6–12 months of life; iron-fortified infant formula is the only acceptable substitute. Those with diabetes will do well following this same schedule and will eventually include strained cereal, fruits, meat, vegetables, and/or vegetable-meat dinners with the formula (see Chapter 4).

Exhibit 20–6 provides a partial food list for infants.[30] Juice may tend to cause an elevated blood glucose level in most infants and should be limited, diluted, or omitted in the diet until the child is eating more solid foods.

When the infant begins eating 2–3 tablespoons of baby foods and/or table food other than low-calorie vegetables, the exchange system or basic carbohydrate counting can be introduced as a guideline to ensure adequate intake. Establishing a feeding schedule despite somewhat erratic eating behaviors in infants is recommended.

1–4 Years of Age

A report that appeared in the *New England Journal of Medicine* in 1992 proposed a possible link between drinking cow's milk as an infant and the development of type 1 diabetes. Upon further investigation, investigators concluded that early exposure to cow's milk was not associated with an elevated risk for type 1 diabetes in individuals who did not have the diabetes susceptibility gene. Although whole cow's milk should not be given during the child's first year, cow's milk should not be removed from the diets of genetically susceptible infants after the first year.

When the infant starts drinking milk from a cup (usually between 12 and 15 months of age), milk intake usually decreases and solid food increases. A total revision of the meal plan is needed at that time. A better acceptance of meat and cheese also occurs, which makes it possible to include the meat group in the meal plan. Although fruits are included in the meal plan, fruit juice should continue to be limited or avoided.

As the toddler develops more mobility and interest in the environment increases, interest in food wanes. In some instances, getting the toddler to eat anything at a meal is an accomplishment. Insulin therapy must be closely monitored when this occurs. In extreme cases, insulin is given after it is known whether and how much the toddler has consumed, so that the dose of insulin can be based on the amount of food eaten and any negative food behaviors can be addressed. Food behavior guidelines for this young group, with or without diabetes, should be firmly established by caregivers at the time the child begins solid foods.

School-Aged Children

Adjusting diabetes around the school schedule, rather than changing PE classes or lunch periods to accommodate an insulin regimen, communicates to the child that the child is more important than the diabetes. It is possible to arrange snacks and injections around most school schedules. Parents should be encouraged to address food and diabetes treatment issues with

Exhibit 20–5 Challenges Facing Parents and/or Children with Diabetes

Parents of infants and toddlers (0–3 yr old)
- Monitoring diabetes control and avoiding hypoglycemia
- Establishing a meal schedule despite the child's normally irregular eating patterns
- Coping with the very young child's inability to understand the need for injections
- Managing the conflicts with older siblings that result from unequal sharing of parental attention

Preschoolers and early elementary school children (4–7 yr old)
- Mastering separation from the family and adapting to the expectations of teachers
- Blaming self for having diabetes; regarding injections and restrictions as punishments
- Educating school personnel, coaches, and scout leaders about diabetes (parents)

Later elementary school children (8–11 yr old)
- Engaging in a wide range of activities with peers
- Understanding long-term benefits of diabetes care
- Becoming involved in diabetes self-care tasks (selecting snacks, selecting and cleaning injection sites, and identifying symptoms of low blood glucose)

Early adolescence (12–15 yr old)
- Integrating physical changes into self-image
- Acknowledging that the young teenager is on the threshold of becoming an adult (parents)
- Assuming increased responsibility for diabetes management in the face of physiologic changes on insulin resistance and sensitivity caused by puberty
- Fitting in with the peer group
- Maintaining good glycemic control while concerned about possible weight gain

Later adolescence (16–19 yr old)
- Making decisions regarding plans after high school
- Living more independently of parents
- Strengthening relationships with fewer friends
- Assuming more independent responsibility for health and health care

Source: Reprinted with permission from H.E. Lebovitz, Psychosocial Adjustment in Children with Type I Diabetes, in *Therapy for Diabetes Mellitus and Related Disorders,* 3rd ed., H.E. Lebovitz, ed., p. 72, © 1998. American Diabetes Association.

school personnel; however, some parents may require assistance from their health care team. School-aged children will ordinarily need three meals and three snacks a day, spaced according to their insulin regimen. However, some children can omit the morning snack without creating a problem, as long as lunch is not delayed. Children should be instructed to carry a fast-acting carbohydrate with them at all times, in case of emergency, as shown in Exhibit 20–7. The use of chocolate candy bars or other high-fat items is discouraged as a treatment for hypoglycemia because fat slows the absorption of the carbohydrate needed to raise the blood glucose to a safe level.

Most schools will substitute lunch items appropriately to meet the needs of children following a meal plan, such as low-fat milk and fresh fruit. If school personnel are unwilling to cooperate, reference can be made to Section 504 of the Rehabilitation Act of 1973 or to the Education for All Handicapped Children Act of 1975, commonly referred to as Public Law No. 94-142, which mandates that handicapped students,

Exhibit 20–6 Food List for Baby Foods Containing about 8 g Carbohydrate

Food	Amount
Cereal	
Dry cereal	3 tbsp
100% Juices—4 fluid oz	
Apple, orange, pear, white grape, mixed fruits	1/2 container
First or Strained Vegetables—2.5-oz jar	
Carrots, green beans, peas, potatoes, squash	1 Jar
First or Strained Fruits—2.5-oz jar	
Applesauce, peaches, pears	1 Jar
Bananas, prunes	1/2 Jar
Second cereals—4-oz jar	
Jarred cereal with fruit	1/3 Jar
Second Vegetables—4-oz jar	
Carrots, creamed spinach, garden vegetables, green beans, mixed vegetables, peas, squash	1 Jar
Sweet potatoes, creamed corn	1/2 Jar
Second Fruits—4-oz jar	
Applesauce, apricots with mixed fruit, peaches, pear pineapple	1/2 Jar
Bananas, pears, plums with apples, prunes with apples	1/3 Jar
Second Dinners—4-oz jar	
Chicken noodle, macaroni cheese, turkey rice, vegetable beef, chicken, ham, or turkey dinner	3/4–1 Jar
Second Desserts—4-oz jar	
Mixed fruit yogurt, peach cobbler, vanilla custard	1/3 Jar
Third Cereals—6-oz jar	
Jarred cereal with fruit	1/3 Jar
Third Vegetables—6-oz jar	
Carrots, squash, broccoli and carrots with cheese	2/3 Jar
Green beans with rice, peas with rice	1/2 Jar
Sweet potatoes	1/3 Jar
Third Fruits—6-oz jar	
Applesauce, apricots with mixed fruit, fruit salad, peaches	1/3 Jar
Bananas, banana pineapple, pears, plums with apples	1/4 Jar

Exhibit 20–6 continued

Third Dinners—6-oz jar	
Beef and egg noodle, chicken noodle, turkey rice, vegetable beef, chicken, ham, or turkey dinner	1/2 Jar
Spaghetti in tomato sauce with beef, vegetables and pasta, vegetable stew dinners	1/3 Jar
Third Desserts—6-oz. jar	
Dutch apple, blueberry buckle, vanilla custard	1/4 Jar

Source: Courtesy of Gerber Product Company, Fremont, Michigan.

Exhibit 20–7 Carbohydrates

The following sources of carbohydrate (equal to 15 g) are ideal for treating low blood sugar:

4 oz orange juice
3 oz regular cranberry juice
3 oz sweetened grape juice
4 oz fruit drinks such as Tang or HiC
6 oz regular ginger ale
5 oz regular soda, such as Coca-Cola or Pepsi
3–4 tsp sugar dissolved in water
8 Life Savers
6 regular-sized jelly beans, or 10 small
9 small gumdrops
3 large marshmallows, or 25 small
1 tbsp marshmallow cream
1 tbsp concentrated syrup such as honey, maple syrup, Karo, Coke
1 small tube cake icing (1/2-oz tube)
1 1/2 portions dried fruits
3 B-D glucose tablets
1/2 tube Glutose (80 g tube)
1 1/2 packages Monojel

Source: From *The Joslin Guide to Diabetes,* page 172, by Richard S. Beaser and Joan V.C. Hill, 1995, Simon & Schuster (Fireside). Copyright © 1995 by The Joslin Diabetes Center. Reprinted with permission.

including children with diabetes, have access to all services necessary to assist in full participation in school.

Adolescents

The advent of adolescence may bring a great deal of conflict into the lives of family members. Adolescents strive for independence and expect parents to trust them to manage their own diabetes. Adolescents may vent their anger about having diabetes for the first time. The key to working successfully with adolescents is for the parents and the health care team to make every effort to provide positive reinforcement and negotiated support. Parents should continue their involvement and supervision of monitoring blood glucose and insulin administration at home. It is often more effective for team members to see teenagers and their parents individually, while at the same time respecting the teenager's confidentiality. More flexibility in food choices and an increase in calories during this period of growth are usually necessary. Food choices may improve in a nonjudgmental atmosphere and with assistance for the teen to work favorite foods into the meal plan. On clinic visits, the teen should be routinely asked if a change in the meal plan is desired. Even if no change is made, the teen will enjoy having some control over the meal plan.

Weight Control

Weight control can become an important issue when children enter adolescence. Concerns about body image must be taken seriously by parents and the health care team. Some weight gain is usually seen prior to growth spurts. The sex maturity ratings (SMRs) developed by Tanner are a useful guide for identifying appropriate weight loss recommendations (see Appendix I). Weight loss before SMR 3 in girls and SMR 4 in boys is not recommended because of the need for calories for continued growth.[31] If a child's weight is too high for height, the weight should be kept stable until the height comes into line with the weight. Calorie reduction and food restriction are not recommended for children at any time during growth and development. Rather, the child should be encouraged to become involved in active play and physical exercise.

Children who are overly concerned about weight gain but who find it difficult to reduce intake may choose to skip insulin injections to promote quick weight loss. When significant weight loss is noted, etiology should be explored. Signs of insulin omission or misuse for weight loss may include:

- weight fluctuations of 10 pounds or more
- uncontrolled diabetes based on glycosylated hemoglobin measures
- controlled diabetes only when hospitalized
- multiple hospital admissions with unexplained diabetic ketoacidosis
- reluctance or refusal to take more insulin
- blaming insulin for weight problems
- preoccupation with body weight or shape
- engagement in excessive exercise
- depression and low self-esteem

Referral to a diabetes nutrition educator is the first line of defense when a child or adolescent exhibits weight dissatisfaction but does not exhibit clinical eating pathology. Strict guidelines regarding food and blood glucose should not be implemented because this may actually promote binge-eating or weight gain. Adolescents should be advised that glucose fluctuations can create increased hunger and result in weight gain. Education should also be provided about serious short- and long-term consequences of destructive food behaviors. Referral to a mental health professional who is knowledgeable about diabetes and disordered eating or hospitalization is often necessary to break the disordered eating cycle.

Growth Maintenance

Routine charting of a child's height, weight, and weight for height is an excellent way to monitor the growth pattern. Deviation from the child's normal growth curve (except for increased height or decreasing weight in a child who has reached full height potential) requires close monitoring.

In a child whose diabetes is poorly controlled, weight percentile will often remain stationary or will decrease. After about 6 months of little or no weight gain, height velocity may also begin to slow. Achieving optimal height potential can be used to motivate boys and girls to strive for better control. Teenagers are more likely to be interested in improved self-care when they understand the relationship between good control, appropriate weight gain, consistent height increase, and/or normal menses.

PREGNANCY

To help ensure a healthy pregnancy and a positive outcome, optimal medical care must begin *before* conception. However, many unplanned pregnancies occur shortly after puberty among young people with and without diabetes, putting those with pregestational diabetes mellitus (PGDM) at a higher risk for early pregnancy loss or congenital malformations in infants. The deterioration of metabolic control, in combination with other obstetric and medical complications during an unplanned pregnancy, can lead to serious complications of diabetes such as retinopathy, nephropathy, hypertension, and neuropathy. It is the responsibility of the health care team to provide prepregnancy counseling, including information on the risk of congenital malformations, to those of child-bearing age who have diabetes.

Unplanned pregnancies should be addressed immediately by a multidisciplinary team approach, including a diabetologist, obstetrician, and diabetes educators, including a nurse, a registered dietitian, a social worker, and possibly an exercise physiologist. The team approach can guide the mother toward a goal of a healthy pregnancy and offspring.[32] Members of the patient's immediate family are encouraged to attend and participate in all learning sessions.

A preconception, interactive care plan outlined by the American Diabetic Association to facilitate reimbursement for all elements of the program by health insurance organizations includes the following:[32]

- *Patient education*—interaction of diabetes, pregnancy, and family planning
- *Training*—diabetes self-management skills
- *Counseling*—professional mental health assistance to reduce stress and improve adherence to the diabetes treatment plan
- *Medical care and laboratory tests*—physician-directed

Practical self-management skills include:[32]

1. using an appropriate meal plan with scheduled meals and snacks
2. planning physical activity
3. choosing the time and site of insulin injections
4. using carbohydrate and glucagon for hypoglycemia
5. reducing stress and coping with denial
6. testing blood glucose and self-adjusting insulin doses

Nutrition management during pregnancy should begin at the earliest possible time. Caloric intake should be evaluated as soon as possible in the first trimester and at the start of each trimester thereafter to ensure adequate intake. For those with PGDM, three meals and three snacks should be spaced no less than 2 hours apart and no more than 4 hours apart. Caloric requirements are based on pregravid weight, height, age, activity level, and usual intake, with distribution of calories as follows: carbohydrate 40–50% of total calories, protein 20–25% of total calories, and fat 30–40% of total calories. In addition, special emphasis should be placed on the following:

1. meal planning to include appropriate calcium, folic acid, and other vitamin intake
2. appropriate modification of the meal plan to address nausea, vomiting, heartburn, and constipation
3. risk assessment and prevention of fasting hypoglycemia
4. adequate carbohydrate and protein intake at bedtime to prevent nocturnal hypoglycemia and or ketones
5. current intake of sweeteners and caffeine
6. adjustment of calories for gestational age:[33]

	first trimester	*second trimester*	*third trimester*
Underweight	30 kcal/kg	36–40	36–40
Desirable Body Weight	30 kcal/kg	36	36–38

Overweight/ Obese	24 kcal/kg present weight	24	24

7. General weight gain goals during pregnancy based on pregravid weight and clinical assessment are as follows:[33]

Underweight:	28–40 pounds
Desirable Body Weight:	25–35 pounds
Overweight/ Obese:	15–25 pounds

General guidelines for rate of weight gain would be 2–5 pounds in the first trimester, followed by 1 pound/week after the first trimester for those at desirable weight, 1.1 pounds/week for those who are underweight, and 0.7 pounds/week for those who are overweight.[33]

Breastfeeding

Breastfeeding is encouraged for mothers with diabetes and provides the same benefits as it does for any mother and infant (insulin is not ingested by the baby through breast milk). Breast milk contains immunoglobulins and antibodies that protect infants from diseases, intestinal distress, and allergic reactions, and the process of breastfeeding encourages mother–infant bonding. Breastfeeding, however, increases the need for fluids, and mothers should be encouraged to drink 2–3 L (8–12 cups) caffeine-free liquids per day to cover the fluid needs of the mother and to replace what is used in breast milk.

Meal planning during breastfeeding requires assistance from a dietitian and a physician. Insulin requirements are usually reduced during breastfeeding; however, caloric intake requires an additional 500 calories per day above what was used before the pregnancy.[33] Extra calories may be added in the form of protein and calcium-rich foods such as milk, yogurt, tofu, and cheese. The calcium requirement for lactating women is 1,200 mg/day. Calcium intake should be routinely assessed by a dietitian to prevent calcium loss from the mother during breastfeeding. If the mother is not able to consume adequate sources of calcium-rich foods, a calcium supplement may be required. It is important to keep a carbohydrate food source (15–20 g) available because hypoglycemia may occur while breastfeeding. To prevent possible nocturnal hypoglycemia, an extra snack containing 20–30 g carbohydrate and a source of protein may be added to the meal plan in the middle of the night.

MONITORING TOOLS

The test for glycosylated hemoglobin measures the average amount of glucose in the blood over a 2- to 3-month period. Used in conjunction with regularly monitored blood glucose results, glycosylated hemoglobin levels can help evaluate the level of control. However, the glycosylated hemoglobin level reflects an average amount of glucose in the blood and can be the result of very high and low blood glucose levels, which is not indicative of good control. Although "excellent control" for an adult with diabetes is 7% or less, the activity levels and eating habits of children and adolescents vary, so reaching a level even under 8% can be unsafe and difficult.[34] It is recommended that glycosylated hemoglobin goals be set by the child's diabetes team and tailored to each child or adolescent.

Home blood glucose monitoring devices provide the child and family with readily available feedback on the effects of food, exercise, insulin, and stress on blood glucose level, allowing for more flexibility in lifestyle and food intake.

A child with diabetes has many responsibilities for self-care. Checking and recording the blood glucose level may be one of the most bothersome because it must be done so often and because others may inappropriately evaluate and judge the results. Blood glucose results are not totally reliable as a monitor of compliance with meal plans. If, by reporting a high blood glucose reading, a child risks accusations of sneaking food or overeating, the child may choose to record more acceptable, but false, levels. This practice may result in poor diabetes management. Establishing a nonjudgmental and honest atmosphere for the exchange of information is imperative for the parent, the dietitian, and other health care providers.

When monitoring blood glucose, use the word *check* rather than *test* and use positive words to describe the results, such as *high* or *low*, rather than *good* or *bad*. Any information received from monitoring provides positive feedback, regardless of the number.[35] High or low blood glucose levels will occur in most children, even when insulin and exercise schedules and the meal plan are followed closely. When a high or low level occurs, it is useful to review the day's activities to see whether there is an obvious explanation for the level.

The extent to which children should monitor blood glucose levels is variable, depending on many factors, such as the type of insulin therapy, increased activity or exercise, sickness or infection, new food choices, change in lifestyle, increased stress, change in insulin type or dose, episodes of hypoglycemia, or overall poor control. A general guideline for blood glucose testing for infants and children is before each meal and before the bedtime snack.

Exercise

Regular exercise is an important element in controlling the blood glucose level, lowering lipid levels, and maintaining appropriate body weight. Aerobic exercise is necessary to maintain a healthy cardiovascular system, as well as to improve glucose control. To prevent obesity in children, emphasis should be placed on the importance of routinely scheduled exercise. An optimum of 30 minutes of uninterrupted daily exercise is a reasonable goal. However, exercising when ketones are present, which may occur when the blood glucose level is above 240 mg/dL, or when the blood glucose is 400 mg/dL or higher without ketones is not recommended.

For prevention of hypoglycemia during exercise, an increase in food or decrease in insulin dose usually needs to be made. Generally, increasing food is the treatment of choice for many children unless the exercise is a continuing, daily routine. If overall activity increases, a child may need less insulin, and the diabetes team should be consulted. Older children may be instructed in how to reduce their insulin dose when participating in sports. It is wise to avoid exercise when insulin is peaking; however, sports events and practices are usually scheduled when the insulin is working hardest. In this instance, a larger snack, including carbohydrate as well as protein, may be needed. However, some find it difficult to eat a large volume of food prior to prolonged activity and plan ahead to reduce their insulin dose.

The amount of reduction depends on the results of blood glucose tests done before and after exercise. Food adjustments will depend on the duration and intensity of the exercise and on the blood glucose level prior to exercise (Exhibit 20–8). A general rule is to add 10–15 g carbohydrate for every hour of extra activity.

Prolonged activity may utilize a majority of the glucose stores in the muscle. The body replaces these stores when blood glucose becomes available. It is very important for the child or adolescent to realize that an adequate snack, probably containing protein as well as carbohydrate, may need to be eaten after prolonged exercise to avoid a low blood glucose level that may occur hours after the activity has stopped.

Hypoglycemia

The most common emergency of insulin-dependent diabetes is hypoglycemia. The exact blood glucose level that produces symptoms of hypoglycemia is an individual response and differs with the level of glucose control. Symptoms may occur when the blood glucose level is 60 mg/dL or below. A rapidly dropping blood glucose level may cause symptoms of hypoglyce-

Exhibit 20–8 Adjustments for Exercise

Types of Exercise and Examples	*If Blood Glucose Is*	*Suggestions of Food To Use*
Exercise of short duration (30 min or less) and of moderate intensity Examples: walking a mile or bicycling for less than 30 min	Less than 100 100–180 180 or more	1 fruit + 1 bread + 1 meat 1 bread or 1 fruit Snack *may* not be necessary
Exercise of intermediate duration (1 hr) and moderate intensity Examples: tennis, swimming, jogging, leisurely bicycling, gardening, golfing, or vacuuming for 1 hr	Less than 100 100–180 180–240 240 or more	1 fruit + 1 bread + 1 meat 1 bread + 1 meat 1 bread or 1 fruit Snack *may* not be necessary
Exercise of long duration (2 hr or more) and high intensity Examples: football, hockey, racquetball, or basketball games; strenuous bicycling or swimming; shoveling heavy snow; skiing; hiking	Consult with your physician or exercise physiologist. Insulin may need to be decreased by 30–75%. Begin with a snack of 2 bread + 2 meat then eat at least 1 bread or 1 fruit per hr of exercise. Test hourly. If blood glucose is 180 or more, an extra snack *may* not be needed for that hour.	

Source: From *The Joslin Guide to Diabetes*, page 79, by Richard S. Beaser and Joan V.C. Hill, 1995, Simon & Schuster (Fireside). Copyright © 1995 by The Joslin Diabetes Center. Reprinted with permission.

mia, even when the level is in the normal range. Exhibit 20–7 lists suggestions for treatment choices for hypoglycemia.

Children with diabetes should be instructed to wear medical alert identification at all times to ensure proper treatment of hypoglycemic reactions, which may render the child unable to communicate.

Sick Days

Illness in the child with diabetes always presents a challenge. Insulin must always be given and may need to be increased during these periods. Monitoring of blood glucose should be done every 3–4 hours. Parents need to know when to call the doctor for assistance in managing illness because prolonged vomiting, as well as fever, can lead to rapid dehydration and diabetic ketoacidosis. During a brief illness, the meal plan should be maintained when possible, using foods that can be tolerated. If the child cannot tolerate food, it is important to replace the usual amount of carbohydrate consumed with sugar-containing liquids that can be easily used by the body for energy. Liquids also help to prevent dehydration. Easily tolerated liquids that contain 15 g carbohydrate may include 4–6 oz of a regular carbonated beverage (with sugar), 4 oz of fruit juice or a frozen fruit bar, or 1/2 cup of regular gelatin. Consuming room-temperature liquids in small sips at a rate of about 15 g carbohydrate/hour is recommended. Sick day guidelines, as shown in Exhibit 20–9, will provide steps to take during the illness of a child to prevent problems with diabetes management.

ORGANIZATIONS AND PUBLICATIONS

There are several national organizations that help families dealing with diabetes in adapting to their new lifestyles. The American Diabetes Association and the Juvenile Diabetes Foundation (JDF) are organizations founded to provide services to persons with diabetes and to fund research in diabetes. Both organizations provide publications for people with diabetes. American Diabetes Association members receive monthly issues of the magazine *Diabetes Forecast*, which contains informative articles on all aspects of diabetes care, including information on new products and the latest research. Summer camps for children with diabetes are sponsored by the American Diabetes Association in many states.

Exhibit 20–9 Sick Day Guidelines

1. NEVER OMIT INSULIN. Continue to give insulin, although the dose may need to be changed.
2. Check the child's blood glucose and urine ketones every 3–4 hours.
3. Prevent dehydration: know the signs and symptoms, such as dry mouth, cracked lips, dry skin, sunken eyes, no tears, and weight loss.
    - 8 ounces of fluid every 1/2–1 hour to prevent dehydration.
    - Use sugar-free drinks if blood sugar remains above 120–150 mg/dL.
    - Fluids with sodium and potassium, such as broth, may be alternated with other fluids.
    - Use sugar-containing fluids if blood sugar is below 80 mg/dL, or below 120–150 and your child is not able to eat the usual meal plan.
    - Keep a scale in your house. A child should be weighed once or twice a day during illness. If a child is losing weight (two or more pounds), CALL YOUR DOCTOR!
4. A Sick Day Nutrition Cupboard should be maintained at home in case a child becomes suddenly ill.
    - A copy of "Sick Day Guidelines".
    - Aspirin-free products, liquid, chewable, and/or suppositories.
    - Broth, bouillon, or noncreamy soups.
    - Cans of soda—sugared and sugar-free.
    - Cans or bottles of juice (do not need refrigeration).
    - Gelatin—sugared and sugar-free.
    - Punch drinks—sugared and sugar-free.
    - Rehydration products for very young children (Pedialyte).
5. When able to eat the usual amount of carbohydrate-containing foods, use foods appropriate for a sick day:

milk	oatmeal	saltines	popsicles
custard	cold cereal	toast	sherbert
yogurt	cream soup	applesauce	eggnog

Source: Adapted from *Caring for Young Children Living with Diabetes,* Parents' Manual, pp. 68–77, by Margaret T. Lawlor, Lori Laffel, Barbara Anderson, and Anna Bertorelli, 1996. Joslin Diabetes Center. Copyright © 1996 by The Joslin Diabetes Center. Adapted with permission.

Numerous other educational materials are available from the American Dietetic Association and the American Diabetes Association for people with diabetes, including a series on ethnic and regional food practices.

Numerous cookbooks containing recipes with information on how to include them in the carbohydrate counting and exchange systems are available in regular book stores and libraries. Several cookbooks have been compiled by the American Dietetic Association, the American Diabetes Association, and the Joslin Diabetes Center. These books help families as they learn to modify and incorporate their own recipes into the meal plan.

CONCLUSION

Nutrition management of the child with diabetes is one of the most important factors in attaining and maintaining good metabolic control. Devising meal plans that provide flexibility while conforming to guidelines based on current research is a challenge to the dietitian. A thorough understanding of all of the components of diabetes management will help the family to adapt diabetes into their lifestyle instead of adapting their lifestyle around the diabetes. It is the job of the diabetes team members to provide the foundation for long-term maintenance of good control.

REFERENCES

1. Lockwood D, Frey ML, Gladish NA, et al. The biggest problem in diabetes. *Diabetes Educ.* 1986;12:30–33.
2. West KM. Diet therapy of diabetes: An analysis of failure. *Ann Intern Med* 1973;79:425–434.
3. Franz MS, Horton ES, Bantle JP, et al. Technical review: Nutrition principles for the management of diabetes and related complications. *Diabetes Care.* 1994;17:490–518.
4. Diabetes Control and Complications Trial Research Group: The effect of intensive treatment of diabetes on the development and progression of long-term complications in insulin-treated diabetes mellitus. *N Engl J Med.* 1993;329:977–986.
5. Drash A. The child, the adolescent, and the diabetes control and complications trial. *Diabetes Care.* 1993;16:1515–1516.
6. US Department of Agriculture, US Department of Health and Human Services. *Nutrition and Your Health: Dietary Guidelines for Americans.* 4th ed. Hyattsville, MD: USDA's Human Nutrition Information Service; 1995.
7. American Diabetes Association. Nutrition recommendations and principles for people with diabetes mellitus. *Diabetes Care.* 1998;21:532–535.
8. Food and Nutrition Board. *Recommended Dietary Allowances.* 10th ed. Washington, DC: National Academy of Sciences; 1989.
9. Mahan LK, Rosebrough RH. Nutritional requirements and nutrition status assessment in adolescence. In: Mahan LK, Rees JM, eds. *Nutrition in Adolescence.* St Louis, MO: Mosby; 1984.
10. Franz MJ. Evaluating the glycemic response to carbohydrates. *Clin Diabetes.* 1986;6(6):129–141.
11. Gillespie S. Implementing liberalized carbohydrate guidelines: Nutrition free-for-all or a more rational approach to carbohydrate consumption? *Diabetes Spectrum.* 1996;9:165–167.
12. Bantle JP, Swanson JE, Thomas W, Laine DC. Metabolic effects of dietary fructose in diabetic subjects. *Diabetes Care.* 1992;15:1468–1476.
13. American Dietetic Association: Use of nutritive and nonnutritive sweeteners (position statement). *J Am Diet Assoc.* 1998;98:580–587.
14. Council on Scientific Affairs. Aspartame: Review of safety issues. *JAMA.* 1985;254:400–402.
15. Saccharin and its salts. *Fed Reg.* 1977 Dec 9;62209.
16. Morrison AS, Buring JE. Artificial sweeteners and cancer of the lower urinary tract. *N Engl J Med.* 1980; 302:537–541.
17. Kay RM. Dietary fiber. *J Lipid Res.* 1982;23:221–242.
18. Alaimo K, McDowell MA, Briefel RR, et al. *Division of Health Statistics: Dietary Intake of Vitamins, Minerals and Fiber of Persons Ages 2 Months and Over in the U.S: Third National Health and Nutrition Examination Survey, Phase 1, 1988–91.* Advance Data from Vital and Health Statistics, No. 258. Hyattsville, MD: National Center for Health Statistics; 1994.
19. Nuttall FQ. Perspectives in diabetes: Dietary fiber in the management of diabetes. *Diabetes.* 1993;42:503–508.
20. Randecker GA, Smiciklas-Wright H, McKenzie JM, et al. The dietary intake of children with IDDM. *Diabetes Care.* 1996;19:1370–1374.
21. Orchard TJ, Dorman JS, Maser RE, et al. Prevalence of complications in IDDM by sex and duration: Pitts-

burgh Epidemiology of Diabetes Complications Study II. *Diabetes*. 1990;39:1116–1124.

22. National Cholesterol Education Program: Report of the expert panel on blood cholesterol in children and adolescents. *Pediatrics*. 1992;89(suppl):525–584.
23. Nakamura T, Higashi A, Nishiyama S, Fujumoto S, Matsuda I. Kinetics of zinc status of children with IDDM. *Diabetes Care*. 1991;14:533–557.
24. Gaudini L, Feingold KR. Alcohol and diabetes: Mix with caution. *Clin Diabetes*. 1984;2:122.
25. Schade DS, Santiago JV, Skyler JS, Rizza RA. In: Travis LB, ed. *Intensive Insulin Therapy*. Princeton, NJ: Excerpta Medica; 1983.
26. Diabetes Care and Education Dietetic Practice Group of the ADA. *Meal Planning Approaches for Diabetes Management*. 2nd ed. Alexandria, VA: American Dietetic Association; 1994:3.
27. Arky RA. Current principles of dietary therapy of diabetes mellitus. *Med Clin North Am*. 1978;62:655.
28. American Diabetes Association and the American Dietetic Association. *Exchange Lists for Meal Planning*. Revised ed. New York: American Diabetes Association; 1995.
29. Anderson BJ. Diabetes and adaptations in family systems. In: Holmes C, ed. *Neuropsychology and Behavioral Aspects of Diabetes*. New York: Springer-Verlag; 1990:85–101.
30. Gerber Products Co. *1998 Nutrient Values*. Fremont, MI: 1998.
31. Behrman RE, Vaughan VC, Nelson Textbook of Pediatrics, 12th ed. Philadelphia: WB Saunders Co; 1983.
32. American Diabetes Association. Preconception care of women with diabetes. *Diabetes Care*. 1998;21:S56–S59.
33. Bertorelli AM. Nutritonal management. In: Brown FM, Hare JW, eds. *Diabetes Complicating Pregnancy: The Joslin Clinic Method*. 2nd ed. New York: Wiley-Liss; 1995:81–97.
34. Beaser RS, Hill JVC. *The Joslin Guide to Diabetes*. New York: Simon & Schuster;1995:199.
35. Lawlor MT, Anderson B, Laffel L. *Blood Sugar Monitoring Owner's Manual Booklet*. Developed with an unrestricted educational grant provided by Boehringer Mannheim Corp. Boston, MA: Joslin Diabetes Center; 1997.

SUGGESTED READING

American Diabetes Association. *Getting Started, Moving On, and Using Carbohydrate/Insulin Ratios*. Alexandria, VA: American Dietetic Association; 1996.

Beaser RS, Hill JVC. *The Joslin Guide to Diabetes*. New York: Simon & Schuster, Joslin Diabetes Center; 1995.

Beaser RS, Joslin Diabetes Center. *Outsmarting Diabetes: A Dynamic Approach for Reducing the Effects of Insulin-Dependent Diabetes*. Minneapolis, MN: Joslin Diabetes Center, Chronimed Publishing; 1994.

Betschart J. *It's Time to Learn About Diabetes: A Workbook on Diabetes for Children*. Minnetonka, MN: Chronimed Publishing; 1991.

Brown FM, Hare JW, eds. *Diabetes Complicating Pregnancy: The Joslin Clinic Method*. 2nd ed. New York: Wiley-Liss; 1995.

Franz M. *Fast Food Facts*. Minnetonka, MN: Chronimed Publishing; 1998.

Hollerorth HJ, Kaplan D, et al. *Everyone Likes to Eat*. 2nd ed. Boston, MA: Joslin Diabetes Center; 1993.

Holzmeister LA. *The Diabetes Carbohydrate and Fat Gram Guide*. The American Diabetes Association, The American Dietetic Association; 1997.

Lawlor MT, Anderson B, Laffel, LM. *Blood Sugar Monitoring Owner's Manual*. Boston, MA: Joslin Diabetes Center; 1997.

Lawlor MT, Laffel LM, Anderson B, Bertorelli A. *Caring for Young Children Living With Diabetes: A Manual for Health Care Professionals*. Boston, MA: Joslin Diabetes Center, 1996.

Lawlor MT, Laffel LM, Anderson B, Bertorelli A. *Caring for Young Children Living With Diabetes: A Manual for Parents*. Boston, MA: Joslin Diabetes Center; 1996.

Powers MA. *Handbook of Diabetes Medical Nutrition Therapy*. 2nd ed. Gaithersburg, MD: Aspen Publishers; 1996.

Satter E. *Child of Mine, Eating with Love and Good Sense*. Palo Alto, CA: Bull Publishing; 1987.

Wolfsdorf JI, Anderson BJ, Pasquarello C. Treatment of the child with diabetes. In: Kahn CR, Weir GC, eds. *Joslin's Diabetes Mellitus*. Philadelphia, PA: Joslin Diabetes Center; 1994:530–551.

Chapter 21

Pediatric Acquired Immunodeficiency Syndrome

Linda Gallagher Olsen, Roseann Cutroni, and Lauren Furuta

The first cases of pediatric acquired immunodeficiency syndrome (AIDS) were reported in 1982, and since that time, over 7,902 cases in children under the age of 13 years have been reported to the Centers for Disease Control (CDC).[1]

Although a leading cause of childhood death, the prognosis of children with AIDS is improving. As of December 1991, 18% of children with AIDS had died; this dropped to 12% in 1996.[1]

The medical, nutritional, and social implications of AIDS are numerous, and effective management requires an approach that is both coordinated and comprehensive. This chapter will provide a brief overview of pediatric AIDS and discuss the goals and strategies of its nutritional management.

AIDS is caused by the human immunodeficiency virus (HIV-1), a type of retrovirus. HIV enters the cell and, after replication, induces cell dysfunction or death. Cells of the immune system are the most commonly affected.

The immune system is comprised of lymphocytes and other white blood cells. Lymphocytes are divided into B cells, which are responsible for humoral immunity (via immunoglobulin production), and T cells, which are necessary for cell-mediated immunity. The T cells can be further classified as either helper (CD4+) or suppressor T cells (CD8+). The helper T cell enhances the operation of the entire immune system, whereas the suppressor T cell shuts down the immune response after the foreign antigens have been destroyed. In healthy individuals, there are twice as many helper T cells as suppressor T cells. AIDS patients commonly have a significant reversal of the helper/suppressor ratio.[2]

HIV preferentially infects the helper T cells. When stimulated by a foreign antigen, the infected lymphocyte will reproduce the virus instead of itself, and this new virus subsequently infects other helper T cells, essentially becoming a part of every cell it infects.

DEFINITIONS FOR AIDS SURVEILLANCE OF CHILDREN

The term *HIV* covers the spectrum of individuals from healthy to very ill. The term *AIDS* is employed by the CDC to refer to those individuals who typically display specific "indicator" diseases as a result of HIV infection.[3]

As indicated in Exhibit 21–1 and Table 21–1, the current CDC definition criteria are based on the results of medical findings and laboratory tests.[4] Only those children who meet the strict diagnostic criteria are classified as having AIDS. The classification categories include a letter designation (eg, N, A, B, C) to indicate the presence of clinical conditions (Exhibit 21–1) and a number designation (eg, 1, 2, 3), indicative of immune status, which is based on CD4 + T= lymphocyte counts and percent of total lymphocytes (Table 21–1).

Exhibit 21–1 Clinical Categories for Children with HIV

CATEGORY N: Not Symptomatic
Children who have no signs or symptoms considered to be the result of HIV infection or who have only one of the conditions listed in Category A.

Category A: Mildly Symptomatic
Children with two or more of the conditions listed below (but none of the conditions listed in Categories B and C):

Lymphadenopathy	Dermatitis
Hepatomegaly	Parotitis
Splenomegaly	Recurrent/persistent upper respiratory infection

Category B: Moderately Symptomatic
Children who have symptomatic conditions other than those listed for Categories A or C that are attributed to HIV infection; examples of conditions include but are not limited to:

Anemia, neutropenia, or thrombocytopenia	Leiomyosarcoma
Bacterial meningitis, pneumonia, or sepsis	Lymphoid interstitial pneumonia or pulmonary lymphoid hyperplasia complex
Candidiasis, oropharyngeal (thrush)	Nephropathy
Cardiomyopathy	Nocardiosis
Cytomegalovirus infection	Persistent fever
Diarrhea, recurrent or chronic	Toxoplasmosis
Hepatitis	Varicella
Herpes simplex virus stomatitis, recurrent	
Herpes zoster	

Category C: Severely Symptomatic
Children who have any condition listed in the 1987 surveillance case definition for acquired immunodeficiency syndrome, with the exception of lymphoid interstitial pneumonia.

- Serious bacterial infections, multiple or recurrent
- Candidiasis: esophageal, tracheal, bronchial
- Coccidioidomycosis, extrapulmonary
- Cryptococcosis, extrapulmonary
- Cryptosporidiosis, chronic intestinal (>1 month)
- Cytomegalovirus in other than liver, spleen, nodes (onset > 1 month)
- HIV Encephalopathy
- Herpes simplex with muccocutaneous ulcer > 1 month, bronchitis, pneumonitis
- Histoplasmosis: disseminated, extrapulmonary
- Kaposi's sarcoma
- Lymphoma: Burkitt's, immunoblastic, primary in brain

Source: Reprinted from *1994 Revised Classification System for Human Immunodeficiency Virus Infection in Children Less than 13 Years of Age,* MMWR, Vol. 43, 1994, Centers for Disease Control and Prevention.

The number of children with seropositive HIV infection, who are at a high risk of developing AIDS, is much greater than the number of AIDS cases actually reported to the CDC. From July 1996 through June 1997, 1,586 cases of pediatric HIV infection were reported to the CDC.[1] However, with only 30 states currently reporting their HIV data to the CDC, the number of in-

Table 21–1 Immune Categories of Pediatric HIV Infection Based on Age-Specific CD4+ Count and T-Lymphocyte Percentage

	<12 months		*1–5 years*		*6–12 years*	
Immune Category	*CD4+ (u/L)*	*T-lymphocyte (%)*	*CD4+ (u/L)*	*T-lymphocyte (%)*	*CD4+ (u/L)*	*T-lymphocyte (%)*
Category 1 No Suppression	≥1,500	≥25	≥1,000	≥25	≥500	≥25
Category 2 Moderate Suppression	750–1,499	15–24	500–999	15–24	200–499	15–24
Category 3 Severe Suppression	<750	15	<500	<15	<200	<15

Source: Reprinted from *1994 Revised Classification System for Human Immunodeficiency Virus Infection in Children Less than 13 Years of Age,* MMWR, Vol. 43, 1994, Centers for Disease Control and Prevention.

fected children is significantly greater than that reflected by available statistics.

DIAGNOSIS

The primary route of HIV transmission in children is perinatal. The exact mechanism for perinatal transfer is unclear, but it appears that the virus can be acquired in utero during any trimester of pregnancy. The transmission rate from a nontreated infected mother to her infant averages 24%.[5–7] Studies indicate a reduction in transmission rate to 8% when HIV-positive women are treated with the antiretroviral drug zidovudine (AZT, now known as ZDV) during pregnancy and labor.[8]

Early diagnosis and prophylaxis enhances the quality and length of life. Infants born to HIV-positive mothers should be closely monitored, beginning immediately after birth. With newer technology, most infected children are diagnosed by 6 months of age. Those children without a definitive diagnosis should have antibody testing performed at 18 months of age. Indications for testing children are found in Exhibit 21–2.[6]

A variety of diagnostic tests is available at selected laboratories. Tests to identify HIV in children younger than 18 months are HIV culture or DNA polymerase chain reaction. For children older than 18 months, standard HIV antibody tests (ELISA and Western blot) are used.[6,9]

EPIDEMIOLOGY

The racial distribution of pediatric AIDS in the United States is 58% black, 23% Hispanic, and 17% white. Blood transfusions represent 5% of childhood-acquired AIDS. Three percent of pediatric AIDS cases can be linked to blood products received as treatment for coagulation disorders.[1]

CLINICAL MANIFESTATIONS

Children with HIV infection display a wide array of clinical features. Presenting symptoms include lymphadenopathy, hepatosplenomegaly, failure to thrive, and bacterial infections.[3] As the clinical course progresses, children become susceptible to more serious infections, including viruses such as herpes simplex virus, cytomega-

Exhibit 21–2 Indicators for HIV Testing in Infants and Children

Failure to thrive
Generalized lymphadenopathy
Recurrent bacterial infections
Chronic diarrhea
Hepatosplenomegaly
Developmental delay
Recurrent oral candidiasis
Radiographic evidence of persistent diffuse lung disease
Maternal risk factors for HIV infection:
- substance abuse
- multiple sexual partners
- history of sexual contact with known infected partner

Source: Reprinted from H.S. Winter and T.L. Miller, Gastrointestinal and nutritional problems in pediatric HIV disease, in *Pediatric AIDS: The Challenge of HIV Infection in Infants, Children and Adolescents,* 2nd ed., P.A. Pizzo and C.M. Wilfert, eds., pp. 513–533, 1994, Lippincott Williams & Wilkins.

lovirus and varicella-zoster; bacteremia; mycobacterium avium complex; and oral-esophageal candidiasis.[10,11] These types of infections, coupled with diagnostic tests, multiple medications, and frequent hospitalizations, may impact the child's desire and ability to consume adequate nutrition and can lead to subsequent nutritional compromise.

Numerous clinical manifestations affecting the gastrointestinal tract may result in diarrhea and the malabsorption of essential nutrients. Diarrhea and malabsorption may be the result of parasitic, fungal, bacterial, and viral infections, small bowel overgrowth, or medication side effects.[6] Children with HIV have an increased probability of developing lactose intolerance, compared with their noninfected counterparts.[12] In cases where no cause for symptoms can be established, the term *HIV enteropathy* has been used to describe bowel injury due to HIV itself.

Other clinical features may also impact a child's desire or ability to eat. For example, oral and esophageal ulcers may result from Candida, herpes simplex virus, or idiopathic causes. Children with AIDS also have a relatively high risk of developing pancreatitis, often requiring the discontinuation of enteral intake.[13]

MEDICATIONS

Antiretroviral therapies for HIV include three major categories: nucleoside reverse transcriptase inhibitors (NRTIs), protease inhibitors, and nonnucleoside reverse transcriptase inhibitors (NNRTIs). Efficacy of drug therapies is based on clinical assessment, CD4+ lymphocyte counts, and on the amount of HIV virus in the blood, commonly referred to as *viral load*. Effective medication therapy decreases the patient's viral load and increases the CD4+ cell counts.

Zidovudine (ZDV) has been the most common antiviral agent used in HIV-infected children. However, recent data from clinical trials in symptomatic children demonstrate that initial therapy using either didanosine (ddI) or lamivudine (3TC) in combination with ZDV is more effective than ZDV or other monotherapy in decreasing viral load and improving the clinical outcome.[14,15] Although combination therapy is now considered the treatment of choice in children, ZDV alone used as chemoprophylaxis for the first 6 weeks of life is still considered appropriate in newborns with indeterminate HIV status born to HIV-positive mothers.

Current recommendations from the CDC working group on antiretroviral therapy and medical management of HIV infection state that Nelfinivir, Ritonavir, or Indinavir, in combination with two NRTIs, are the most effective therapies. This is supported by evidence that it suppresses viral load in adults.[16] Treatment trials in children are underway. Most of the clinical evidence in children is available on the combinations of ZDV and 3TC or ZDV and ddI. Clinical trials with other combination therapies are ongoing.

Many of the anti-HIV drugs have side effects, including nausea, vomiting, and diarrhea, all of which can negatively impact the child's nutritional state. Examples of these drugs and their relevant side effects are listed in Table 21–2. Other medications used for the prophylaxis or treatment of secondary infections may also have similar gastrointestinal side effects. Some of

Table 21–2 Antiretroviral Medications and Common Side Effects

Generic Name (Trade Name)	*Side Effects (Most Common)*
Nucleoside Reverse Transcriptase Inhibitor	
zidovudine, AZT, ZDV (Retrovir)	nausea
didanosine, ddI (Videx)	nausea, vomiting, abdominal pain, diarrhea
zalcitabine, ddC (Hivid)	gastrointestinal disturbances, oral ulcers
stavudine, d4T (Zerit)	gastrointestinal disturbances
lamivudine, 3TC (Epivir)	nausea, diarrhea, abdominal pain, pancreatitis
Non-Nucleoside Reverse Transcriptase Inhibitor	
nevirapine, NVP (Viramune)	diarrhea, nausea
delavirdine, DLV (Rescriptor)	GI complaints
Protease Inhibitor	
saquinavir (Invirase—hard gel) (Fortovase—soft gel)	diarrhea, nausea, abdominal discomfort
indinavir (Crixivan)	nausea, abdominal pain, metallic taste
ritonavir (Norvir)	nausea, vomiting, abdominal pain, diarrhea, anorexia
nelfinavir (Viracept)	diarrhea

Source: Reprinted from *Guidelines for the Use of Antiretroviral Agents in Pediatric HIV Infection. MMWR* vol. 47, pp. 18, 19, 34–43, 1998, Centers for Disease Control and Prevention.

these medicines include acyclovir, amphotericin B, erythromycin, ketoconazole, pentamidine, and rifampin.

NUTRITIONAL IMPLICATIONS

The nutritional status of HIV-infected children impacts their growth and cellular immune function. Studies are emerging that link the importance of nutrition in predicting and improving clinical outcomes.[17] In combination with effective drug therapies, nutrition support enhances the quality of life and survival in children infected with HIV.[18]

The majority of children infected with HIV will experience nutritional deficits during the course of their illness.[17] Weight loss and malnutrition are common and may be the result of several factors, including impaired absorption, decreased dietary intake, and increased nutrient requirements (see Exhibit 21–3). It has been proposed that malnutrition influences both the child's susceptibility to HIV infection and the progression of the disease.[17] In addition, malnutrition has a deleterious effect on immune function, compromising the ability to produce effective antibodies and, thereby, increasing the risk of life-threatening infections.[19] Micronutrient deficiencies leading to depressed immune function are common, as well.[17]

Improving the nutritional status of the HIV-infected child may functionally improve immune status and augment overall health and survival.[17]

GROWTH AND BODY COMPOSITION

Research demonstrates a variety of growth patterns in HIV-infected children, reflecting a broad spectrum of clinical course and disease activity. It appears that HIV does not significantly affect the infant's birth weight, but significant postnatal growth abnormalities, even in the asymptomatic child, can occur quickly.[17] Studies reflect impairments in growth by at least 2 years of age, with one study showing such deficits by 4 months in some infected infants.[20,21] The Women and Infants Transmission Study (WITS), a natural history HIV investigation, has revealed that infected children experience deficits in growth and body mass in an early and progressive manner.[17,22]

Failure to thrive is a common identifying component of HIV infection. Because diarrhea, vomiting, and hydration status may all acutely impact weight, tracking serial anthropometric measurements is particularly important in assessing the HIV-infected child. Z-scores can be useful in detecting small changes in both weight and height, and in characterizing degrees

Exhibit 21–3 Causes of Malnutrition

1. Decreased Intake
   (etiology: nausea, anorexia, oral ulceration, esophagitis, chewing difficulties, pain, dementia, depression)
2. Increased Losses
   (etiology: lactose intolerance, pancreatic insufficiency, malabsorption)
3. Increased Requirements
   (etiology: fever, opportunistic infections, metabolic abnormalities)

of deviation from the norm in children who fall below the fifth percentile for age (see Chapter 18 for further details about Z scores).

In children infected with HIV, there is a preferential loss of lean body tissue over that of fat mass, sometimes without an associated weight loss.[17] This contrasts to typical starvation, where the body responds by initially depleting fat stores, then draws on lean body mass. The evaluation of body cell mass identifies changes in body composition and is a good indicator of the child's state of nutritional health. Dual energy X-ray absorptiometry (DEXA) is the most accurate means of determining body composition but is prohibitively expensive in many clinical settings. Bioelectrical impedance (BIA) and arm circumference and skinfold measurements are relatively inexpensive and clinically useful in assessing body composition status. When evaluated together, body composition and anthropometry measurements provide insight into the extent of a nutritional compromise so that appropriate nutritional interventions can be implemented.

NUTRITIONAL ASSESSMENT

Nutritional assessment should be an integral component of care provided to all HIV-infected children (see Exhibit 21–4). A baseline nutrition assessment should be determined as soon as the infected child is identified because early nutritional intervention can help prevent malnutrition and growth failure. Nutritional reassessment by the dietitian should be done at least every 6 months. More frequent evaluation and intervention are warranted when clinical symptoms or growth abnormalities are present.

Anthropometrics

Height, weight, head circumference (until 36 months of age), triceps skinfold, and a calculated midarm muscle area are among the anthropometric measurements that should be obtained at initial presentation and at least every 6 months thereafter. Children who are showing deceleration in weight or height by declining across percentiles on the growth chart should be evaluated quickly for nutritional intervention. Changes in skinfold measurements will reflect any preferential use of muscle tissue for energy needs (see Appendix H for standards).

Biochemical and Clinical

A positive correlation has been established between albumin status and length of life.[18] However, due to albumin's lack of sensitivity, prealbumin is a much more reliable marker of visceral protein status and should be a standard component of biochemical evaluation. Other biochemical studies should include those directed toward the evaluation of anemia and those that will identify micronutrient deficiencies. A number of serum micronutrient abnormalities has been identified in patients with HIV infection, but there is little information to establish the impact of these deficiencies on clinical manifestations in pediatric patients.

Because micronutrient deficiencies may be associated with disease progression, serum status should be assessed and nutrients repleted in any malnourished or wasted HIV-infected child. Deficiencies of zinc, selenium, iron, folate, and vitamins A, E, B_6, B_{12}, and C have been reported, even when seemingly adequate nutrient intake has been observed.[18]

Children with documented fat malabsorption, liver disease, or pancreatic dysfunction should be assessed for fat-soluble vitamin status, and children experiencing diarrhea should be evaluated for deficiencies of electrolytes, magnesium, and zinc. Symptoms of cheilosis, dermatitis, and peripheral neuropathy may also signal micronutrient deficiencies.

Dietary Intake

A comprehensive review of the child's dietary consumption should be included in the nutritional assessment. Incorporated into the review should be an evaluation of the child's typical in-

Exhibit 21–4 Nutritional Evaluation and Management of the HIV-Infected Child

Nutritional Assessment
- Dietary Intake
- Diet Analysis (calories, macro- and micronutrient sufficiency)
- Anthropometrics and Body Composition Measurements
- Biochemical Evaluation
- Medical History
- Drug–Nutrient Interactions

Nutritional Intervention
- Enhanced-Calorie Diet (nutrient-dense foods, commercial supplements)
- Diet Modifications (due to malabsorptive conditions, intolerances, or if at high risk for aspiration)
- Nutrition Education (caloric enhancement, food safety)
- Vitamin/Mineral Supplementation
- Tube Feedings/Total parenteral nutrition (TPN)

take; an investigation of any gastrointestinal abnormalities, such as vomiting, diarrhea, or early satiety; and a review of the availability and access to nourishing and safe food. The nutritional adequacy of the diet should be analyzed using a 24-hour recall, food record, and/or food frequency questionnaire. Dietary intake can then be compared to expected nutrient requirements and correlated with growth and biochemical parameters to develop and implement the appropriate nutrition intervention or care plan.

CALORIC REQUIREMENTS

Caloric requirements of HIV-infected children are not well defined. Although children with HIV were once thought to have an increased resting metabolic rate caused by viral infection, subsequent research suggests that clinically stable children have normal caloric needs.[23] Weight loss is linked to inadequate intake by the child or increased caloric requirements imposed by opportunistic infections or malabsorptive losses.[24] Caloric requirements should be calculated according to additional needs subsequent to stress, fever, increased respiratory needs, and growth.

Infants and young children who are failing to thrive should have their caloric needs calculated using the catch-up growth formula (see Chapter 18, Table 18–4). For older children and adolescents, basal energy requirements should be adjusted, based on the increased needs mentioned above.[25] As a general guideline, providing approximately 150% of the daily recommended intake (DRI) for energy can promote weight gain if malabsorption and diarrhea are not significant. Frequent weight and height measurements will help determine adequacy of caloric estimations.

NUTRITIONAL INTERVENTION

There is no one formula or special diet that is universally appropriate for HIV-infected children. The most appropriate nutrition plan for an HIV-infected child is one tailored to his or her clinical manifestations, growth, dietary history, gastrointestinal function, and social situation (Exhibit 21–4).

It is typical for HIV-infected children to be prescribed a high-calorie, high-protein, nutrient-dense diet. If enhancement of the typical diet is not sufficient to promote desired growth, oral nutritional supplementation, including shakes and commercial formulas, should be considered. When oral measures alone cannot achieve the nutritional goals, enteral tube supplementation should be incorporated. If enteral feedings are contraindicated, parenteral nutrition can be utilized.

Oral Feedings and Supplementation

Nutritional therapy in the HIV-infected child should be proactive to prevent malnutrition. When signs of growth or clinical dysfunction are present, nutrition intervention should be comprehensive and aggressive. The child's caretakers should receive ongoing education pertaining to nutrient-dense diets, supplements, safe food handling, and any special dietary modifications. Because of the risk of micronutrient deficiency in the HIV-infected child, it is prudent to consider a complete multivitamin/mineral supplement that provides one to two times the DRI.[18,26]

In infants, standard formulas are generally well tolerated. When growth acceleration is needed, formulas can be concentrated or calorically enhanced with the addition of carbohydrate or fat modulars to optimize caloric intake. Because HIV can be transmitted in breast milk, formula feeding is currently recommended for all infants born to HIV-infected mothers in the United States and in industrialized countries where clean water and sterile formulas are readily available.[5,6]

For children eating solids, a high-calorie diet that includes nutrient-dense feedings and small, frequent meals should be emphasized. Oral nutritional supplements should be utilized when indicated and selected based on clinical presentation. Children who are experiencing diarrhea and malabsorption may need to eliminate certain foods or ingredients from their diets. In the presence of symptoms such as diarrhea, abdominal pain, distention, or poor weight gain, a child with documented lactose malabsorption may benefit from dietary restriction of lactose-containing foods. The use of lactose-free formulas (eg, Pediasure, Kindercal, Resource Just for Kids, and Nutren Jr.), lactose-reduced dairy products, and enzyme substitutes help to provide a more varied and nutritionally adequate diet to the lactose-intolerant child. Use of a strict diet is generally counterproductive because it may result in restricted food choices and subsequent poor intake. Fortunately, many children with lactose malabsorption are asymptomatic and do not require a lactose-modified diet.

In the presence of enteropathy, fat and/or protein malabsorption may occur. Formulas or enteral products made with hydrolyzed protein or altered fat, such as medium-chain triglyceride (MCT) oil, may be effective in normalizing absorption. Examples of such formulas include Peptamen Jr., Optimental, and Neocate 1+.

For children experiencing oroesophageal ulcers, soreness, or inflammation, care should be given to selecting foods that are soft, nutrient dense, and not highly spiced or acidic. The side effects of many drugs (see Table 21–2) may lead to anorexia, nausea/vomiting, epigastric distress, diarrhea, and/or glossitis, and could result in a child's refusal to eat. Appetite stimulants, such as megestrol acetate (Megace), may be used to increase oral intake in some anorectic children. Megace has been associated with improvements in weight gain, although primarily by increasing fat mass and generally without concurrent improvements in linear growth. Although further studies using this progestational hormone in children are needed, it appears that the weight gain effects may not be sustained once the medication is discontinued.[27,28]

Dysphagia, developmental delay, and poor gross motor control secondary to neurologic complications associated with HIV may also contribute to poor intake. Neurologically impaired children should be closely monitored to ensure adequate intake and to prevent aspiration.

Enteral Supplementation

If a child's oral intake is inadequate, it may be necessary to place a nasogastric tube to achieve nutritional goals and promote desired growth. Once weight gain with nasogastric feedings is established, children anticipated to require long-term supplementation should be evaluated for placement of a gastrostomy tube.

Nocturnal tube feedings are often the preferred schedule because they allow the child to eat normally during the day. Formula selection should be determined as noted in the oral feedings section above. Studies show improvements in weight gain (primarily as increased fat mass) in response to the increased caloric provisions and suggest an improvement in morbidity and survival as a result of such nutritional rehabilitation.[29]

Parenteral Nutrition

Total parenteral nutrition, despite its associated infection risks, may be warranted if hydration, electrolyte balance, or weight gain cannot be achieved through enteral means. Children with intractable diarrhea with accompanying weight loss, or severe recurrent or chronic pancreatic or biliary tract dysfunction may be candidates for parenteral nutrition.[17]

CONCLUSION

Optimal nutritional status has been associated with improvements in immune function and morbidity in the HIV-infected child. Close nutrition surveillance and intervention results in improved clinical outcome and quality of life. Malnutrition in HIV-infected children is a serious complication. Early and aggressive nutritional support is indicated in all children infected with HIV and should include nutrient-dense oral feedings and enteral supplementation when necessary. Anthropometric and body composition changes should be serially monitored, and biochemical parameters should be assessed so that necessary nutrition intervention can occur. Ongoing research continues to augment the understanding of the interrelationship between nutrition and HIV, and will elucidate more definitive nutrition intervention strategies.

REFERENCES

1. Centers for Disease Control, Division of HIV/AIDS. *HIV/AIDS Surveillance*. Atlanta GA: Centers for Disease Control;1997;19:1–30.
2. Rogers MF. AIDS in children: A review of the clinical, epidemiological, and public health aspects. *J Pediatr Infect Dis*. 1985;4:230–236.
3. Falloon J, Eddy J, Pizzo P. Human immunodeficiency virus infection in children. *J Pediatr*. 1989;114:1–30.
4. Centers for Disease Control. 1994 Revised classification system for human immunodeficiency virus infection in children less than 13 years of age. *MMWR*. September 1994;43:PR-12.
5. European Collaborative Study. Risk factors for mother-child transmission of HIV-1. *Lancet*. 1992; 339:1007–1012.
6. Winter HS, Miller TL. Gastrointestinal and nutritional problems in pediatric HIV disease. In: Pizzo PA, Wilfert CM, eds. *Pediatric AIDS: The challenge of HIV infection in infants, children and adolescents*. 2nd edition. Baltimore: Williams & Wilkins; 1994:513–533.
7. Tovo PA, De Martino M, Gabiano C. Prognostic factors and survival in children with perinatal HIV-1 infection. *Lancet*.1992;339:1249–1253.
8. Connor EM, Sperling RS, Gelber R, et al. Reduction of maternal-infant transmission of human immunovirus type 1 with zidovudine treatment. *N Engl J Med*. 1994;331:1173–1180.
9. McIntosh K, Pitt J, Brambilla D. Blood culture in the first six months of life for the diagnosis of vertically transmitted immunodeficiency virus infection. *J Infect Dis*.1994;170:996–1000.
10. Johann-Liang R, Cervia J, Noel GJ. Characteristics of human immunodeficiency virus-infected children at the time of death: An experience in the 1990s. *Pediatr Infect Dis J*. 1997;16:1145–1150.
11. Morris Cr, Araba-Owoyele L, Spector SA, Maldonado YA. Disease patterns and survival after acquired immunodeficiency syndrome diagnosis in human immunodeficiency virus-infected children. *Pediatr Infect Dis J*. 1996;15:321–328.
12. Miller TL, Orav EJ, Martin SR, Cooper ER, McIntosh K, Winter HS. Malnutrition and carbohydrate malabsorption in children with vertically transmitted human immunodeficiency virus 1-infection. *Gastroenterol*. 1991;100:1296–1302.
13. Miller TL, Winter HS, Luginbuhl LM, Orav EJ, McIntosh K. Pancreatitis in pediatric human immunodeficiency virus infection. *J Pediatr*. 1992;120:223–227.
14. McKinney RE, PACTG Protocol 300 Team. Pediatric ACTG Trial 300: Clinical efficacy of ZDV/3TC vs ddI

vs ZDV/ddI in symptomatic HIV-infected children. In: *Program and Abstracts of the 35th Annual Meeting of the Infectious Diseases Society of America.* San Francisco, CA. September 13–16, 1997: Abstract 768.

15. Englund JA, Baker CJ, Raskino C, et al. Zidovudine, didanosine or both as the initial treatment for symptomatic HIV-infected children. AIDS clinical trials group (ACTG) Study 152 Team. *N Engl J Med.* 1997; 336:1704–1712.
16. Centers for Disease Control and Prevention. Guidelines for the use of antiretroviral agents in pediatric HIV infection. *MMWR.* 1998;47 (RR-4):18,19,34–43.
17. Miller TL. Nutritional aspects of pediatric HIV infection. In: Walker WA, Watkins JB, eds. *Nutrition in Pediatrics.* 2nd edition. Hamilton, Ontario: C. Decker; 1996:534–550.
18. Heller LS, Shattuck D. Nutrition support for children with HIV/AIDS. *J Am Diet Assoc.* 1997;97:473–474.
19. Chandra RK. Mucosal immune responses in malnutrition. *Ann NY Acad Sci.* 1983;409:345–352.
20. Miller TL, Evans S, Orav EJ, Morris V, McIntosh K, Winter HS. Growth and body composition in children with human immunodeficiency virus-1. *Am J Clin Nutr.* 1993;57:588–592.
21. McKinney RE, Robertson JR. Effect of human immunodeficiency virus infection on the growth of young children. Duke Pediatric AIDS Clinical Trials Unit. *J Pediatr.* 1993;123:579–582.
22. Sheon RK, Diaz C, Cooper E. *Natural History of Somatic Growth in Pediatric HIV Infection: Preliminary data of the Women and Infants Transmission Study (WITS).* First National Conference on Human Retroviruses and Related Infections; December 1993:Abstract 695.
23. Alfaro MP, Siegel RM, Baker RC. Resting energy expenditure and body composition in pediatric HIV infection. *Pediatr AIDS HIV Infect.* 1995;6:276–280.
24. Coodley GO, Loveless MO, Merrill TM. The HIV wasting syndrome: A review. *J Acquir Immune Defic Syndr.* 1994;7:681–694.
25. Long CL, Schaffel N, Geiger JW, Schiller WR, Blakemore WS. Metabolic response to injury and illness: Estimation of energy and protein needs from indirect calorimetry and nitrogen balance. *J Parenter Enteral Nutr.* 1979;3:452–456.
26. Galvin T. Micronutrients: Implications in human immunodeficiency virus disease. *Top Clin Nutr.* 1992: 7(3):63–73.
27. Clarick RH, Hanekom WA, Yoger R, Chadwick EG. Megestrol acetate treatment of growth failure in children infected with human immunodeficiency virus. *Pediatrics.* 1997;99:354–357.
28. Antiretroviral therapy and medical management of pediatric HIV infection and 1997 USPHS/IDSA report on the prevention of opportunistic infections in persons infected with human immunodeficiency virus. *Pediatrics.* 1998;102,4(suppl):1047–1062.
29. Miller TL, Awnetwant EL, Evans S, Morris VM, Vazquez IM, McIntosh K. Gastrostomy tube supplementation for HIV-infected children. *Pediatrics.* 1995; 96:696–702.

Chapter 22

Oncology and Marrow Transplantation

Karen V. Barale and Paula M. Charuhas

Childhood cancer is the most common cause of death from disease in children between the ages of 1 and 14 years.[1] The incidence of malignancies in children under the age of 15 is 13.6 per 100,000 population among whites and 10.8 per 100,000 among blacks.[2] Table 22–1 lists the common childhood tumors with their standard treatment. Approximately 50% of the cases are leukemia and lymphomas.

Prognosis depends on tumor histology, tumor stage, age of patient, and certain laboratory indexes. Treatment may include chemotherapy, surgery, irradiation, and marrow, stem cell, or cord blood transplantation. In many instances, initial treatment is curative because of excellent response to multimodal therapy. Advances in nutrition support have paralleled improvements in treatment, making optimum care of these patients possible. Pediatric nutrition support goals in oncology are to prevent or reverse nutritional deficits, promote normal growth and development, minimize morbidity and mortality, and maximize quality of life.[3,4] The disease, its therapy, and any complications will affect the nutritional status of the child.

NUTRITIONAL EFFECTS OF CANCER

Protein-Energy Malnutrition

Protein-energy malnutrition (PEM) is a common secondary diagnosis in pediatric patients with cancer.[3] At diagnosis, the incidence ranges from 6% in children with newly diagnosed leukemia to as high as 50% in children with stage IV neuroblastoma.[5] Certain populations of children with neoplastic disease are at high risk of developing PEM. In general, patients with advanced disease during initial intense treatment and those who relapse or do not respond to treatment are most likely to develop PEM.[6] Additionally, certain types of treatment promote the development of PEM: major abdominal surgery; irradiation of the head, neck, esophagus, abdomen, or pelvis; or intense, frequent courses of chemotherapy (3-week intervals or less). Finally, complications such as pain, fever, and frequent or severe infections decrease appetite and may increase energy requirements.

PEM ultimately results from decreased energy intake, increased energy requirements, and malabsorption.[5] Organ systems most readily affected by PEM (hematopoietic, gastrointestinal,

Note: This work was supported in part by Grant Number DK35816 US Department of Health and Human Services for the Clinical Nutrition Research Unit, Fred Hutchinson Cancer Research Center.

Table 22–1 Cancers in Childhood

Malignancy	*% of Cases*	*Standard Treatment*	*Comment*
Hematologic			
Leukemia	42.8		
Acute lymphoblastic leukemia (ALL)		Induction chemo Consolidation chemo CNS prophylaxis (RT or IT chemo) Oral maintenance chemo with intermittent IV Rx lasts about 3 years BMT for persistent relapse or second remission	65–70% 5-year disease-free survival
Acute nonlymphoblastic leukemia (ANL)		Remission induction with intensive chemo Continuation therapy up to 18 mo CNS prophylaxis BMT for persistent relapse or first remission	30–50% 3-year continuous complete remission
Chronic myelocytic leukemia (CML)		Chronic phase: oral chemo for symptomatic relief, BMT Length of Rx based on symptoms & phase Blast crisis: aggressive chemo, BMT	<5% incidence in children Blast crisis <20% survival
Juvenile chronic myelocytic leukemia (JCML)		Oral chemo BMT	Usually diagnosed before 2 years of age Median survival <9 mo
Hodgkin's disease and lymphoma	11.3		
Hodgkin's disease			
Stages I–IV, with involvement ranging from single node region to diffuse or		Chemo vs. RT controversial for all stages; multimodal therapy often used Autologous BMT for failure to achieve remission or relapse	In children <10 years, male incidence higher Chemo has the advantage of avoiding high-dose radiation to the growing spine

Source: Data from references 1, 2, and 87.

disseminated involvement to extralymphatic organs			70–96% survival
Nonlymphoblastic lymphoma		Chemo with/without RT for 6–18 mo	Therapy depends on extent of disease Cure rate 10%–40% with bone marrow involvement; to 90% with limited disease
Lymphoblastic lymphoma		Aggressive chemo, autologous or allogeneic BMT during early remission, plus whole-brain RT, IT chemo	Adverse prognostic factors: extensive marrow or CNS involvement
Brain tumors Astrocytoma (most prevalent) Medulloblastoma Brain stem glioma Ependymomas	20.7	Surgical removal/debulking Chemo and RT	Survival based on tumor type & location 5-year survival 15–70% Brain stem gliomas lead to CNS dysfunction and swallowing problems Can have cranial nerve palsies or paresis
Neuroblastoma Stages I–IV, with involvement ranging from localized disease to metastatic disease	7.3	Surgical resection of local disease Palliative RT to shrink tumor size Chemo BMT, allogeneic or autologous, for advanced disease	2 years = median age at diagnosis 50–90% survival, depending on stage & location Most common primary site is adrenal gland, which produces an abdominal mass, metastatic disease Most common extracranial solid tumor in childhood; comprises up to 50% of malignancies in infants
Wilms' tumor Stages I–V, with involvement ranging from well-encapsulated tumor to bilateral disease and metastases	6.1	All stages: surgery for staging and tumor removal Chemo—preferred therapy Metastatic disease to bone, liver, or lung: RT	Usually seen between ages 1 and 5 years 59–90% survival, stages I–III Survival dependent on stage at presentation

continues

Table 22–1 continued

Malignancy	*% of Cases*	*Standard Treatment*	*Comment*
Bone tumors Rhabdomyosarcoma Stages I–IV, with involvement ranging from localized disease to distant metastasis	6.0	Surgery—total excision if possible Chemo RT 5000–6000 cGy to primary tumor with wide ports	Most common soft tissue sarcoma in children 28–71% survival, depending on stage
Osteogenic sarcoma		Surgery: amputation or limb salvage Chemo to prevent metastasis	Resistant to RT Common sites: around knee joint and below shoulder Primary malignant tumor of bone Peak incidence during adolescent growing spurt 60% survival
Ewing's sarcoma	2.1	RT, based on site and leg length growth: if length discrepancy won't be excessive, 6000–7000 cGy; if it will be excessive, amputation and chemo or salvage procedures	Males predominate 2:1 Peak age of incidence: 11–12 years, female; 15–16 years, male Small-cell bone tumor 2-year disease-free survival 70%
Retinoblastoma Stages I–V, based on number and size of lesions	2.9	Surgery RT Chemo for advanced disease	90% < 5 years of age; average age is 18 mo Increased risk for other sarcoma, secondary to therapy 90% survival

Note: BMT, bone marrow transplant; chemo, chemotherapy; CNS, central nervous system; IV, intravenous; IT, intrathecal; RT, radiation therapy; Rx, treatment.

and immunologic) are also the most sensitive to oncologic treatment. Thus, the prevention or reversal of PEM to maximize the function of these organ systems seems prudent in childhood cancer.[5]

Cachexia

Cancer cachexia is a poorly understood syndrome that includes tissue wasting, anorexia, weakness, anemia, hypoalbuminemia, hypoglycemia, lactic acidosis, hyperlipidemia, impaired liver function, glucose intolerance, accelerated gluconeogenesis, skeletal muscle atrophy, visceral organ atrophy, and anergy.[6] The particular combination of features varies with tumor type and patient (Exhibit 22–1). Additionally, poor utilization of nutrients, either absorbed or infused, can contribute to cachexia.[6] It is a major source of morbidity for young cancer patients.[8] Children with progressive and metastatic disease have an incidence of cachexia as high as 40%.[9]

NUTRITIONAL EFFECTS OF CANCER THERAPY

Multimodal treatments can have an additional adverse effect on nutritional status.[4] Antitumor therapies may produce only mild, transient nutritional disturbances or may lead to severe, permanent problems.

Chemotherapy

The nutritional consequences of chemotherapeutic agents are shown in Table 22–2. These drugs affect normal as well as malignant cells, targeting rapidly dividing cells, such as the epithelial cells of the gastrointestinal tract. The degree to which gastrointestinal function is altered depends on the particular drug, dosage, duration of the treatment, rate of metabolism, and the child's susceptibility.

Nausea and vomiting are the most common problems interfering with adequate oral intake.[10] These occur as a result of a direct central nervous system effect as drugs are administered. Complications of chemotherapy-induced emesis include weight loss, dehydration, fluid and electrolyte imbalances, and metabolic alkalosis.[11] Management of chemotherapy-induced nausea and vomiting includes the judicious use of antiemetics. Single-agent or combination antiemetics are frequently used and can decrease the child's discomfort. Antiemetics such as ondansetron, metoclopramide, and diphenhydramine assist in controlling symptoms of nausea and vomiting. Nonpharmacologic interventions such as music therapy, hypnosis, and muscle relaxation have also been described as effective techniques of treating nausea and vomiting.[12]

Alterations in taste and smell as a result of chemotherapy may persist well beyond periods of nausea and vomiting, and result in prolonged

Exhibit 22–1 Major Contributors to Cachexia in Young Cancer Patients

Abnormal host metabolism of macronutrients
Tumor consumption of nutrients for tumor growth
Host requirement of adequate nutrients for normal growth
Anticancer therapy
Inadequate intake of nutrients to meet expenditures

Source: Data from references 5, 7, 8, 9, and 40.

Table 22–2 Chemotherapeutic Agents and Toxicities Affecting Nutritional Status

Drug	*Synonyms*	*Antitumor Spectrum*	*Toxicities*
Alkylating agents			
Cyclophosphamide	Cytoxan, CTX	Lymphomas, leukemias, sarcomas, neuroblastoma	N&V, cystitis, water retention; cardiac (HD)
Ifosfamide	IFOS	Sarcomas	N&V, cystitis, NT, renal
Cisplatin	Platinol, CDDP	Testicular and other germ cell, osteosarcoma, brain tumors, neuroblastoma	N&V, renal, NT
Busulfan	Myleran	Leukemia (CML) Used in conditioning regimens for MT	N&V, mucositis Do not eat for one hr before or after taking medication
Dacarbazine	DTIC	Neuroblastoma, sarcomas	N&V, flulike syndrome, hepatic
Melphalan	Akeran, L-PAM	Rhabdomyosarcoma, sarcomas, neuroblastoma, and leukemias	N&V, mucositis & diarrhea (HD)
Mechlorethamine	Mustargen, HN_2, nitrogen mustard	Hodgkin's, brain tumors	N&V, mucositis; NT (HD)
Procarbazine	Matulan, PCZ	Hodgkin's, brain tumors	N&V, NT, rash, mucositis; low tyramine diet indicated
Lomustine	CCNU	Brain tumors, lymphomas	N&V, renal & pulmonary toxicity
Antimetabolites			
Methotrexate	MTX	Leukemia, lymphoma, osteosarcoma	Mucositis, rash, hepatic; renal (HD), NT
6-Mercaptopurine	Purinethal, 6-MP	Leukemia (ALL, CML)	Hepatic, mucositis
6-Thioguanine	6-TG	Leukemia (ANL)	N&V, mucositis, hepatic
Cytarabine	Cytosine arabinoside, Cytosar, Ara-C	Leukemia, lymphoma	N&V, mucositis, GI; NT, ocular, skin (HD)
Antibiotics			
Adriamycin	Doxorubicin, ADR	Leukemia (ALL, ANL), lymphoma, most solid tumors	Mucositis, N&V, cardiac (acute and chronic)
Daunomycin	Daunorubicin, DNR	Leukemia (ALL, ANL)	Same as adriamycin
Bleomycin	Blenoxane, BLEO	Lymphoma, testicular cancer	Lung, skin, hypersensitivity; Raynaud's
Dactinomycin	Cosmegen, ACT-D, actinomycin D	Wilms' tumor, sarcomas	N&V, mucositis

Plant alkaloids			
Vincristine	Oncovin, VCR	Leukemia (ALL), lymphomas, most solid tumors	NT, SIADH, hypotension, constipation
Vinblastine	Velban, VLB	Histiocytosis, Hodgkin's, testicular	Mucositis, mild NT
Etoposide	VePesid, VP-16, VP-16-213	Leukemias (ALL, ANL), lymphomas, neuroblastoma, sarcomas, brain tumors	N&V, mucositis, mild NT, hypotension, allergic
Miscellaneous			
Prednisone (po)	Deltasone, PRED	Leukemia, lymphoma	Increased appetite, centripetal obesity, myopathy, osteoporosis, aseptic necrosis of hip, peptic ulceration, pancreatitis, hyperactivity, hypertension, diabetes, growth failure, amenorrhea, impaired wound healing, atrophy of subcutaneous tissue
Prednisolone (IV)		Leukemia, lymphoma	
Dexamethasone	Decadron, DEX	Leukemia, lymphoma, brain tumors	
L-Asparaginase	Elspar, L-ASP	Leukemia (ALL), lymphoma	N&V, acute pancreatitis, decreased serum albumin, insulin & lipoproteins

Note: ALL, acute lymphoblastic leukemia; ANL, acute nonlymphoblastic leukemia; CML, chronic myelogenous leukemia; GI, gastrointestinal toxicity; HD, high-dose; IV, intravenous; N&V, nausea and vomiting; NT, neurotoxicity.

Source: Adapted with permission from F.M. Balis, J.S. Holcenberg and D.G. Poplack. General Principles of Chemotherapy, in *Principles and Practice of Pediatric Oncology*, D.H. Pizzo and D.G. Poplack, eds., © 1989, Lippincott Williams & Wilkins.

anorexia. In addition, children may develop food aversions that can limit intake.

Mucositis is a major gastrointestinal complication and is usually intensified by concurrent radiation therapy. Mucositis may affect any part of the gastrointestinal tract and lead to ulceration, bleeding, and malabsorption. Chemotherapy-induced neutropenia accentuates these complications. Rigorous mouth care prevents additional oral breakdown.[5] Fortunately, the renewal rate of the gastrointestinal tract mucosa is rapid, so that mucositis from chemotherapy is usually short-lived.

Certain chemotherapy and antibiotic agents cause malabsorption and alterations in the gut flora, with associated weight loss and intractable diarrhea.[5] Constipation related to use of vincristine or narcotics or inactivity may result in significant abdominal discomfort and loss of appetite.

Surgery

Surgical removal of a tumor may lead to insufficient oral intake over several days during a time of increased requirements. Radical surgery of the head and neck can lead to chewing and swallowing problems. Massive intestinal resection may cause malabsorption of vitamin B_{12} or bile acids.[13]

Radiation

Complications of radiation (Table 22–3) may develop acutely or become chronic and progress after completion of therapy.[13] Side effects and their intensity vary according to the (1) region of the body irradiated; (2) dose, fractionation, length of time, and field size of the radiation administered; (3) concurrent use of other antitumor therapy, such as surgery or chemotherapy; and (4) the child's initial nutritional status.[13]

Table 22–3 Radiation Effects in Pediatric Patients

Head and neck
- Nausea, anorexia
- Mucositis, esophagitis
- Decreased taste and smell
- Damage to developing teeth
- Decreased salivation → thick, viscous mucus
- Decreased jaw mobility

Thoracic
- Pharyngeal and esophageal inflammation and cell damage
- Sore throat, dysphagia

Abdominal or pelvic
- Nausea, vomiting, diarrhea
- Ulceration
- Colitis
- Malabsorption
- Fluid, electrolyte imbalance

Total body
- Nausea, vomiting, diarrhea
- Mucositis, esophagitis
- Decreased taste and salivation
- Anorexia
- Delayed growth and development

Source: Data from references 5, 7, and 13.

Marrow Transplantation

Marrow transplantation (MT) has become an established treatment modality for certain pediatric hematologic and oncologic disorders (Exhibit 22–2). Children receiving an MT are prepared with a conditioning regimen consisting of high doses of chemotherapy, with or without total body irradiation (TBI). An intravenous infusion of marrow follows. The source of the marrow may be the patient (autologous), an identical twin (syngeneic) or other family member, or a suitably matched, unrelated donor (allogeneic).[14] Bone marrow is obtained from the donor under general anesthesia in the operating room and infused directly into the patient through an indwelling venous catheter.

Autologous and allogeneic peripheral blood stem cell transplants are being used with increased frequency as an effective alternative to MT and provide prompt hematopoietic recovery

Exhibit 22–2 Conditions for Application of Marrow Transplantation in the Pediatric Population

Hematologic Malignancies
Acute Myeloid Leukemia (AML)
Acute Lymphocytic Leukemia (ALL)
Chronic Myelogenous Leukemia (CML)
Juvenile Chronic Myelogenous Leukemia
Recurrent Lymphoma
Myelodysplastic Syndrome

Malignant Solid Tumors
Advanced-Stage Neuroblastoma
Refractory Ewing's Sarcoma
Recurrent Hodgkin's Disease

Immunologic Disorders
Severe Combined Immundeficiency Disease
Wiskott-Aldrich Syndrome
Other Cellular Immunodeficiencies

Non-Neoplastic Disorders of the Bone Marrow
Severe Aplastic Anemia
B-thalassemia Major
Fanconi's Anemia
Congenital Hypoplastic Anemia (Blackfan-Diamond Syndrome)
Sickle-Cell Anemia

Genetic Storage Diseases
Mucopolysaccharidoses (Hurler's Disease, Hunter's Disease)
Metachromatic Leukodystrophy
Niemann-Pick Disease
Infantile Osteopetrosis

Source: Data from references 14 and 15.

following myeloablative conditioning regimens.[16] Umbilical cord blood transplants, rich in hematopoietic stem cells, are also being explored and have the potential to make transplantation available to children without suitable donors.[17]

Conditioning Regimen

The bone marrow infusion is preceded by multimodal chemotherapy or high-dose chemoradiotherapy administered over a 4- to 10-day period. TBI is used for patients with aggressive malignancies or unrelated donors. This intense conditioning regimen is designed to eliminate active and residual malignant cells or a defective hematopoietic system, as well as to facilitate immunosuppression of the patient to allow acceptance of the marrow graft.[18]

Posttransplantation Course

Severe pancytopenia lasts from 2 to 6 weeks posttransplant. Patients are at the greatest risk for bacterial and fungal infections until the marrow engrafts. During this period, some institutions may place patients in protective isolation rooms or in laminar airflow rooms. Supportive care includes frequent red blood cell and platelet transfusions and systemic antibiotic therapy, as well as aggressive parenteral nutrition (PN) support.

Nutritional effects of MT are due to conditioning therapy, infections, graft-versus-host disease (GVHD), and medications, including anti-infectious and immunosuppressive agents.[19] Complications interfering with nutrient intake include mucositis, esophagitis, altered taste, xerostomia, viscous saliva, nausea, vomiting, anorexia, diarrhea, steatorrhea, and multiple-organ dysfunction.[20–25] The duration and intensity of symptoms, as well as the stress of treatment, preclude oral intake for a period of 1–7 weeks posttransplantation and necessitate the use of PN support.

Oral intake is encouraged as soon as tolerated. Protein and calorie goals should be defined for the patient and family. Some facilities restrict certain foods or require a modified diet for neutropenic patients.[26] No other restrictions are needed unless gastrointestinal symptoms occur. At hospital discharge, many patients are still unable to eat an adequate amount of nutrients, and partial PN or tube feeding may be prescribed.[27] Although enteral feedings are not commonly used in the immediate posttransplant period, they may be an option for children with chronic food aversions and long-term anorexia posttransplant. Supplemental intravenous hydration may also be necessary. Follow-up nutrition counseling and assessment are imperative to prevent PEM.[19,27]

Graft-versus-Host Disease (GVHD)

Patients who receive allogeneic transplants are at risk for the development of GVHD following marrow engraftment. GVHD is an immunologic reaction in which the newly engrafted marrow recognizes the host's cells as foreign; the ensuing immunologic response can cause multiple-organ damage.[14,19] It may occur as an acute reaction early posttransplantation or progress to a chronic condition. Because of its potentially devastating effects, efforts are directed at prevention of GVHD. Medications and therapy used for prophylaxis and treatment of GVHD are shown in Table 22–4.

Acute GVHD can affect the skin, liver, or gastrointestinal tract. Clinical symptoms include maculopapular rash, cholestatic liver dysfunction, or diarrhea. Gastrointestinal GVHD can involve either the upper or lower gastrointestinal tract.[23] Upper gastrointestinal GVHD symptoms include anorexia, dyspepsia, and inability to eat. In lower gastrointestinal GVHD, diarrhea may be severe and, at its worst, associated with bleeding, crampy abdominal pain that requires narcotics, and refractory nausea or vomiting.[21,22] Patients with severe disease often require a period of bowel rest with PN support. Refeeding guidelines[19] include slow diet progression and feeding one new food at a time, as illustrated in Table 22–5.

Table 22–4 Medications and Therapy for Prophylaxis and Treatment of GVHD

Medication	*Nutritional Implications*
Antithymocyte Globulin	Nausea, vomiting, diarrhea, stomatitis
Azathioprine (Imuran)	Nausea, vomiting, anorexia, diarrhea, mucosal ulceration, esophagitis, steatorrhea
Beclomethasone dipropionate	Xerostomia, dysgeusia, nausea
Corticosteroids (Methylprednisone) (Prednisone) (Dexamethasone)	Sodium and fluid rentention resulting in weight gain or hypertension; hyperphagia; weight gain; hypokalemia; skeletal muscle catabolism and atrophy; gastric irritation and peptic ulceration; osteoporosis; growth retardation in children; decreased insulin sensitivity and impaired glucose tolerance; hypertriglyceridemia
Cyclosporine (Neoral or Sandimmune)	Nausea and vomiting; renal insufficiency; magnesium wasting, hyperkalemia. Should not take cyclosporine with grapefruit, papaya, pineapple juice, or carbonated beverages. Neoral preparation does not require lipid vehicle for absorption.
Tacrolimust (Prograf or FK-506)	Nephrotoxicity; hyperglycemia; hyperkalemia; hypomagnesemia
Methotrexate	Nausea and vomiting (mild to moderate), anorexia, mucositis and esophagitis, diarrhea, renal and hepatic changes, decreased absorption of Vitamin B_{12}, fat, and D-xylose; hepatic fibrosis; change in taste acuity
Mycophenolate mofetil	Vomiting and diarrhea
PUVA (Psoralen with Ultraviolet A)	Nausea; hepatotoxicity
Sirolimus (Rapamycin) (Investigational)	Weight loss; hyperglycemia; anorexia; hypertriglyceridemia
Thalidomide (Investigational)	Constipation, nausea, xerostomia
Ursodeoxycholic acid (UDCA) (Actigall)	Nausea and vomiting; diarrhea, dyspepsia

Source: Adapted with permission from P.M. Charuhas, *Introduction to marrow transplantation, Oncology Nutrition Dietetic Practice Group Newsletter,* vol. 2, no. 3, pp. 2–9, © 1994, American Dietetic Association.

Table 22–5 Gastrointestinal GVHD Diet Progression

Phase	*Clinical Symptoms*	*Diet*	*Clinical Symptoms of Diet Intolerance*
1. Bowel rest	GI cramping Large-volume watery diarrhea Depressed serum albumin Severely reduced transit time Small bowel obstruction or diminished bowel sounds Nausea and vomiting	Oral: NPO IV: stress energy and protein requirements	
2. Introduction of oral feeding	Minimal GI cramping Diarrhea less than 500 mL/day Guaiac-negative stools Improved transit time (minimum 1.5 hours) Infrequent nausea and vomiting	Oral: isosmotic, low-residue, low-lactose beverages, initially 60 mL every 2–3 hours, for several days IV: as for Phase 1	Increased stool volume or diarrhea Increased emesis Increased abdominal cramping
3. Introduction of solids	Minimal or no GI cramping Formed stool	Oral: allow introduction of solid food, once every 3-4 hours: minimal lactose*, low fiber, low fat (20–40 gm/day)†, low total acidity, no gastric irritants IV: as for Phase 1	As in Phase 2
4. Expansion of diet	Minimal or no GI cramping Formed stool	Oral: minimal lactose*, low fiber, low total acidity, no gastric irritants; if stools indicate fat malabsorption: low fat† IV: as needed to meet nutritional requirements	As in Phase 2
5. Resumption of regular diet	No GI cramping Normal stool Normal transit time Normal albumin	Oral: progress to regular diet by introducing one restricted food per day: acid foods with meals, fiber-containing foods, lactose-containing foods Order of addition will vary, depending on individual tolerances and preferences	As in Phase 2

Table 22–5 continued

Phase	*Clinical Symptoms*	*Diet*	*Clinical Symptoms of Diet Intolerance*
		Patients no longer exhibiting steatorrhea should have the fat restriction liberalized slowly IV: discontinue when oral nutritional intake meets estimated needs	

* Lactose is one of the last disaccharidases to return following villous atrophy. A commercially prepared lactose solution (Lactaid[R]) is used to reduce the lactose content of milk by >90%. Lactaid milk (100% lactose free) is also commercially available.

† Additional calories may be provided by commercially available medium-chain triglycerides, which do not exacerbate symptoms.

Source: Reprinted with permission from J. Darbinian and M.M. Schubert, Special Management Problems in *Nutritional Assessment and Management During Marrow Transplantation,* P. Lenssen and S.N. Aker, eds., pp. 65–66, © 1985, Fred Hutchinson Cancer Research Center.

NUTRITIONAL ASSESSMENT

Nutritional status at diagnosis has been associated with treatment outcome in children with cancer.[3,28–30] Nutrition assessment should begin at diagnosis and continue through and following treatment.[3] Techniques for the newly diagnosed patient do not differ from normal assessment recommendations as presented in Chapter 2. Table 22–6 provides guidelines for ongoing assessment in the pediatric cancer patient.

Anthropometry

Initial measurements should include age, height (recumbent length in children less than two years of age), weight, and, in children younger than 3 years of age, head circumference. Any measurement below the tenth percentile should be investigated as a sign of growth impairment due to inadequate nutrition. Weight for height percentile is believed to be the most reliable anthropometric indicator of nutritional status in the child with cancer.[3,31] It can be used reliably to predict nutritional status because of its high direct correlation with triceps skinfold and midarm muscle circumference measurements. In the pediatric cancer patient, current or previous chemoradiotherapy may depress growth. Catch-up growth has been observed in these patients.[32] However, patients who receive cranial irradiation may develop long-term growth disturbances.[33] Growth increments should be plotted yearly to detect deviations from normal growth patterns in children receiving long-term therapy, or after MT (Appendix B).[34]

Evaluation of Nutrient Intake

For a thorough evaluation of intake, daily food intake records provide a basis for decisions regarding supplemental or nonvolitional feeding. Parenteral or enteral nutrient solutions, other intravenous fluids, and oral intake must all be included when evaluating intake. Patients and family members may assist with record-keeping and provide valuable intake information.

Determination of feeding skills in the young child will facilitate choices for self-feeding. Many children's feeding skills will regress during acute illness.[35]

Table 22–6 Ongoing Nutrition Assessment Measurements that Identify Real or Impending Nutritional Depletion in Children with Cancer

Measurements	*Risk Criteria and Interpretation*	*Comments*
Nutrient intakes		
Energy (kcal/kg) % of healthy children	<80% of median intake: low intake	Energy intakes calculated from records kept by trained parents or personnel and reviewed by a dietitian for completeness, explicitness, and use of acceptable measures. Adjust for emesis: emesis within half hour—do not include in calculations; emesis 1–2 hours after eating—calculate as half intake; emesis 3–4 hours later—calculate as all intake. Energy intakes >80% of medium intake may be low when diarrhea occurs.
Anthropometric		
Height		
Height for age	<5th percentile: growth stunting which may be due to chronic PEM*	
Weight		
% change	>5% loss: acute PEM (with adequate hydration state)	Percentage weight loss derived from highest previous weight. Weight is inaccurate when child has edema, large tumor masses and organs extensively infiltrated with tumor, effusions or organ congestion, solid mass, or excess fluid administration (twice maintenance) for chemotherapy.
Weight for age	<5th percentile: acute or chronic PEM	Weight losses of >2% a day suggest dehydration.
Weight for height	<5th percentile: acute PEM when height for age is <10th percentile	
Skinfold thickness measurements		Steroid therapy may increase fat deposition. Measurements are inaccurate when child has edema.
Triceps	<10th percentile: depleted body fat stores	
Subscapular	>0.3 mm decrease: subclinical PEM†	

Table 22–6 Continued

Measurements	*Risk Criteria and Interpretation*	*Comments*
Biochemical		
Albumin	<3.2 gm/dL:[‡] acute or chronic PEM	Biological half-life of 14 days. May be decreased in presence of overhydration, severe liver dysfunction, or zinc deficiency.
% change	>10% decrease:[§] subclinical PEM	
Transferrin	<200 mg/dL: subclinical PEM	Biological half-life of 8 days. May be decreased in the presence of liver dysfunction; may be elevated in the presence of infection or iron deficiency.
% change	>20% decrease:[§] subclinical PEM	
Prealbumin	<20 mg/dL: subclinical PEM	Biological half-life of 2 days. May be decreased in the presence of severe liver dysfunction, vitamin A deficiency, or zinc deficiency; can be useful in assessing adequacy of nutrition support regimens.
% change	>20% decrease:[§] subclinical PEM	
Retinol-binding protein	<4 mg/dL: subclinical PEM	Biological half-life of 12 hours. May be elevated in the presence of renal failure; can be useful in assessing adequacy of nutrition support regimens.
% change	>20% decrease:[§] subclinical PEM	

* PEM, protein-energy malnutrition.

† More than twice coefficient of variation (method error) determined from 265 data sets of measurements obtained by two trained examiners.

‡ Lowest percentile of healthy children.

§ More than twice coefficient of variation.

Source: From Rickard KA, Grosfeld JL, Coates TD, Weetman R and Baehner RL, Advances in nutrition care of children with neoplastic disease: a review of treatment, research and application. Copyright The American Dietetic Association. Reprinted by permission from *Journal of The American Dietetic Association* (1986;86:1666).

Biochemistry

The disease or treatment may affect laboratory data used for nutritional assessment. Hemoglobin and hematocrit values in children with leukemia, lymphoma, and Hodgkin's disease reflect the disease state, rather than nutritional status.[3] Many chemotherapeutic agents cause bone marrow suppression and decreased total lymphocyte count. The complete blood count must also be interpreted cautiously in patients with solid tumors or hematologic malignancies because once therapy begins, complete blood counts primarily reflect treatment effects.

A concentration of serum albumin of less than 3 g/dL may reflect PEM; however, infection, excessive GI or renal losses, impaired liver function, certain chemotherapy agents, and overhydration can all depress serum albumin level. Furthermore, serum albumin level does not clearly reflect weight for height percentiles, calorie intake, or dietary protein intake in pediatric cancer patients.[36] Biochemical indices on visceral protein status, as well as renal and hepatic function, serum lipids, glucose, and electrolytes, should be reviewed for detection of nutrient deficiencies.

NUTRIENT REQUIREMENTS

Energy and Protein

The Recommended Dietary Allowances (RDAs) of the National Academy of Sciences can serve as an initial estimation of calorie and protein needs (Appendix K). Although the RDAs include factors for activity that may not apply to hospitalized children, the factor increase may approximate the additional calorie levels required by a child with cancer due to fever, active tumor metabolism, or host metabolism demands. Nitrogen balance and actual energy balance can be measured to ensure that desired results have been achieved. The best long-term indicator of adequate nutrient intake is growth (refer to Chapter 1 for additional information).

The Harris-Benedict formula and other equations have been used to estimate calorie needs in adults and may be appropriate for children who have completed their growth. Estimates of basal metabolic rate in children have been published by Altman[37] and the Mayo Clinic.[38] When these figures are used as a basis to determine energy needs, factors must be added for growth, infection, and stress. Multiplying basal metabolic rate by a factor of 1.6 to 1.8 for very young or malnourished children will allow for growth, stress, and light activity.[39]

Bacterial sepsis and fever secondary to neutropenia are other problems that increase metabolic demands in the child. Secondary complications, such as neutropenic enterocolitis, can further impair ability to absorb nutrients.

Vitamin and Mineral Requirements

Marginal nutrient deficiencies can occur in the pediatric patient with cancer. Patients who (1) are receiving PN and have no gastrointestinal function for an extended period, (2) have sustained radiation or surgical damage to an area of the intestine, or (3) are receiving antibiotics for chronic infections are especially susceptible to nutrient deficiencies due to malabsorption or inadequate supplementation.[6] Specific nutrient deficiencies can be masked by therapy effects and are difficult to identify. For example, thiamin deficiency has been noted in children maintained on long-term PN. The peripheral neuropathy that can accompany this deficiency mimics chemotherapy toxicity.[6]

NUTRITIONAL SUPPORT

Suboptimal oral intake of short duration during treatment is of less concern if the child is initially well nourished and can compensate when feeling well. These children may benefit from high-density foods that increase energy and other nutrient levels of the diet. Suggestions for boosting nutrient density of foods consumed are shown in Exhibit 22–3. Dietary guidelines for common problems seen during and following therapy are listed in Exhibit 22–4.

Oral Supplementation

The greatest limitation of nutritional supplements in the pediatric population is patient acceptance.[40] Milkshakes made with familiar products and supplemented by glucose polymers or other nondetectable modular components are usually best tolerated. Supplements are often acceptable if offered in an unobtrusive manner as part of the regular meal or snack pattern.[41] For the lactose-intolerant child, lactose-reduced or soy-based products can be useful. Oral and esophageal lesions may limit tolerance for oral supplements. Hyperosmolar or lactose-containing products may aggravate diarrhea. Encouragement from staff, patient education, and nutrition classes can help improve acceptance of supplements.

Tube Feeding

Children who cannot or will not eat may benefit from tube feeding (TF). Enteral nutrition has several practical advantages over PN. These include lower risk of infection or other catheter-related complications, more normal play activities, an opportunity for parent and child to become involved in the child's care, and decreased cost.[40] The utility and safety of gastrostomy feedings in pediatric cancer patients have been demonstrated. Gastrostomy tube feeding used in 25 malnourished children with cancer provided a safe and cost-effective method of reversing malnutrition.[42] Gastrostomy feedings were assessed in 33 pediatric cancer patients, primarily with solid tumors. Although minor complications occurred in 90% of the patients, gastrostomy feedings permitted effective nutrition support.[43]

Nasogastric TF may not be appropriate in the older infant, toddler, and preschool-age groups because of psychologic trauma associated with insertion and maintenance of tubes. In addition, nausea and vomiting, as well as decreased intestinal motility and absorption secondary to oncologic therapy, make TF less favorable and less effective.

The most common complications of TF are diarrhea and delayed gastric emptying.[44] In determining the cause of diarrhea, it is important to decide whether the problem occurred prior to initiation of the feeding, because the diarrhea may be related to an underlying infection or to medications. Constipation can occur with long-term use of a low-residue product but is rarely a problem.

Enteral feedings for children undergoing MT have been used infrequently because of more severe regimen-related toxicities, thrombocytopenia, and neutropenia. Szeluga et al[45] compared parenteral and enteral feeding programs in the first month posttransplant in 57 (adult and pediatric) allogeneic patients. Although there was improved body weight maintenance in the group receiving PN, there was no difference in the rate of hematopoietic recovery, length of hospitalization, or short-term survival between the groups. The investigators concluded that PN was not superior to an enteral feeding program. Several anecdotal case studies utilizing enteral feedings during MT have been reported;[46–50] however, further research exploring optimal time for initiation of feedings, types of tubes, methods of delivery, and appropriate formulas is vital.

Parenteral Nutrition

PN serves as a reliable source of nutrients for the patient who cannot ingest, digest, or absorb food via the gastrointestinal tract.[6] Nutritional support has been demonstrated to improve treatment tolerance in children with advanced neoplastic disease.[51] Fewer treatment delays[52] and the ability to provide planned courses of chemotherapy[53] have been reported in children maintained on PN. Accelerated recovery of bone marrow function has also been reported in children with acute nonlymphocytic leukemia receiving PN.[54] Finally, the use of PN was associated with improved adherence to chemotherapy schedules in children with solid tumors requiring both abdominal radiation and chemotherapy.[55]

Due to intensive treatment regimens, PN is standard supportive care for children undergoing MT.[56] Improved visceral protein status,[57] maintenance of body weight,[58] and earlier engraftment following cytoreductive therapy[59] have also been reported in pediatric transplant patients. Improved disease-free survival has been reported in allogeneic transplant patients who received prophylactic parenteral nutrition.[60]

The decision to use central or peripheral PN is based on nutritional status, expected duration of nutrition therapy, and availability of peripheral veins. Central venous catheters are often placed for chemotherapy, making central PN the logical choice.[6] Multiple-lumen catheters help simplify the delivery of medications, blood products, and nutrient solutions (see also Chapter 25). Cyclic/

Exhibit 22–3 Suggestions for Increasing Nutrient Density of Children's Diets

- Add cooked and diced meat, shrimp, tuna, or crab meat to soups, casseroles, and baked potatoes, or add to sauces and serve over rice, cooked noodles, toast, or hot biscuits.
- Add chopped, hard-cooked eggs to salads and casseroles. Add an extra egg to French toast or pancake batter.
- Cooked, dried peas and beans and bean curd (tofu) can be added to soups, pastas, casseroles, and grain dishes.
- Choose dessert recipes that contain eggs, such as sponge cake, bread pudding, or pudding made with milk substitute.
- Add peanut butter and margarine to bread, crackers, celery sticks, or pancakes and waffles.
- Add margarine or corn oil to hot foods such as soups, vegetables, mashed potatoes, cooked cereal, rice, or pasta. Meat, poultry, and fish that are breaded and fried are higher in calories than when baked or broiled.
- Mayonnaise has 100 calories per tablespoon—almost twice as much as salad dressing. Use it in salads and on sandwiches.
- Top pudding, pies, hot chocolate, fruit, and jello with a nondairy whipped topping (eg, Cool Whip).
- Add raisins, dates, chopped nuts, and brown sugar or maple syrup to hot or cold cereals.
- Add granola to cookie, muffin, or bread batters and sprinkle on pudding and ice cream.
- Instead of drinking water, select beverages that contain calories, such as fruit juice.
- Eat small, frequently scheduled meals throughout the day. Six feedings a day may help to meet caloric requirements without too much effort.
- Notice the time of day when appetite is best and plan for higher-calorie foods then. Eat a good snack before bedtime.
- Serve raw vegetables with a sour cream or yogurt dip.
- Spread cream cheese on crackers or fruit.
- Use cream or Half & Half in place of regular milk and water in hot cocoa, soups, or puddings.
- Powdered milk can be added to hot cereal, cream sauces, and gravies. It can also be added to milk.

Source: Adapted from L.M. Gallagher et al., Pediatric Acquired Immunodeficiency Syndrome, in *Handbook of Pediatric Nutrition,* P.M. Queen and C.E. Lang, eds., pp. 384–399, © 1993, Aspen Publishers, Inc.

Exhibit 22–4 Guidelines for Managing Common Nutrition Problems of Pediatric Oncology Patients

Tooth Decay
- If the child is not having a problem with loss of appetite or weight loss, limit the amount of sugar offered in the diet
- Avoid giving children foods that tend to stick to the teeth such as caramels or chewy candy bars
- Avoid giving small children bottles at night to prevent "baby bottle syndrome"

Dysgeusia (taste alterations)
- Flavored poultry, fish, eggs, dairy products
- Herbs, spices, flavor extracts, and marinades may enhance food taste
- Cold, non-odorous foods
- Fruit-flavored beverages
- Highly aromatic foods
- Tart foods, such as oranges or lemonade, may have more taste
- Good oral hygiene
- Drinking fluids with meals may help to take away a bad taste in the mouth

Xerostomia (oral dryness)
- Moist foods (stews, casseroles, canned fruit) and liquids
- Add extra sauces, gravies, margarine, butter, and broth to foods
- Encourage liquids with meals
- Adding vinegar and pickles to foods may help lessen xerostomia
- Sucking lemon-flavored, sugarless candy may stimulate saliva
- Good oral hygiene
- Commercial saliva substitutes may help

Thick, viscous saliva and mucous
- Adequate fluid intake
- Clear liquids (tea, popsicles, slushes, warm broth)
- Good oral hygiene

Oral and esophageal mucositis (inflammation of oral and esophageal mucosa)
- Soft/puree-textured or blenderized liquid diet
- Smooth, bland, moist foods (custard, cream soups, mashed potatoes)
- Soft, nonirritating, cold foods (popsicles, ice cream, frozen yogurt, slushes)
- Use a straw to drink beverages and liquids
- Encourage frequent mouth rinsing to remove food and bacteria and to promote healing

Nausea and Vomiting
- High-carbohydrate foods and fluids (crackers, toast, gelatin); nonacidic juices
- Small, frequent feedings

continues

Source: Adapted with permission from P.M. Charuhas. Introduction to marrow transplantation, *Oncology Nutrition Dietetic Practice Group Newsletter* vol. 2, no. 3, pp. 2–9, © 1994, American Dietetic Association; and *Managing Your Child's Eating Problems During Cancer Treatment*, NIH Publication No. 94-2038, 1994, National Cancer Institute.

Exhibit 22–4 continued

- Cold, clear liquids and solids
- Avoid overly sweet or high fat foods
- Avoid feeding the child in a stuffy, too-warm room or one filled with cooking odors or other odors that might be disagreeable
- Encourage drinking or sipping liquids frequently throughout the day; using a straw may help
- Encourage rest periods after meals
- Don't force the child to eat favorite foods when nauseated; it may cause a permanent dislike of the food
- Observe whether there is a pattern or regularity to when the child becomes nauseated or what causes it (specific foods, events, surroundings); suggest appropriate changes in the child's diet or schedule.

Diarrhea
- Low-fat, low-fiber diet
- Avoid caffeine
- Cold or room-temperature foods and beverages may be better tolerated
- Low-lactose intake
- Encourage adequate fluids to prevent dehydration

Constipation
- Encourage adequate fluids
- A hot beverage in the morning or evening may stimulate a bowel movement
- Offer the child high-fiber foods
- Encourage regular exercise, if tolerated

Anorexia
- Small, frequent meals of foods high in calories and protein
- Use carbohydrate supplements and protein powders
- Create a pleasant mealtime atmosphere with enhancing food aromas, colorful place settings, varied color and textures of foods
- Involve the child in grocery shopping, meal planning, and simple meal preparation
- Relaxation techniques and light exercise before meals may help improve food intake
- Therapeutic play with food models, food coloring book, food stickers, and other food-related activities may help to increase interest in eating
- Avoid forcing foods
- Avoid strong odors

Heartburn (Reflux)
- Limit high-fat foods
- Avoid highly seasoned foods
- Avoid caffeine, chocolate, and peppermint

Early Satiety
- Offer frequent, small meals
- Limit high-fat foods
- Avoids liquids at mealtime
- Encourage regular exercise, if tolerated

home PN can be used to reverse malnutrition while allowing the patient time out of the hospital. A home health care agency can work with the family to provide PN solutions, education, and monitoring.[6]

Troubleshooting

Lipid clearance may be impaired in sepsis, cachexia, or during corticosteroid or cyclosporine therapy.[61,62] Serum triglyceride should be checked weekly to verify normal lipid clearance.[63] Lipids should be discontinued at least 5 hours prior to checking triglyceride. Actual lipid clearance can be measured during infusion of lipids. A carbohydrate load of 15–16 mg/kg/min should be considered the maximum.[64,65]

SPECIAL CONSIDERATIONS

Long-Term Nutritional Sequelae

The growing child receiving antineoplastic therapy is susceptible to adverse effects of the treatment modalities, which may not become apparent until the child matures. Endocrine complications such as gonadal dysfunction, hypothyroidism, and impaired growth have been described.[66]

Growth hormone deficiency with decreased growth velocity and delayed onset of puberty have been observed in children treated with MT.[67] Children who have received cranial irradiation prior to MT show growth hormone deficiency with deceleration of normal growth rates.[68] Regular evaluations to determine occurrence of endocrine gland dysfunction are recommended.

Neuropsychologic complications, cardiac complications, and dental abnormalities are other consequences of cancer therapy.[66,69,70]

Clinical Pathways

In recent years, clinical pathways have been developed for pediatric oncology patients. The clinical pathways enable standardization of care for children, especially those receiving nutritional support, by mapping the management course to achieve specific outcomes. Nutrition care is streamlined with planned time lines for initiation and monitoring of nutritional support.[71] Benefits of pediatric oncology clinical pathways include assurance of standardized, optimal care; improved interdisciplinary communication; and enhanced patient education.

Alternative Nutrition Therapies

Alternative nutrition therapies such as the use of botanicals and megavitamin therapy in the treatment of childhood cancer raise great concern. Parents may use alternative treatment out of desperation to cure their child, to ease pain, or to augment conventional treatment.[72] Areas of concern regarding these nutrition-related therapies include:

1. Unexpected or undesirable interactions between preparations and prescribed medications may affect the action of drugs routinely used during the course of chemotherapy and MT.
2. Potential contamination of preparations derived from plants poses the risk of bacterial, fungal, or parasitic infections, which may cause life-threatening infections in immunosuppressed children.[73] A few specific preparations have been associated with serious toxic side effects or infections.[74,75]
3. Alternative nutrition therapy may be chosen as the sole source of treatment.

Herbals and botanicals are frequently explored as alternative therapies. These preparations are derived directly from plants and may be sold as tablets, capsules, liquid extracts, teas, powders, and topical preparations. A common herbal taken by cancer patients to boost immune function is echinacea. This herb acts as an immunostimulant by increasing phagocytosis and promoting the activity of lymphocytes, which results in the increase of tumor necrosis factor production.[76] It is available in tincture, capsule, or liquid form; however, the dose is dependent on the potency of the preparation. Side effects may include nausea and vomiting, and infrequent allergic reactions may occur in children allergic to members of the sunflower family (Asteraceae).[76] Recommendations regarding the effectiveness of echinacea as an adjunct to traditional childhood cancer therapy cannot be made at this time because no studies in the pediatric population have been reported (see Chapter 26).

Some herbals are contraindicated in children with cancer because of their association with serious side effects. Garlic and gingko biloba may reduce blood clotting factors.[74,76] Other botanicals containing pyrrolizidine alkaloids, such as comfrey and mate tea, may induce hepatotoxicity.[74] Dietitians must be sensitive to the family's views and biases and must educate the family and health care team appropriately.

Guidelines for Oral Intake

Diet for the Immunosuppressed Patient

The goal of the diet for the immunosuppressed patient is to minimize the introduction of pathogenic organisms into the gastrointestinal tract by food while maximizing healthy food options.[19,26,77] Diets vary from facility to facility and range from no raw fresh fruits or vegetables to a specific low-microbial diet for patients in laminar air flow rooms.[26,77] No empirical research exists on the relative benefits of restricting specific food groups.[20,29]

Exhibit 22–5 describes the diet restrictions recommended by the Fred Hutchinson Cancer Research Center, Seattle, Washington, for marrow and stem cell transplant patients undergoing treatment in the hospital and at home. High-risk foods, identified as potential sources of organisms known to cause infection in immunosuppressed patients, are restricted. The diet suggests foods that have been shown by culture to be safe when properly prepared in the home and hospital kitchen. Patients are counseled to follow these guidelines for 3 months after chemotherapy or autologous transplant. For patients receiving an allogeneic transplant, the guidelines are recommended until all immunosuppressive therapy is completed.

Food Safety

Immunocompromised patients are at increased risk for food-borne infections.[78,79] Center for Disease Control has targeted four bacterial pathogens— *E. coli 0157:H7, Salmonella enteritidis, Listeria monocytogenes,* and *Campylobacter jejuni*—as those of greatest concern. Improper holding temperatures and poor personal hygiene of food handlers contribute most to disease incidence.[80] Education for patients and caregivers is essential in preventing food-borne infections. Emphasis should be placed on hand washing, high-risk foods, proper temperatures for storage, defrosting, and cooking, cross-contamination issues, correct cooling and reheating procedures, and sanitation. In addition, water from wells or private water systems should be tested yearly for coliforms.

Food Service Concepts

The food service for oncology patients must be designed to provide a variety of foods served at frequent intervals to meet patient tolerance. A review of food items ordered by MT patients during the 2 weeks prior to discharge showed that nonacidic beverages were ordered most frequently, followed by bread products and cooked fruits.[81] Traditional hospital food services with set menus, tray line service, rigid meal hours, and 24-hour advance menu selection may fail to meet the needs of many oncology and transplant patients. A more flexible food service, such as unit nourishment centers or satellite kitchens, will provide opportunities for oral intake.[82]

A few facilities have implemented hotel-style room service with extended hours (up to 24 hours/day), telephone ordering systems, short delivery times, and elimination of wasted trays.[83,84] This system requires reorganization of the traditional food service department. The changes in traditional culinary mix of staff, diverse diet orders, kitchen equipment requirements, and staff education make this an immense undertaking. The main goals of this type of system are improved patient satisfaction and decreased waste.

Promoting Oral Intake during Hospitalization

Encouraging oral intake in the pediatric cancer patient can be a challenge.[41] Anxious, scared, or depressed children do not feel like eating. Chronic pain may also decrease the child's interest in eating. Providing a calm, relaxed hospital atmosphere for eating with uninterrupted time for feeding (door closed, sign posted) may improve intake. Small children require a secure feeding position (high chair or toddler feeding table), a bib, a towel, and a covered floor area to limit anxiety over spills.

Children should not be forced to eat; a maximum mealtime of 20–30 minutes should be adequate. Food texture and portion size appropriate for age should be provided. Older children may benefit from group eating situations, such as a playroom area, or participatory food preparation times, as well as knowing their oral intake goals for hospital discharge.

For patients refusing to eat, behavior modification techniques may be necessary.[85] Children transitioning from tube to oral feeding may exhibit oral, motor, sensory, and developmental feeding problems that make weaning difficult. A weaning process based on developmental stages is recommended.[86]

Many facilities implement some type of outside food policy, allowing the patient's family or caregivers to bring food into the hospital. Outside food items must conform to the medical diet order. These items are usually not stored on the unit; perishable foods must be consumed immediately. Family education in food safety is important.

Exhibit 22–5 Food Restrictions for Immunosuppressed Patients

Raw and undercooked meat (including game), fish, shellfish, poultry, eggs, hot dogs, tofu, sausage, bacon
Cold smoked fish (salmon) and lox; pickled fish
Unpasteurized and raw milk and raw milk products, including cheese and yogurt
Aged cheese (eg, brie, camembert, blue, Roquefort, sharp cheddar, Stilton, etc.)
Refrigerated cheese-based salad dressings (eg, blue cheese), not shelf-stable
Mexican hot cheese (eg, hot chili pepper) and farmer's cheese; Feta cheese
Unwashed raw vegetables and fruits, and those with visible mold; alfalfa sprouts
Unpasteurized commercial fruit and vegetable juices
Raw or unpasteurized honey
All miso products, including soup; tempe (tempeh); maté tea
All moldy and out-dated food products
Unpasteurized beer
Well water, unless tested yearly and found safe
Herbal and nontraditional (health food store) nutrient supplements

Source: Reprinted with permission from Diet for Immunosuppressed Patients, in *Standard of Practice Manual*, © 1997, Fred Hutchinson Cancer Research Center.

ADDITIONAL RESOURCES

Additional educational resources pertinent to both patients and health care professionals working in the nutrition care of children with cancer are listed after the References.

REFERENCES

1. Ross JA, Severson RK, Pollock HB, Robison LL. Childhood cancer in the United States. A geographical analysis of cases from the Pediatric Cooperative Clinical Trials Group. *Cancer*. 1996;77:201–207.
2. Gurney JG, Severson RK, Davis S, Robison LL. Incidence of cancer in children in the United States. Sex-, race-, and 1-year age-specific rates by histologic type. *Cancer*. 1995;75:2186–2195.
3. Novy MA, Saavedra JM. Nutrition therapy for the pediatric cancer patient. *Top Clin Nutr*. 1997;12:16–25.
4. Mauer AM, Burgess JB, Donaldson SS, et al. Special nutritional needs of children with malignancies: A review. *J Parenter Enter Nutr*. 1990;14:315–324.
5. Coates TD, Rickard KA, Grosfeld JL, et al. Nutritional support of children with neoplastic diseases. *Surg Clin North Am*. 1986;66:1197–1212.
6. Alexander HR, Rickard KA, Godshall B. Nutritional supportive care. In: Pizzo PA, Poplack DG, eds. *Principles and Practice of Pediatric Oncology*. Philadelphia: JB Lippincott Co; 1997:1167–1182.
7. Rickard KA, Grosfeld JL, Coates TD, et al. Advances in nutrition care of children with neoplastic diseases: A review of treatment, research and application. *J Am Diet Assoc*. 1986;86:1666–1676.
8. Kern KA, Norton JA. Cancer cachexia. *J Parenter Enter Nutr*. 1988;12:286–298.
9. Van Eys J. Nutrition and cancer: Physiological interrelationships. *Annu Rev Nutr*. 1985;5:435–461.
10. Sallan SE, Billett AL. Nausea and vomiting. In: Pizzo PA, Poplack DG, eds. *Principles and Practice of Pediatric Oncology*. Philadelphia, PA: JB Lippincott Co; 1997:1201–1208.
11. Charuhas PM, Aker SN. Nutritional implications of antineoplastic chemotherapeutic agents. *Clin Appl Nutr*. 1992;2:20–33.
12. Keller VE. Management of nausea and vomiting in children. *J Pediatr Nurs*. 1995;10:280–286.
13. Donaldson SS, Lenon RA. Alterations of nutritional status. Impact of chemotherapy and radiotherapy. *Cancer*. 1979;43:2036–2052.
14. Pinkel D. Bone marrow transplantation in children. *J Pediatr*. 1993;122:331–341.
15. Abramovitz LA, Senner AM. Pediatric bone marrow transplantation update. *Oncol Nurs Forum*. 1995;22: 107–117.
16. Secola R. Pediatric blood cell transplantation. *Semin Oncol Nurs*. 1997;13:184–193.
17. Kelly P, Kurtzberg J, Vichinsky E, Lubin B. Umbilical cord blood stem cells: Application for the treatment of patients with hemoglobinopathies. *J Pediatr*. 1997;130: 695–703.
18. Peterson FB, Bearman SI. Preparative regimens and their toxicity. In: Forman, SJ, Blue KG, Thomas, ED, eds. *Bone Marrow Transplantation*. Boston: Blackwell Scientific Publications; 1994.
19. Lenssen P. Bone marrow and stem cell transplantation. In: Matarese LE, Gottschlich MM, eds. *Contemporary Nutrition Support Practice: A Clinical Guideline*. Philadelphia: WB Saunders Co; 1998:561–581.
20. McDonald GB, Sharma P, Hackman RD, et al. Esophageal infections in immunosuppressed patients after marrow transplantation. *Gastroenterology*. 1985;88: 1111–1117.
21. McDonald GB, Shulman HM, Sullivan KM, Spencer GD. Intestinal and hepatic complications of human bone marrow transplantation, part I. *Gastroenterology*. 1986;90:460–477.
22. McDonald GB, Shulman HM, Sullivan KM, Spencer GD. Intestinal and hepatic complications of human bone marrow transplantation, part II. *Gastroenterology*. 1986;90:770–784.
23. Weisdorf DJ, Snover DC, Haake R, et al. Acute upper gastrointestinal graft-versus-host-disease: Clinical significance and response to immunosuppressive therapy. *Blood*. 1990;76:624–629.
24. Shubert MM, Williams BE, Lloid ME, et al. Clinical assessment scale for the rating of oral mucosal changes associated with bone marrow transplantation. *Cancer*. 1992;69:2469–2477.
25. Shubert MM, Sullivan KM, Truelove EL. Head and neck complications of bone marrow transplantation. In: Peterson DE, Sonis ST, eds. *Head and Neck Management of the Cancer Patient*. The Hague: Martinus Nijhoff Publishing; 1986:92–112.
26. Moe GL. The low microbial diets for patients with granulocytopenia. In: Bloch A, ed. *Nutritional Management of the Cancer Patient.* Gaithersburg, MD: Aspen Publishers; 1990:125–134.
27. Lenssen P, Moe GL, Cheney CL, et al. Parenteral nutrition in marrow transplant recipients after discharge from the hospital. *Exp Hematol*. 1983;11:974–981.
28. Donaldson SS, Wesley MN, DeWys WD, et al. A study of the nutritional status of pediatric cancer patients. *Am J Dis Child*. 1981;135:1107–1112.

29. Rickard KA, Detamore CM, Coates TD, et al. Effect of nutrition staging on treatment delays and outcome in stage IV neuroblastoma. *Cancer*. 1983;52:587–598.
30. Deeg HJ, Sediel K, Bruemmer B, et al. Impact of patient weight on non-relapse mortality after marrow transplantation. *Bone Marrow Transplant*. 1995;15:461–468.
31. Carter P, Carr D, Van Eys J, Coddy D. Nutritional parameters in children with cancer. *J Am Diet Assoc*. 1983;82:616–622.
32. Katz JA, Chambers B, Everhart C, et al. Linear growth in children with acute lymphoblastic leukemia treated without cranial irradiation. *J Pediatr*. 1991;118:575–578.
33. Moshang T Jr, Grimberg A. The effects of irradiation and chemotherapy on growth. *Endocrinol Metab Clin North Am*. 1996;25:731–741.
34. Tanner JM, Davies PW. Clinical longitudinal standards for height and height velocity for North American children. *J Pediatr*. 1985;107:317–329.
35. Pipes P. *Nutrition in Childhood*. St Louis, MO: CV Mosby; 1977.
36. Merritt RJ, Kalsch M, Roux, LD, et al. Significance of hypoalbuminemia in pediatric oncology patients: Malnutrition or infections? *J Parenter Enter Nutr*. 1983; 9:303–306.
37. Altman PL, Dittmer DS. *Metabolism*. Bethesda, MD: Federation of American Societies for Experimental Biology; 1968:344.
38. Pemberton CM, Moxness KE, German MJ, Nelson JK, Gastineau CF. *Mayo Clinical Diet Manual, A Handbook of Dietary Practices*. Burlington, Ontario: BC Decker, Inc; 1988.
39. Fred Hutchinson Cancer Research Center, Swedish Medical Center, Veterans Administration Medical Center. *BMT/PBSCT Nutrition Care Criteria*. Seattle, WA: Fred Hutchinson Cancer Research Center; 1995.
40. Norton JA, Peter J. Nutritional supportive care. In: Pizzo PA, Poplack DG, eds. *Principles and Practice of Pediatric Oncology*. 2nd ed. Philadelphia, PA: JB Lippincott Co; 1993:1021–1038.
41. Sherry ME, Aker SN, Cheney CL. Nutrition assessment and management of the pediatric cancer patient. *Top Clin Nutr*. 1987;2:38–48.
42. Aquino VM, Smyrl CB, Hagg R, et al. Enteral nutritional support by gastrostomy tube in children with cancer. *J Pediatr*. 1995;127:58–62.
43. Mathew P, Bowman L, Williams R, et al. Complications and effectiveness of gastrostomy feedings in pediatric cancer patients. *J Pediatr Hematol Oncol*. 1996;18:81–85.
44. Holden D, Sexton E, Paul L. Enteral nutrition. *Pediatric Nurs*. 1996;8:28–33.
45. Szeluga DJ, Stuart RK, Brookmeyer R, et al. Nutritional support of bone marrow transplant recipients: A prospective, randomized clinical trial comparing total parenteral nutrition to an enteral feeding program. *Cancer Res*. 1987;47:3309–3316.
46. Davies S, McCorkle N. *A Retrospective Review of Pediatric Bone Marrow Transplant Patients' Transition to Oral Feeds Using Enteral Nutrition in the Early Posttransplant Phase*. Presented at American Society for Parenteral and Enteral Nutrition, 18th Clinical Congress; San Antonio, TX: February 1, 1994.
47. Ringwald-Smith K, Krance R, Sticklin L. Enteral nutrition support in a child after bone marrow transplantation. *Nutr Clin Pract*. 1995;10:140–143.
48. Barron MA. *Successful Use of Percutaneous Endoscopic Gastrostomy (PEG) Tube Feeding Pre- and Post-Bone Marrow Transplant (BMT)*. Presented at 19th Clinical Congress of the American Society for Parenteral and Enteral Nutrition; Miami, FL: January 17, 1995.
49. Pietsch JB, Ford C, Whitlock J. *Nasogastric Tube Feedings in Children Receiving Intensive Chemotherapy or Bone Marrow Transplant: A Pilot Study*. Presented at the 22nd Clinical Congress of the American Society of Parenteral and Enteral Nutrition; Orlando, FL: January 20, 1998.
50. O'Leary E, House J, Mogul M, et al. *Nasogastric Tube Feeding for Nutrition Support in Pediatric Bone Marrow Transplant Patients*. Presented at the 22nd Clinical Congress of the American Society of Parenteral and Enteral Nutrition; Orlando, FL: January 20, 1998.
51. Rickard KA, Coates TD, Grosfeld JL, Weetman RM, Baehner RL. The value of nutrition support in children with cancer. *Cancer*. 1986;58:1904–1910.
52. Rickard KA, Detamore CM, Coates TD, et al. Effect of nutrition staging on treatment delays and outcome in stage IV neuroblastoma. *Cancer*. 1983;52:587–598.
53. Van Eys J. Malnutrition in children with cancer. Incidence and consequence. *Cancer*. 1979;43:2030–2035.
54. Hays DM, Merritt RJ, White L, et al. Effect of total parenteral nutrition on marrow recovery during induction therapy for acute nonlymphocytic leukemia in childhood. *Med Pediatr Oncol*. 1983;11:134–140.
55. Ghavimi F, Shils ME, Scott BF, et al. Comparison of morbidity in children requiring abdominal radiation and chemotherapy, with and without total parenteral nutrition. *J Pediatr*. 1982;101:530–537.
56. American Society for Parenteral and Enteral Nutrition. Guidelines for the use of parenteral and enteral nutrition in adult and pediatric patients: Nutrition support for infants and children with specific diseases and conditions. *J Parenter Enter Nutr*. 1993;7(suppl):39SA–41SA.

57. Uderzo C, Rovelli A, Bonomi M, et al. Total parenteral nutrition and nutritional assessment in leukemia children undergoing bone marrow transplantation. *Eur J Cancer*. 1991;27:758–762.

58. Yokoyama S, Fujimoto T, Mitomi T, et al. Use of total parenteral nutrition in pediatric bone marrow transplantation. *Nutrition*. 1989;5:27–30.

59. Weisdorf S, Hofland C, Sharp HL, et al. Total parenteral nutrition in bone marrow transplantation: A clinical evaluation. *J Pediatr Gastroenterol Nutr*. 1984;3:95–100.

60. Weisdorf SA, Lynse J, Wind D. Positive effect of prophylactic total parenteral nutrition on long-term outcome of bone marrow transplantation. *Transplantation*. 1987;43:833–838.

61. Neumanitis J, Deeg HJ, Yee GC. High cyclosporine levels after bone marrow transplantation associated with hypertriglyceridemia. *Lancet*. 1986;2:744–745.

62. Darbinian J, Schubert MM. Special management problems. In: Lenssen P, Aker SN, eds. *Nutrition Assessment and Management During Marrow Transplantation. A Resource Manual*. Fred Hutchinson Cancer Research Center; 1985:63–80.

63. Seashore JH. Nutritional support of children in the intensive care unit. *Yale J Biol Med*. 1984;57:111–134.

64. Khalidi N, Coran AG, Wesley JR. Guidelines for parenteral nutrition in children. *Nutr Supp Serv*. 1984;12:27–28.

65. American Academy of Pediatrics Committee on Nutrition. Commentary on parenteral nutrition. *Pediatrics*. 1983;71:547–552.

66. DeLaat CA, Lampkin BC. Long-term survivors of childhood cancer: Evaluation and identification of sequelae of treatment. *Ca Cancer J Clin*. 1992;42:263–282.

67. Sanders JE. Growth and development after bone marrow transplantation. In: Forman SJ, Blume KG, Thomas ED, eds. *Bone Marrow Transplantation*. Boston, MA: Blackwell Scientific Publications; 1994:527–537.

68. Sanders JE, Pritchard S, Mahoney P, et al . Growth and development following marrow transplantation for leukemia. *Blood*. 1986;68:1129–1135.

69. Copeland DR. Neuropsychological and psychosocial effects of childhood leukemia and its treatment. *Ca Cancer J Clin*. 1992;42:283–295.

70. Uderzo C, Fraschini D, Balduzzi A, et al. Long-term effects of bone marrow transplantation on dental status in children with leukemia. *Bone Marrow Transplant*. 1997;20:865–869.

71. Holeck RA, Sellards SM. Use of a detailed clinical pathway for bone marrow transplant patients. *J Pediatr Oncol Nurs*. 1997;14:252–257.

72. Pendergrass TW. Alternative therapies in the treatment of childhood cancer. In: Forman SJ, Blume KG, Thomas ED, eds. *Bone Marrow Transplantation*. Boston, MA: Blackwell Scientific Publications; 1994:1383–1393.

73. Fred Hutchinson Cancer Research Center. Naturopathic remedies: Guidelines for the use of herbal and nutrient supplement preparations during transplantation and high dose chemotherapy. *Standard Practice Guidelines*. Seattle, WA: Fred Hutchinson Cancer Research Center; 1997.

74. Tyler VE. *The Honest Herbal: A Sensible Guide to the Use of Herbs and Related Remedies*. New York: Pharmaceutical Products Press; 1993.

75. McGee J, Patrick RS, Wood CB, Blumgart LH. A case of veno-occlusive disease of the liver in Britain associated with herbal tea consumption. *J Clin Pathol*. 1976;29:788–794.

76. Tyler VE. *Herbs of Choice: The Therapeutic Use of Phytomedicinals*. New York: Pharmaceutic Products Press; 1994.

77. Henry L. Immunocompromised patients and nutrition. *Prof Nurse*. 1997;12:655–659.

78. Altekruse SF, Swerdlow DL. The changing epidemiology of foodborne disease. *Am J Med Sci*. 1996; 311(1):23–29.

79. Newman KA, Schimpff SC. Hospital hotel services as risk factor for infection among immunocompromised patients. *Rev Infect Dis*. 1987;9:206–213.

80. Collins JE. Impact of changing consumer lifestyles on the emergence/reemergence of foodborne pathogens. *Emerging Infect Dis*. 1997;3:471–479.

81. Gauvreau-Stern J, Cheney CL, Aker SN, Lenssen P. Food intake patterns and food service requirements on a marrow transplant unit. *J Am Diet Assoc*. 1989; 89:367–372.

82. Dezenhall A, Curry-Bartley K, Blackburn SA, et al. Food and nutrition services in bone marrow transplant centers. *J Am Diet Assoc*. 1987;87:1351–1353.

83. Schroeder K, Lopeman C, McBeth C, Barale K. Reengineering food service: From trayline to hotel-style a la carte dining. *J Am Diet Assoc*. 1997; 97(suppl):A82.

84. Lowe M, Mortensen S. "Room service"—feeding on demand succeeds for cancer patients. *J Am Diet Assoc*. 1995;95(suppl):A82.

85. Handen BL, Mandell F, Russo DC. Feeding induction in children who refuse to eat. *Am J Dis Child*. 1986; 140:52–54.

86. Schauster H, Dwyer J. Transition from tube feedings to feeding by mouth in children: Preventing eating dysfunction. *J Am Diet Assoc*. 1996;96:277–281.

87. Pizzo PA, Poplack DG, eds. *Principles and Practice of Pediatric Oncology*. Philadelphia, PA: JB Lippincott Co; 1997.

RESOURCES

Available, at no charge, from the National Cancer Institute: (800) 4-CANCER

Managing Your Child's Eating Problems During Cancer Treatment. NIH Publication No. 94-2038, 1994.

Talking With Your Child About Cancer. NIH Publication No. 94-2761, 1994.

Young People With Cancer. A Handbook for Parents. NIH Publication No. 93-2378, 1993.

From the Leukemia Society of America: (800) 955-4572

Emotional Aspects of Childhood Leukemia. A Handbook for Parents. (P-14 40M, 6/96).

Internet Resource

Nutrition for Children website and *Feeding Kids* Newsletter:
http://www.teleport.com/~eversc/NFC.htm.

Newsletters of Interest

Blood and Marrow Transplant Newsletter, written and published by a former BMT patient, for patients. For information contact: Blood and Marrow Transplant Newsletter, 1985 Spruce Ave., Highland Park, IL 60035, (847) 831-1913.

Friends Network Funletter, a national activities letter for children and families living with cancer. For subscription information contact: Friends Network, PO Box 4545, Santa Barbara, CA 93140.

The Candlelighters Childhood Cancer Foundation, 7910 Woodmont Avenue, Bethesda, MD 20814, (800) 366-2223, is a mutual support and self-help group of parents of children with cancer dedicated to improved communication, information, and treatment. The Candelighters Childhood Cancer Foundation quarterly newsletter is also available to professionals working with children with cancer, at no charge.

Tiny Tummies Newsletter. Nutrition news aimed at children. Monthly newsletter provides practical tips for feeding children, current childhood nutrition information, good nutrition and practical feeding ideas, tips, and recipes. For subscription information contact: Sanna James, MS, RD, Tiny Tummies, PO Box 2171, Sausalito, CA 94966-2171, (415) 389-6494.

CHAPTER 23

Nutrition in the Burned Pediatric Patient

Michele Morath Gottschlich

Trauma is a major cause of mortality in children, and a significant number of these deaths are from burns. Burn injury poses a complex metabolic challenge that is directly related to subsequent morbidity and mortality. As such, an important determinant of outcome is adequacy of energy and nutrient provision. If nutriture becomes impaired, wound healing and organ function will suffer. In addition, malnutrition will induce deterioration of immune defenses and profound catabolism.

The purpose of this chapter is to point out special metabolic changes in and physiologic deficiencies and nutritional requirements of burned infants and children. Because the common denominator to which all nutrients are related is adequacy of energy intake, methods for evaluating caloric requirements will be emphasized. The basis for selecting the safest and most efficacious route of support and ratio of nutrients will be addressed. This section will also review enteral and parenteral hyperalimentation techniques, as well as present options available for assessing and monitoring the nutrition rehabilitation program.

ANATOMIC AND PHYSIOLOGIC CONSIDERATIONS

Pediatric burn injury has a high mortality rate, compared with that of adults with equivalent burns,[1,2] although outcome has clearly improved with advancements in burn care.[3] The higher incidence of complications in pediatric burn patients is partially attributable to the fact that the unique physical and metabolic features of infants and children are frequently overlooked. It is important to recognize that the burned youngster in need of medical and nutritional therapy presents a separate and often much more complex therapeutic problem than does his or her adult counterpart.

Although the older child rapidly approaches the physical and metabolic makeup of the adult and responds to injury and treatment in a corresponding fashion, specialized nutritional care is required by younger age groups, due to their anatomic and physiologic immaturity (Table 23–1). All burned children, however, pose a special challenge to meet obligatory growth needs; burn injuries represent a particular threat to growth through imposition of a catabolic state. Bone growth is slowed during the acute phase postburn.[4] Furthermore, height and weight gain velocities have been documented during the first 3 years following the burn injury without a subsequent period of significant catch-up growth.[5]

A burned child, with both more limited endogenous reserves and greater caloric and protein requirements than an adult, quickly reaches negative nitrogen balance with a smaller area of burn than an adult does. Furthermore, the functional immaturity of the infant's gastrointestinal tract and renal system[6–8] poses a unique challenge to his or her ability to tolerate nonvoli-

Table 23–1 Anatomic and Physiologic Immaturities of Children of Various Ages

System	*Deficit*	*Clinical Implications*	*Age Maturation*
Temperature regulation	Labile system Surface area/body weight ratio greatly increased	Increased radiant and evaporative heat loss Increased metabolic rate in an attempt to maintain core temperature	10–12 years
Integument	Thin skin	Heat penetrates more rapidly, with resultant deeper burn	16–18 years
Gastrointestinal	Immature tract Limited surface area of the small intestinal mucosa Decreased gastric volume capacity	Limited capacity to digest or assimilate some nutrients Prone to antigen absorption High incidence of diarrhea	1–2 years
Renal	Glomerular immaturity Young kidneys inefficient in excretion of sodium chloride and other ions, as well as in water resorption	Renal concentrating ability low; therefore, more water required to excrete the renal solute load produced by the metabolism of protein and electrolytes Susceptible to dehydration	1–2 years

tional feeding regimens and nutrient-dense products. They are extremely susceptible to diarrhea, dehydration, and malnutrition, which only worsen the degree of catabolism.

METABOLIC MANIFESTATIONS OF THERMAL INJURY

In addition to developmental immaturities, the burned child must respond to the metabolic challenges associated with thermal injury. Extensive burn injury initiates the most marked alterations in body metabolism that can be associated with any illness. The pattern of physiologic events following thermal injury falls into two phases, the ebb and the flow responses.[9,10] The initial, or ebb, response of the burn syndrome is short, lasting 3–5 days postinjury. This phase is characterized by general hypometabolism and is manifested by reductions in oxygen consumption, cardiac output, blood pressure, and body temperature (Table 23–2). Fluid resuscitation is conducted during this time in response to the tremendous fluid losses that occur during the early postburn period.

With the resuscitative restoration of circulatory blood volume, the body advances to a prolonged state of hypermetabolism and increased nutrient turnover, termed the *flow phase.* This second phase is influenced by elevations in circulating levels of catecholamines,[11,12] glucocorticoids,[13–15] and glucagon.[16–19] Insulin levels are usually in the normal range or even elevated. However, the rise in the glucagon/insulin

Table 23–2 Metabolic Alterations Following Burns

		Flow Response	
	Ebb Response	*Acute Phase*	*Adaptive Phase*
Dominant factors	Loss of plasma volume Shock Low plasma insulin levels	Elevated catecholamines Elevated glucagon Elevated glucocorticoids Normal or elevated insulin High glucagon to insulin ratio	Stress hormone response subsiding
Symptoms	Hyperglycemia Decreased oxygen consumption Depressed resting energy expenditure Decreased blood pressure Reduced cardiac output Decreased body temperature	Catabolism Hyperglycemia Increased respiratory rate Increased oxygen consumption Hypermetabolism Increased body temperature Increased cardiac output Redistribution of polyvalent cations, such as zinc and iron Mobilization of metabolic reserves Increased urinary excretion of nitrogen, sulphur, magnesium, phosphorus, and potassium Accelerated gluconeogenesis	Anabolism Normoglycemia Energy turnover diminished Convalescence

Source: Adapted from Gottschlich MM, Alexander JW, Bower RH, Enteral nutrition in patients with burns or trauma, in *Enteral and Tube Feeding*, JL Rombeau and MD Caldwell (eds), with permission of WB Saunders Co, 1990.

ratio,[19,20] in combination with the other hormonal derangement, initiates gluconeogenesis, lipolysis, and protein degradation. Hypermetabolism and hypercatabolism also vary with the time postburn. The classic studies of Wilmore et al[12,21] show that, following the ebb phase, catabolic hormone production and oxygen consumption increase dramatically, peaking between the sixth and tenth day following burns.[12,21] Thereafter, metabolic rate slowly begins to decrease, and a gradual recession of catabolism occurs. These metabolic and hormonal sequelae have important implications from a nutritional perspective.

FLUID REQUIREMENTS

Water is the most critical of all nutrients. It is an essential component of all cellular structures and is the medium in which all chemical reactions of the host take place. The body composition of the infant is 70–75% water, compared with that of an adult, which is 60–65% water. The extracellular fluids of the infant constitute approximately 50% of the total body weight, compared with 20–25% in the adult. Excesses or deficits in water of more than 5% of the optimal value produce measurable effects, and large deviations may lead to death.

Immediately after burns, altered capillary permeability results in the escape of fluid, electrolytes, and protein from the vascular compartment to the interstitial area surrounding the burn wound. The injured area also loses its ability to act as a barrier to water evaporation. In children, with their relatively larger surface area per weight, the insensible water loss is of critical magnitude. Infants and young children are particularly susceptible to a lack of sufficient water intake because of their considerably higher obligatory urinary and insensible water losses, compared with those of adults. Hemodynamic dysfunction as a consequence of fluid shifts necessitates prompt provision of intravenous fluid resuscitation to restore tissue blood flow and to prevent shock following burns. Children require more fluid per square meter of body surface area than do adults with burns.[22]

The most popular pediatric fluid replacement formula in use is the Parkland formula,[23] modified for children (Exhibit 23–1). The modified Parkland formula includes a factor for basal fluid needs, in addition to compensation for losses from the burn wound. Lactated Ringer's solution is currently the fluid of choice in resuscitation regimens because its concentration of electrolytes most closely resembles that of extracellular fluid. Fluid replacement formulas serve as guidelines. The patient's vital signs, blood pressure, and urinary output should be constantly evaluated to determine adequacy of replacement.

CALORIC NEEDS

Increases in energy expenditure accompany burn injury. The degree of hypermetabolism is generally related to the size of the burn,[21] with burns of approximately 50% body surface area encountering a peak in energy expenditure, generally twice that of preinjury. It was once thought that the increase in metabolic rate was a response to the tremendous evaporative heat loss from the wound,[24,25] supported by the finding that raising ambient temperature partially reduced the hypermetabolic response. However, even in very warm environments, burn patients remained hypermetabolic, and their core and skin temperatures persisted. Other causes of hypermetabolism were sought after Zawacki and associates[26] demonstrated that blocking evaporation by application of impermeable dressings to the burn wound

Exhibit 23–1 Pediatric Fluid Calculations for Resuscitation and Maintenance

Modified Parkland Formula

Total resuscitation fluids (mL/24 hr) = [4 mL × % burn × weight (kg)] + [basal fluid requirements (1500 × m^2)]

1/2 of calculated fluid volume given in the first 8 hours
1/2 of calculated fluid volume given in the next 16 hours

Maintenance Fluid Calculation

Total maintenance fluids (mL/hr) = basal fluids + evaporative losses

$$= \frac{1500 \text{ ml} \times \text{m}^2}{24 \text{ hr}} + (35 + \% \text{ burn}) \times \text{m}^2$$

Source: Courtesy of the Shriners Hospital Burn Institute, Cincinnati, Ohio.

produced only a modest reduction in metabolic rate. The root cause of hypermetabolism continues to be an active area of investigation; it presently appears to be primarily driven by catecholamines.[12,27,28] Metabolic rate slows with wound healing and convalescence, although reactivation of hypermetabolism can occur, with complications such as infection or organ failure.

The substantial energy demands imposed by rapid growth and development during infancy and childhood are well documented. The caloric requirements of pediatric patients may be two to three times as great as those of adults in terms of body weight. Furthermore, youngsters' caloric reserves are usually small, particularly during infancy, and deficiencies develop more rapidly as a consequence. Every effort should be made to minimize energy demands by reducing external stresses such as pain, anxiety, and fear. The pediatric burn patient also has a major problem with temperature control. Therefore, when operative procedures or tubing and dressing changes are warranted, attention should be given to maintaining a warm environment.

The provision of sufficient calories to meet the increased metabolic expenditure is a critical factor in the management of the burned child. Energy needs may be estimated or measured. Numerous formulas exist for estimating the daily metabolic expenditure of burn patients; however, most of the popular equations have been predicated on data obtained from adults.[29,30] Recently, various equations that specifically address metabolic differences in children have appeared in the literature.[31–37] The pediatric formula proposed by Hildreth and colleagues[32,33] estimates maintenance caloric requirement obtained from the Recommended Dietary Allowances (RDAs) for normal children, expressed in terms of body surface area rather than age or weight. The formula also considers energy needs relative to burns by taking into account the heat loss associated with the predicted fluid losses that occur as a result of evaporation and exudation of the burn wound:

Caloric Requirements = (1800 kcal/m^2 body surface area) + (2200 kcal/m^2 body surface area burned)

Long's modification[36] of the Harris-Benedict equation[39] has also been used to estimate energy expenditure of burned children. Developed in 1919, the Harris-Benedict equation estimates basal metabolic rate (BMR) with reasonable accuracy. The Harris-Benedict equation for BMR was derived by multiple-regression analysis, using indirect calorimetry measurements performed on healthy volunteers, and it includes a factor for age. Long proposed that BMR be adjusted for hospitalized patients by taking into account activity and injury factors. An injury factor of 2.1 was recommended for burns:

Men

BMR = (66.47 + 13.75 W + 5.0 H – 6.76 A) × (activity factor) × (injury factor)

Women

BMR = (655.10 + 9.56 W + 1.85 H– 4.68 A) × (activity factor) × (injury factor)

W = weight in kg; H = height in cm; and A = age in years.

Activity Factor	*Injury Factor*
a. Confined to bed = 1.2	a. Severe thermal burn = 2.1
b. Out of bed = 1.3	

Curreri et al[29] proposed calculating caloric needs of the burned adult on the basis of 25 kcal/kg of body weight plus 40 kcal/% total body surface area burned. This formula has subsequently been modified for pediatrics,[38] using balance studies of weight in burned children:

Ages 0–1: Basal calories + 15 kcal/% burn
Ages 1–3: Basal calories + 25 kcal/% burn
Ages 3–15: Basal calories + 40 kcal/% burn

The aforementioned Curreri junior formula is designed for burns of less than 50% total body surface area. It typically overestimates caloric requirements in burns exceeding 50%.[32]

Studies in burned children at the Shriners Hospitals for Children, Boston, show that energy intake approximates the RDAs with generous protein intake and aggressive early excision and grafting procedures. Their data suggest that the elevated energy needs due to burns (without sepsis) are offset by reduced physical activity; thus, energy needs approximate those for healthy children of the same age.[40] The contribution of physical activity to total energy expenditure becomes more pronounced after the burn is healed and activity is resumed.

The wide range of formulas for calculating energy needs is an indication of the uncertainties of this approach. Most mathematic derivations utilize body weight, age, and burn size as the only determinants of caloric requirements. Although these three factors represent significant effectors of metabolic rate, energy expenditure is also influenced by surgery, pain, anxiety, sepsis, body composition, sex, thermal effect of food, sleep deprivation, and physical activity.[41] Therefore, mathematic formulas could derive fairly inaccurate caloric goals, considering the variability among individuals. If caloric needs are underestimated, some tissues, as well as exogenous substrates, will be consumed for energy. Although it is important to provide pediatric burn patients with the energy needed to compensate for hypermetabolism, as well as for growth and development, reports also caution against the delivery of an overabundance of calories.[42] Administering a surfeit of calories has been associated with increased metabolic rate, hyperglycemia, and liver abnormalities, and can cause an increase in carbon dioxide production.[43,44]

Portable indirect calorimetry represents a recent technological advance in terms of energy assessment of the pediatric burn patient. The use of indirect calorimetry in burn care has been extensively reviewed elsewhere.[45,46] In general, the patient's caloric goal should be calculated at 120–130% of the measured resting energy expenditure (REE).[45,47] Although there is some degree of error possible with this extrapolation, it is more accurate than estimates based solely on weight, age, burn size, sex, and/or height. To ensure the clinical validity of this goal, tests must be repeated regularly. Because hypermetabolism undergoes transient variation during the recovery phase, it is recommended that indirect calorimetry be conducted twice weekly, at minimum (Table 23–3), for proper adjustment of the nutritional support regimen.

CARBOHYDRATE NEEDS

Metabolic changes that occur following thermal injury include deranged carbohydrate metabolism. Early in the response to burns, glycosuria and hyperglycemia frequently occur. A similar response is observed in patients with supervening sepsis. Predisposition to glucose intolerance is correlated with the severity of the burn injury. Elevated blood glucose is also modulated by the phase of injury. During the shock phase, hyperglycemia is primarily caused by decreased peripheral tissue utilization in lieu of impaired tissue perfusion and low insulin levels.[48–50] Glucose intolerance typically persists during the flow phase, but it appears to be the result of enhanced hepatic glucose production and gluconeogenesis.[27,51]

Carbohydrate plays an important role in the nutritional support of the burned child. It appears to be the most important nonprotein calorie source in terms of nitrogen retention in burned patients,[52–55] although a limit exists to its effectiveness as an energy source.[43] Excessive glucose loads—which can increase carbon dioxide production, heighten glucose intolerance, and induce hepatic fat deposition—should be avoided.[40,44,53,56,57] Therefore, all burn patients should be monitored for hypercapnia and hyperglycemia. When these symptoms are present, the intake of total calories or carbohydrate may need to be reduced. Exogenous insulin administration is often necessary to improve blood glucose levels and to achieve maximal glucose utilization.

Table 23–3 Nutritional Assessment Protocol

Parameter	*Frequency*	*Comments*
Diet history	On admission	Obtain usual food intake history. Look for evidence of preinjury malnutrition, food allergies, intolerances, and chewing or swallowing difficulties.
Indirect calorimetry	Biweekly	Valuable indicator of severity of hypermetabolism, as well as the progression of convalescence. Nutrition support is inadequate when REE × 1.3 exceeds caloric intake or when RQ is less than 0.83.
Weight	Daily	Admission weight and height measurements should be compared to NCHS percentiles. In addition, daily weight monitoring can provide a means of assessing the adequacy of nutrition support. However, a weight change greater than 1 lb/d indicates fluid imbalances and will skew interpretation of visceral proteins. Corrections must be made for amputations, occlusive dressings, and major escharotomies.
Nitrogen balance	Daily	Amount of urine urea nitrogen excreted per 24 hours is a valuable index of severity of hypercatabolism. Nitrogen balance indicates whether nitrogen intake is exceeding body mass breakdown. Nutrition support is considered inadequate if nitrogen balance is negative.
Serum albumin, transferrin, prealbumin, retinol-binding protein levels	Weekly	Deficits of serum protein levels occur rapidly as a result of protein losses through the wound and altered protein metabolism. Repletion of visceral proteins occurs when adequate nutrients are provided. These parameters also are helpful in identifying burn patients at risk of infection.
Serum glucose level	Daily	Some patients with previously normal glucose tolerance may require sliding-scale insulin therapy during aggressive nutritional support following burns.
BUN and serum creatinine levels	Daily until stable, then twice weekly	If azotemia develops, increase the delivery of free water and/or decrease protein content of nutrient substrate.
Calorie and protein intake	Daily	Daily monitoring of oral, tube feeding, and parenteral intake can identify nutritional deficits or excesses before weight and laboratory values reveal an imbalance. Modification in nutrition support should be made if deviation of actual intake from goal is detected.
Delayed hypersensitivity skin testing, total lymphocyte count, C_3 and IgG levels	Optional	Suboptimal nutritional status can cause deficits in immune function.

Note: BUN, blood urea nitrogen; NCHS, National Center for Health Statistics; RQ, respiratory quotient.

Source: Data from references 102–105.

PROTEIN NEEDS

Thermal injury also brings about momentous changes in protein metabolism. There is increased proteolysis as energy needs are met by deamination of amino acids in the generation of carbon skeletons for glucose.[48,51] Transamination of amino acids likewise occurs as an intermediary step in the formation of nonessential amino acids and priority proteins associated with host defense, wound healing, and survival.[58] Reservoirs of amino acids that are mobilized to the liver include skeletal muscle, connective tissue, and gastrointestinal mucosa. The degree of amino acid mobilization is related to the size of the burn and adequacy of protein intake.

The protein requirements of the burned infant and child are elevated because of accelerated tissue breakdown and exudative losses during a period of rapid repair and growth. Failure to meet heightened protein needs can be expected to yield suboptimal clinical results in terms of wound healing and resistance to infection. The infant and child further adapt to inadequate protein intake by curtailing growth of cells, conceivably sacrificing genetic potential.

Studies have shown that enteral fortification using large quantities of protein can accelerate the synthesis of visceral proteins and promote positive nitrogen balance and host defense factors.[47,59–64] For example, Alexander et al[59] demonstrated that severely burned children on enteral diets containing approximately 22% of calories as protein had higher levels of total serum protein, retinol-binding protein, prealbumin, transferrin, C3, and immunoglobulin G (IgG), and better nitrogen balance, compared with patients receiving 15% of calories as protein. In addition, the high-protein group had improved survival and fewer episodes of bacteremia. Therefore, in planning a nutritional intervention strategy for a burned youngster, an important goal is the provision of a sufficient quantity of protein. It is recommended that 20–23% of calories be delivered as protein,[9,59,65] which translates to 2.5–4.0 g/kg, for a nonprotein calorie/nitrogen ratio of 80:1. Other factors that influence protein repletion, assuming an adequate intake of energy, include the quality of dietary protein and the source of nonprotein energy that the patient receives.

Of the 20 amino acids, 8 are essential in healthy adults, 9 are considered essential in infants, and several others are conditionally essential in the presence of stressors such as burns, prematurity, and extremely rapid growth (Table 23–4). Such changes in amino acid metabolism are illustrated by the alterations in plasma amino acids following burns.[47,59,66–69] It appears that many reparative and immunologic functions are dependent on the availability of specific amino acids. Improvements in aminograms and outcome in burned patients receiving supplemental arginine, histidine, cysteine, and glutamine suggest that the percentage of nitrogen needed for semi-essential amino acids may be significantly increased.[47,69]

Close monitoring of protein intake (see Table 23–3) is necessary because excessive protein loads or amino acid imbalances may result in azotemia, hyperammonemia, or acidosis. Particular care must be taken when administering high-protein feedings to children younger than 12 months of age, because excessive amounts can have adverse effects on immature or compromised kidneys. Ongoing assessment of fluid status, blood urea nitrogen (BUN) level, levels of plasma proteins, and nitrogen balance is recommended for individual evaluation of tolerance and adequacy. However, when fluid intake is not restricted, renal or hepatic dysfunction does not exist, and pathways of intermediary metabolism are relatively mature, a high-protein diet is usually well tolerated.

FAT NEEDS

During the flow phase, burn-mediated increases in catecholamine and glucagon levels stimulate an accelerated rate of fat mobilization and oxidation. It is recognized, however, that

Table 23–4 Essential and Conditionally Essential Amino Acids

Amino Acid	*Condition*
Threonine	Adult and infant
Leucine	Adult and infant
Isoleucine	Adult and infant
Valine	Adult and infant
Lysine	Adult and infant
Methionine	Adult and infant
Phenylalanine	Adult and infant
Tryptophan	Adult and infant
Histidine	Infants, burn patients
Cystine/cysteine	Premature infants, burns
Arginine	Premature infants, burns
Tyrosine	Premature infants
Glutamine	Catabolic states

Source: Data from references 47, 62, 106, 107.

lipid is important to the diet of the burned child because of its high caloric density, its role in myelination of nerve cells and brain development, the palatability it imparts to food, and its role as a carrier for the fat-soluble vitamins. In addition, fat in the form of the essential fatty acid linoleate provides vital components for cellular membranes and is a precursor for dienoic prostaglandin synthesis.

The minimum requirement for linoleic acid needed to prevent omega-6 fatty acid deficiency is considered to be approximately 2–3% of the calories consumed. This requirement is usually not difficult to accomplish because most enteral feeding supplements and intravenous fat emulsions contain high levels of fat and linoleic acid.[47,65,70] An overabundance of dietary lipid, however, can be detrimental to recovery from burns.[71] Complications ascribed to excessive fat intake have been reported. These include lipemia, fatty liver, diarrhea, and decreased resistance to infection.[70–72] Furthermore, lipid appears to represent an inefficient source of calories for the maintenance of nitrogen equilibrium and lean body mass following major injury.[53,55,73] Therefore, conservative administration of fat (at the 2–3% of calories level), particularly linoleic acid, is recommended.[47] Providing some fat in the form of omega-3 fatty acids also appears to be warranted.[47,72]

MICRONUTRIENT NEEDS

The functions of vitamins and trace elements pertinent to burn injury have been summarized elsewhere.[65,74,75] Optimal vitamin and mineral intake of the burned child remains to be determined, because few satisfactory data are available in this area of nutrition. Nevertheless, several facts are indisputable and bring to mind the importance of micronutrient supplementation. First, vitamin and mineral requirements increase with severity of thermal injury, related to heightened protein synthesis, enhanced caloric expenditure, and increased micronutrient losses. Second, individual vitamin and mineral needs are also dependent on preburn status. Finally, micronutrient stores are low in the young.

Undoubtedly, a deficiency of vitamins and minerals would compromise reparative processes. However, oral, tube feeding, and intravenous hyperalimentation regimens frequently do not meet the needs for certain micronutrients in a burned patient. Thus, it is recommended that additional supplementation be provided,[65,70,74–80] especially of those vitamins and trace elements associated with energy expenditure, wound healing, immune function, and those likely to have enhanced urinary and wound losses. Thiamine, riboflavin, niacin, folate, biotin, vitamin K, magnesium, phosphorus, chromium, and manganese are all cofactors for energy-dependent processes. The requirement for pyridoxine is closely related to dietary protein intake and protein metabolism. Vitamin B_{12}, folate, and zinc are cofactors necessary for collagen synthesis. Furthermore, inadequacy of many micronutrients, particularly vitamins A, C, E, and pyridoxine, as well as zinc, copper, and iron inadequacies, can adversely affect immune function. Iron supplementation, however, remains controversial,[47] because excessive iron also appears to enhance susceptibility to infection.[81]

Daily intakes of a multivitamin and supplemental vitamin A, vitamin C, and zinc (Table 23–5) are usually suggested. Many centers administer folate and vitamin E as well, although there is much less information on which to base levels of intake at this time. Although select vitamin and mineral replacement in excess of RDAs appears to be justified in burned children, some micronutrients, particularly fat-soluble vitamins, are toxic in large amounts. Thus, all micronutrients should be administered judiciously.

NUTRITIONAL INTERVENTION STRATEGIES

Nowhere is specialized nutritional support more important than in the rehabilitation of the infant and child who has sustained a burn injury. A decade ago, many children with thermal injuries died from malnutrition and sepsis because nutritional support was not possible or was inadequate. More recently, there have been exceptional clinical advances in applied nutritional

Table 23–5 Vitamin and Trace Mineral Recommendations

Children and adolescents (3 years or older)

1. Major burn
   - One multivitamin daily
   - 500 mg ascorbic acid twice daily*
   - 10,000 IU vitamin A daily
   - 220 mg zinc sulfate daily*
2. Minor burn (<20%) or reconstructive patient
   - One multivitamin daily

Children (< 3 years of age)

1. Major burn
   - One children's multivitamin daily
   - 250 mg ascorbic acid twice daily*
   - 5000 IU vitamin A daily
   - 100 mg zinc sulfate daily*
2. Minor burn (<20%) or reconstructive patient
   - One multivitamin daily

*Recommended delivery in suspension for tube feeding because oral vitamin C and zinc in large doses may precipitate nausea or vomiting.

support, with the marketing of oral supplements and improvements in enteral and parenteral hyperalimentation techniques. This technological progress has had a significant positive impact on the survival of extensively burned victims.

The goal of nutritional support for the pediatric burn patient is to provide adequate calories and nutrients to offset the increased metabolic demands induced by injury and growth. Ideally, nutrition intervention should be aimed at facilitating wound healing, maximizing immunocompetence, maintaining or improving organ function, and preventing loss of lean body mass. Specific objectives vary, however, according to the underlying metabolic and nutritional status of each patient. Special consideration is indicated whenever fluid restriction, organ failure, septicemia, mechanical ventilation, or any other presenting condition limits the ability to obtain vital nutrients.

Small burns (< 20% surface area) not complicated by facial injury, psychologic problems, inhalation injury, or preburn malnutrition can usually be supported by an oral high-protein, high-calorie diet if time is allocated for individual menu selection. Experience has shown that common food preferences among pediatric burn patients include hamburgers, hot dogs, spaghetti, chicken, and beef barbeque.[82] Vitamins and mineral supplements should be provided for the pediatric burn victim, as noted in Table 23–5. Between-meal snacks should be encouraged. Commercial meal replacement beverages or the addition of nutrient modules to menu selections may be helpful in boosting a marginal intake of calories or protein.

Collaboration between burn center departments, such as child life and nutrition, has led to the implementation of various creative, nutritious, food-related activities, including group dining, family picnics, bedside snack cart, edible adventures with new and unique foods, cooking and food preparation activities, restaurant meals, nutrition lessons, and skits (see Figure 23–1). The programs have proven useful in terms of promoting hospital adjustment for the child, encouraging patient–family unit development, and improving dietary intake. Additional suggestions for improving food consumption are listed in Exhibit 23–2.

Children with burns covering a larger surface area (20%) generally cannot meet their nutrient requirements by oral intake alone.[3] In these cases, alternative forms of feeding must be implemented. Nutrients should be provided to

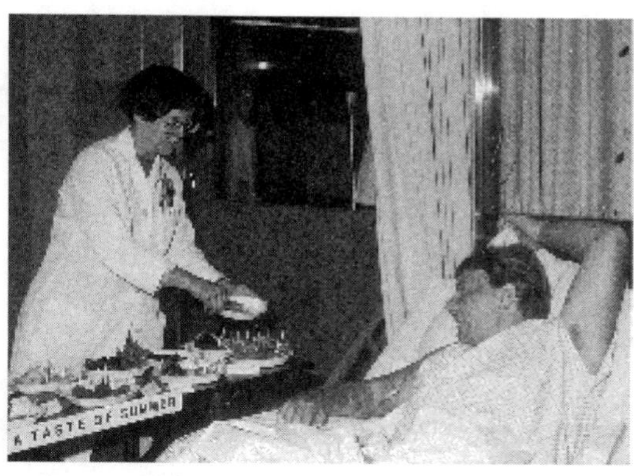

Figure 23–1 An edible adventure taking place at bedside.

Exhibit 23–2 Dietary Interventions Frequently Helpful in Improving Appetite

- Provide small, frequent meals and snacks
- Serve food in an attractive or creative manner
- Incorporate variety into the meals
- Avoid scheduling painful procedures shortly before mealtimes
- Hold tube feedings 1–2 hours before meals

the burned youngster by the enteral route whenever possible. The enteral route is preferred over intravenous because it is safer, gastrointestinal function is preserved, and the integrity of the small intestinal mucosal surface is better maintained,[70,83,84] thus possibly minimizing bacterial translocation from the gastrointestinal tract.[83,85]

Ordinarily, patients with thermal injuries can be successfully fed enterally.[9,65,86–88] The most common tube feeding routes are nasogastric and nasoenteric. Burn severity and projected frequency of surgeries are factors that can be used to gauge which enteral route is clinically indicated. In general, the stomach is the more traditional area of placement. It is appropriate in alert patients with an intact gag reflex who are presenting with a mild injury. A functional gastrointestinal tract is a prerequisite for nasogastric feedings. Continuous infusions using a tube feeding pump are recommended, with hourly monitoring of gastric residuals. Aspirates in excess of the previous hour's feeding are considered significant and warrant holding the tube feeding for 1 hour. Other tube feeding problems and solutions are reviewed in Exhibit 23–3.

In the more critically injured burn patient, stomach motility is diminished, resulting in acute gastric dilation and paralytic ileus, which limits the usefulness of the stomach for nutritional support. Other contraindications for nasogastric tube feedings include intractable vomiting, as well as required preoperative, perioperative, and postoperative periods of fasting.

Owing to the grave concern for possible aspiration, enteral alimentation that bypasses the stomach and uses the functional small intestine is desirable. Fluoroscopically or endoscopically placing feeding tubes into the third portion of the duodenum can be a safe means of enteral nutritional support, even during critical periods such as resuscitation, surgery, anesthesia for major dressing changes, or septic ileus.[89,90] Care must be taken that the duodenal tube remains in the small bowel. This can be accomplished by measuring the portion of the feeding tube that is left outside, from the nares to the end of the tube, once enteric placement is verified, then repeating this measurement at frequent intervals. Securing the feeding tube with staples or sutures can be done as a safeguard against accidental displacement. Gastric decompression can be simultaneously maintained using a nasogastric tube connected to intermittent suction. Once

Exhibit 23–3 Common Tube-Feeding Problems and Solutions

Diarrhea	May develop upon initiation of enteral alimentation following a period of parenteral support, which is associated with gut mucosal atrophy. Diarrhea may also result from lactose or fat intolerance, as well as from altered gut flora secondary to antibiotic therapy. Enteric feeding tubes positioned significantly beyond the ligament of Treitz can bring about malabsorption due to diminished absorptive surface area. Early enteral administration of moderate fat regimens, vitamin A supplementation, and proper positioning of feeding tubes can help decrease the incidence of diarrhea.
Gastric ileus	Is an indicator for nasoduodenal or nasojejunal tube feedings. Enteric feeding can be a safe means of alimentation during surgical, postburn, or septic ileus. Gastric decompression is essential.
Poor appetite	Can be minimized if tube feeding is held at mealtime. As appetite improves, nocturnal tube feeding may be sufficient.

Source: Reprinted with permission from M.M. Gottschlich et al., Diarrhea in Tube-fed Burn Patients: Incidence, Etiology, Nutritional Impact, and Prevention, *Journal of Parenteral and Enteral Nutrition,* vol. 12, pp. 338–345, © 1988, American Society for Parenteral and Enteral Nutrition.

bowel sounds are present, the nasogastric tube can be removed.

The question regarding the correct time for initiating a tube feeding program requires consideration. In general, enteral nutritional support should commence as soon as possible. The obvious reasons include the fact that a significant nutrient deficit can develop when alimentation is delayed following thermal injury, which has a direct bearing on morbidity and mortality. In addition, aggressive enteral support has been associated with improved tube feeding tolerance and sustained bowel mucosal integrity.[70,84,91] Furthermore, when tube feeding is initiated within the first few hours postburn, the hypermetabolic response can be partially suppressed, as evidenced by decreased energy expenditure and improvements in measurements of nitrogen balance, visceral proteins, and catabolic hormones.[60,84,87,88]

Because burn patients usually have unscathed digestive and absorptive capabilities, products containing intact nutrients should be used. Elemental or dipeptide formulations are unnecessary, unless dictated by concomitant disease or anatomic anomalies,[92] and appear to yield less favorable results in burns.[93] Most tube feedings can be started at full strength. The initial hourly infusion rate should begin at approximately half of the final desired volume and be increased by 5 mL/hour in the child and 10 mL/hour in the adolescent, as tolerated, until the final hourly rate is achieved. As oral intake improves and nutrient needs decrease, the child can be gradually weaned from the tube feeding regimen. Initially, tube feedings can be held at mealtime to stimulate appetite. Once the patient demonstrates the ability to consume 25–50% of caloric needs by mouth, the tube feeding program may be necessary only at night. Eventually, when the patient is able to meet approximately 90% or greater of his or her caloric needs orally, tube feedings can be discontinued.

The composition of the enteral infusate should take into account the unique metabolic and age-related alterations in nutrient utilization that accompany an extensive burn injury. Suggested tube feeding regimens for pediatric burn patients can be divided into two major categories: those appropriate for children younger than 12 months of age and those for patients 1 year of age or older.

To date, no one has examined in a randomized, controlled study the unique nutritional needs of the burned infant. Consequently, enteral protocols for infants up to 1 year old are generally conservative, relying on commercial infant formulas. The normal dilution of infant formula is 20 kcal/oz (0.66 kcal/mL). Gradually advancing the concentration to 24 kcal/oz is routinely safe. Further progression to 27–30 kcal/oz to meet the infant's energy needs must be monitored carefully, due to the resulting increased renal solute load.

The protein content of infant formulas ranges from 9% to 12% of total calories. This level is sometimes insufficient in those with large surface area burns. The addition of a protein module to the infant formula may be indicated in such cases if, once again, the patient is carefully monitored. Infant formulas derived from soy protein should not be used unless casein or whey intolerances have been confirmed, because the biologic value of soy protein is less than that of animal protein. Nutritional support regimens containing significantly reduced fat content are likewise not routinely recommended during infancy, because fat is an extremely important nutrient during the period of central nervous system maturation.

Tube feeding products for children over 12 months of age can generally be selected from formularies established for adults. The coincident fluid needs and energy requirements normally result in utilizing a tube feeding concentration of 30 kcal/oz or 1 kcal/mL. If the tube feeding product selected is low in protein, according to the guidelines established for burn patients,[8,59,65,94] products should be enriched with protein modules to yield 20–23% of their energy content as protein, using recipes such as that illustrated in Exhibit 23–4.

To date, there are no commercially manufactured tube feeding formulas specifically

Exhibit 23–4 Recipe Card for Modular Protein Enrichment of Commercial Tube Feeding Product

No.: Formula 1

Equipment: Waring Blender, Gram Scale, Graduated Cylinder

Date: 1/87
Rev.: 1/99

Note: (1) Wash and sanitize all utensils and equipment prior to preparation
(2) Discard after 24 hours.
(3) Label contains Item, Amount, Patient's Name, Date, and Initials of Preparer.

Diet: Osmolite/Promix Tube Feeding

Ingredients	*1000 mL*	*2000 mL*	*3000 mL*	*4000 mL*	*Method*
Sterile Water	175 mL	350 mL	525 mL	700 mL	1. Measure sterile water and pour into Waring blender.
Osmolite*	3 bottles plus 105 mL Osmolite	6 bottles plus 210 mL Osmolite	10 bottles plus 75 mL Osmolite	13 bottles plus 180 mL Osmolite	2. Measure Osmolite using graduated cylinder.
Promix RDP†	34 g	68 g	102 g	136 g	3. Weigh Promix. Add to liquids in blender.
Centrum Liquid‡	30 mL	60 mL	90 mL	120 mL	4. Measure Centrum Liquid using graduated cylinder. Add to blender.
Vitamin A§	0.1 mL	0.2 mL	0.3 mL	0.4 mL	5. Add Aquasol-A preparation. (Note: Aquasol-A contains 5,000 USP units of vitamin A/0.1 mL) Mix all ingredients in blender on low speed for 30 seconds. Do not overmix. Pour into one-liter paper cartons. DO NOT WAIT for foam to settle. The foam will create additional volume, so you may end up with an additional carton. (Example—recipe for 4,000 cc = 5 cartons). Label each container. Deliver to nursing unit. Refrigerate immediately.

*Ross Laboratories, Columbus, OH
†Corpak, Inc., Wheeling, IL
‡Lederle Laboratories, Pearl River, NY
§Astra Pharmaceuticals, Westborough, MA

Source: Courtesy of Shriners Hospital Burn Institute, Cincinnati, Ohio.

designed for the burn patient. However, it is clear from recent studies that this patient population has atypical nutritional needs that transcend traditional recommendations for a high-calorie, high-protein solution. Modular tube feeding recipes have evolved that not only take into consideration energy and quantitative protein guidelines but also offer the only means of currently incorporating findings regarding their unique fat, amino acid, vitamin, and mineral requirements.[47,70,88,95,96] Employment of modular tube feeding prescriptions has been correlated with statistically significant reductions in infection rates and length of hospital stay.[14] However, because complex recipes are not feasible at many institutions, due to the laborious, complicated preparation procedures involved, protein enrichment of commercial substrates is recommended as a practical alternative.

PARENTERAL HYPERALIMENTATION

During the late 1960s, when intravenous feeding was shown to permit growth and development, it became possible to provide nutritional support to virtually any child.[97] This technique has subsequently been incorporated into the care plans of many burned children.[98,99] Although the gastrointestinal tract is the preferred route of nutritional support, under certain circumstances, intravenous feeding can become a necessary, and even lifesaving, part of burn management.

Appropriate indications for intravenous feeding in burns are listed in Exhibit 23–5. There are two general categories of pediatric patients for whom parenteral nutrition is indicated. The first major category includes youngsters with protracted diarrhea or serious tube feeding intolerance, resulting in caloric insufficiency. If at all possible, however, at least some nutrients should be administered enterally during episodes of diarrhea. Children with gastrointestinal disease or injury form a second group that frequently requires total parenteral nutrition (TPN).

In general, peripheral parenteral support does not provide adequate calories and nitrogen in and of itself, and the delivery of intravenous nutrients via a central line is necessary to promote anabolism in the presence of burns.[100] Standard central venous regimens for the thermally injured patient usually consist of a final concentration of 25% dextrose and 5% crystalline amino acids, although individualized balancing is often warranted. Patients receiving 100% of their energy needs via the parenteral route will also require the administration of modest amounts of intravenous fat. Five hundred milliliters of 10% lipid emulsion (or 250 mL of 20% lipid emulsion) infused two to three times weekly will suffice in meeting essential fatty acid requirements.

The application of parenteral nutrition has undoubtedly contributed to improved outcome in pediatric burn victims unable to be supported enterally. No longer does the thermally injured

Exhibit 23–5 Indications for Total Parenteral Nutrition in Burns

- Gastrointestinal trauma
- Curling's ulcer
- Severe pancreatitis
- Superior mesenteric artery syndrome
- Obstructions of the gastrointestinal tract
- Severe vomiting or abdominal distention
- Intractable diarrhea
- Adjunct to insufficient enteral support

patient need to deteriorate when enteral feeding is insufficient or contraindicated. However, the metabolic and mechanical complications of parenteral hyperalimentation and the high incidence of septic complications in burns speak for reserving TPN for those whose nutritional needs cannot be met by the enteral route. Adherence to strict protocols of infection control, along with continuous monitoring of tolerance, will most often promote a successful intravenous feeding program in burns.[100]

NUTRITIONAL ASSESSMENT

Nutritional assessment is the process of identifying an individual's energy and nutrient requirements and evaluating the adequacy of enteral or parenteral nutrition support programs in meeting these needs. Because there is little specific information regarding the precise nutritional requirements of the burned child, assessment and monitoring patient response to diet therapy are especially important so that the clinician can react to alterations in metabolism that occur over time and reduce the opportunity for complications. At a minimum, this should include plotting of growth charts, daily evaluation of caloric and protein intake, clinical inspection of feeding lines, records of bowel function, determination of changes in body weight, and laboratory monitoring of serum albumin, glucose, BUN, and creatinine levels. Table 23–3 outlines parameters that can aid in the evaluation of nutritional status in burns. Interpretation of these data has been extensively reviewed elsewhere.[30,45,101]

CONCLUSION

Burn injury in pediatrics has important ramifications for nutrition. Decisions regarding what and how to feed patients continue to pose perplexing problems. Prompt provision of individually tailored diet therapy is of paramount importance in preventing malnutrition in burned children. This nutritional challenge is complicated by the fact that our knowledge of these patients' precise nutrient requirements remains incomplete. Burned infants and children represent separate and much more complex diet therapy problems, compared with their adult counterparts, because requirements for growth and development must be considered, as well as the increased nutrient needs imposed by burns. It is obvious that we have much to learn regarding optimal feeding practices in pediatric burn patients. Further research is needed to establish more definitive guidelines for nutritional intervention in burned children.

REFERENCES

1. Curreri PW, Luterman A, Braun DW, et al. Burn injury: Analysis of survival and hospitalization time for 937 patients. *Ann Surg*. 1980;192:472–478.
2. Feller I, Jones CA. The national burn information exchange. *Surg Clin North Am*. 1987;67:167–189.
3. Tompkins RG, Remensnyder JP, Burke JF, et al. Significant reductions in mortality for children with burn injuries through the use of prompt eschar excision. *Ann Surg*. 1988;208:577–585.
4. Klein GL, Herndon DN, Rutan TC, et al. Bone diseases in burn patients. *J Bone Miner Res*. 1993;8(3):337–345.
5. Rutan RL, Herndon DN. Growth delay in postburn pediatric patients. *Arch Surg*. 1990;125:392–395.
6. Grybowski JD. Gastrointestinal function in the infant and young child. *Clin Gastroenterol*. 1977;6:253–265.
7. Lebenthal E, Lee PC. Development of functional response in human exocrine pancreas. *Pediatrics*. 1980; 66:556–560.
8. Spitzer A. The role of the kidney in sodium homeostasis during maturation. *Kidney Int*. 1982;21:539–545.
9. Gottschlich M, Alexander JW, Bower RH. Enteral nutrition in patients with burns or trauma. In: Rombeau JL, Caldwell MD, eds. *Enteral and Tube Feeding*. 2nd ed. Philadelphia: WB Saunders Co; 1990:306–324.
10. Cuthbertson DP, Zagreb H. The metabolic response to injury and its nutritional implications: Retrospect and prospect. *J Parenter Enter Nutr*. 1979;3:108–130.
11. Aikawa N, Caulfield JB, Thomas RJS, et al. Postburn hypermetabolism: Relation to evaporative heat loss and catecholamine level. *Surg Forum*. 1975;26:74–76.
12. Wilmore DW, Long JM, Mason AD, et al. Catecholamines: Mediators of the hypermetabolic response to thermal injury. *Ann Surg*. 1974;180:653–669.

13. Bane JW, McCaa RE, McCaa CS. The pattern of aldosterone and cortisone blood levels in thermal burn patients. *J Trauma*. 1974;14:605–611.
14. Dolocek R, Adamkova M, Sotornikova T. Endocrine response after burn. *Scand J Plast Reconstr Surg*. 1979;13:9–16.
15. Vaughn GM, Becker RA, Allen JP, et al. Cortisol and corticotrophin in burned patients. *J Trauma*. 1982; 22:263–273.
16. Wilmore DW, Lindsey CA, Moylan JA, et al. Hyperglucagonemia after burns. *Lancet*. 1974;1:73–75.
17. Johoor F, Herndon DH, and Wolfe RR. Role of insulin and glucagon in the response of glucose and alanine kinetics in burn-injured patients. *J Clin Invest*. 1986; 78:807–814.
18. Orton CI, Segal AW, Bloom SR, et al. Hypersecretion of glucagon and gastrin in severely burned patients. *Br Med J*. 1975;2:170–172.
19. Shuck JM, Eaton RP, Shuck LW, et al. Dynamics of insulin and glucagon secretions in severely burned patients. *J Trauma*. 1977;17:706–713.
20. Shuck JM. Insulin-glucagon ratios and catabolic state. *J Trauma*. 1979;19:909–910.
21. Wilmore DW. Nutrition and metabolism following thermal injury. *Clin Plast Surg*. 1974;1:603–619.
22. Merrell SW, Saffle JR, Sullivan JJ, et al. Fluid resuscitation in thermally injured children. *Am J Surg*. 1986; 152:664–669.
23. Baxter CR, Shires T. Physiological response to crystalloid resuscitation of severe burns. *Ann NY Acad Sci*. 1968;150:874–894.
24. Caldwell FT. Energy metabolism following thermal burns. *Arch Surg*. 1976;111:181–185.
25. Caldwell FT, Bowser BH, Crabtree JH. The effect of occlusive dressings on the energy metabolism of severely burned children. *Ann Surg*. 1981;193:579–591.
26. Zawacki BE, Spitzer KW, Mason AD, et al. Does increased evaporative water loss cause hypermetabolism in burn patients? *Ann Surg*. 1970;171:236–240.
27. Wilmore DW, Orcutt TW, Mason AD, et al. Alterations in hypothalamic function following thermal injury. *J Trauma*. 1975;15:697–703.
28. Harrison TS, Seaton JF, Feller I. Relationship of increased oxygen consumption to catecholamine excretion in thermal burns. *Ann Surg*. 1967;165:169–172.
29. Curreri PW, Richmond D, Marvin J, et al. Dietary requirements of patients with major burns. *J Am Diet Assoc*. 1974;65:415–417.
30. Morath MA, Miller SF, Finley RK, et al. Interpretation of nutritional parameters in burn patients. *J Burn Care Rehabil*. 1983;4:361–366.
31. Solomon JR. Nutrition in the severely burned child. *Prog Pediatr Surg*. 1981;14:63–79.
32. Hildreth MA, Herndon DN, Desai MH, et al. Reassessing caloric needs in pediatric burn patients. *J Burn Care Rehabil*. 1988;9:616–618.
33. Hildreth MA, Carvajal HF. Caloric requirements in burned children: A simple formula to estimate daily caloric requirements. *J Burn Care Rehabil*. 1982;3:78–80.
34. Sutherland AB, Batchelor ADR. Nitrogen balance in burned children. *Ann NY Acad Sci*. 1968;150:700–710.
35. Pleban WE. Nutritional support of burn patients. *Conn Med*. 1979;43:767–768.
36. Long CL, Schaffel N, Geiger JW, et al. Metabolic response to injury and illness: Estimation of energy and protein needs from indirect calorimetry and nitrogen balance. *J Parenter Enter Nutr*. 1979;3:452–456.
37. Mayes T, Gottschlich MM, Khoury J, Warden GD. Evaluation of predicted and measured energy requirements in burned children. *J Am Diet Assoc*. 1996: 96:24–29.
38. Day T, Dean P, Adams MC, et al. Nutritional requirements of the burned child: The Curreri junior formula. *Proc Burn Assoc*. 1986;18:86.
39. Harris JA, Benedict FG. *Biometric Studies of Basal Metabolism in Man*. Carnegie Institute of Washington, Publ No. 279, 1919.
40. Young VR, Motil KJ, Burke JF. Energy and protein metabolism in relation to requirements of the burned pediatric patient. In: Suskind RM, ed. *Textbook of Pediatric Nutrition*. New York: Raven Press; 1981:309–340.
41. Gottschlich MM, Jenkins M, Mayes T, et al. Lack of effect of sleep on energy expenditure and physiologic measures in critically ill burn patients. *J Am Diet Assoc*. 1997;97:131–136,139.
42. Wolfe RR. Burn injury and increased glucose production. *J Trauma*. 1979;19:898–899.
43. Burke JF, Wolfe RR, Mullany CJ, et al. Glucose requirements following the burn injury: Parameters of optimal glucose infusion and possible hepatic and respiratory abnormalities following excessive glucose intake. *Ann Surg*. 1979;190:274–283.
44. Askanazi J, Elwyn DH, Silverberg PA, et al. Respiratory distress secondary to high carbohydrate load. *Surgery*. 1980;87:596–598.
45. Saffle JR, Medina E, Raymond J, et al. Use of indirect calorimetry in the nutritional management of burned patients. *J Trauma*. 1985;25:32–39.
46. Ireton-Jones CS. Use of indirect calorimetry in burn care. *J Burn Care Rehabil*. 1988;9:526–529.
47. Gottschlich MM, Jenkins M, Warden GD, et al. Differential effects of three enteral regimens on selected outcome parameters. *J Parenter Enter Nutr*. 1990;14: 225–236.

48. Wilmore DW, Goodwin CW, Aulick LH, et al. Effect of injury and infection on visceral metabolism and circulation. *Ann Surg.* 1980;192:491–500.
49. Wilmore DW, Mason AD, Pruitt BA. Insulin response to glucose in hypermetabolic burn patients. *Ann Surg.* 1976;183:314–320.
50. Wolfe RR, Burke JF. Effect of burn trauma on glucose turnover, oxidation and recycling in guinea pigs. *Am J Physiol.* 1977;223:80–85.
51. Wolfe RR, Durkot MJ, Allsop JR, et al. Glucose metabolism in severely burned patients. *Metabolism.* 1979;28:1031–1039.
52. McDougal WS, Wilmore DW, Pruitt BA. Effect of intravenous near isosmotic nutrient infusions on nitrogen balance in critically ill injured patients. *Surg Gynecol Obstet.* 1977;145:408–414.
53. Long JM, Wilmore DW, Mason AD, et al. Effect of carbohydrate and fat intake on nitrogen excretion during total intravenous feeding. *Ann Surg.* 1977;185: 417–422.
54. Pearson E, Soroff HS. Burns. In: Schneider HA, Anderson CE, Coursin DB, eds. *Nutritional Support of Medical Practice.* New York, NY: Harper & Row; 1977:222–235.
55. Souba WW, Long JM, Dudrick SJ. Energy intake and stress as determinants of nitrogen excretion in rats. *Surg Forum.* 1978;29:76–77.
56. Barrocas A, Tretola R, Alonso A. Nutrition and the critically ill pulmonary patient. *Respir Care.* 1983;28: 50–61.
57. Askanazi J, Rosenbaum SH, Hyman AI, et al. Respiratory changes induced by large glucose loads of total parenteral nutrition. *JAMA.* 1980;243:1444–1447.
58. Blackburn GL, Bistrian BR. Protein metabolism and nutritional support. *J Trauma.* 1981;21:707–711.
59. Alexander JW, MacMillan BG, Stinnett JD, et al. Beneficial effects of aggressive protein feeding in severely burned children. *Ann Surg.* 1980;192:505–517.
60. Dominioni L, Trocki O, Mochizuki H, et al. Prevention of severe postburn hypermetabolism and catabolism by immediate intragastric feeding. *J Burn Care Rehabil.* 1984;5:106–112.
61. Serog P, Baigts F, Apfelbaum M, et al. Energy and nitrogen balances in 24 severely burned patients receiving 4 isocaloric diets of about 10 MJ/m²/day (2392 kcal/m²/day). *Burns.* 1983;9:422–427.
62. Saito H, Trocki O, Wang S, et al. Metabolic and immune effects of dietary arginine supplementation after burn. *Arch Surg.* 1987;122:784–789.
63. Dominioni L, Trocki O, Fang CH, et al. Nitrogen balance and liver changes in burned guinea pigs undergoing prolonged high-protein enteral feeding. *Surg Forum.* 1983;34:99–101.
64. Dominioni L, Trocki O, Fang CH, et al. Enteral feeding in burn hypermetabolism: Nutritional and metabolic effects of different levels of calorie and protein intake. *J Parenter Enter Nutr.* 1985;9:269–279.
65. Gottschlich MM. Acute thermal injury. In: Lang CE, ed. *Nutritional Support in Critical Care.* Gaithersburg, MD: Aspen Publishers; 1987;159–181.
66. Cynober L, Nguyen Dinh F, Blonde F, et al. Plasma and urinary amino acid pattern in severe burn patients: Evolution throughout the healing period. *Am J Clin Nutr.* 1982;36:416–425.
67. Groves AC, Moore JP, Woolf LI, et al. Arterial plasma amino acids in patients with severe burns. *Surgery.* 1978;83:138–143.
68. Herndon DN, Wilmore DW, Mason AD, et al. Abnormalities in phenylalanine and tyrosine kinetics: Significance in septic and nonseptic burned patients. *Arch Surg.* 1978;113:133–135.
69. Gottschlich MM, Powers C, Khoury J, Warden GD. Incidence and effects of glutamine depletion in burn patients. *J Parenter Enter Nutr.* 1993;17:23(S).
70. Gottschlich MM, Warden GD, Michel MA, et al. Diarrhea in tube-fed burn patients: Incidence, etiology, nutritional impact and prevention. *J Parenter Enter Nutr.* 1988;12:338–345.
71. Mochizuki H, Trocki O, Dominioni L, et al. Optimal lipid content for enteral diets following thermal injury. *J Parenter Enter Nutr.* 1984;8:638–646.
72. Gottschlich MM, Alexander JW. Fat kinetics and recommended dietary intake in burns. *J Parenter Enter Nutr.* 1987;11:85–89.
73. Freund H, Yoshimura N, Fischer JE. Does intravenous fat spare nitrogen in the injured rat? *Am J Surg.* 1980; 140:377–383.
74. Gottschlich MM, Warden GD. Vitamin supplementation in the burn patient. *J Burn Care Rehabil.* 1990; 11:275–279.
75. Gamliel Z, DeBiasse MA, Demling RH. Essential microminerals and their response to burn injury. *J Burn Care Rehabil.* 1996;17:264–272.
76. Pochon JP. Zinc and copper replacement therapy: A must in burns and scalds in children? *Prog Pediatr Surg.* 1981;14:151–172.
77. King N, Goodwin CW. Use of vitamin supplements for burned patients: A national survey. *J Am Diet Assoc.* 1984;84:923–925.
78. Council on Scientific Affairs. Vitamin preparations as dietary supplements and as therapeutic agents. *JAMA.* 1987;257:1929–1936.
79. Shippee RL, Wilson SW, King N. Trace mineral supplementation of burn patients: A national survey. *J Am Diet Assoc.* 1987;87:300–303.

80. Jenkins ME, Gottschlich MM, Kopcha R, et al. A prospective analysis of serum vitamin K and dietary intake in severely burned pediatric patients. *J Burn Care Rehabil.* 1998;19:75–81.
81. Weinberg ED. Iron and susceptibility to infectious disease. *Science.* 1974;184:952–956.
82. Holli BB, Oakes JB. Feeding the burned child. *J Am Diet Assoc.* 1975;67:240–242.
83. Saito H, Trocki O, Alexander JW, et al. The effect of route of nutrient administration on the nutritional state, catabolic hormone secretion, and gut mucosal integrity after burn injury. *J Parenter Enter Nutr.* 1987;11:1–7.
84. Saito H, Trocki O, Alexander JW. Comparison of immediate postburn enteral versus parenteral nutrition. *J Parenter Enter Nutr.* 1985;9:115.
85. Deitch EA, Maejima K, Berg R. Effect of oral antibiotics and bacterial overgrowth on the translocation of the gastrointestinal tract microflora in burned rats. *J Trauma.* 1985;25:385–392.
86. Kravitz M, Woodruff J, Petersen S, et al. The use of the Dobhoff tube to provide additional nutritional support in thermally injured patients. *J Burn Care Rehabil.* 1982;3:226–228.
87. Jenkins M, Gottschlich M, Waymack JP, et al. An evaluation of the effect of immediate enteral feeding on the hypermetabolic response following severe burn injury. *Proc Am Burn Assoc.* 1988;20.
88. Jenkins M, Gottschlich MM, Alexander JW, et al. Enteral alimentation in the early postburn phase. In: Blackburn GL, Bell SJ, Mullen JL, eds. *Nutritional Medicine: A Case Management Approach.* Philadelphia: WB Saunders Co; 1989:1–5.
89. Gottschlich MM. Early and perioperative nutrition support. In: Matarese L, Gottschlich MM, eds. *Contemporary Nutrition Support Practice.* Philadelphia: WB Saunders Co; 1998:265–278.
90. Jenkins M, Gottschlich M, Baumer T, et al. Enteral feeding during operative procedures. *J Burn Care Rehabil.* 1994;15:199–205.
91. Mochizuki H, Trocki O, Dominioni L, et al. Mechanism of prevention of postburn hypermetabolism and catabolism by early enteral feeding. *Ann Surg.* 1984; 200:297–310.
92. Gottschlich MM. Managing chylothorax in a pediatric burn patient. *RD.* 1987;7:10–12.
93. Trocki O, Mochizuki H, Dominioni L, et al. Intact protein versus free amino acids in the nutritional support of thermally injured animals. *J Parenter Enter Nutr.* 1986;10:139–145.
94. Gottschlich MM, Alexander JW, Jenkins M, et al. Burns. In: Blackburn GL, Bell SJ, Mullen JL, eds. *Nutritional Medicine: A Case Management Approach.* Philadelphia: WB Saunders Co; 1989:6–9.
95. Bell SJ, Molnar JA, Carey M, et al. Adequacy of a modular tube feeding diet for burned patients. *J Am Diet Assoc.* 1986;86:1386–1391.
96. Gottschlich MM, Stone M, Havens P, et al. Therapeutic effects of a modular tube feeding recipe in pediatric burn patients. *Proc Am Burn Assoc.* 1986;18:84.
97. Dudrick SJ, Wilmore DW, Vars HM, et al. Can intravenous feeding as the sole means of nutrition support growth in the child and restore weight loss in an adult? *Ann Surg.* 1969;169:974–984.
98. Derganc M. Parenteral nutrition in severely burned children. *Scand J Plast Reconstr Surg.* 1979;13:195–200.
99. Popp MB, Law EJ, MacMillan BG. Parenteral nutrition in the burned child: A study of twenty-six patients. *Ann Surg.* 1974;179:219–225.
100. Gottschlich MM, Warden GD. Parenteral nutrition in the burned patient. In: Fischer JE, ed. *Total Parenteral Nutrition.* Boston: Little Brown & Co; 1991:270–298.
101. Bell SJ, Molnar JA, Krasker WS, et al. Prediction of total urinary nitrogen from urea nitrogen for burned patients. *J Am Diet Assoc.* 1985;85:1100–1104.
102. Kagan RJ, Matsuda T, Hanumadass M, et al. The effect of burn wound size on ureagenesis and nitrogen balance. *Ann Surg.* 1982;195:70–74.
103. Jensen TG, Long JM, Dudrick SJ, et al. Nutritional assessment indications of postburn complications. *J Am Diet Assoc.* 1985;85:68–72.
104. Morath MA, Miller SF, Finley RK. Nutritional indicators of postburn bacteremic sepsis. *J Parenter Enter Nutr.* 1981;5:488–491.
105. Ogle CK, Alexander JW. The relationship of bacteremia to levels of transferrin, albumin and total serum protein in burn patients. *Burns.* 1981;8:32–38.
106. Snyderman SE, Boyer A, Roitman E, et al. The histidine requirement of the infant. *Pediatrics.* 1963;31: 786–801.
107. Pohland F. Cystine: A semi-essential amino acid in the newborn infant. *Acta Pediatr Scand.* 1974;63:801–804.

CHAPTER 24

Enteral Nutrition

Nancy Nevin-Folino and Myrna Miller

Healthy infants and children possess the capacity to consume a diet voluntarily that provides adequate nutrients. Unfortunately, this may not be possible for a number of pediatric patients with a variety of acute and/or chronic conditions. Infants and children who are unwilling or unable to ingest, digest, or absorb an adequate amount of nutrients orally are candidates for supplemental feedings and/or an alternate route of nutritional support. If the patient's gastrointestinal tract is functioning, enteral nutrition is indicated.

Enteral nutritional support (ENS) refers to the nonvolitional delivery of nutrients by a tube to the gastrointestinal tract. Enteral nutrition is preferred over parenteral feeding because it is more physiologic, is associated with fewer technical and infectious complications, and is also less expensive.[1–3] Additionally, enteral feedings may be nutritionally superior to parenteral feedings because more is known about enteral nutrient requirements and utilization.[4] Advances in commercial formulas and equipment for their delivery have made enteral feeding safe and efficacious to administer to pediatric patients in either the hospital or home setting.

This chapter provides practical guidelines for: (1) selecting appropriate candidates for enteral nutrition, ranging in age from birth to 18 years; (2) selecting specific products; (3) administering and monitoring enteral feedings; and (4) considering specific factors of the pediatric population. Note that enteral feeding of the premature infant is addressed in Chapter 3 of this text.

PATIENT SELECTION

In the inpatient setting, candidates for ENS or patients admitted with enteral feedings should be identified through a hospital screening program within 24 hours of hospital admission.[5,6] An example of a pediatric nutrition screening form is included in Exhibit 24–1. This type of screening can be used hospital-wide and can utilize the joint expertise of clinical dietitians, nurses, and physicians. Using specific high-risk criteria, a customized screen can be developed and utilized for all inpatient units or for specific specialty conditions, such as the neonatal intensive care unit[7] or oncology,[8] by the clinical dietitians to identify risks specific to a patient population. As hospitals move toward computerized patient information systems, the nutrition screen could be included in the computerized admission data. (See Chapter 2 for additional information on nutritional screening.)

The health care team should establish outpatient criteria for consideration of ENS. An outpatient screening should identify patients who are failing to thrive or progress by self-initiated hunger or consumption of oral feeds. Factors to evaluate would include:

1. usual calorie intake of < 80% of needs
2. weight maintenance or loss

Exhibit 24–1 Nutrition Screening Form

the children's medical center

Nutritional Screen

Present Diagnosis: ______

Previous Illness/Surgery: ______

Age ______ Months/years

Admission: Length/Ht: ______ cm Wt ______ kg HC ______ cm Wt/Ht ______ % of standard

______ %ile ______ %ile ______ %ile

Nutritional Screening on admission can facilitate the identification of patients at nutritional risk; and patients who are normal on admission but are at risk of subsequent depletion can also be identified.

The following criteria are used to identify patients at nutritional risk:

Circle or insert correct points.

Growth Pattern

	Criterion	Points
______	> 5% body weight loss in past month	2 pts.
______	Length/height for age < 5th percentile	2 pts.
______	Weight/height < 5th percentile, or < 90% of standard	1 pt.
______	Weight/height < 80% of standard	4 pts.
______	Weight/height > 120% of standard	2 pts.
______	Weight/height > 160% of standard	4 pts.

Disease/Condition (1 point each)

		Points
Acute/chronic renal failure	Gastrointestinal Disorder	______ pts.
Carcinoma/Leukemia	Metabolic Disorder	______ pts.
Cystic Fibrosis	Prematurity/Low Birth Weight	______ pts.
Diabetes Mellitus	Trauma	______ pts.
Failure to Thrive	Other ______	______ pts.

HISTORICAL/Dietary data: other factors effecting nutrition, growth, dietary intake, digestion, utilization (1 point each) ______ pts.

Laboratory Data (if available)

	Criterion	Points
______	Hgb/Hct below standard	2 pts.
______	Total lymphocyte count: < 1500 mm³	1 pt.
	< 1000 mm³	2 pts.
	(exclusive of patients on chemoradiotherapy)	
______	Serum albumin < 3.0 g/dl	2 pts.
______	Serum albumin < 2.5 g/dl	4 pts.

Present Diet Order: ______ (1, 2, 3 pts.) ______ pts.

Comments ______

Total points ______

☐ DATA insufficient to give an accurate point evaluation.

Screen completed by: ______ (Clinical Dietitian) ______ (Date)

Point Evaluation:
> 10 points - Nutritional Support Service or Nutrition consult recommended.
8-10 points - Nutritional Consult recommended.
4-8 points - Nutrition follow-up by dietitian.

DTY-0019-M (3/96)

Source: Courtesy of The Children's Medical Center, Dayton, Ohio.

3. weight/length or /height ratio < 5 percentile
4. excessive feeding time or physical inability to keep liquids from dribbling out of the mouth
5. oral aversion
6. mechanical problems with mastication, swallowing or peristalsis[9,10]

Again, specific screens can be developed for a particular disease state or condition.[11–14]

After the screen is completed, the dietitian should review patients identified to be at nutritional risk and coordinate a medical nutrition therapy plan with the health care team for the patient who will possibly require or is receiving ENS.

Malnutrition has been well documented in pediatric hospital settings[15] and is most frequently observed in critically ill infants and children who are diagnosed with various acute and chronic diseases. Using a nutrition screen can provide early identification of patients who are at nutritional risk and make subsequent intervention possible to prevent malnutrition and its associated complications.

To summarize, pediatric patients with a variety of diseases are at nutritional risk and have been shown to benefit from ENS (Exhibit 24–2). However, when enteral nutrition is contraindicated, due to severe intestinal dysfunction (Exhibit 24–3), parenteral nutrition constitutes the appropriate route for specific nutritional support (see Chapter 25).

Exhibit 24–2 Indications for Enteral Nutrition in the Pediatric Patient

Functional:
1. Neurologic disorders
2. Neuromuscular
3. Prematurity
4. Inability to take in adequate nutrition
5. Genetic/metabolic

Structural
1. Congenital anomalies
   A. Tracheoesophageal fistula
   B. Esophageal atresia
   C. Cleft palate
   D. Pierre Robin syndrome
2. Obstruction
   A. Cancer of head/neck
   B. Intubation
3. Injury
   A. Ingestions
   B. Trauma
   C. Sepsis
4. Surgery

Exhibit 24–3 Potential Contraindications for Enteral Nutrition in Pediatric Patients

Necrotizing enterocolitis
Gastrointestinal obstruction
Intestinal atresia
Severe inflammatory bowel disease
Severe gastrointestinal side effects of cancer therapy
Severe acute pancreatitis

Source: Reprinted from C.D. Lingard, Enteral Nutrition, in *Handbook of Pediatric Nutrition,* P.M. Queen and C.E. Lang, eds., © 1993, Aspen Publishers, Inc.

PRODUCT SELECTION

There is a wide variety of commercial infant, pediatric, and adult enteral formulas that can be utilized for pediatric patients. However, proper product selection is contingent on a number of factors related to the specific medical and nutritional status of the patient. Patient-specific factors include age, gastrointestinal function, history of feeding tolerance, nutrient requirements, and feeding route. Other important factors to take into consideration are formula-specific. These factors include osmolality, renal solute load, nutrient complexity, product availability and cost, and caloric density. Select patient- and formula-specific factors will be explored in greater detail below.

Infants Less Than 1 Year of Age

Human milk and/or commercial infant formulas constitute the most appropriate feedings for infants who are less than 1 year of age. Proposed standards specifying the nutrient content of infant formulas have been established by both the American Academy of Pediatrics[16] and the 1986 revision of the Infant Formula Act of 1980.[17,18] These standards are based on estimated requirements that will promote optimal growth in infants from birth to 12 months.

General categories of commercial infant formulas include standard cow's milk-based (CMB), CMB lactose-free, soy formulas (lactose-free), casein hydrolysates (semi-elemental), elemental, and those modified in fat (Table 24–1). The available formula choices contain macronutrients in either complex or semi-elemental forms, which are suited for a variety of medical problems found in infants and are listed in Table 24–1. Most manufacturers' product guides have detailed information about the indicated use of formulas and absorption/utilization routes.[19,20] The use of highly specialized formulas for infants and children with inborn errors of metabolism is addressed in Chapter 13.

The standard dilution for infant formulas is 20 kcal/oz. However, infants who have increased metabolic needs and/or a decreased fluid tolerance may not be able to consume an adequate volume of standard formulas to promote growth. In this instance, a more concentrated formula may be needed. Formulas with a caloric density greater than 20 kcal/oz are most commonly provided to infants with chronic lung disease and congenital heart disease or to those infants with chronic renal failure who require continuous ambulatory peritoneal dialysis. Concentrated infant formulas may also be useful for infants with nonorganic failure to thrive during periods of catch-up growth.

Infant formulas can be concentrated to a maximum of 30 kcal/oz (without modular additives) by adding less water to a concentrated liquid or powdered formula base.[21] If human milk is used in lieu of infant formulas, it can be "concentrated" with the addition of powdered infant formula. When this formula base (or human milk) is concentrated, the infant's water balance in relation to renal solute load should also be monitored (see Exhibit 24–4). Patients on formulas concentrated to > 120% (24 kcal/oz)[22] should be monitored frequently for signs of:

- dehydration
- irregular output (urine, stool, or emesis)
- urine specific gravity
- renal solute load
- serum electrolytes
- intolerance or nutrient toxicity

For initial fluid prescription, it is general practice to use 100 mL/kg for the first 10 kg of body weight; for weight between 10–20 kg, use 1000 mL plus 50 mL/kg for each kg > 10 kg; and for weight > 20 kg, use 1500 mL plus 20 mL/kg for each kg > 20 kg.[23,24] Adjust fluid delivery frequently based on weight gain changes. Insensible water loss should be factored, as well as additional needs caused by any medical condition.

If insensible water losses are increased, it would be advisable to concentrate only the base formula (or human milk) to 24 kcal/oz. The caloric density can be then increased by utilizing modular additives of carbohydrate (glucose polymers) or fat (vegetable oil or medium-chain triglycerides). Carbohydrate and fat additives do not increase the renal solute load. However, carbohydrate additives can cause a moderate increase in osmolality. With the addition of a long-chain triglyceride, the gastric emptying time may also be decreased. This effect may be clinically significant for only those infants who are at risk for aspiration and already have delayed gastric emptying.

Increases in caloric density are best tolerated by the patient when advanced gradually in increments of 2–4 kcal/oz/day. Formulas that consist of a base concentration of 24–26 kcal/oz and also contain modular additives of fat (eg, 0.25–0.50 g corn oil/oz, 2.5–5.0 kcal/oz, re-

Table 24–1 Characteristics of Selected Enteral Formulas

Formula Classification	Product Characteristics	Possible Indications for Use	Infant Formula (Manufacturer)	Pediatric Formula (Manufacturer)	Adult Formula (Manufacturer)
Standard milk-based (SMB)	Intact protein Contains lactose Long-chain triglycerides Moderate residue Low to moderate osmolality	Normally functioning gastrointestinal tract Lactose tolerant	Human milk Similac (Ross) Enfamil (Mead Johnson)		Compleat* (Sandoz)
Standard milk broad, altered	Intact protein Electrolyte manipulation (low iron)	Renal	Prn 60:40† (Ross)	Pediasure‡§ (Ross)	Ensure (Ross) Osmolite‡ (Ross) Isocal‡ (Mead Johnson)
	SMB Lactose free	Ex-premie, lactose intolerant	Lactofree (Mead Johnson)	Resource Just for Kids§ (Sandoz)	
	Added rice starch	Mild reflux	Enfamil AR (Mead Johnson)		
Standard soy, lactose free	Intact protein Low to moderate residue Low to moderate osmolality	Primary lactase deficiency Secondary lactase deficiency (intestinal injury or PEM) Galactosemia	Isomil (Ross) Prosobee (Mead Johnson)		
Standard fiber-containing¶	Intact protein Lactose free 4.3–14 g fiber per 1,000 mL Low to moderate osmolality	Constipation Diarrhea Normal digestive and absorptive capacity		Pediasure with fiber§ (Ross) Kindercal § (Mead Johnson)	Ensure with fiber Jevity‡ (Ross) Boost with fiber (Mead Johnson) Compleat-Modified* (Sandoz)

Source: Data from references 88–91; product information guidelines.

continues

Table 24–1 continued

Formula Classification	*Product Characteristics*	*Possible Indications for Use*	*Infant Formula (Manufacturer)*	*Pediatric Formula (Manufacturer)*	*Adult Formula (Manufacturer)*
Lactose free/ modified fat	Intact protein Fat content is 88% medium-chain triglycerides and 12% long-chain triglycerides	Chylothorax Intestinal lymphangiecatasia Severe steatorrhea Choleo stasis Liver disease	Portagen[‡,‖] (Mead Johnson)		Portagen[‡,‖] (Mead Johnson)
Semi-elemental	Hydrolyzed protein (peptides and amino acids) Lactose free Low to moderate osmolality Partial medium-chain triglyceride content	Steatorrhea Intestinal resection Cystic fibrosis Chronic liver disease Inflammatory bowel disease Diarrhea associated with hypoalbuminemia Allergy to cow's milk and soy proteins Not needed for jejunal feedings in patients with normal gastrointestinal function	Pregestimil[‡] (Mead Johnson) Alimentum[‡] (Ross) Nutramigen[¶] (Mead Johnson)		Vital HN[‡] (Ross) Reabilan[‡] (O'Brien) Subdue (Mead Johnson)
Elemental	Protein in form of free amino acids Lactose free High osmolality Low fat Carbohydrate in form of glucose oligosaccharides	Intestinal fistula Glycogen storage disease Chylothorax or intestinal lymphangiectasia not responsive to Portagen Short gut syndrome HIV+ Inflammatory bowel disease	Neocate (SHS) Ele-Care (Ross)	Neocate One+[§] (SHS) Vivonex Pediatric[§] (Sandoz) Peptamen Junior[§] (Nestles)	Vivonex (Sandoz) Peptamen (Nestles) Perative (Nestles)

Calorically dense	Intact protein Lactose free High renal solute load High osmolality 1.5–2.0 kcal/mL	Fluid restriction Increased metabolic needs Not recommended for transpyloric feedings			Ensure Plus (Ross) Magnacal (Sherwood Medical)
Follow-up	Increased nutrients Increased calories	Expremature babies for first year of life	Neocare (Ross) Enfamil 22 (Mead Johnson)		
	Over 1 year of age Iron fortified Balanced formulation with vitamins and minerals			Toddie's Best (Ross) milk and soy Next Step and Next Step Soy (Mead Johnson)	

* Blenderized feedings, contain 4.3 g dietary fiber per 100 kcal
† Low in phosphorus
‡ Contains medium-chain triglycerides as part of its total fat
§ Designed for children from ages 1 to 10
‖ Standardly prepared from powder at a 20 kcal/oz dilution for infants and a 30 kcal/oz dilution for children and adults. Essential fatty acid deficiency may occur with long-term use in infants with chronic liver disease. See reference 92.
¶ Does not contain medium-chain triglycerides

Exhibit 24–4 Physical Signs and Symptoms of Dehydration

Weight loss > 1% per day
Increased thirst
Decreased skin turgor
Dry oral membranes
Increased urine specific gravity (>1.030)
Decreased urine output (<1–2 mL/kg/h)
Increased hematocrit, serum sodium, and blood urea nitrogen levels
Fever
Depressed anterior fontanel in an infant

Source: Reprinted from C.D. Lingard, Enteral Nutrition, in *Handbook of Pediatric Nutrition,* P.M. Queen and C.E. Lang, eds., © 1993, Aspen Publishers, Inc.

spectively) and/or carbohydrates (eg, 0.5–1.0 g glucose polymer/oz, 2–4 kcal/oz, respectively). These recipes, which equal 30–32 kcal/oz, are generally tolerated by infants. Adding modulars to increase calories will change the percentage of calories from carbohydrate and fat, and the ratio of protein/100 calories.

In Table 24–2, there are three comparisons of nutrient percentages. The 20-kcal/oz formula has 43% of calories from carbohydrate, 9% of calories from protein, and 48% of calories from fat. This does not change with concentration to 24 kcal/oz. However, adding 4 kcal/oz corn oil skews the nutrient values so that there is a much higher percentage of calories from fat. Patients on nutrient-skewed formula recipes should be monitored closely and changed to a more appropriate distribution of macronutrients, as tolerated.

Foman recommends the following caloric distribution for infants: 7–16% of calories from protein, 30–55% of calories from fat, and 35–65% of calories from carbohydrate. It is important to note that when the protein intake provides for less than 6% of the caloric intake, protein deficiency may result.[25] Protein intakes accounting for more than 16% of calories could contribute to azotemia and negative water balance if associated fluid intakes are low. Foman has established protein needs per 100 calories. A minimum of 2.2 g/kg is recommended for infants younger than 3 months and a minimum of 1.8 g/kg for infants older than 3 months.[26] Additionally, high carbohydrate intakes may

Table 24–2 Nutrients in Different Concentrations and Formula Recipes

Formula	*20 kcal/oz Standard Dilution*	*24 kcal/oz from Formula Power or Liquid Concentrates*	*24 kcal/oz from 20 kcal/oz + 4 kcal/oz Corn Oil*
Oz per 100 calories	5	4.16	3.57
CHO (g/oz)	2.4	2.5	2.5
% calories	43	43	36
Pro g/oz	0.43	0.51	0.51
% calories	9	9	7
Fat (g/oz)	1.08	1.3	1.82
% calories	48	48	57
Protein (g per 100 kcal)	2.14	2.14	1.82

contribute to osmotic diarrhea, and fat intakes that exceed 60% of the formula calories could lead to ketosis.

Diluting formula to less than 20 kcal/oz should be done only with careful consideration and monitoring because of the risk of hyponatremia, diluted or insufficient nutrients, and/or excess fluid.[1,22] It is important to explain the exact amount of water to use without variance when giving formula recipe instructions to caregivers.

Children Older than 1 Year

Feedings for children who are older than 1 year of age include a choice of concentrated infant formulas, pediatric follow-up formulas, pediatric enteral formulas, various homemade blenderized feedings, and/or a number of commercial adult formulas. The caloric density of feedings utilized for children in this age group is approximately 30 kcal/oz. Once again, the caloric density may need to be increased further if the patients have increased metabolic needs and/or decreased fluid tolerance.

Formulas designed for pediatric enteral feedings meet the daily Recommended Dietary Allowances (RDAs) for children who are younger than 11 years of age in approximately 1,000–1,100 mL per day (see Appendix K). These enteral products are isotonic and lactose free, with a partial medium-chain triglyceride content to facilitate absorption.

Under specific conditions, infant formulas can be continued through 4 years of age. These formulas can be concentrated to provide higher levels of nutrients. Additional vitamin or mineral supplementation may also be needed, depending on the specific volume provided. Altered formulas have not been tested in vitro or processed by the manufacturer to be absorbed or used by the body as the original product. Adding nutrient supplementation, such as calcium or phosphorus, to a formula does not guarantee that the patient will be able to utilize the extra nutrients. Infant formulas have a lower renal solute load than do products designed for patients who are older than 1 year of age. These formulas may be more appropriate for malnourished toddlers who may actually be infant size.

Adolescents

For children between 10 and 18 years, many factors require consideration, such as maturation level, physical ability or limitations, calorie requirements, and volume tolerance. Adolescent nutrient needs increase with this last growth phase. Their calorie and protein needs may be met in a pediatric formula but not other nutrients, such as calcium and iron. Micronutrient analysis is helpful in matching a formula or combination of pediatric and adult formulas to meet the unique needs of the teen. There are a variety of computer nutrition assessment programs available, and when selecting one, pediatric parameters and pediatric formulas within the database should be considered in the selection criteria.

Blenderized Feedings

Blenderized feedings consist of a mixture of various meats, fruits, vegetables, milk (or formula), carbohydrates, fats, water, vitamins, and minerals. These blenderized feeding recipes can be made for use in an institution or in the home setting. Blenderized feedings are moderate in residue and moderate to high in osmolality and viscosity. Because their high viscosity hinders flow through small feeding tubes, these feedings are most often administered as gastrostomy tube feedings. Other disadvantages of blenderized feedings include a potentially high bacteria count[27–29] and the additional labor required for preparation. Homemade blenderized feedings 1) provide a more variable nutrient content than do commercially manufactured products, 2) are not emulsified, 3) can be used only when enteral feeding is delivered into the stomach, and 4) do not necessarily contain all essential nutrients in the level that a pediatric patient requires.

Blenderized feedings are considered for use today in the health care arena when third-party reimbursement or support is not provided. Although homemade formulas seem to be more economic in the home setting using food products, nutrient adequacy or variety is not taken into account. Economics becomes particularly important to families of children with chronic diseases, and blenderized concoctions will continue to represent a viable feeding alternative when a pediatric specific product is not covered.

Because inappropriate homemade tube feedings can result in hypernatremic dehydration[30] and a number of nutrient deficiencies, it is important to perform a periodic analysis of the recipe, including verification of how the family is making the formula at home, the adequacy of the nutrients, and the associated fluids. It is equally important to monitor the intake of protein and electrolytes because excess may lead to a negative water balance in the patient. Guidelines for the safe use of homemade blenderized feedings for children with gastrostomy tubes are available.[30]

Commercial Adult Formulas

A large variety of adult enteral products is commercially available. These products contain macronutrients in various forms and percentages (Table 24–3). They can be divided into several general categories: standard milk-based, lactose-free, elemental, fiber-containing, and calorically dense. General characteristics of selected adult enteral products with possible indications for use are covered in Table 24–1. This list is not inclusive of all products that are commercially available but is intended to provide examples of products that are available in each general category. Information regarding the complete nutrient composition of commercial adult and infant formulas is readily available from various manufacturers.

It should be noted that adult enteral products have not been designed for use in children, nor have they been extensively tested in the pediatric population. Specific concerns regarding the use of these products in children are addressed in the upcoming discussions of renal solute load and nutrient requirements.

Renal Solute Load and Fluid Balance

The renal solute load of a formula consists primarily of electrolytes and metabolic end products of protein metabolism that must be excreted in the urine.[21] These solutes require water for urinary excretion. Infants have an immature renal system, with limited concentrating ability, and they require more free water to excrete solutes than do older children and adults. Therefore, infants are at particular risk for negative water balance and subsequent dehydration. Potential renal solute load (PRSL) does not need to be calculated routinely but is important with patients who have medical problems or formula prescriptions that would influence renal metabolism. Equations for PRSL vary in the units of measurement for solute load.[1] An example equation is as follows:

$$\text{PRSL (mOsm/L)} = \text{mEq sodium/L} + \text{mEq potassium/L} + \text{mEq chloride/L} + [4 \times \text{protein(g)/L}]$$

The renal solute load and fluid balance should be closely monitored when infants have a low fluid intake, are receiving calorically dense feedings, and have increased extrarenal fluid losses (ie, fever, diarrhea, sweating) or impaired renal concentrating ability.[21] Neurologically impaired infants and children who are unable to indicate thirst may also be at risk for dehydration.

Infant formulas at standard dilution contain approximately 95% water[27] (preformed water plus water of oxidation). In contrast, standard adult enteral formulas contain approximately 85% water. Because adult formulas are also higher in protein and electrolytes, this contributes to a higher renal solute load. Therefore, when administering adult products to infants and toddlers, proper precautions should be taken. For example, additional water may be required and can usually be given while flushing the feeding tube.

Osmolality

Osmolality refers to the number of particles in a kilogram of solution. The osmolality of a for-

Table 24–3 Macronutrient Content of Infant and Adult Formulas

	Carbohydrate	*Protein*	*Fat*
Caloric Distribution (standard products)			
Infant formulas	40–54%	9–14%	35–50%
Adult formulas	45–60%	12–20%	30–40%
Intact sources	Modified food starch* Vegetables Corn syrup solids Tapioca starch Hydrolyzed cereal solids	Milk† Casein isolate† Soy isolate† Lactalbumin† Beef† Sodium caseinate† Calcium caseinate† Egg white solids†	Long-chain triglycerides:‡ corn oil, soy oil, sunflower oil, safflower oil, butterfat
Semi-elemental sources	Glucose oligosaccharides§ Maltodextrins Lactose‖ Sucrose‖	Partially hydrolyzed casein, whey, lactalbumin, meat, soy, fish¶	Medium-chain triglycerides: fractionated coconut oil#
Elemental forms**	Glucose	Crystalline amino acids††	Short-chain triglycerides‡‡

* Starch is well tolerated in most disease states.
† Pancreatic enzymes are required for digestion.
‡ Long-chain triglycerides contain essential fatty acids (EFAs). The EFA requirement for infants is 3% of calories. Bile acids and pancreatic lipase are required for digestion and absorption. A trophic effect on bowel mucosa has been observed following intestinal resection. See reference 96.
§ Glucose polymers from 2 to 10 units, which are rapidly hydrolyzed by the brush border enzyme maltase.
‖ Require disaccharidases in the brush border for hydrolysis prior to absorption.
¶ Enzymatically hydrolyzed to oligopeptides, dipeptides, tripeptides, and free amino acids. There is a reduced allergenic response following mucosal injury; see reference 97.
\# Fatty acid chains of 8–12 carbon atoms, which require less bile salts and pancreatic lipase than do long-chain triglycerides for digestion and absorption. They are absorbed directly into the portal vein without micelle or chylomicron formation and do not contain essential fatty acids. See reference 98.
**Contribute significantly to osmolality, due to their small particle size.
††Short peptide chains have a more efficient absorption system than do free amino acids; see reference 99.
‡‡Less practical for use because of chemical instability.

Source: Reprinted from C.D. Lingard, Enteral Nutrition, in *Handbook of Pediatric Nutrition,* P.M. Queen and C.E. Lang, eds., © 1993, Aspen Publishers, Inc.

mula may affect the tolerance. Feeding intolerances associated with delivering a hyperosmolar formula may include delayed gastric emptying, abdominal distention, vomiting, or diarrhea.

Carbohydrates, electrolytes, and amino acids are the major factors that determine the gastrointestinal osmotic load of a formula. Smaller particles, such as glucose and free amino acids, contribute more to a higher osmolality than do larger particles, such as polysaccharides or intact protein molecules. Thus, formulas that contain hydrolyzed protein and monosaccharides will tend to have a higher osmolality than will formulas with intact protein and glucose polymers.

Recommendations for infant formulas are an osmolality less than 460 mOsm/kg.[35] Therefore, the osmolality in formulas given to infants and children younger than 4 years should be < 400 mOsm/kg and for older children < 600 mOsm/kg.[1,35] The osmolality of infant formulas at a caloric density of 20 kcal/oz generally falls below this suggested limit (range of 150–380 mOsm/kg). However, several of the adult enteral products exceed this limit at a caloric density of 30 kcal/oz and may require a dilution to two-thirds strength prior to use in infants. Medications can increase osmolality significantly and should be evaluated.[31] The osmolality of Pregestimil concentrated to 27 kcal/oz is 496 mOsm/kg, where a multivitamin with iron (Poly-vi-sol with Iron) at 10 mg/1mL Fe is 10,683 mOsm/kg.[31]

Nutrient Requirements

The RDAs published by the National Academy of Sciences (Food and Nutrition Board) are the standards most frequently used for the assessment of enteral intakes of children.[32] It should be noted that the RDAs were intended to be recommendations for a healthy population and may not reflect the needs imposed by specific disease states or treatment modalities. In addition, the RDAs (with the exception of energy) include a safety factor that exceeds the requirements of most people to ensure that the specific needs of the majority of the population will be met.

Dietary reference intakes (DRI) have been established to give values to be used as goals for actual consumption.[33] Using RDAs and DRIs with a nonambulatory, ill, or physically delayed child must be done with consideration. Values for specific conditions, such as spina bifida, Down syndrome, and bronchopulmonary dysplasia, have been established.[34–36] Calorie levels are based on cm/height or percentage of RDAs.

The DRI and the RDA may both be lower than potential therapeutic needs dictated by specific disease or deficiency states. In specific circumstances, both infant and adult formulas may require vitamin and/or mineral supplementation. Again, supplements may not be absorbed or utilized in the body as desired and should be evaluated frequently. Infant formulas that contain iron generally provide adequate amounts of vitamins and minerals with a volume of 1 quart. However, infants who have restricted fluid intakes may require vitamin and mineral supplementation (eg, infants with congenital heart disease).

Adult enteral formulas are designed to provide the adult RDAs for vitamins and minerals when a volume of 1,500–2,000 mL/day is administered. However, when these adult enteral products are administered to children at lower volumes, some nutrients may not be adequate. When using adult formulas, the specific supplementation of vitamin D, calcium, phosphorus, iron, and zinc is frequently required.

PRODUCT AVAILABILITY AND COST

The cost of commercial enteral formulas may exceed the financial resources of some families. Therefore, whenever medically possible, the least specialized enteral product should be considered. The more specialized the feedings are (ie, hydrolyzed protein and medium-chain triglyceride oil), the higher will be the cost.

Formula costs do not necessarily constitute a socioeconomic barrier. Infants and children who range in age from birth to 5 years may be enrolled in the Women, Infant, and Children (WIC) nutrition program if their family income falls below a certain level. A variety of infant formulas is available through this program. The Medicaid program and private insurance companies may cover enteral formulas and needed tubes, bags, or pumps. Coverage varies; the health care team should work closely with home care companies and insurers to ensure that the patient obtains the best coverage possible.

Selection of Specific Feeding Routes

Common routes for enteral nutrition in pediatric patients include nasogastric, nasoduodenal, nasojejunal, gastrostomy, and jejunostomy feedings. The risk of aspiration becomes a major consideration when determining whether the tube should be placed in the stomach or small intestine. Evaluation process for gastroesophageal reflux (GER) may include UGI, modified barium swallow, pH probe, and occasional esophageal motility. See Figure 24–1 for a decision tree as to the use of nasogastric or enterostomy feeding routes. If the patient is determined to have a high risk of aspiration due to GER, surgical placement of a gastrostomy is done, along with a fundoplication (surgical repair for GER).

The expected duration of the enteral feeding also is a factor when determining whether a nasoenteral or a surgically placed tube will be used. Figure 24–1 gives criteria for making a decision to use a nasogastric or enterostomy feeding route.[37]

Gastric Feeding

A direct gastric feeding is preferable to an intestinal feeding because it allows for a more normal digestive process. This is generally true because the stomach serves as a reservoir and provides for a gradual release of nutrients into the small bowel. Gastric feedings are associated with a larger osmotic and volume tolerance, a more flexible feeding schedule, easier tube insertions, and a lower frequency of diarrhea and dumping syndrome. In addition, gastric acid has a bactericidal effect that may be an important factor in decreasing the patient's susceptibility to various infections. See Table 24–4 for enteral feeding sites and routes.

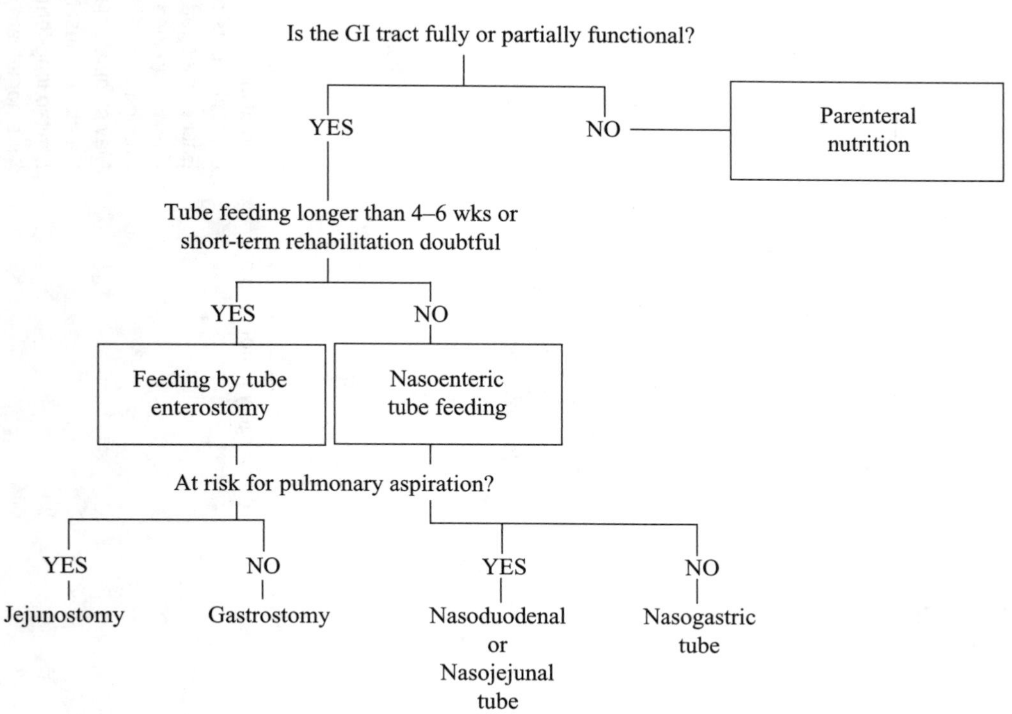

Figure 24–1 Decision-making for selecting feeding site. *Source:* Adapted with permission from J.L. Rombeau and M.D. Caldwell, eds, Enteral and Tube Feeding, in *Clinical Nutrition,* Vol. 1, © 1984, W.B. Saunders Company.

Table 24–4 Enteral Feeding Sites and Routes

Site	*Route*	*Advantage*	*Disadvantages*	*Indications*	*Contraindication*
Stomach		Antiinfective mechanism Allows for normal digestive processes and hormonal responses Tolerances of larger osmotic loads Decreased incidence of dumping syndrome Greater mobility between feedings Greater flexibility in feeding schedule and formula choice		As the first consideration for enteral nutrition	Delayed gastric emptying Pulmonary aspiration GER Intractable vomiting Impaired or absent gag reflex
	Orogatstric	Does not obstruct nasal passage	May increase salivary flow and make clearance more difficult	< 34-wk gestation with gag; doesn't obstruct nasal passage	> 34-wk gestation or when patient acquires a gag
	Nasogastric	Easy intubation Surgery is not required	Nasal esophageal, or tracheal irritation Local skin care required Easily dislodged by a toddler Easily dislodged by a forceful cough May stimulate gag Caretaker must be well trained Limited long-term compliance in the home care setting	For short-term use	Same as for the stomach

Source: Copyright © 1990, K. Hendricks and W. Walker.

	Gastrostomy	Allows patient greater mobility Feedings are generally well tolerated Larger diameter feeding tube lessens changes of obstruction/clogged feeding tube Doesn't obstruct the airway	Requires a surgical procedure for placement May result in increased GER Occasional leakage around the insertion site Skin irritation and infection Difficulty hiding the external portion of the tube under clothing Risk of intra-abdominal leak with peritonitis	Prolonged enteral nutrition support	Same as for the stomach
Small Bowel		Can feed enterally despite poor gastric motility and persistent high gastric residuals Lessens the changes of gastric distention	Less mixing of formula with pancreatic enzymes Tube is easily malpositioned Greater exposure to radiation when checking placement Greater risk of bacterial overgrowth Changes small bowel intestinal flora May limit choices of feeding schedule and formula selection	Congenital upper GI anomalies Inadequate gastric motility Alter upper GI surgery Patients with increased risk of aspiration	Nonfunctioning GI tract
	Nasojejunal		Requires radiographic proof of adequate placement Takes a long time to pass without radiographic placement The tube is easily displaced during peristalsis	For short-term nutrition support	

continues

Table 24–5 continued

Site	*Route*	*Advantage*	*Disadvantages*	*Indications*	*Contraindication*
	Jejunostomy		Technically difficult to place	Jejunal feedings for > 6 mo For postop nutritional management of abdominal surgery while an ileus exists	Patients at operative risk

Nasogastric feeding tubes are used for the short term (6–8 weeks). Patients requiring long-term enteral nutrition are then evaluated to determine the best enteral device to meet their needs. Nasogastric tubes range in length from 22 inches to 43 inches and in French sizes from 5FR–12FR. Some have weighted tips; others have stylets to assist with placement. When choosing the size of the tube, consider the size of the patient, the viscosity of the formula, and the volume of formula to be delivered.

Nasogastric feeding is contraindicated in patients with severe esophagitis or who have an obstruction between the nose and stomach. In addition, nasogastric tubes may not be tolerated in neonates, who are obligate nose breathers. To prevent airway occlusion in this instance, orogastric tubes are often used when tube feeding is indicated.

A variety of small-bore, soft nasogastric tubes are available for use in pediatric patients. Desirable features of pediatric nasogastric tubes are outlined in Exhibit 24–5. When selecting a feeding tube, considerations should be given to the child's age and size, the viscosity of the formula, and whether an infusion device will be used.[38] By selecting the tube with the smallest bore possible, the child's comfort will be increased, and associated trauma will be minimized. Note that longer tubes may be required for nasoduodenal or nasojejunal intubation.

Specific guidelines referring to tube insertion and placement verification have been published.[39,40] Improper tube insertion or placement can lead to a number of potentially serious complications. Any nasally placed tube may be inadvertently inserted into the trachea.[41] Practitioners should verify the correct placement of the nasogastric tube by utilizing auscultation, pH-guided techniques, aspiration techniques, and/or a combination of methods.[40,42–44] If a gastric aspirate is not obtained, tube placement confirmation by radiography is mandatory in many institutions before feedings are initiated. Proper placement is an important aspect for ENS, and many institutions have policies and procedures established for consistency.

Transpyloric Feedings

Nasoduodenal, nasojejunal, or gastrojejunal feeding is desirable for patients who are at risk of aspiration. Typically, this includes patients who have a diminished gag reflex, delayed gastric emptying, frequent vomiting, or severe gastroesophageal reflux.

Exhibit 24–5 Desirable Features of a Pediatric Nasogastric Tube

1. Made of Silastic or polyurethane
2. Available in small diameters (no. 10 French or smaller)
3. Available in variety of lengths with markings to facilitate measuring depth of tube insertion
4. Weighted tip to prevent dislodgement
5. Smooth bolus to facilitate easy insertion and removal
6. Stylet that remains in place during insertion, is prelubricated for easy removal, and is flow-through to determine proper tube placement with stylet still in place
7. Radiopaque for placement verification
8. Compatible with administration sets and with feeding containers in a variety of sizes to accommodate use in neonates and older children

Source: Reprinted from S.W. Cooning, "Unique Aspects in Pediatric Care," in *Nutrition Support in Critical Care*, C.E. Lang, ed., © 1987, Aspen Publishers, Inc.

Nasojejunal feeding may be more efficacious than nasoduodenal feeding in preventing aspiration. Gastric reflux of duodenally administered solutions can be a problem. Additionally, nasoduodenal tubes may fail to enter or stay in the duodenum, resulting in aspiration.[45] Thus, aspiration precautions should be used during nasoduodenal feedings. Nasojejunal tubes may also be less likely than nasoduodenal tubes to become dislodged in children with cystic fibrosis, who may experience severe coughing episodes. This is also true for children with cancer, who may have vomiting associated with chemotherapy. Specific procedures for nasoduodenal or nasojejunal intubation have been outlined by Wesley.[46] The enteric position of the tube requires radiographic verification before feeding is initiated. A potential complication of transpyloric feeding is intestinal perforation with use of stiff, large-bore tubes.[46] Use of small-bore tubes made of polyurethane or silicone might decrease the incidence of this complication; however, there may be an increase in tube clogging.

Jejunostomy Feeding

There are many enteral feeding devices currently available. Endoscopically placed gastrostomies or jejunostomies (PEG/PEJ) are becoming very popular because they are less invasive and require less anesthesia time or even conscious sedation.[40]

Low-profile gastrostomy devices are frequently used as replacement devices after the stoma tract is well healed (usually 6–8 weeks). There are also low-profile devices that can be placed initially as a one-step procedure.[39,40] Enteral feedings, although safer than parenteral nutrition, are not without complications (see Table 24–5).

ADMINISTRATION OF FEEDING

Methods of Delivery

The specific method utilized for feeding delivery is contingent on the clinical condition of the patient and the anatomic location of the tube (gastric or transpyloric). Continuous drip and intermittent bolus administration are the two methods most often used for delivery of enteral feedings to infants and children. Intermittent bolus feedings are generally delivered to the stomach by gravity over 15–30 minutes on a schedule of every 2–4 hours. In contrast, the continuous drip method provides an infusion of nutrients at a constant rate over several hours. Continuous drip feedings are beneficial for patients with altered gastrointestinal function and essential for those receiving enteral transpyloric or nocturnal feedings. Each method of delivery provides a number of specific advantages and disadvantages (see Exhibit 24–6). In practice, the individual patient's tolerance ultimately dictates the method of delivery. Exhibit 24–7 lists considerations in selecting enteral feeding delivery systems.

Pumps

Enteral feeding pumps are typically utilized to control the rate of delivery of continuous drip feedings. A number of enteral feeding pumps is available for use in pediatric patients.[48] Portable enteral pumps allow for greater patient mobility.

Important features of enteral pumps for use in the pediatric population include the ability to provide low delivery rates (< 5 mL/hour) and to advance in small increments (1–5 mL/hour). Other desirable features of pediatric pumps include tamper-proof controls, an occlusion alarm, and a low-battery indicator.[49] These features all contribute to the safe and efficient delivery of continuous tube feedings for the pediatric population. Exhibit 24–8 gives considerations for pump selection in the pediatric population, and Exhibit 24–9 indicates desirable characteristics in the feeding containers used for enteral feedings.

Initiation and Advancement of Feedings

Many clinicians have published recommendations for advancing enteral nutrition in pediatric patients.[50–52] These recommendations are based on institutional practices and modification of adult regimens. Generally, the rate

Table 24–5 Complications of Enteral Feeding

Complication	*Possible Cause*	*Management/Prevention*
	Gastrointestinal	
Aspiration Pneumonia	Aspiration of feedings Emesis Displacement or migration Supine position during feeds Gastroesophageal reflux	Confirm tube placement prior to administration of feedings Elevate head 30 to 45 degrees
	Presence of nasogastric tube preventing complete closure of esophagus	Tube placement into the duodenum
	Delayed gastric emptying	Use of prokinetics
Bloating/Cramps/Gas	Air in tubing	Remove as much air as possible when setting up feeding
Diarrhea	Bacterial contamination of formula	Proper storage, preparation and administration of feedings
	Food allergies	Consider changing to formula that is lactose free
	Hyperosmolar formulas	Consider changing formula to an isotonic product
	Too rapid infusion	Slow down rate of infusion to previously tolerated rate
	Low fiber intake	Consider using a fiber-containing product
	Fat malabsorption	Consider changing formula to a product with partial medium-chain triglyceride content
	Medications (antibiotics), antacids, sorbitol, magnesium, antineoplatic agents	
Dumping Syndrome	Cold formula	Administer formula at room temperature
	Rapid feeding	Slow down rate of feeding
Vomiting	Hyperosmolar formulas	Consider changing formula to an isotonic product
	Delayed gastric emptying	Consider transpyloric route for feeding Consider continuous infusion Elevate head of bed 45 degrees during feeding administration Check residuals prior to feedings Consider utilizing prokinetics

continues

Source: Data from references 93–95.

Table 24–5 continued

Complication	*Possible Cause*	*Management/Prevention*
	Obstruction	Discontinue feedings
	Too rapid advancement of volume and/or concentration	Return to previously tolerated strength and volume, and advance more slowly
	Mechanical	
Clogged Tube	Inadequate flushing	Flush tube before and after aspirating residuals, after bolus feedings, and every 4–8 hours during continuous feedings
	Inadequate crushing of medications	Dissolve crushed tablets in warm water
		Use liquid form of medication instead of crushed tablet whenever possible
	Formula and medication residue	Flush tube before and after medication administration
		Avoid mixing formula with medication
	Kinking of the feeding tube	Replace feeding tube
	Highly viscous fiber-rich formulas	
Tube Displacement	Coughing	Replace the tube
	Vomiting	
	Inadvertent dislodgment	
	Removal of tube by patient	
	Metabolic	
Dehydration	Inadequate free water	Monitor intake and output
		Monitor hydration status of patient routinely
	Hyperosmolar formulas	Assess renal solute load of formula
Overhydration	Excessive fluid administration	Advance feedings slowly
	Too rapid refeeding or patients with moderate to severe PEM	Allow a 5- to 7-day period to meet nutritional goals
Electrolyte imbalance	Formula components	Evaluate electrolyte adequacy of specific formula and appropriateness of formula dilution
	Medical condition/diagnosis	Monitor electrolytes, phosphorus, BUN, creatinine, glucose

Table 24–5 continued

Complication	*Possible Cause*	*Management/Prevention*
Failure to achieve appropriate weight gain	Inadequate nutrient intake	Evaluate adequacy of nutrient intake Perform routine nutritional assessments
	Psychologic	
Fear of tube insertion	Psychologic trauma associated with insertion of nasogastric tube/gastrostomy tube	Utilize relaxation techniques Medical play—child to handle tube and insert tube in doll Comfort child after tube insertion Consider sedation prior to replacement of gastrostomy tube
Altered body image	Visible presence of nasogastric tube or gastrostomy tube	Consider nocturnal feedings and removal of tube during the day Consider use of low-profile gastrostomy device
Food refusal	Deprivation of normal oral feeding experiences	Initiate oral feedings when medically possible Provide positive oral experiences during tube feedings Referral to speech therapist

of advancement of a feeding regimen (Exhibit 24–10) is contingent on the structure and function of the patient's gastrointestinal tract. Long-term parenteral nutrition support or malnutrition can cause a number of physiologic alterations of the gastrointestinal tract that may affect a child's ability to digest and absorb nutrients. The various functional and histologic changes generally associated with malnutrition include:

1. shortened microvilli
2. decreased production of a number of pancreatic enzymes, including lipase, trypsin, and amylase
3. decreased brush border enzyme activities of maltase, sucrase, and lactase[49,50]

Parenteral nutrition support without concomitant enteral feeding also has been shown to lead to a decrease in enteric mucosal mass and associated brush border enzymes.[2] Therefore, children who are being weaned from parenteral nutrition and/or who are malnourished generally require a more conservative feeding progression than what is typically administered to children who have normal gastrointestinal function.

Breast Milk Tube Feedings

Human milk provides the optimal feeding for infants and offers many immunologic and nutritional benefits. Infants who are unable to nurse at the breast can receive pumped breast milk through a feeding tube. However, the delivery of breast milk by tube requires some unique considerations. First of all, the mother must be taught safe methods for the collection and storage of her milk.[53] Breast milk adminis-

Exhibit 24–6 Methods of Delivering Enteral Feedings

Continuous Drip Feedings

Advantages	*Disadvantages*
1. Ability to increase volume of formula more rapidly 2. Improved absorption of major nutrients in infants with intestinal diseases 3. Reduced stool output in hypermetabolic patients 4. Associated with a reduced incidence of vomiting in infants with gastroesophageal reflux 5. Greater caloric intake when volume tolerance may be a problem	1. More expensive feeding method because a pump is required for delivery 2. Restricts patient ambulation 3. Less physiologic

Intermittent Feedings

Advantages	*Disadvantages*
1. More physiologic because a normal feeding schedule is mimicked 2. Less expensive because an enteral pump is not required 3. Greater flexibility in feeding schedule 4. Freedom from infusion equipment 5. Improved nitrogen retention with less fat and fluid accumulation 6. Allows the gastric acidity to increase	1. Associated with a longer time to reach nutritional goals 2. Reduced weight gain and nutrient absorption in infants with malabsorption 3. Larger-bore tube may be required for gravity administration 4. More time required for administration than for pump-delivered feedings

Exhibit 24–7 Factors in Selection of an Enteral Feeding Delivery System

Enteral access route
Rate of feeding
Volume of feeding
Stability of patient (critical or noncritical illness)
Gastric emptying rate
GI tolerance of tube feeding
Age of patient
Type of formula
Calorie and protein needs
Ease of administration
Patient cooperation and mobility

Source: Reprinted with permission from L.K. Lysen and P.Q. Samour, Enteral Equipment, *Principles of Nutrition Support*, p. 202, © 1998, W.B. Saunders Company.

tration techniques also should be devised and implemented.

Continuous drip feedings of human milk have been associated with appreciable fat losses, which result in a significant reduction of energy delivered to the infant.[54,55] These losses occur because the fat in human milk separates and collects in the infusion system. A caloric loss of approximately 20% is typical. The delivery of essential fatty acids, phospholipids, cholesterol, and associated fat-soluble vitamins may also be diminished.[51]

It should be noted that when residual milk is flushed from the tubing, a large fat bolus may be delivered to the patient. Patients with impaired gastrointestinal function may not tolerate a fat bolus.

Short-term refrigeration of human milk has been shown to increase the delivery of fat during continuous feedings.[56] Unfortunately, signifi-

Exhibit 24–8 Considerations for Pump Selection

Simple to use
Alarm system
Lightweight
Long battery life
Portable
Quiet
Intravenous pole attachment
Clear instructions on pump use
Easy to read
Volume-infused indicator
Inexpensive
Compact
Easy to clean
Flow rate accurate to within ± 10%
Ability to advance in small increments

Source: Reprinted with permission from L.K. Lysen and P.Q. Samour, Enteral Equipment, *Principles of Nutrition Support,* p. 211, © 1998, W.B. Saunders Company.

Exhibit 24–9 Important Characterists of Enteral Feeding Containers

Easy to fill, close and handle
Easy-to-read calibrations and directions
Appropriate size
Adaptable tubing port
Compatible with pump
Easy to clean
Leakproof
Requires minimal storage space
Recyclable

Source: Reprinted with permission from L.K. Lysen and P.Q. Samour, Enteral Equipment, *Principles of Nutrition Support,* p. 211, © 1998, W.B. Saunders Company.

cant fat losses still occur. Therefore, when delivering a continuous feeding of breast milk, the use of refrigerated milk may be advantageous. If continuous feedings of expressed breast milk are required, blending the expressed breast milk with a liquid fortifier or other liquid formulas can promote more efficient delivery of breast milk nutrients via tube.[57]

Intermittent bolus feeding of human milk, in contrast, does not result in a significant loss of fat in the tubing or the terminal delivery of a large fat bolus.[54,55] Therefore, intermittent bolus feeding is the preferred method of delivery for the tube feeding of human milk, whenever possible.

PREVENTION AND TREATMENT OF COMPLICATIONS

Complications associated with enteral nutritional support can be minimized by properly monitoring the patient.[41,58] Potential complications are generally classified into gastrointestinal, mechanical (tube-related), metabolic, and psychologic categories. Some pediatric studies have reported complications that include various mechanical problems related to gastrostomy[59,60] and to nasogastric tubes,[61,62] metabolic disturbances,[27] and feeding disorders that are related to the delayed introduction of oral feedings.[63] Additionally, gastrointestinal complications have been associated with low serum albumin levels in pediatric surgical patients,[64] delayed enteral support in pediatric burn patients,[65] and with contaminated feedings.[66] A summary of the most common complications and associated management suggestions is presented in Table 24–5.

Enteral Feeding Contamination

Gastrointestinal complications can potentially result from the bacterial contamination of continuous drip enteral feedings. Contamination from gram-negative bacilli has been found to cause abdominal distention in both pediatric and adult patients who were receiving continuous drip feedings.[66]

Various practitioners have reported an incidence of feeding contamination ranging from 5%[63] to 90%.[66] Feeding contamination generally occurs during the preparation, delivery, handling, or storage of the product.[67,68]

Exhibit 24–10 Initiation and Advancement of Feedings

General Considerations

1. Plan for a 2- to 5-day period to meet nutritional goals.
2. Use isotonic feedings initially.
3. Avoid making a simultaneous change in volume and concentration.
4. Consider initial use of dilute feedings in patients with altered gastrointestinal function or when beginning transitional feeding following parenteral nutrition.
5. Advance more cautiously in patients who are critically ill and malnourished, and those with histories of feeding intolerances.
6. Increase volume before concentration when administering transpyloric feedings.
7. Advance concentration before volume when administering gastric feedings.
8. If a feeding intolerance develops, return to the previously tolerated concentration and volume, and progress more slowly.

Continuous Drip Feeding

1. Begin at a rate of 1–2 mL/kg/h.
2. Advance in increments of 0.5–1.0 mL/kg/h every 8–24 hours, as tolerated, until nutritional goal is achieved.
3. Typical feeding rates for various age groups:

Age	*Weight (kg)*	*Initial Rate (mL/h)*	*Maximum Rate (mL/h)*
Infant	3–10	3–10	25–50
Toddler/preschool	10–20	10–20	60–70
School age	20–40	20–40	80–100
Teenage	>40	40–50	100–150

Intermittent Feeding

1. Determine the total volume of formula needed to provide nutritional goal.
2. Begin delivery at 25% of the volume goal on the first day.
3. Divide the formula volume equally between 5 and 8 feedings.
4. Increase formula volume by 25% per day as tolerated, with total volume equally divided between number of feedings.
5. Administer by gravity over 15–30 minutes.

Source: Reprinted from C.D. Lingard, Enteral Nutrition, in *Handbook of Pediatric Nutrition,* P.M. Queen and C.E. Lang, eds., © 1993, Aspen Publishers, Inc.

Formulas that require reconstitution or manipulation (dilution or additives) are at the greatest risk for bacterial contamination.[66,68] In contrast, the use of sterile, undiluted "ready-to-feed" products minimizes the risk of contamination.

Precautions that should be taken to guard against the contamination of enteral feedings include the daily changing of the feeding bag and tubing, careful attention to clean technique during handling of the feedings, and limiting of the hang time of the formulas. Specific recommendations for preparation, administration, and monitoring of enteral feedings to maximize bacteriologic safety have been published.[69]

A hang time of 8–12 hours should be safe for commercially manufactured products, provided that both a closed delivery system and clean technique are used in the transfer process.[70] In contrast, blenderized feedings[63] and breast milk should not remain in the feeding container for more than 4 hours. Guidelines for storage and administration of feedings are outlined in Exhibit 24–11.

It is important to note that disposable enteral feeding bags should not be reused in the hospital setting.[69,71] However, for stable patients in the home setting, where nosocomial pathogens are less common, it may be safe to wash feeding containers and reuse them.[69] In this instance, containers intended for reuse at home should be carefully washed with warm water and soap, thoroughly rinsed, and hung to dry.[71]

Exhibit 24–11 Guidelines for Storage and Administration of Feedings

Storage	*Recommendation*
Sterile* canned/bottled liquid products	Store at temperatures <30.5°C (85°F). Cover and refrigerate opened, unused product, labeled with date and time opened. Use/discard within 24 to 48 hours or in accordance with manufacturer's recommendation, and/or hospital policy.
Powdered products†	Store in cool, dry area. Cover opened, unused product labeled with date, time, and nature of preparation. Use/discard according to hospital policy.

Administration	*Recommendation*
Container and pump set	Change every 24 hr or in accordance with gavage or pump-set manufacturer's recommendations, and/or hospital policy. Consider more frequent changes when nonsterile feedings are given. Rinse with water between feedings. Do not add new formula to that already in container.
Hang time	Sterile feedings* may be hung for 8–12 hours or in accordance with manufacturer's recommendations and/or hospital policy. Nonsterile feedings† should not remain in feeding container for >6–8 hours (or for >2–4 hours, if blenderized).
Feeding-tube irrigation	Rinse with water (eg, 20–30 mL) before and after each intermittent feeding or every 3–4 hours during continuous feeding.

* Sterile feedings include industrially produced prepacked liquid formulas that are "commercially sterile."

† Nonsterile feedings are those that may contain live bacteria and include hospital- or home-prepared (blenderized) formulas, reconstituted powdered feedings, and commercial liquid formulas to which nutrients and/or other supplements have been added in the kitchen, pharmacy, home, or ward.

Source: Used with permission of Ross Products Division, Abbott Laboratories, Columbus, OH 43216 from *Enteral Nutrition Support of Children,* © 1988 Ross Products Division, Abbott Laboratories.

WEANING

When the patient's medical condition allows for normal oral feedings, weaning from tube feedings can be initiated. The management of the transition back to oral feedings is multifaceted and involves the medical team, the patient, and the caregivers.[72] A complete weaning from ENS should not be considered until the patient has achieved a satisfactory nutritional status, because the patient may stop gaining weight for a time during the transition.

The weaning time may vary from a few days to several months. Records of the patient's oral intake should be kept during this time because it is important to maintain an adequate intake. Tube feedings should be continued until the patient can demonstrate that nutrient requirements can be met consistently by the oral intake. There is a certain amount of patients who use enteral nutrition with a combination of parenteral nutrition and/or oral intake.[73] A combination of enteral and cycled parenteral nutrition is controlled on the basis of patient tolerance. Monitoring for intolerance or complications would be completed similarly to any nutrition delivery that is provided and not patient-initiated. A combination of enteral and oral feedings is more difficult to project. Total daily requirements in fluid and calories are calculated, then enteral feedings complete what the oral feedings lack. To stimulate hunger, the enteral feeds will need to be decreased. A guideline is to begin with a 25% decrease in the caloric intake by tube, then start to offer oral feeds. This transition will require evaluation frequently because of the risk of decrease in growth with a lower caloric intake or if the child has trouble or delay in progressing. If the oral intake varies from day to day, a sliding scale for supplemental enteral feeds should be created. To summarize the recommendations at the time of transition, Glass and Lucas[74] suggest normalizing tube feeding schedules to approximate meals/snacks timing, altering feeding schedule to promote hunger, reducing the calories from tube feedings, providing adequate fluids, and, as oral intake increases, adjusting the tube feedings accordingly.

Feeding Disorders

Infant and toddler feeding disorders constitute a tube-feeding complication that is unique to the pediatric population. Many times, when a chronically ill infant is medically ready to begin oral feedings, the infant or toddler may display no interest in eating or actual hysteria when food, liquid, or utensils are near the face. When offered feedings, the child typically refuses, cries, gags, or vomits. This oral aversion can occur in children with or without mechanical eating problems.

Due to the emotional component of eating/feeding, a dysfunctional or uninformed family may further the trauma of eating by force-feeding. Children who have been given ENS often do not have normal hunger cycles, normal eating experiences at a table, or a mealtime routine. All of these points should be addressed when the transition to oral feeding occurs. Severe cases of oral aversion require intervention and behavior modification from pediatric psychologic professionals, as well as other health professionals, such as speech pathologists, dietitians, and occupational therapists.[75]

Illingsworth[76] suggests that resistant feeding behavior may be due to missing a "critical period" in the development of the child's feeding skills. He indicates that the critical period for the development of chewing skills is 6–7 months of age; if solids are not introduced during this time, the child typically will have difficulty accepting them later.

Other important oral experiences during the first year of life include the development of the rooting and sucking reflexes, the oral exploration of objects, and the association of hunger with feeding.[76] When a child is deprived of these normal oral feeding experiences during the first year of life, he or she may subsequently experience feeding difficulties that last throughout the toddler and preschool years. These children may also demonstrate significant delays in gross motor and personality development.[63] Daily oral therapy or "mouth play" can help to eliminate or reduce the problems that typically occur in the patient with nonoral nutrition support.[77]

Initiating oral feedings as soon as medically possible can minimize feeding disorders. Concomitant speech or feeding therapy with ENS can help to alleviate oral aversion.[78] Nonnutritive sucking during tube feedings in infancy can help to stimulate oral sucking and swallowing behavior. Pediatric occupational therapists or speech pathologists are the health professionals most qualified to assess an infant's feeding potential and to design an appropriate, ongoing oral motor stimulation program. Intervention should be considered during enteral feeding, versus at the termination of enteral feeding. Lastly, textured foods ideally should be offered, if medically feasible, when the infant is at a developmental age of 6–7 months.

Swallowing Disorders

Recently, there has been an increase in recommendations to thicken liquids for therapy in the management of an infant or child who has been diagnosed with misswallowing by modified barium swallow studies using videofluoroscopy. This diagnosis means that, on regular fluid consistency, the patient is at risk for aspiration or actually aspirates. Several disease states or conditions contribute to misswallowing.[79]

Swallowing dysfunction is compounded in infants or young children who have not learned the act of swallowing. A behavioral eating plan is a complicated process because the family and/or medical team are often trying to avoid an alternative feeding delivery. Developmental progress, therapy, and nutrition all must be considered as the patient's plan is developed.[80]

Adding a thickening agent or food to the formula or liquid changes the fluid so that the patient can swallow liquid with decreased risk of aspiration. However, thickening has nutritional consequences. The more thickener that is required, the more effect this will have on nutrition content of the intake. Most clinical commercial products available for thickening agents are carbohydrate-based, with little to no other nutrients. Adding a carbohydrate product will skew the nutrients, add calories, and increase free water needs in a medically unstable patient or one who is at risk for dehydration. The recipe for thickened consistency is included with the package label, and the categories for thickening generally are nectar, honey, and pudding consistencies. An example of the nutrition effect is a baby who is 3 months old, taking 22 oz of 20 kcal/oz formula, growing well, and is diagnosed with misswallowing. The recommended therapy is liquid thickened to honey consistency. The thickener is 15 calories per tablespoon. The recipe for this consistency is one tablespoon + one teaspoon (4 teaspoons or 1 teaspoon/oz) of thickener per 4 oz of fluid. The baby previously was receiving 440 calories and 660 mL of fluid. Now, with the thickener (7 tablespoons + 1 teaspoon), the calories are 553 (126% of the original) and 660 mL of fluid, with the free water needs varying by status of patient, in addition. For patients who are at fluid risk, it has been suggested to use 1 mL of water for every kilocalorie consumed.[81] Added calories will increase the gain per day for this infant if the formula amount continues at 22 oz per day. It is a paradox as to whether to add calories and risk rapid weight gain or to decrease the formula intake to match the previous caloric intake.[82] There is an option of using baby rice cereal as a thickener, which will provide some nutrients other than carbohydrate. However, the product is difficult to blend with the formula in a liquid form, does not thicken evenly, is not an exact measured substitute for thickener, and varies in the amount of time that it takes to thicken. In older children, a variety of other food products may be used as a thickening agent.[81] In all situations, there may be an increased need for fluid/free water with no method of delivery unless ENS is considered as a means of alternative delivery. Because of these factors, judicious prescription and follow-up must be made. Time frames for trial therapy should be established. A well-developed behavioral and skill progression feeding plan is helpful and should include a multidisciplinary team familiar with pediatric dysphagia. Oral intake is important to encourage—as much as is medically safe. At the conclusion of the trial therapy, the patient should be evaluated for progress and/or level of rehabilitation. If there has been no change in ability, a different modality for fluid delivery should be established, with swallowing therapy to work with oral skills. Lefton-Greif has published a detailed skill list matched with nutrition modality recommendations that is helpful to use as an evaluation tool.[80]

For a growing infant, 3–4 weeks on an altered regime would be the maximum for a trial period, as would 2–3 months for a toddler or older child.

In summary, the management plan for dysphagia should focus on reduction or elimination of factors that potentially contribute to airway compromise, provide adequate nutrition and hydration, and facilitate a workable interaction between the caregiver and the child.[80]

PLANNING FOR HOME ENTERAL SUPPORT

Whenever possible, ENS should be provided in the home, rather than in the hospital. Advantages of home enteral support include a number of psychosocial benefits for the child and the family, and an economic benefit is also provided because the costly hospital stay is minimized. Often, third-party payers are making the decision of home enteral support because of the much-reduced cost of home management. A patient who is a candidate for home enteral feedings should be evaluated on the following criteria:[83,84]

1. The patient must be medically stable and have demonstrated a tolerance to the feeding regimen in the hospital.
2. A safe home environment is required, with available running water, electricity, refrigeration, and adequate storage space.
3. The family (or patient) must be willing and capable of administering the feedings at home.
4. A payment source is needed for the formula and associated tube-feeding equipment.
5. A home care agency should be available to service the patient in his/her home locale. If an agency is not available, a hospital team that takes responsibility for home monitoring must be identified (pediatric nurse, dietitian, and pharmacist).
6. A physician must be willing to assume responsibility for following the patient after discharge from the hospital.

Once the above criteria are met, discharge planning must be coordinated and thorough. Availability of supplies and equipment, discharge communication with medical monitoring, and patient/caregiver education must be arranged. The patient's discharge should be accompanied by information from a medical/nursing prospective, as well as a nutrition plan.[85] For an example of communication from the inpatient setting to community care, see Exhibit 24–12 for a nutrition discharge summary.

Discharge teaching for the family/caregivers is also required. The instructional plan should focus on the preparation, administration, and monitoring of the feeding. The family will need a social support system to deal successfully with problems associated with ENS in the home environment.[86] Feeding tube care and problem-solving techniques should also be addressed. See Table 24–6 for a detailed education checklist. Monitoring forms should be used for these patients to document data collected between medical evaluations (see Exhibit 24–13). Any forms used or developed should allow for quality improvement monitoring or the collection of data to measure outcomes.[87] Lastly, arrangements should be made for outpatient follow-up. Initially, the hospital team following the patient (not the team guiding the primary caregiver)

Exhibit 24–12 Nutrition Discharge Summary

the children's medical center

INFANT NUTRITION SCREEN TO IDENTIFY NUTRITION RISK

PATIENT NAME	CAREGIVER'S NAME	PHONE	D.O.B.
DIAGNOSIS		BIRTH WEIGHT	GESTATIONAL AGE

DISCHARGE INFORMATION ☐ Growth Chart Attached

CORRECTED AGE AT DISCHARGE	DISCHARGE WEIGHT	LENGTH	OFC
	kg	cm	cm

NICU Nutrition History / Course: ____________________

NUTRITION CONCERNS / GOALS

FORMULA CONCERNS

☐ Tolerance
☐ Adequacy / rate advancement
Formula Goals: ☐ ______ Kcal / kg / day
Comments:

☐ Special Formula need for medical problem
☐ Short-term need of special formula
Recommenation: ____________________

INTAKE ABILITY CONCERNS

☐ Volume ☐ Skill ☐ Tube Fed
☐ Calories ☐ High Needs ☐ Combination PO / Tube Fed
Intake Goals: ☐ ______ cc / kg / day
Comments:

GROWTH CONCERNS

☐ Slow weight gain
☐ Just established weight gain goal
Growth Goals: ☐ gain 15-20gms / day ☐ gain 20-30 gms / day
Comments:

☐ Different growth expectation than growth chart curve
Comments: ____________________

NUTRITION INSTRUCTION AT DISCHARGE

☐ Regular formula ____________________ Volume / FDG Schedule ____________________
☐ High calorie formula ☐ Infant Nutrition Clinic Appointment Scheduled
Recipe: ____________________ Date ____________
☐ WIC referral made to ____________________ County ____________
Comments:

FOLLOW-UP RECOMMENDATIONS

☐ Weight Check
☐ Q 2 weeks ☐ Q month
☐ Check-up 2 to 3 days after discharge to assure adequate breastfeeding
Other: ____________________

If this patient fails to meet the nutrition goals, a referral for indepth nutrition assessment and therapy can be made to Infant Nutrition Clinic at The Children's Medical Center, Dayton, OH by calling 1-937-226-8383.

Screen completed by: ____________________
From: ____________________
For nutrition questions or concerns, contact:
Name: ____________________
Phone: ____________________

NIC0071M (8/97)

Source: Courtesy of The Children's Medical Center, Dayton, Ohio.

Table 24–6 Home Enteral Education Checklist

Patient Outcome	*Invervention*
A. Patient will state understanding of feeding therapy and equipment	1. Provide education materials 2. Discuss reason for enteral nutrition 3. Show and discuss function of equipment 4. Identify brand and size of patient's feeding tube and record 5. Record and explain feeding schedule, rate of delivery, and total volume required 6. Have patient state reason for therapy and function of equipment
B. Patient will demonstrate checking of tube placement	Instruct and observe in: 1. Demonstration of tube placement check (residual check or tube marking)
C. Patient will demonstrate correct procedure for feeding administration	Instruct and observe in: 1. Hand washing 2. Formula preparation 3. Equipment setup 4. Patient position for feeding 5. Priming of tubing 6. Connection to feeding tube 7. Rate control with flow regulator or pump
D. Patient will demonstrate correct procedure for discontinuation of administration	Instruct and observe in: 1. Stopping pump or clamping set 2. Disconnecting tubing from feeding tube 3. Flushing tube 4. Clamping of feeding tube 5. Positioning of tube when off feedings 6. Care and storage of feeding equipment
E. Patient will demonstrate medication administration through feeding tube	Instruct and observe in: 1. Crushing of medications or liquid preparations 2. Medications to not use in feeding tube 3. Dosage and time of medications 4. Tube flushing before and after each medication 5. Potential side effects and/or drug–nutrient interactions
F. Patient will demonstrate correct tube site care	Instruct and observe in: 1. Dressing removal 2. Cleansing of skin 3. Removal of crusts with dilute hydrogen peroxide 4. Observing of signs of irritation or infection 5. Applying clean dressing 6. Retaping procedure

Source: Weckwerth and Ireton-Jones, Nutrition Support in Home Care, in *Contemporary Nutrition Support Practice: A Clinical Guide,* Matarese and Gottschlich, eds., p. 614, © 1998, W.B. Saunders Company.

Table 24–6 continued

Patient Outcome	*Invervention*
G. Patient will state potential complications and interventions	Explain procedure and actions to take for: 1. Tube dislodgment 2. Tube clogging 3. Intolerance to enteral feedings: diarrhea, nausea, vomiting, constipation, bloating 4. Weight changes 5. Method for recording oral and tube intake 6. Procedure for contacting home health nurse, dietitian, or physician

should assign follow-up for nutrition[88] and medical assessment. Babies should be nutritionally assessed every month at the minimum; children younger than 5 years should be seen every 6 months, minimally, for a medical nutrition assessment and prescription. Children older than 5 years should be assessed every year, as a minimum. Teens should be assessed and assigned follow-up individually, due to the variance in the age of maturation.

Successful ENS can be delivered in the medical or home environment to provide for a patient's nutritional needs. The improvement in products, supplies, and complications of ENS has enabled many ill children improved nutrition and health outcomes.

Exhibit 24–13 An Example of a Pediatric Home Care Monitoring Form

Date ________

Patient DOB
Caregiver
Address

Phone #

Primary Care Physician
Hospital RD
Monitoring Comments ______________________
____
Nutrition Support Contact Person ______________

Age: Last measurements, date: ________ Last nutrition Rx: Date ________
Wt: Wt: Formula:
Ht: Ht: Total Volume
OFC OFC Delivery Schedule

Procurement Enteral ☐ Parenteral ☐ **Supporting Medical Equipment**

Formula ________________ Provider __________ Monitor ☐ provider ______________
Equipment ________________ Provider __________ Oxygen ☐ provider ______________
Supplies ________________ Provider __________ Other ☐ provider ______________
Problems __________________________ Problems __________________________
__________________________ __________________________

Formula and Delivery ☐ Same ☐ Change to ______________________

Formula Concentration
Vol/day Substitute Formula

Infusion and Schedule

☐ By mouth (po) - attach diet history
☐ PO in combination with - attach diet history
☐ Intermittent Infuse _______ ml over _____ minutes _______ times per day
☐ Continuous Infuse _______ ml/hr for _____ hours from _______ to ________
☐ Parenteral Infuse _______ ml/hr for _____ hours from _______ to ________
(See formula next page)

Feeding Tube Type: ________________________ Size: ___________
☐ Nasogastric ☐ PEG ☐ Gastrostomy ☐ Jejunostomy ☐ Other ______________

Water Flushes: Vol/day ___________ ml _________ ml water per flush ________ flushes/day

Medications and methods of delivery: ______________________________________
____
____

Exhibit 24–13 continued

Monitoring Instructions (labs, anthropometrics, nutrition, specialists, etc)

Referral Recommendations:

Care Giver Issues:

Home Nutrition`Support Information given to

Signature

Home Care Staff
Telephone:

Comments:

Problems: ☐ Vomiting ☐ Reflux ☐ Aspiration ☐ Gagging ☐ Diarrhea ☐ Illness ☐ Constipation ☐ Weight loss ☐ Behavioral ☐ Sepsis ☐ Equip. Malfunction ☐ Other

Parenteral Rx Date

Dextrose
Amino Acid
NaCl
KCl
Kphos
CaClu
Mg
Na Acetate
Other

Calories provided
Amt. Protein

PLAN OF CARE

signature

REFERENCES

1. Klawitter BM. Pediatric Nutrition Support. In: Williams CP, ed. *Pediatric Manual of Clinical Dietetics*. Chicago, IL: The American Dietetic Association; 1998.
2. ASPEN Board of Directors: Guidelines of the use of parenteral and enteral nutrition in adult and pediatric patients. *J Parenter Enter Nutr.* 1993;17(supp):1SA–11SA.
3. Minard GM, Kudsk KA. Is early feeding beneficial? How early is early? *New Horizons.* 1994;2(2):156–163.
4. Trijillo EB. Enteral Nutrition: A comprehensive overview. In: Matarese LE, Gottschlich MM, eds. *Contemporary Nutrition Support Practice A Clinical Guide.* Philadelphia, PA: WB Saunders Co; 1998.
5. Joint Commission on Accreditation of Healthcare Organizations. *Assessment of Patients, Comprehensive Accreditation Manual for Hospitals; 1998.* Oakbrook Terrace, IL: JCAHO; 1998.
6. Mezoff A, Gamm L, Konek S, Beal KG, Hitch D. Validation of a nutritional screen in children with respiratory syncytial virus admitted to an intensive care complex. *Pediatrics.* 1996;97:543–546.
7. Nevin-Folino NL. Nutrition assessment of premature infants. In: Williams CP, ed. *Pediatric Manual of Clinical Dietetics.* Chicago, IL: The American Dietetic Association; 1998:13–15.
8. Bloch AS, Cancer. In: Materese LE, Gottschlich MM, ed. *Contemporary Nutrition Support Practice: A Clinical Guide.* Philadelphia, PA: WB Saunders Co; 1998: 476.
9. Klawitter BM. Pediatric nutrition support. In: Williams CP, ed. *Pediatric Manual of Clinical Dietetics.* Chicago, IL: The American Dietetic Association; 1998:480.
10. Issacs JS, Cialone J, Horsley JW, et al. *Children With Special Health Care Needs: A Community Nutrition Pocket Guide.* Columbus, OH: Ross Products, a division of Abbott Laboratories; 1997:50.
11. Cox JH, ed. *Nutrition Manual for At-Risk Infants and Toddlers.* Appendix B. 1997:183–186.
12. Stice J. Routine nutrition care during follow-up. In: Groh-Wargo S, Thompson M, Cox JH, eds. *Nutritional Care for High-Risk Newborns.* Chicago, IL: Precept Press; 1994:385.
13. Campbell MK, Kelsey KS. The PEACH survey: A nutrition screening tool for use in early intervention programs. *J Am Diet Assoc.* 1994;94(10):1156–1158.
14. Feldhausen J, Thomson C, Duncan B, Taren D. *Referral Criteria in Pediatric Nutrition Handbook.* New York: Chapman & Hall; 1996:65.
15. Pennington CR, Powell-Tuck J, Shaffer J. Review article: Artificial nutritional support of improved patient care. *Aliment Pharmacol Ther.* 1995;9:471–481.
16. Committee on Nutrition, American Academy of Pediatrics. Commentary on breast-feeding and infant formulas, including proposed standards for formulas. *Pediatrics.* 1979;63:52.
17. United States Congress. *Infant Formula Act of 1980.* Public Law 96–359. Sept. 26, 1980. Revision 1986.
18. The American Acadamy of Pediatrics. *Pediatric Nutrition Handbook.* Appendix D. Elk Grove Village, IL: The American Academy of Pediatrics; 1998:653.
19. *Composition of Feedings for Infants and Young Children: Ross Ready Reference.* Columbus, OH: Ross Products, a division of Abbott Laboratories; 1996.
20. Mead Johnson Nutritionals. *Pediatric Products Handbook.* Evansville, IN: Mead Johnson Company; 1996.
21. Bergmann KE, Ziegler EE, Fomon SJ. Water and renal solute load. In: Fomon SJ, ed. *Infant Nutrition.* 2nd ed. Philadelphia, PA: WB Saunders Co; 1974:245–266.
22. Fomon SJ. *Nutrition of Normal Infants.* St. Louis, MO: Mosby-Year Book; 1993:100.
23. Kerner JA Jr, ed. Manual of Pediatric Parenteral Nutrition. New York: John Wiley & Sons; 1983:71.
24. Behrman RE, et al. eds. *Nelson Textbook of Pediatrics.* 15th ed. Philadelphia, PA: WB Saunders Co; 1995:143.
25. Fomon SJ, Ziegler EE, O'Donnell AM. Infant feeding in health and disease. In: Fomon SJ, ed. *Infant Nutrition.* 2nd ed. Philadelphia, PA: WB Saunders Co; 1974;472–519.
26. Foman SJ. *Nutrition of Normal Infants.* St. Louis, MO: Mosby-Year Book; 1993:138.
27. Gallagher-Allred CR. Comparison of institutionally and commercially prepared formulas. *Nutr Supp Serv.* 1983; 3:32.
28. Listernick R, Sidransky E. Hypernatremic dehydration in children with severe psychomotor retardation. *Clin Pediatr.* 1985;24:440.
29. Fink MJ. Ban the blender. In: *ONN News, The Newsletter of the Ohio Neonatal Nutritionists.* Spring 1998.
30. Cowen SL. Feeding gastrostomy: nutritional management of the infant or young child. *J Pediatr Perinat Nutr.* 1987;1:51.
31. Jew RK, Owen D, Kaufman D, Balmer D. Osmolality of commonly used medications and formulas in the neonatal intensive care unit. *Nutr Clin Pract.* August 1997;12:158–163.
32. Food and Nutrition Board. *Recommended Dietary Allowances.* 9th ed. Washington, DC: National Academy of Sciences; 1989.
33. Food and Nutrition Board. *Dietary Reference Intakes,* Washington, DC: National Academy of Sciences; 1997.
34. Ekvall SW, ed. *Pediatric Nutrition in Chronic Diseases and Developmental Disorders.* New York: Oxford University Press; 1993.

35. Cox JH, ed. *Nutrition Manual for At-Risk Infants and Toddlers*. Chicago, IL: Precept Press; 1997.
36. Issacs JS, Cialone J, Horsley JW, et al. *Children With Special Health Care Needs: A Community Nutrition Pocket Guide*. Columbus, OH: Ross Products, a division of Abbott Laboratories; 1997:22.
37. Walker WA, Hendricks KM, eds. Enteral nutrition: Support of the pediatric patient. In: *Manual of Pediatric Nutrition*. Philadelphia, PA: WB Saunders Co; 1990.
38. Paine JS. Practical aspects of nasogastric feeding in pediatric patients from a ward nursing perspective. *Nutr Supp Serv*. 1986;6:11.
39. Bowers S. Tubes: A nurse's guide to enteral feeding devices. *Med Surg Nurs*. Oct 1996;5(5):313–325.
40. Lord LM. Enteral access devices. *Nurs Clin North Am*. Dec 1997;32(4):685–702.
41. Bernard M, Forlaw L. Complications and their prevention. In: Rombeau RL, Caldwell MD, eds. *Enteral and Tube Feeding*. Philadelphia, PA: WB Saunders Co; 1984:542–569.
42. Lysen LL, Samour PQ. Enteral equipment. In: Materese LE, Gottschlich MM, eds. *Contemporary Nutrition Support Practice: A Clinical Guide*. Philadelphia, PA. WB Saunders Co; 1998:202–215.
43. Ackerman MH, Ciechoski MJ, Marx L. Current trends in enteral feeding. *Soc Gastroenterol Nurs Assoc*. Apr 1992;233–236.
44. Eisenburg PG. Nasoenteral tubes. *RN*. Oct 1994;62–70.
45. Kiver KF, Hays DP, Fortin DF, et al. Pre- and post-pyloric enteral feeding: Analysis of safety and complications. *J Pediatr Enter Nutr*. (Abstract 87) 1984;8:95.
46. Wesley JR. Special access to the intestinal tract. In: Balistreri WF, Farrell MK, eds. *Enteral Feeding: Scientific Basis and Clinical Applications*. Report of the 94th Ross Conference on Pediatric Research. Columbus, OH: Ross Products, a division of Abbott Laboratories; 1988: 57–62.
47. American Academy of Pediatrics. *Pediatric Nutrition Handbook*. Elk Grove Village, IL; 1998:30.
48. Walker WA, Hendricks KM, eds. Enteral nutrition support of the pediatric patient. In: *Manual of Pediatric Nutrition*. Philadelphia, PA: WB Saunders Co; 1985.
49. Cooning SW. Unique aspects in pediatric care. In: Lang C, ed. *Nutrition Support in Critical Care*. Gaithersburg, MD: Aspen Publishers; 1987:395–404.
50. Braunschweig CL, Wesley JR, Clark SF, et al. Rationale and guidelines for parenteral and enteral transition feeding of the 3- to 30-kg child. *J Am Diet Assoc*. 1988; 88:479.
51. Wilson SE, Dietz WH Jr, Grand RJ. An algorithm for pediatric enteral alimentation. *Pediatr Ann*. 1987;16: 233.
52. Hohenbrink K, Oddleifson N. Pediatric nutrition support. In: Shronts EP, ed. *Nutrition Support Dietetics, Core Curriculum*. Silver Spring, MD: ASPEN; 1989: 231–272.
53. Lawrence R. The storage of human milk and cross-nursing. In: Lawrence RA, ed. *Breastfeeding, a Guide for the Medical Profession*. 3rd ed. St Louis, MO: CV Mosby Co; 1994.
54. Narayanan I, Singh B, Harvey D. Fat loss during feeding of human milk. *Arch Dis Child*. 1984;59:475.
55. Greer FR, McCormick A, Loker J. Changes in fat concentration of human milk during delivery by intermittent bolus and continuous mechanical pump infusion. *J Pediatr*. 1984;105:745.
56. Lavine M, Clark RM. The effect of short-term refrigeration of milk and addition of breast milk fortifier on the delivery of lipids during tube feeding. *J Pediatr Gastroenterol Nutr*. 1989;8:496.
57. Wessel JJ, Feeding methodologies. In: Groh-Wargo S, Thompson M, Cox JH, eds. *Nutritional Care for High-Risk Newborns*. Chicago, IL: Precept Press; 1994:213–214.
58. Krey S, Porcelli K, Lockett G, et al. Enteral nutrition. In: Shronts EP, ed. *Nutrition Support Dietetics, Core Curriculum*. Silver Spring, MD: ASPEN; 1989:63–81.
59. Grumow JE, Al-Hafidh AS, Tunell WP. Gastroesophageal reflux following percutaneous endoscopic gastrostomy in children. *J Pediatr Surg*.1989;24:42.
60. Canal DF, Vane DW, Goto S, et al. Reduction of lower esophageal sphincter pressure with Stamm gastrostomy. *J Pediatr Surg*. 1987;22:54.
61. Kellie SJ, Fitch SJ, Kovnar EH, et al. A hazard of using adult-sized weighted-tip enteral feeding catheters in infants. *Am J Dis Child*. 1988;142:916.
62. Allen DB. Postprandial hypoglycemia resulting from nasogastric tube malposition. *Pediatrics*. 1988;81:582.
63. Beratis M, Kolb R, Sperling E, et al. Development of a child with long lasting deprivation of oral feeding. *J Am Acad Child Psychiatr*. 1984;20:53.
64. Ford EG, Jennings M, Andrassy RJ. Serum albumin (oncotic pressure) correlates with enteral feeding tolerance in the pediatric surgical patient. *J Pediatr Surg*. 1987;22:597.
65. Gottschlich MM, Warden GD, Michel M, et al. Diarrhea in tube-fed burn patients: Incidence, etiology, nutritional impact, and prevention. *Parenter Enter Nutr*. 1988;12:388.
66. Freedland CP, Roller RD, Wolfe BM. Microbial contamination of continuous drip feedings. *J Parenter Enter Nutr*. 1989;13:18.
67. Beyer PL. Complications of enteral nutrition. In: Materese LE, Gottschlich MM, eds. *Contemporary Nutrition Support Practice*. Philadelphia, PA: WB Saunders Co; 1998:216–226.

68. Patchell CJ, Anderton A, MacDonald A, George RH, Booth JW. Bacterial contamination of enteral feeds. *Arch Dis Child*. 1994;70:327–330.

69. Guidelines for preventing contamination of enteric feedings. In: Cameron A, Redfern DE, eds. *Report of the Ross Workshop on Contamination of Enteral Feeding Products during Clinical Usage*. Columbus, OH: Ross Products, a division of Abbott Laboratories; 1983:40–42.

70. ASPEN Board of Directors. Guidelines of the use of parenteral and enteral nutrition. *J Parenter Enter Nutr*. 1989.

71. Groschel DHM. Disposable enteral feeding bags should not be reused. *JAMA*. 1982;248:2536.

72. Issacs JS, Cialone J, Horsley JW, et al. *Children with Special Health Care Needs: A Community Nutrition Pocket Guide*, Columbus, OH. Ross Products, a division of Abbott Laboratories; 1997:54.

73. Issacs JS. Nutritional care for the gastrostomy-fed child with neurological impairments. *Top Clin Nutr*. 1993;8(4):58–65.

74. Glass RP, Lucas B. *Making the Transition from Tube Feeding to Oral Feeding. Nutrition Focus for Children with Special Health Care Needs*. Seattle, WA: Children's Development and Mental Retardation Center, University of Washington; 5:1–4.

75. Schauster H, Dwyer J. Transition from tube feedings to feedings by mouth in children: Preventing eating dysfunction. *J Am Diet Assoc*. 1996;96:277–281.

76. Illingsworth RS, Lister J. The critical or sensitive period, with special reference to certain feeding problems in infants and children. *J Pediatr*. 1964;65:8.

77. Therapy Skill Builders. *Oral Play When the Doctor Says Tastes Are Okay*. Communication Skill Builders, Inc; 1994:523–524.

78. Camp KM, Kalscheur MC. Nutritional approach to diagnosis and management of pediatric feeding and swallowing disorders. In: Tuchman DN, Walter RS, eds. *Disorders of Feeding and Swallowing in Infants and Children: Pathophysiology, Diagnosis, and Treatment*. San Diego, CA: Singular Publishing Group; 1994:153–185.

79. American Academy of Pediatrics. *Pediatric Nutrition Handbook*. 4th ed. Elk Grove, IL; 1998:108.

80. Lefton-Grief MA. Diagnosis and management of pediatric feeding and swallowing disorders: Role of the speech-language pathologist. In: Tuchman DN, Walter RS, eds. *Disorders of Feeding and Swallowing in Infants and Children: Pathophysiology, Diagnosis, and Treatment*. San Diego, CA: Singular Publishing Group; 1994:97–113.

81. Feucht S. Guidelines for the use of thickeners in foods and liquids. In: *Nutrition Focus for Children with Special Health Care Needs*. Seattle, WA: Children's Developmental and Mental Retardation Center, University of Washington; 10(6):1–6.

82. Rokusek C, Heinrichs E, eds. *Tube Feeding and an Introduction to Solids in Nutrition and Feeding for Persons with Special Needs: A Practical Guide and Resource Manual*. Pierre, SD: South Dakota Department of Education and Cultural Affairs, Child and Nutrition Services; 1992:185–198.

83. McCrae JD, Hall NH. Current practices for home enteral nutrition. *J Am Diet Assoc*. 1989;89:233.

84. ASPEN Board of Directors. Standards for home nutrition support. *Nutr Clin Pract*. 1992;7:65–69.

85. Weckworth J, Ireton-Jones C. Nutrition support in home care. In: Materese LE, Gottschlich MM, eds., *Contemporary Nutrition Support Practice: A Clinical Guide*. Philadelphia, PA: WB Saunders Co; 1998:611–623.

86. Michaelis CA, Warzak WJ, Stanek K, Van Riper C. Parental and professional perceptions of problems associated with long-term pediatric home tube feeding. *J Am Diet Assoc*. 1992;92:1235–1238.

87. Gallagher AL, Onda RM. Using quality assurance procedures to improve compliance with standards to nutrition care for patients receiving isotonic tube feeding. *J Am Diet Assoc*. 1993;93:678–679.

88. American Dietetic Association. Position of the American Dietetic Association: Nutrition monitoring of the home parenteral and enteral patient. *J Am Diet Assoc*. 1994;94:664–666.

89. Green HL. Response of the bowel to injury and the transition from parenteral to enteral feedings. *Acta Chir Scand Suppl*. 1983;517:21.

90. Brinson R, Kolts BE. Diarrhea associated with severe hypoalbuminemia: A comparison of a peptide-based chemically defined diet and standard enteral alimentation. *Crit Care Med*. 1988;16:130.

91. Heymsfield SB, Bleier J, Whitmire L, et al. Nutrient bioavailability from nasojejunally administered formulas: Comparison to solid food. *Am J Clin Nutr*. 1984; 39:243.

92. Gourley GR, Farrell PM, Odell GB. Essential fatty acid deficiency after portoenterostomy for biliary atresia. *Am J Clin Nutr*. 1982;36:1194.

93. Rickard KA, Baehner RL, Coates TD, et al. Supportive nutritional intervention in pediatric cancer. *Cancer Res* 1982;42:766s–773s.

94. Listernick R, Sidransky E. Hypernatremic dehydration in children with severe psychomotor retardation. *Clin Pediatr*. 1985;24:440.

95. Cowan SL. Feeding gastrostomy: Nutritional management of the infant or young child. *J Pediatr Perinat Nutr*. 1987;1:51.

96. Vanderhoff JA, Grandjean CJ, Kaufman SS, et al. Effect of high percentage medium-chain triglyceride diet on mucosal adaptation following massive bowel resection in rats. *J Parenter Enter Nutr.* 1984;8:685.

97. Lifschitz C. Intestinal permeability. *J Pediatr Gastroenterol Nutr.* 1985;4:520.

98. Koretz RL, Meyer JH. Elemental diets–facts and fantasies. *Gastroenterology.* 1980;78:393.

99. Silk DBA, Fairlough PD, Clark ML, et al. Use of a peptide rather than free amino acid nitrogen source in chemically defined elemental diets. *J Parenter Enter Nutr.* 1980;4:548.

CHAPTER 25

Parenteral Nutrition

Janice Hovasi Cox and Ingrida Mara Melbardis

The use of parenteral nutrition (PN) in pediatrics has greatly evolved over the past years. It has been viewed as an almost routine aspect of care in the treatment of a wide variety of conditions. Technologic advances and refinements in delivery systems that have made PN so commonplace in the hospital setting have propelled this complex form of nutritional support into the home setting. In more recent years, enteral feedings have been found to be beneficial and cost-effective in a variety of settings, where PN was once readily provided. These advances require us to rethink the circumstances under which we currently utilize PN.[1–3] This chapter summarizes the complexities of pediatric PN as it is utilized in the hospital and in the home.

Parenteral nutrition is the intravenous delivery of nutrients, including water, carbohydrates, protein, fat, electrolytes, vitamins, minerals, and trace elements. The proportions of these nutrients are individualized based on an assessment of the child's clinical and nutritional needs. The goal of PN is to support normal growth and development, as well as to promote tissue repair and maintenance when oral/enteral feedings are precluded or limited.

CLINICAL INDICATIONS

Parenteral nutrition is indicated when an infant or child is unable to meet ongoing nutrition needs with an oral diet and/or enteral feedings. In extremely premature infants, gastrointestinal (GI) tract immaturity may prevent sufficient enteral feedings for several weeks. Because premature infants have low nutritional stores, PN should be started within 1–3 days of birth. Undernourished infants and children require nutritional support within 1–2 days if they will not be able to consume adequate feedings. Initially well-nourished infants and children are better able to tolerate longer periods without nutrition intervention, up to 3–5 and 5–7 days, respectively.[4,5] Intravenous solutions (dextrose/sodium chloride/potassium chloride) are usually provided during this time to meet fluid needs and to prevent hypoglycemia.

It is important to ensure that PN is used appropriately and that the infants and children who receive PN are managed effectively to support the best outcome at the lowest cost. Policies/decision algorithms can help practitioners choose the most suitable form of nutrition support[5] (see Figure 25–1). Conditions that may require PN are listed in Exhibit 25–1. Some hospitals utilize interdisciplinary nutritional support teams (physicians, dietitians, nurses, and pharmacists)[6] and/or clinical pathways [7] to help evaluate and manage patients requiring enteral or parenteral nutrition.

GI tract dysfunction can occur at any age due to disease, injury, or radiation/chemotherapy.[4,8] In GI conditions requiring surgical resection, the extent of macronutrient and micronutrient malabsorption depends on the amount of bowel

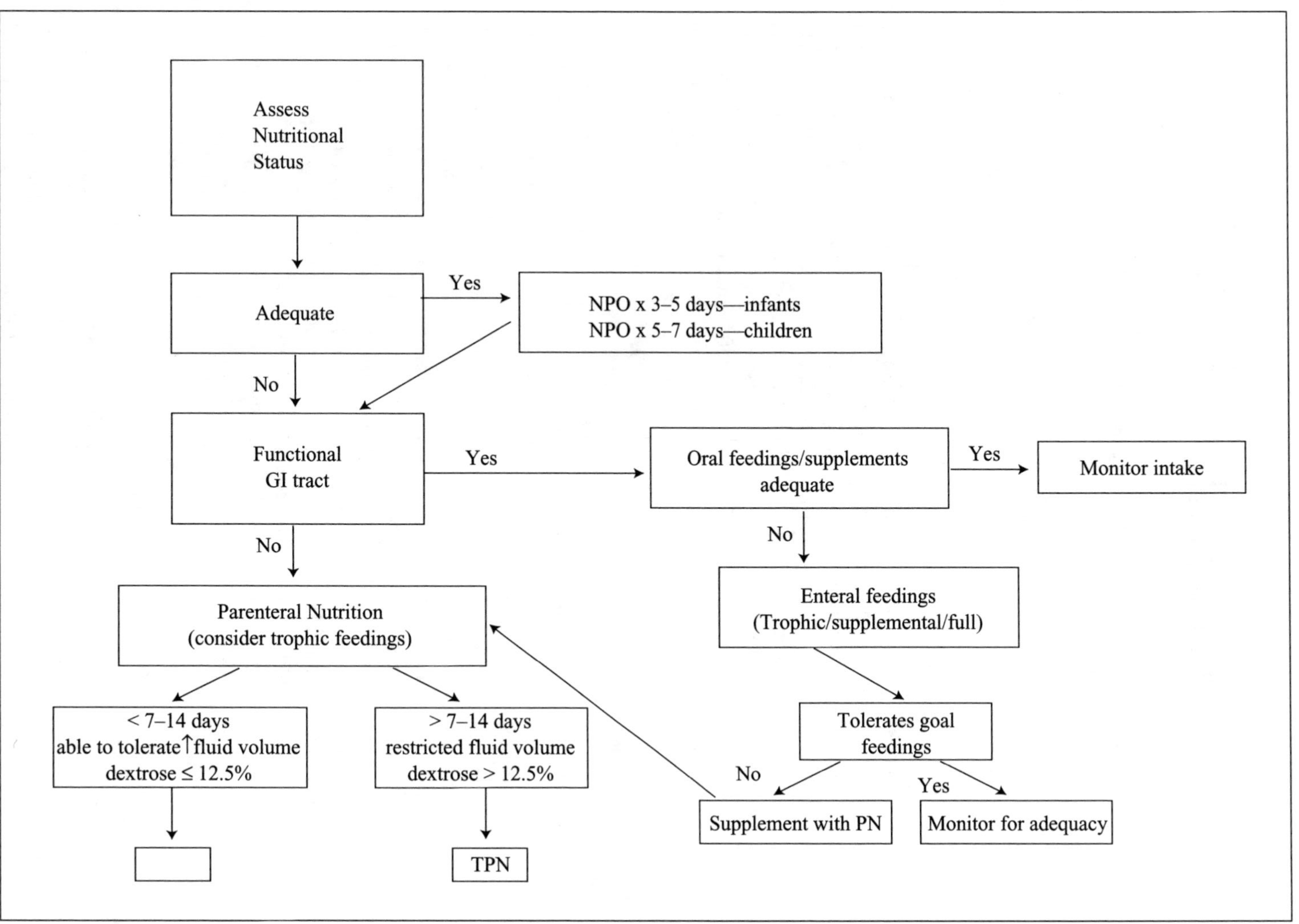

Figure 25–1 Pediatric nutrition support algorithim.

Exhibit 25–1 Conditions that May Require Parenteral Nutrition

GI Conditions		*Other Circumstances*
bowel obstruction	meconium ileus	anorexia nervosa
Crohn's disease	necrotizing enterocolitis	bronchopulmonary dysplasia
diaphragmatic hernia	neuromuscular intestinal disorders	cancer cachexia
gastroschisis	omphalocele	chylothorax
high-output fistulas	radiation enteritis	low-birth-weight neonate (<1,500 g)
intestinal atresia	severe Hirshprung's disease	
intractable diarrhea	short bowel syndrome	
intussusception	ulcerative colitis	
malrotation/volvulus		

resected, the presence or absence of the ileocecal valve, and the function of the remaining bowel. Often, children with short gut syndrome are able to tolerate at least partial enteral feedings. When the ileocecal valve is absent, the rapid transit time of enteral formulas through the bowel may require a greater dependence on PN.[9] The extent of the resection, paired with the tolerance of enteral feedings, can help predict the duration of a neonate's dependence on PN.[10]

Although PN may help bring about disease remission in children with irritable bowel disease (IBD), ulcerative colitis, or Crohn's disease, relapse occurs soon after a normal diet is resumed.[11] Elemental enteral feedings may be more beneficial for inducing remission of IBD, improving nutritional status, and reversing growth failure.[12] Parenteral nutrition should be reserved for only those children who are unable to tolerate enteral feedings. Gastrointestinal disorders requiring nutritional support are discussed in detail in Chapter 16.

Children with cancer are at increased risk for malnutrition. The causes for cancer cachexia seem to be multifaceted and include anorexia, anxiety, and increased metabolic needs.[8] Whether enteral feeding has been impeded by the side effects of radiation and chemotherapy or by surgical procedures, the child with cancer may have an improved quality of life with PN.[13–16] Helping children to maintain optimal nutrition during therapy may promote improved growth and better tolerance of therapies.[17] Some children may be able to tolerate small amounts of gastric feedings along with PN to meet nutrition needs. Most practitioners agree that children receiving aggressive cancer therapy should also receive supportive nutrition therapy, but the benefits of PN should be weighed against the potential risks, which include increased infection rates and metabolic abnormalities.[18,19]

Parenteral nutrition may be used in the refeeding process for children with anorexia nervosa simply because it has less resemblance to food than does the enteral feeding. The use of PN in these patients depends on the severity of malnutrition and on the patient's tendency to interfere with the infusion apparatus.[20,21]

VASCULAR ACCESS

Peripheral Venous Access

Parenteral nutrition needs may be met through a peripheral or central venous route, depending on the anticipated length of therapy, nutrition needs, and the volume of the solution to be given. Because a final concentration of no more than 12.5% dextrose and a maximum solution osmolarity of < 900 mOsm/L is recommended in the administration of peripheral PN (PPN), it is difficult to provide sufficient calories to meet the long-term nutritional needs of most children using this route. Because PPN solutions are not as calorically dense as total PN (TPN) solutions, greater fluid volumes are required to provide comparable calories. Peripheral parenteral nutrition is typically feasible when the anticipated length of therapy will be less than 2 weeks. The major complications associated with PPN are soft tissue sloughs and phlebitis (this is more common with solutions with an osmolarity > 900 mOsm/L). The peripheral delivery route may be more restrictive to normal activity, depending on the site and stability of venous access.

Central Venous Access

Providing TPN through a central vein is indicated when the child requires fluid restriction or long-term nutrition therapy, or when the child is a candidate for home PN. Total parenteral nutrition solutions are more safely infused into central veins because the high blood flow rapidly dilutes the hypertonic solutions. The major complications associated with central venous catheter (CVC) insertion and use include infection and thrombosis.[22,23] Please see Exhibit 25–2 for additional complications.

Central venous catheters are used to provide PN, chemotherapy, prolonged antibiotic therapy, and blood components. Blood sampling can also be done from a CVC site. Central venous access can be temporary or permanent.

Exhibit 25–2 Potential Physical Complications in Pediatric Parenteral Nutrition

CVC Insertion Complications	*CVC Postinsertion Complications*	*Septic Complications*
Pneumothorax	Venous thrombosis	Catheter-related sepsis (site infection, bacteremia, fungemia)
Hemothorax	Superior vena cava syndrome	Solution-related sepsis
Hydrothorax	Thrombophlebitis	Septic thrombosis
Brachial nerve plexus injury	Catheter erosion through vein	
Phrenic nerve injury	Aseptic phlebitis (PICC lines)	
Horner's syndrome	Catheter embolism	
Carotid artery injury	Air embolism	
Arteriovenous fistula	Catheter occlusion	
Arterial cannulation	Extravasation	
Subclavian artery injury	Exsanguination	
Subclavian or innominate vein laceration		
Thoracic duct laceration		
Cardiac perforation and tamponade		
Arrhythmias		
Tracheal puncture		
Catheter embolism		
Air embolism		
Catheter malposition		

Source: Reprinted from J.H. Cox and S.W. Cooning, Parenteral Nutrition, in *Handbook of Pediatric Nutrition,* P.M. Queen and C.E. Lang, eds., © 1993, Aspen Publishers, Inc.

Permanent catheters are indicated when long-term access (> 3 weeks) is needed.[23] The surgically placed right atrial catheter (eg, Broviac, Hickman) is the most suitable CVC for pediatric patients who require long-term or home TPN. The catheter is placed in the external jugular or facial vein and threaded through the internal jugular vein and down into the superior vena cava. The distal end of the catheter is tunneled subcutaneously and exits midchest. The Dacron cuff affixed to the tunneled portion of the catheter helps secure the catheter because subcutaneous fibrous tissue adheres to the cuff. The peripherally inserted central catheter (PICC line), provides reliable central venous access and may be inserted at the bedside using strict sterile techniques.[24–27] Many of the insertion-related complications inherent in the surgically placed CVC, such as pneumothorax and hemothorax, are virtually eliminated with the PICC line. Some studies have also found that sepsis rates tend to be lower in neonates and children with PICC lines compared with surgically placed central catheters.[28,29] PICC lines are being used in increasing numbers in both neonates and older children because they provide central venous access less invasively, with lower risks and at lower cost than surgically placed CVCs.[23,30]

Although a single-lumen CVC is the venous access device most often used for the pediatric PN patient, two- and three-lumen CVCs have also been developed for the pediatric population. The double- and triple-lumen catheters are particularly useful in patients who require frequent infusions of blood products and medications in addition to the nutrition solution. Any lumens not in use must be heparinized and capped. Multilumen catheters may be more suitable for the larger child rather than the neonate because of total catheter size. Strict aseptic technique is critical when a multilumen CVC is in place.[31,32]

To avoid some of the problems associated with the externalized CVC, a totally implantable vascular device consisting of a catheter connected to a chamber or port was developed.[33] The advantages of the implantable port are that it eliminates the daily dressing change when not in use, and it is not as disruptive to body image.

For the child on home PN, the implanted CVC requires daily access. Daily percutaneous punctures or leaving a Huber needle in place with a dressing for days at a time may negate the overall benefits of the implanted device. Skin irritation and breakdown have been associated with frequent port access, and other CVC-related complications, such as occlusion and infection, remain risks with the implanted CVC.[23]

SOLUTION ADMINISTRATION METHODS AND EQUIPMENT

Parenteral nutrition can be ordered in various ways. Nutrients can be ordered based on the infant's or child's weight (per kg), per liter, or in combinations of both. Standard ranges for the various nutrients can be included on order forms to help the prescriber design an appropriate, nutritionally complete solution[34] (see Exhibits 25–3 through 25–6 for sample order forms). Computerized programs are also available to simplify order entry for PN.[35]

Parenteral nutrition solutions should be initiated slowly and advanced gradually as the child's fluid and glucose tolerance permits. Infusion pumps are used to maintain a constant flow rate, thereby maintaining steady glucose delivery. If the PN infusion is interrupted or discontinued abruptly, a 10% dextrose solution may be infused to maintain euglycemia (or to prevent hypoglycemia) until the PN solution can be replaced (see Exhibit 25–7 for recommended features of infusion devices).

There are two ways of preparing PN solutions. In 2-in-1 solutions, dextrose and amino acids are combined, and this solution is infused through one arm of a Y-connector while lipids are infused in the other. A 3-in-1 or total nutrient admixture (TNA) combines the lipid emulsion, amino acid, and dextrose solutions in the same container. Although the TNA is more convenient to use, there has been concern about the stability and safety of these solutions. TNAs,

Exhibit 25–3 Pediatric Parenteral Nutrition Order Form

SPARROW HOSPITAL LANSING, MICHIGAN

PEDIATRIC NUTRITIONAL SUPPORT SOLUTION

DATE	TIME	BAG NO.	☐ REFILL AS PREVIOUSLY ORDERED
WEIGHT Kg	☐ PERIPHERAL ☐ CENTRAL	VOLUME mL	RATE mL/hr

DAILY AMOUNT	ITEM	TOTAL AMOUNT
gm/kg	AMINO ACIDS	
%	DEXTROSE	
gm/kg	FAT	
mEq/kg	SODIUM CHLORIDE	
mEq/kg	SODIUM ACETATE	
mEq/kg	POTASSIUM CHLORIDE	
mEq/kg	POTASSIUM PHOSPHATE (1.5 mEq K/mM; 1 mg P/mM)	
mEq/kg	CALCIUM GLUCONATE	
mEq/kg	MAGNESIUM SULFATE	
ml	MVI ☐ PEDIATRIC ☐ ADULT	
ml	TRACE ELEMENT ☐ PEDIATRIC ☐ ADULT	

SPECIAL INSTRUCTIONS

PHYSICIAN

TIME NEEDED A.M. P.M. NOTED BY:

FLUIDS AND ELECTROLYTES

_______ ml/kg/d x______ kg = _________ ml

-IV's ml/d = _________ ml

TPN ml/d = _________ ml

CALORIE COUNT

PROTEIN

__________ gm/kg/day x____________ kg wt x 4 kcal/gm = ____________ kcal

DEXTROSE

__________ total ml/day x $\frac{\text{\% dextrose}}{100}$ x 3.4 kcal/gm = ____________ kcal

FAT

20%____________ gm/kg/day x___________ kg x 9 kcal/gm = ___________ kcal

TOTAL DAILY CALORIES

$\frac{\text{\_\_\_\_\_\_ protein kcal + \_\_\_\_\_\_ dextrose kcal + \_\_\_\_\_\_ fat kcal = \_\_\_\_\_\_}}{\text{kg weight}}$ = kcal/Kg/day

Use Adult Form for patients > 100 lbs

NORMAL DAILY REQUIREMENTS

ADDITIVE	PEDIATRIC	ADULT
AMINO ACIDS	1.5-3 gm/kg	0.5-2 gm/kg
DEXTROSE	7-14 mg/kg/min	
FAT	2-4 gm/kg	
SODIUM	2-4 mEq/kg	60-150 mEq
ACETATE	2-4 mEq/kg	60-150 mEq
POTASSIUM	2-3 mEq/kg	60-150 mEq
PHOSPHATE	< 15 kg 0.5-2 mM/kg; > 15 kg 0.3-0.8 mM/kg	40-50 mEq
CALCIUM	< 15 kg 1-1.6 mEq/kg; > 15 kg 0.5-0.7 mEq/kg	10-15 mEq
MAGNESIUM	0.2-0.5 mEq/kg	8-24 mEq
VITAMINS	MVI-Pediatric	MVI-Adult
	< 3 kg: 3 ml	> 11 yr: 10 ml
	> 3 kg - 11yrs; 5 ml	
TRACE ELEMENTS	Trace Element - Pediatric	Trace element - Adult
	< 20 kg: 0.2 ml/kg	> 20 kg: 5 ml
MVI	amt/ 5 ml	amt/10 ml vial
ASCORBIC ACID	80 mg	100 mg
VITAMIN A (RETINOL)	0.7 mg	1 mg
VITAMIN D	10 mcg	5 mcg
THIAMINE (B_1)	1.2 mg	3 mg
RIBOFLAVIN (B_2)	1.4 mg	3.6 mg
PYRIDOXINE (B_6)	1 mg	4 mg
NIACIN	17 mg	40 mg
PANTOTHENIC ACID	5 mg	15 mg
VITAMIN E	7 mg	10 mg
FOLIC ACID	140 mcg	400 mcg
VITAMIN B_{12} (Cyanocoabalamin)	1 mcg	5 mcg
VITAMIN K_1	200 mcg	___
BIOTIN	20 mcg	60 mcg
TRACE ELEMENT	amt/ ml	amt/ ml
ZINC	0.5 mg	0.8 mg
COPPER	0.1 mg	0.1 mg
MANGANESE	.3 mg	0.03 mg
CHROMIUM	1 mcg	0.03 mg

HELPFUL HINTS

1. TPN must be reordered daily.
2. TPN orders must be received by 2 p.m.
3. PERIPHERAL SOLUTION: Do not exceed 10% dextrose final concentration.
4. WEIGHT: Write daily weight...necessary for Pharmacy calculations.
5. AMINO ACIDS: Order gm/kg/day; Travasol dispensed unless ordered otherwise.
6. DEXTROSE: Order desired final concentration.
7. ELECTROLYTES: Order mEq/kg/day; note requirements of ions listed - in most cases no need to exceed adult requirements.
8. OPTIMAL Calcium/Phosphorus ratio = 1.7 mg/1 mg.
9. MVI/TRACE ELEMENTS: order ml/day; note requirements listed.
10. TOTAL AMOUNT: if needed may calculate total daily amount of additives in middle column. (Optional)

F-10207 (8/96) WHITE - Chart Copy CANARY - Pharmacy Copy

Source: Courtesy of Sparrow Health System, Lansing, Michigan.

Exhibit 25–4 Neonatal Parenteral Nutrition Order Form

SPARROW HEALTH SYSTEM LANSING, MICHIGAN

NEONATAL NUTRITIONAL SUPPORT SOLUTION

DATE	TIME	BAG NO.	☐ REFILL AS PREVIOUSLY ORDERED
WEIGHT Kg	☐ PERIPHERAL ☐ CENTRAL	VOLUME mL	RATE mL/hr

DAILY AMOUNT	ITEM	TOTAL AMOUNT
gm/kg	AMINO ACIDS (Trophamine)	
%	DEXTROSE	
gm/kg	FAT	
mM/kg	CYSTEINE	
mEq/kg	SODIUM CHLORIDE	
mEq/kg	SODIUM ACETATE	
mEq/kg	POTASSIUM CHLORIDE	
mM/kg	POTASSIUM PHOSPHATE 31 mg P/mM 1.5 mEq K/mM	
mEq/kg	CALCIUM GLUCONATE 19mg Ca/mEq	
mEq/kg	MAGNESIUM SULFATE	
UNITS/ml	HEPARIN	
ml	MVI-PEDIATRIC *	
ml/kg	TRACE-ELEMENT SOLUTION **	

SPECIAL INSTRUCTIONS

PHYSICIAN

TIME NEEDED A.M. P.M. NOTED BY:

FLUIDS AND ELECTROLYTES

_______ ml/kg/d x______ kg = _________ ml

-IV's ml/d = _________ ml

TPN ml/d = _________ ml

CALORIE COUNT

PROTEIN

__________ gm/kg/day x____________ kg wt x 4 kcal/gm = ____________ kcal

DEXTROSE

__________ total ml/day x $\frac{\%\ \text{dextrose}}{100}$ x 3.4 kcal/gm = ____________ kcal

FAT

20%__________ gm/kg/day x__________ kg x 9 kcal/gm = ____________ kcal

TOTAL DAILY CALORIES

$\frac{\text{\_\_\_\_\_ protein kcal + \_\_\_\_\_ dextrose kcal + \_\_\_\_\_ fat kcal = \_\_\_\_\_}}{\text{kg weight}}$ = kcal/Kg/day

Use for RNICU patients only

NORMAL DAILY REQUIREMENTS

ELEMENT	
AMINO ACIDS	0.5-3.0 gm/kg
DEXTROSE	5-8 mg/kg/min
FAT	0.5-3 gm/kg
CYSTEINE	1.0 mM/kg
SODIUM	2-3 mEq/kg
POTASSIUM	2-3 mEq/kg
PHOSPHORUS	0.5-1.5 mM/kg
CALCIUM	0.5-2.5 mEq/kg
MAGNESIUM	0.5 mEq/kg
HEPARIN	1 UNITS/ml
MVI-PEDIATRIC	2.5-5.0 ml
TRACE ELEMENT SOLUTION	1 ml/kg

*** MVI-PEDIATRIC Each 5 ml contains:**

- ASCORBIC ACID .... 80 mg
- A (RETINOL) .... 0.7 mg
- D (ERGOCAL CIFEROL) .... 10 mcg
- THIAMINE (B_1) .... 1.2 mg
- RIBOFLAVIN (B_2) .... 1.4 mg
- PYRIDOXINE (B_6) .... 1 mg
- NIACIN (B_2) .... 17 mg
- PANTOTHENIC ACID .... 5 mg
- E .... 7 mg
- FOLIC ACID .... 140 mcg
- CYANOCOBALAMIN (B_{12}) .... 1 mcg
- K_1 (PHYTONADIONE) .... 200 mcg
- BIOTIN .... 20 mcg

**** TRACE ELEMENT SOLUTION Each ml contains:**

- Zn .... 0.5 mg
- C .... 0.1 mg
- Mn .... 0.03 mg
- Cr .... 1.0 mcg

HELPFUL HINTS

1. TPN must be reordered daily.
2. TPN orders must be received by 12N.
3. WEIGHT: record weight...necessary for Pharmacy calculations.
4. DAILY VOLUME:_____ ml/kg/day x________ kg = __________ml.
5. AMINO ACIDS: Order gm/kg/day; Trophamine dispensed unless ordered otherwise.
6. DEXTROSE: Order desired final concentration.
7. Fat:_________gm/kg/day x_______kg x 5 = _________mL
8. ELECTROLYTES: Order mEq/kg/day; note normal requirements.
9. TOTAL AMOUNT: may calculate total daily amount of additives in center if needed. (Optional)

F-10215 (12/97) WHITE - Chart Copy CANARY - Pharmacy Copy

Source: Courtesy of Sparrow Health System, Lansing, Michigan.

Exhibit 25–5 Pediatric Parenteral Nutrition Pharmacy Request Form

BRONSON METHODIST HOSPITAL
Kalamazoo, Michigan

PEDIATRIC PARENTERAL NUTRITION

PHARMACY REQUEST FORM

DATE	TIME	ORDERS
		(for children in PICU and Peds Unit) RATE: ____________ ml/hr (____________ hr/day) WEIGHT: ____________ kg

Generally recommended dose range is given in parentheses after each nutrient.
The clinical condition of an individual patient may require doses outside these ranges.

1. Final Base Concentration
   ___% Liposyn (0.5 - 3.5 gm%)
   ___% Protein - Standard Amino Acids (2.0 - 3.5%)
   ___% Protein - Other specialty formula ____________________
   ___% Dextrose (10 - 25% depending upon route of venous access)

2. Individual Additives (order per 1000 ml unit)
   ___ mEq (NaCl) Sodium Chloride (20 - 60 mEq/L)
   ___ mM (Na Phos) Sodium Phosphate (0 - 15 mM/L) * (1 mM Na Phos = 1.33 mEq Na)
   ___ mEq (Na Ac) Sodium Acetate (0 - 30 mEq/L)
   ___ mM (K Phos) Potassium Phosphate (0 - 15 mM/L) * (1 mM K Phos = 1.47 mEq K)
   ___ mEq (K Ac) Potassium Acetate (20 - 50 mEq/L)
   ___ mEq (K Cl) Potassium Chloride (0 - 40 mEq/L)
   ___ ml (50% $MgSO_4$) Magnesium Sulfate (0.6 - 2.0 ml/L)
   ___ mg (Ca Glu) Calcium Gluconate (1000 - 2000 mg/L)*
   ___

* Total PO_4 should generally be 5 - 15 mM/L.
Ca (mEq) + PO_4 (mM) < 30 to avoid precipitation
1000 mg Ca Gluconate = 4.7 mEq Ca

3. Routine Additives per 24° bag unless ordered otherwise
   - Pediatric multivitamin 1 vial
   - Pediatric trace mineral 1 ml

4. Other Additives
   ___ mg Famotidine per 24 hours (max = 40mg)
   ___ mg Cimetidine per 24 hours
   ___ units Regular Human Insulin per 24 hours
   ___ units Heparin per 24 hours
   ___

Physician's signature ______________________________

PHYSICIAN'S ORDER FORM
NS 532-3409 (4/93)
(SO422) 11/93, 2/94, 2/96

PLEASE PRINT, USE BALL POINT PEN, PRESS HARD
WHITE-CHART YELLOW-PHARMACY PINK-NURSING

Source: Courtesy of Bronson Methodist Hospital, Kalamazoo, Michigan.

Exhibit 25–6 Neonatal Parenteral Nutrition Pharmacy Request Form

BRONSON METHODIST HOSPITAL
Kalamazoo, Michigan

NEONATAL PARENTERAL NUTRITION

PHARMACY REQUEST FORM

DATE	TIME	ORDERS
		(may be used for infants under one year of age) RATE: ____________ ml/hr WEIGHT: ____________ kg

1. FINAL BASE CONCENTRATION
   - ______% Protein - Standard Amino Acids
   - ______% Protein Neonatal Formula (L-cysteine 0.6 mMol/% added by Pharmacy)
   - ______% Dextrose
   - ______% Liposyn (0.5% - 2.5%)*

2. INDIVIDUAL ADDITIVES (ordering per 1000 ml concentration)
   - ______ mEq (NaCl) Sodium Chloride (15-40 mEq)*
   - ______ mEq (Na Ac) Sodium Acetate (0-20 mEq)*
   - ______ mM (K Phos) Potassium Phosphate (5-15 mM)*
   - ______ mEq (KCl) Potassium Chloride (0-40 mEq)*
   - ______ mEq (K Ac) Potassium Acetate (0-20 mEq)*
   - ______ ml (50% $MgSO_4$) Magnesium Sulfate (.4-1.2 ml)*
   - ______ mg (Ca Glu) Calcium Gluconate (700-4000 mg)*
   - ______ units Heparin
   - ______ mg Zinc (1 mg/L for infants < 1.5 kg)*
   - ______

Ca (mEq) + PO_4 (mM) < 30 to avoid precipitation Ca Gluconate 1000 mg = 4.7 mEq

3. Other Additives
   ______mg Cimetidine per 24 hrs.

4. Routine Additives/24° bag
   Unless Deleted/Changed
   - Peds - MVI (2.5 vials/Liter ratio up to 14 ml/hr, then 1 vial/24 hr. bag ratio)
   - Peds - trace minerals (1.3 ml/Liter ratio)

* suggested ranges adjust as clinically necessary.

Physician's signature ______________________________

PHYSICIAN'S ORDER FORM
10/93, 12/93
955016

PLEASE PRINT, USE BALL POINT PEN, PRESS HARD

WHITE-CHART YELLOW-PHARMACY

Source: Courtesy of Bronson Methodist Hospital, Kalamazoo, Michigan.

Exhibit 25–7 Pediatric Parenteral Infusion Device—Desirable Features

1. Inexpensive
2. Suitable for use with clear and opaque solutions
3. Equipped with tamper-proof controls
4. Small and lightweight for ambulatory patients
5. Equipped with sturdy, wheeled stand or pole with a wide base of support to prevent overturning
6. Has audible and visual alarms for
   - Low battery
   - Occlusion
   - Infusion complete
   - Air in line
7. Easy to operate and set up
8. Pump pressure compatible for use with in-line filter devices
9. Delivers known fluid volume via peristaltic or volumetric syringe pump methods
10. Has flow rate that is accurate, with delivery rates as low as 1 mL/h, which can be increased in 0.1 mL increments
11. Can be programmed to taper infusion rate for patient on cyclic infusion
12. Can operate accurately on long-life battery (12 to 24 hours)

Source: Reprinted from J.H. Cox and S.W. Cooning, Parenteral Nutrition, in *Handbook of Pediatric Nutrition,* P.M. Queen and C.E. Lang, eds., © 1993, Aspen Publishers, Inc.

unlike 2-in-1 solutions, are emulsions and, therefore, are more significantly influenced by pH and temperature.[36] Of concern has also been the potential peroxidation of lipid emulsions by phototherapy lights.[37] Shielding the bag and the tubing from phototherapy lights with aluminum foil or a blanket can prevent this from occurring.

In TNAs, three main variables affect the overall stability of the final product: the final concentration of the macronutrients, the amount of added cations (especially polyvalent cations such as iron, magnesium, calcium, and zinc), and the compounding order.[38,39] Care must be taken to identify any precipitates or emulsion breakdown in the TNA before infusion occurs. The most commonly found precipitate is calcium phosphate. Emulsion breakdown or creaming (liberation of free oil) can result when higher amounts of cations are used in the mixture. The presence of yellow-brown oil droplets at or near the TNA surface is an indicator that the solution is unsafe for administration.[39] Various methods of in-process end-product testing are described in the American Society for Parenteral and Enteral Nutrition (ASPEN) guidelines to ensure and document the safety of the end TNAs.[39]

Of greatest concern with neonatal and pediatric PN solutions is the solubility of calcium and phosphorus.[38] Although the addition of lipids to the PN solution does not directly affect the solubility of calcium and phosphorus, the opacity of the admixture makes visual detection of precipitates very difficult. Computer programs are available to help maximize the amount of calcium and phosphorus that can be provided safely in PN solutions.[38]

For neonates and children receiving home PN, the stability of the PN should be assured for longer periods of time. Using dual-chamber bags to separate the lipid from the rest of the solution and adding vitamins just before infusion helps improve the shelf-life of TNAs used in this setting.[39] Caretakers administering PN in the home need to be trained how to visually assess the stability of the emulsion.

The use of filters with PN provides additional safety.[39,40] Filters can prevent the infusion of particulate matter, air, and microorganisms. Different types of filters are used for 2-in-1 and 3-in-1 solutions. Positively charged filters and 0.2-mm filters can be used with 2-in-1 solutions. These filters remove microorganisms and pyrogens (gram-negative endotoxin) and reduce the risk of air embolism. For TNAs, larger 1.2-mm filters are used to allow administration of lipid droplets. These can filter out particulate matter and larger organisms, such as *Candida albicans*, but are unable to filter out common smaller bacterial contaminants.

CYCLING

Administration of PN in cycles provides for planned interruption of the nutrient infusion. Cycling more closely simulates normal patterns of food ingestion and fasting, and may help prevent PN-associated hepatic complications.[41] Whether at home or in the hospital, cyclic PN allows the child a more normal daytime routine, enhancing mobility and activity patterns and leaving a "window" of time for lipid clearance.

The nutrition needs of the child, compared with the ability to tolerate oral/enteral feedings, should be taken into consideration when deciding on cyclic PN. Infants younger than 4–6 months old who are receiving all of their nutrition parenterally may be able to tolerate breaks from PN up to only 4 hours in duration. Older infants and children may tolerate interruptions of up to 6–8 hours. Infants and children who are receiving enteral feedings or are eating in addition to their PN may receive adequate PN in shorter spans of time. Supplemental PN can usually be provided over 8–12 hours. Children who are more tolerant of the necessary fluid load can receive their total required caloric and fluid loads condensed into 10- to 16-hour cycles.

Gradually increasing the rate when starting the infusion and slowly weaning the rate at the end of the infusion may lessen the likelihood of hyper/hypoglycemia. The rate should be adjusted over a period of 1–2 hours (ie, run at half rate for the first and last hour) to maintain euglycemia. Infusion pumps that can be programmed to accomplish the gradual introduction and weaning of PN are available.

As an infant or child is able to transition to enteral/oral feedings, the volume of PN should be gradually decreased (decreased hourly rate and/or decreased infusion time). Total energy needs must be adjusted as the percentage of nutrition provided by an enteral route is increased (PN needs are usually lower than enteral needs because energy is not required for digestion and there are no absorptive losses). Providing PN at night provides supplemental nutrition with limited suppression of appetite during the day, which may better support a transition to oral feedings.

FLUID AND ELECTROLYTES

Guidelines for the administration of parenteral fluids to infants and children are based on normal maintenance estimates, with adjustments for increased or decreased losses due to disease or environmental conditions (see Table 25–1). During the first week of life, infants experience three phases of fluid and electrolyte homeostasis.[44] Renal excretion of fluid, sodium, and potassium is minimal, and insensible water loss (IWL) may be high during the first 12–36 hours of life or prediuretic phase. The onset of the diuretic phase usually occurs within the first 2 days and accounts for most of the weight, sodium, and potassium loss that occurs during the first week of life. The postdiuretic phase usually begins between 3 and 5 days of age and is characterized by improved homeostasis of fluid, sodium, and potassium.[44]

Although fluid losses through urine and the GI tract may be relatively easy to measure, IWL through the respiratory tract and skin is more elusive and may be affected by environmental conditions. Prematurely born infants may lose 10–25% of their body weight during the first

Table 25–1 Daily Maintenance Fluid Requirements

Clinical Condition	*Fluids Required per Day*	
Sick newborn, day 1	40–80	mL/kg
Sick newborn, week 1	100–150	mL/kg
Anuria, extreme oliguria	45	mL/kg
Diabetes insipidus	up to 400	mL/100 kcal
1–10 kg body weight	100	mL/kg
11–20 kg body weight	1000 ml + 50	mL/kg above 10 kg
Body weight above 20 kg	1500 ml + 20	mL/kg above 20 kg
Body surface area	1500–1800	mL/m^2

Source: Data from references 42 and 43.

week of life, primarily due to their greater percentage of total body water as extracellular water and increased IWL associated with their relatively large body surface area/body mass ratio and their more permeable epidermis.[42] Radiant heat warmers and ultraviolet light therapy may increase IWL by 20–25%.[45,46] Use of double-walled isolettes may prevent this increase in water loss.[47] Use of mist tents and humidified air may decrease IWL.[48] In older infants and children, hyperventilation and visible sweating, often associated with fever, may increase IWL by 20–25%.

Low-birth-weight infants may require up to 200 mL/kg/day, due to their renal immaturity and increased IWL. They may also be intolerant of excessive fluid intake. Patent ductus arteriosus, bronchopulmonary dysplasia, intraventricular hemorrhage, and necrotizing enterocolitis have each been linked with excessive fluid administration.[49–53] Frequent monitoring of fluid and electrolyte intake, serum and urine electrolyte levels, weight changes, and urine output may be needed to appropriately manage fluid and electrolyte balance during the neonatal period.

Beyond the first week of life and throughout childhood, maintenance fluid and electrolyte requirements are directly related to metabolic rate.[54] Infants and children generally require at least 115 mL of fluid for every 100 kcal of energy provided[55] (see Table 25–1). The amount of fluid needed to maintain adequate hydration often does not provide adequate nutrition when using peripheral venous access, though administration of fluids 30–50% above maintenance levels is usually well tolerated. Changes in metabolic rate, respiratory rate, IWL, and water production from the oxidation of protein, carbohydrate, and fat also affect fluid needs. Older infants and children may initially require fluids and electrolytes in excess of maintenance requirements to establish normal hydration if they have had prolonged or excessive vomiting or diarrhea.

Losses of fluid and electrolytes through the GI tract in disease states may be measured directly for replacement or estimated by monitoring changes in body weight every 8 or 24 hours. Gastrointestinal losses may be due to vomiting, nasogastric suctioning, diarrhea, or ostomy drainage. Due to the wide range in electrolyte composition of various GI fluids, direct measurement may be required to provide adequate replacement.

Urinary losses of fluid and electrolytes depend largely on intake and renal maturity. Infants younger than 1 year of age can dilute urine to 50 mOsm/kg of water, and concentrating ability at birth is about 600 mOsm/kg of water, which gradually increases to 1,000–1,200 mOsm/kg of water during the first year. During periods of growth, the renal solute load is lower, because nitrogen, phosphorus, sodium, potassium, and chloride are retained as constituents of body tissues. During periods of stress and tissue catabolism, the renal solute load is higher.

Various conditions may alter urinary losses of fluid and electrolytes. Preterm infants have an immature capacity to either excrete or retain electrolytes and maintain acid-base balance.[56,57] Excessive sodium losses are common and may require up to 12 mmol/kg/day of sodium. Inappropriate or excessive antidiuretic hormone (ADH) secretion, often associated with hypoxia, hemorrhage, central nervous system insult, hypotension, anesthesia, pneumothorax, or pain requires fluid restriction and sodium supplementation to maintain normal extracellular fluid volumes and to prevent hyponatremia.[56] However, hyperchloremic acidosis in preterm infants is associated with excessive chloride intake when sodium is provided solely as sodium chloride. Using sodium acetate (up to 14.2 mmol/kg/day) has been shown to reduce the incidence of metabolic acidosis and hyperchloremia.[57] If IWL (which is all free water) is high in prematurely born infants—particularly during the diuretic phase of initial fluid and electrolyte homeostasis—hypernatremia may develop.[44,58]

Fluid and electrolyte restriction may be necessary in some disease states, such as congestive heart failure, head trauma, and renal insufficiency. Medications may be a significant source of fluid and/or electrolytes. Saline flushes used in routine care of intravenous lines may be a significant source of sodium and chloride.[59] Some medications may cause increased excretion or retention of some electrolytes. Direct measurement of urine volume and electrolytes may be necessary to provide appropriate replacement.

ENERGY

Parenteral energy needs are approximately 10–15% lower than estimated enteral needs for most infants and children, due to reduced fecal losses and reduced energy required for digestion and absorption (see Table 25–2). Although meeting basal energy needs prevents catabolism and weight loss, energy needs to support catch-up growth or even normal growth and activity levels may be nearly double.[65] Energy requirements for postoperative infants and children may be closer to basal needs, possibly due to administration of sedative medications and temporary interruption of growth, although energy needs generally return to normal within 1–3 days of surgery and may even exceed normal levels.[4,66] Energy needs during the acute phase of critical illness, sedation, or paralysis may be lower than normal. As indirect calorimetry becomes more readily available for infants and children, energy can be given and doses adjusted to meet individual needs.[1,4,67]

The percentage contribution of protein, carbohydrate, and fat to total energy intake varies with individual tolerance to fluid, carbohydrate, lipid infusion, and the route of delivery. General guidelines for energy distribution are 8–15% protein, 45–60% carbohydrate, and 25–40% fat.[42] Positive nitrogen balance is best achieved when the nonprotein calorie/nitrogen ratio is 150–300:1.[68,69]

CARBOHYDRATE

Glucose (dextrose monohydrate, 3.4 kcal/g) is the primary source of parenterally administered carbohydrate. Glycerol, found in parenterally administered fat emulsions, is also a source of carbohydrate. Dose recommendations for infants and children are found in Table 25–3. Glucose infusions of less than 2 mg/kg/min (3 g/kg/day) may be insufficient to prevent ketosis caused by mobilization of fat stores as a source of energy. Glucose in excess of 16 mg/kg/min (24 g/kg/day) is not recommended, because this may be associated with hyperglycemia, hepatic steatosis, and/or excess carbon dioxide production.[1,69]

Insulin is not generally added to parenteral nutrient admixtures because dose response varies widely, particularly in the low-birth-weight

Table 25–2 Daily Recommendations for Parenteral Administration of Nutrients

					Age			
		Premature Infants	*Term Infants*	*1–3 Years*	*4–6 Years*	*7–10 Years*	*11–18 Years*	*Maximum Dose*
Basal Energy	kcal/kg[1]	46–55	55	40–55	38–40	25–38	23–25	
Total Energy	kcal/kg[2]	80–105	95	75–90	65–80	55–75	40–55	
Carbohydrate	g/kg	4–18	8–23	8–20	8–16	8–14	8–12	see text
Protein[3]	g/kg	2.5–3.5	2.5–3.5	1.5–2.5	1.5–2.5	1.5–2.5	1.5–2.5	4.0
Fat	g/kg	0.5–3.0	0.5–3.5	0.5–2.5	0.5–2.5	0.5–2.5	0.5–2.5	4.0
Pediatric Vitamins[4]	5 mL dose	2 mL/kg	5 mL	5 mL	5 mL	5 mL	—	5 mL
Adult Vitamins[4]	10 mL dose	—	—	—	—	—	10 mL	10 mL
Sodium	mEq/kg	2–4	2–4	2–4	2–4	2–4	60–150 mEq/d	
Potassium	mEq/kg	2–4	2–4	2–4	2–4	2–4	70–180 mEq/d	
Chloride	mEq/kg	2–4	2–4	2–4	2–4	2–4	60–150 mEq/d	
Magnesium[5]	mEq/kg	0.3–0.5	0.25–1.0	0.25–1.0	0.25–1.0	0.25–1.0	8–32 mEq/d	see text
Calcium[6]	mEq/kg	2.0–4.0	2.0–3.0	0.6–2.0	0.6–2.0	0.6–2.0	10–40 mEq/d	see text
Phosphorus[7]	mMol/kg	1.3–2.0	1.3–1.5	0.5–1.3	0.5–1.3	0.5–1.3	9–30 mMol	see text
Zinc	mcg/kg	325–400	250 < 3 mo 100 > 3 mo	100	100	50	50	5000 mcg/d
Copper[8]	mcg/kg	20	20	20	20	20	300–500 mcg/d	500 mcg/d
Chromium	mcg/kg	0.14–0.2	0.14–0.2	0.14–0.2	0.14–0.2	0.14–0.2	0.14–0.2	15 mcg/d
Manganese[8]	mcg/kg	1	1	1	1	1	1	50–150 mcg/d
Selenium	mcg/kg	2	2	2	2	30–40 mcg/d	30–40 mcg/d	40 mcg/d
Iron[9]	mg/kg	see text	0.1	see text	see text	see text	see text	see text

[1] Basal calories ↑ 12% for every degree of fever; ↑ 15–25% in cardiac failure; ↑ 20–30% in traumatic injury or major surgery; ↑ 25–30% in severe respiratory distress or bronchopulmonary dysplasia; ↑ 40–50% in severe sepsis; ↑ 6 kcal/g weight gain for catch-up growth.
[2] Total parenteral energy needs do not include calories required for digestion or stool losses that are normally included in estimating enteral energy needs.
[3] Protein needs are 0.8–2.0 g/kg/d in renal failure; 3 g/kg/d for necrotizing enterocolitis, major surgery, traumatic injury, sepsis; 4-8 g/kg/d for thermal injury. Most efficient protein utilization occurs when nonprotein/calorie ratio is 150–250:1 (100–150:1 in burns, multiple trauma).
[4] MVI Pediatric and MVI-12, Astra USA, Inc., Westborough MA 01581. See Table 25–9.
[5] Magnesium sulfate 50% contains 500 mg magnesium sulfate heptahydrate or 4.1 mEq magnesium/mL.
[6] Calcium gluconate 10% contains 100 mg calcium gluconate or 10 mg of elemental calcium (0.5 mEq or 0.25 mmol of calcium) per mL.
[7] Potassium phosphate contains 93 mg (3 mmol) phosphorus and 4.4 mEq potassium per mL; sodium phosphate contains 93 mg (3 mmol) phosphorus and 4 mEq sodium per mL.
[8] As copper and manganese are excreted primarily through bile, decrease or temporarily omit these trace minerals in patients with cholestasis.
[9] Iron is not routinely included in parenteral admixtures. See text.

Source: Data from references 4, 42, 45, 60-64.

Table 25–3 Parenteral Glucose Dose Recommendations

	mg/kg/min	*g/kg/d*
Very-low-birth-weight infants		
Initial dose	3–4	4–6
Dose during first few days	6–8	8.5–11.5
Dose after first week	8–12	12–18
Term infant or child		
Initial dose	6–8	8.5–11.5
Dose after first week	12–14	19–23

Source: Data from references 42, 69, and 70.

infant. Insulin, when needed, may be given in a separate infusion starting at 0.1 U/kg/hour and increased or decreased as needed to maintain euglycemia.[70,71] Small glycogen stores in low-birth-weight and undernourished infants and children place them at a greater risk of developing hypoglycemia following abrupt cessation of parenteral glucose. Gradual weaning from parenteral glucose and adequate enteral feeding help prevent the development of hypoglycemia.

The recommended dose of carbohydrate may be delivered while meeting normal fluid requirements by using a 10–12.5% dextrose solution. This concentration is compatible with peripheral intravenous infusion. Greater concentrations of carbohydrate are given by central venous infusion, generally up to a maximum concentration of 25%.[72] These may be needed when caloric needs are greater than normal, when parenterally administered fat is poorly tolerated, or when fluid restriction is necessary. Excess carbohydrate intake, if converted to and stored as fat, may increase carbon dioxide production and retention that may compromise respiratory management.[65]

PROTEIN

Several studies have estimated the optimal protein intake for infants,[73–76] though recommendations beyond infancy are more empirical or disease related.[69,76] General recommendations for protein administration for infants and children are given in Table 25–2. Protein usually comprises about 10–15% of total energy intake. Individual protein needs can be determined from nitrogen balance studies, though protein status is generally evaluated by monitoring serum total protein and albumin levels. Changes in serum prealbumin, transferrin, or retinol-binding protein levels may identify changes in protein status more quickly. Monitoring blood urea nitrogen or ammonia levels helps to identify excess protein intake. Recommendations concerning monitoring and complications of protein administration are found in Tables 25–4 and 25–5.

Unlike energy needs during periods of acute stress, protein needs do not decrease.[77] Administering amino acids as soon as possible after birth, even in the smallest of neonates and during periods of acute stress, along with enough energy to meet basal requirements, helps to maintain normal plasma amino acid concentrations, increases nitrogen retention, and may stimulate endogenous insulin secretion to improve glucose tolerance.[4,65]

Crystalline amino acid (CAA) products have been developed for infants, reflecting the amino acid composition of human milk or plasma aminograms of healthy term infants fed mature human milk (see Tables 25–6 and 25–7). Metabolic immaturity has also been considered,

Table 25–4 Suggested Laboratory Monitoring During Pediatric Parenteral Nutrition

Laboratory Index	*Initial*	*Stable*	*Home Monitoring*
Blood glucose	Daily	Daily to 3x/week	Daily to 3x/week
Acid-base status	Daily to weekly	Every other week	Monthly < 6 months Every 3 months < 1 year Every 6 months > 1 year
Electrolytes Na, K, Cl, CO_2	Daily	Weekly or Every other week	
Chemistry profile: total protein albumin BUN, creatinine Ca, Phos, Mg triglyceride	Weekly	Weekly or Every other week	Monthly < 6 months Every 3 months < 1 year Every 6 months > 1 year
Liver profile: total bilirubin alk phos LDH, ALT, AST PTT	Weekly	Monthly	Monthly < 6 months Every 3 months < 1 year Every 6 months > 1 year
Hematology profile: HBG/HCT platelet count	Baseline	Weekly	Monthly < 6 months Every 3 months < 1 year Every 6 months > 1 year
CBC w/ diff	Weekly	Monthly or as indicated*	As above or as indicated*
iron/TIBC/ferritin	As indicated*	As indicated*	As indicated*
Other: Trace minerals Vitamins Carnitine	As indicated*	As indicated*	As indicated*
Urine glucose specific gravity pH	2-4 times a day	Daily to weekly	As indicated*

*as indicated = clinical condition or symptoms indicating deficiency, imbalance, or abnormality

Note: BUN = blood urea nitrogen; LDH = lactic dehydrogenase; ALT = alanine amino transferase; AST = aspartate amino transferase; PTT = prothrombin time; HGB = hemoglobin; HCT = hematocrit; CBC = complete blood count; TIBC = total iron binding capacity

Table 25-5 Metabolic Complications of Pediatric Parenteral Nutrition

Complication	*Cause*	*Treatment*
Hyperglycemia, glycosuria, osmotic diuresis, hyperosmolar nonketotic dehydration, coma	Excessive dose or rate of glucose infusion	Decrease rate, concentration of glucose; use insulin with caution, results are often erratic in the very low birth weight infant
Hypoglycemia	Abrupt discontinuation of glucose infusion; excess insulin	Maintain constant glucose infusion; decrease glucose infusion rates slowly; decrease insulin
Metabolic acidosis, hyperammonemia, prerenal azotemia	Excessive amino acid infusion, inappropriate protein/calorie ratio	Decrease amino acids, increase nonprotein calories
Hyperchloremic metabolic acidosis	Excessive chloride administration causing cation gap	Provide equal amount of sodium and chloride in infusate; neutralize cation gap with lactate or acetate if respiratory status allows
Hypokalemia	Inadequate potassium infusion relative to increased requirements for protein anabolism	If potassium needs are greater than the potassium provided by potassium phosphate, potassium acetate is generally recommended
Hyperkalemia	Excessive potassium administration; especially in metabolic acidosis	Decrease potassium in infusate
Volume overload, congestive heart failure	Excessive rate of fluid administration	Monitor weight daily; monitor intake and output daily to prevent volume overload; do not attempt to "catch up" by increasing rate of infusion; to treat, decrease rate of infusion
Hypocalcemia	Inadequate calcium administration or phosphorus administration without simultaneous calcium infusion; hypomagnesemia or hypoalbuminemia	Increase calcium infusion, maintaining appropriate phosphorus and magnesium infusion
Hypophosphatemia	Inadequate phosphorus administration especially relative to increased needs of protein anabolism	Increase phosphorus infusion, maintaining appropriate calcium/ phosphorus precipitation

Table 25-5 continued

Complication	*Cause*	*Treatment*
Hypomagnesemia	Inadequate magnesium infusion relative to increased gastrointestinal losses in chronic diarrhea or increased needs for protein anabolism	Increase magnesium infusion
Essential fatty acid deficiency	Inadequate linoleic acid infusion	Provide at least 4–8% of total calories as intravenous fat emulsion to provide 1–4% of total calories as linoleic acid
Hypertriglyceridemia, hypercholesterolemia	Lipids infused at a rate greater than the capacity to metabolize	Decrease or interrupt lipid infusion; add heparin to infusate*
Anemia	Deficiency of iron, folic acid, vitamin B_{12}, or copper	Administer appropriate nutrient
Cholestatic jaundice	Sepsis, prematurity, starvation, essential fatty acid deficiency, lipid infusion, amino acid deficiency, amino acid excess, carbohydrate excess, decreased bile flow, bowel obstruction, lack of enteral feedings	Begin enteral feedings as soon as possible, maintain adequate but not excessive intake; liver function generally returns to normal within 6–9 months after cessation of therapy, but may progress to chronic liver disease

* Data from reference 43, chapter 7.

Source: Adapted with permission from S. Groh-Wargo, et al., *Nutritional Care for High-Risk Newborns,* pp. 56–58, © 1994, Precept Press, Inc.

because cystine, taurine, tyrosine, and histidine may be essential amino acids for the neonate. Methionine, phenylalanine, and glycine concentrations have been decreased in these solutions, whereas histidine, tyrosine, taurine, arginine, glutamic acid, and aspartic acid may be added or their concentrations increased. Although glutamine is not routinely added to PN solutions due to solubility problems, this amino acid may be conditionally essential during periods of sepsis, trauma, surgery, or shock, when circulating levels decrease and needs are increased—particularly in maintaining GI mucosal cell integrity.[4,82] For extremely low-birth-weight infants, glutamine added to PN in amounts of 0.28–0.5 g/kg/day (or 20% of amino acid intake) appears safe and may support earlier achievement of full enteral feedings.[83]

Although cysteine may be a conditionally essential amino acid in the young neonate, it is not included in CAA solutions because it is unstable in solution for prolonged periods of time. It is available as L-cysteine hydrochloride to be added separately at the time of administration. However, cystathionase activity matures to 70% of adult activity by 9 days

Table 25–6 Amino Acid Content of Parenteral Products (mg/dL of 2% Amino Acid Solution)

Amino Acid	*Aminosyn*	*Freamine III*	*Travasol*	*Aminosyn PF*	*Trophamine*	*Novamine*
Isoleucine	146	138	96	153	163	97
Leucine	189	182	124	237	280	139
Lysine	146	146	116	135	163	157
Methionine	80	106	116	36	67	100
Phenylalanine	89	112	124	86	97	139
Threonine	106	80	84	103	83	100
Tryptophan	34	30	36	36	40	33
Valine	161	132	92	129	157	128
Alanine	258	142	415	140	106	289
Arginine	198	190	207	246	243	196
Histidine	60	56	88	63	97	119
Proline	175	224	84	163	137	119
Serine	86	118	—	99	77	79
Tyrosine	11	—	8	13	47	5
Glycine	258	280	415	77	73	139
Cysteine	—	<5	—	—	<3	—
Glutamic Acid	—	—	—	165	100	100
Aspartic Acid	—	—	—	106	64	58
Taurine	—	—	—	14	5	—

Note: Aminosyn and Aminosyn PF: Abbott Laboratories, North Chicago, IL; Freamine III and Trophamine: Kendall-McGaw Laboratories, Irvine, CA; Travasol and Novamine: Travenol, Clintec, North Chicago, IL.

Source: Adapted from J.H. Cox and S.W. Cooning, Parenteral Nutrition, in *Handbook of Pediatric Nutrition,* P.M. Queen and C.E. Lang, eds., © 1993, Aspen Publishers, Inc.

of age in preterm infants and by 3 days of age in term infants.[84,85]

Cysteine supplementation does not increase overall nitrogen retention or improve growth in neonates when 120 mg/kg/day methionine is provided. The most commonly recommended dose for cysteine is 40 mg/g of protein for pediatric CAA products, but cysteine may not be needed for standard solutions, due to higher methionine content.[86–88] Adding L-cysteine hydrochloride decreases the solution's pH, which increases calcium and phosphorus solubility, thus increasing mineral delivery.[89]

Most of the studies evaluating the efficacy or comparing pediatric and standard CAA products have been done in small numbers of patients over a relatively short duration (5–21 days).[70,78–80,90] Although greater weight gain and nitrogen balance with pediatric products may be statistically significant, these differences may not be clinically significant. The greatest advantage seems to be that plasma amino acid patterns are similar to those of healthy breastfed neonates. What implications this has for use with older infants or children has not been clearly identified. Although the data are inconclusive, there may be a decreased incidence of cholestatic liver disease during pediatric CAA product administration.[88,91]

Practically, based on current literature, pediatric CAA products may be of benefit to the prematurely born infant or to the infant who requires long-term PN. Pediatric CAA products may require cysteine supplementation for

Table 25–7 Plasma Aminograms of Pediatric Patients on Parenteral Nutrition Compared to Plasma Aminograms of Healthy Breastfed Infants (mmol/dL)

Amino Acid	*Breast Milk*	*Aminosyn*		*Freamine III*		*Travasol*		*Aminosyn PF*		*Trophamine*	
		Mean	*SD*	*Mean*	*SD*	*Mean*	*SD*	*Mean*	*SD*	*Mean*	*SD*
Isoleucine	24–100	97	20	62	5	70	16	39	2	67	6
Leucine	53–169	125	24	78	18	71	18	59	2	113	10
Lysine	80–231	**299**	**54**	140	15	103	39	83	4	161	15
Methionine	19–50	**64**	**17**	**58**	**5**	**114**	**49**	**12**	1	44	4
Phenylalanine	22–71	**84**	**29**	**76**	**5**	**92**	**19**	28	1	71	3
Threonine	70–197	**288**	**78**	138	18	**279**	**67**	137	7	190	14
Tryptophan	18–101			43	3			20	1	30	2
Valine	88–222	**288**	**53**	155	11	130	26	**83**	**4**	177	15
Alanine	125–647	376	81	218	18	359	84	173	10	195	19
Arginine	42–148	140	50	79	5	124	46	44	3	86	8
Histidine	34–119	98	16	73	5	83	36	42	3	72	5
Proline	82–319	284	66	238	21	165	30	136	7	177	15
Serine	43–326	271	84	183	23	196	41	116	5	162	11
Tyrosine	38–119	**27**	**9**	**21**	**4**	71	33	**9**	**1**	75	8
Glycine	60–376	**699**	**142**	**532**	**40**	**993**	**266**	188	7	311	23
Cysteine	35–69	**5**	**5**	35	5	**34**	**11**	**5**	**1**	**44**	**3**
Glutamic Acid	24–243	**282**	**98**	70	9	509	133	189	16	63	6
Glutamine	142–850	304	138	366	34			**129**	**9**	386	43
Aspartic Acid	21–132	43	11	42	4	59	14	30	2	48	6
Taurine	1–167	97	57	50	11	82	44			73	6

Note: Mean protein intake range: 2.59–2.75 grams protein/per kilogram per day; mean caloric intake range 80–100 kcal/kg/d. SD = +/– 1 standard deviation. Bold print values indicate plasma amino acid levels outside target range.

Aminosyn and Aminosyn PF: Abbott Laboratories, North Chicago, IL; Freamine III and Trophamine: Kendall-McGaw Laboratories, Irvine, CA; Travasol: Travenol, Baxter Healthcare Corporation, North Chicago, IL.

Data from references 70, and 78–81.

Source: Reprinted from J.H. Cox and S.W. Cooning, Parenteral Nutrition, in *Handbook of Pediatric Nutrition,* P.M. Queen and C.E. Lang, eds., © 1993, Aspen Publishers, Inc.

infants younger than 4 months of age (55–77 mg/kg/day), due to inadequate cystathionase activity, and for all other infants and children (3–22 mg cysteine per gram of total amino acid content), due to reduced methionine concentration.[70,84,86–88]

Special solutions of L-isomer CAA, formulated for adults with severe hepatic or renal failure, appear to be efficacious also in children with severe hepatic or chronic renal failure, though standard CAA solutions may better meet the amino acid needs of children with acute renal failure.[92–96] Older children with sepsis or traumatic injury may benefit from using formulations with increased amounts of branched-chain amino acids.[97]

FAT

Fat is included in PN regimens for infants and children as a source of essential fatty acids and energy. Linoleic acid deficiency is clinically manifested as dry, flaky skin, dry hair, poor growth, decreased platelets, and impaired wound healing. Biochemical deficiency of linoleic acid precedes these clinical manifestations. Plasma levels of linoleic, arachidonic, and eicosatrienoic acids are low, and the ratio of plasma eicosatrienoic acid (triene/tetraene) is elevated. Numbness, paresthesia, weakness, inability to walk, and blurring of vision may occur if linolenic acid deficiency is present.[4,98] Very low-birth-weight infants or infants and children with depleted body stores of fat or with a chronic history of fat malabsorption are at greatest risk of developing essential fatty acid deficiencies.[99]

Providing as little as 1–2% of the total daily caloric intake as linoleic acid and 0.54% of the total daily caloric intake as linolenic acid can prevent deficiency.[42] The fatty acid content of parenteral lipid emulsion products is given in Table 25–8. Although products vary in their essential fatty acid content, providing 4% of total calories as lipid (0.5 g of fat or 2.5 mL of 20% lipid emulsion per kilogram per day) prevents essential fatty acid deficiency in most infants and children. Intravenous products made with medium-chain triglyceride (MCT) oil are not available in the United States but are available in Europe. Theoretically, products containing MCT oil may provide advantages of more rapid hydrolyzation and oxidation, with improved tolerance and better energy delivery, but they also contain lower amounts of essential fatty acids.[65]

Limitations of glucose or fluid tolerance and high energy needs usually dictate a greater intake of lipid than that which prevents deficiency. Fifty percent of energy intake is derived from fat in the breastfed infant. Parenteral lipid doses of 2.5–3.0 g/kg/day provide infants with only 25–30% of total energy intake as fat, but higher doses may be poorly tolerated, especially in premature or small-for-gestational-age infants.[42,69,100,101] In children over 2 years of age, it may be advisable to limit fat to 30% of total calories (generally, 1.5–2.5 g/kg/day), as recommended by the American Academy of Pediatrics.[102] Fat should not provide more than 60% of total calories in any patient because ketotic acidosis may occur.[103]

Adverse effects of intravenous fat, when given in boluses or in doses exceeding 3.6 g/kg/day, have been reported, including altered pulmonary function, impaired neutrophil function, and an increased risk of kernicterus in infants with elevated serum bilirubin level.[104–106] Preterm or malnourished infants and children may be at greater risk for impaired fat tolerance, due to decreased adipose tissue mass, reduced lipoprotein lipase activity, hepatic immaturity, or carnitine deficiency. Whereas heparin stimulates the release of lipoprotein lipase, it may not significantly affect lipid clearance over time and is not routinely recommended for that purpose.

Intravenous fat may be safely given if: (1) the initial dose is 0.5 g/kg/day and it is gradually increased by 0.25–0.5 g/kg/day; (2) the highest dose is < 0.12 g/kg/hour (3 g/kg/day) or < 0.08 g/kg/hour (2 mg/kg/day) during periods of acute sepsis; (3) it is given over 24 hours whenever possible; and (4) serum triglycerides are monitored and kept within the normal range, although

Table 25–8 Composition of Intravenous Fat Emulsions

	Intralipid 10% (Intralipid 20%)*	*Liposyn† II 10% (Liposyn II 20%)*	*Liposyn† III 10% (Liposyn III 20%)*	*Soyacal‡ 10% (Soyacal 20%)*	*Nutrilipid§ 10% (Nutrilipid 20%)*
Concentration (g/dL)	10 (20)	10 (20)	10 (20)	10 (20)	10 (20)
Fat source (g/dL)					
Soybean oil	10 (20)	5 (10)	10 (20)	10 (20)	10 (20)
Safflower oil		5 (10)			
Fatty acid content (Percent of total fat)					
Linoleic	50	65.8	54.5	49–60	49–60
Oleic	26	17.7	22.4	21–26	21–26
Palmitic	10	8.8	10.5	9–13	9–13
Stearic	3.5	3.4	4.2	3–5	3–5
Linolenic	9	4.2	8.3	6–9	6–9
Egg phosphatides (g/dL)	1.2	1.2	1.2	1.2	1.2
Glycerol (g/dL)	2.25	2.5	2.5	2.21	2.21
Osmolality (mOsm/L)	260	276 (258)	284 (292)	280 (315)	280 (315)
pH	6–8.9	6–9	6–9	6–7.9	6–7.9
Calories (kcal/mL)	1.1 (2.0)	1.1 (2.0)	1.1 (2.0)	1.1 (2.0)	1.1 (2.0)

* Clintec Nutrition Company, Deerfield, IL.
† Abbott Laboratories, North Chicago, IL.
‡ Alpha Therapeutic Corporation, Los Angeles, CA.
§ Kendall-McGaw Laboratories, Santa Ana, CA.

Source: Reprinted from J. H. Cox and S.W. Cooning, Parenteral Nutrition, in *Handbook of Pediatric Nutrition,* P.M. Queen and C.E. Lang, eds., © 1993, Aspen Publishers, Inc.

there are various recommendations given in the literature for the acceptable upper limit of normal, from 150 to 250 mg/dL.[104,105]

If serum bilirubin levels are greater than 8–10 mg/dL (while the serum albumin level is 2.5 to 3 g/dL), lipids should be given only in amounts adequate to prevent essential fatty acid deficiency.[106] If intravenous fat is given in greater amounts or given in bolus doses, the free fatty acid/serum albumin molar ratio should be maintained at less than 6 while bilirubin levels remain elevated[42] (see Chapter 3 for further discussion on this issue).

Studies are somewhat conflicting regarding whether carnitine supplementation facilitates parenteral lipid utilization.[107–110] Carnitine is normally synthesized by the liver from methionine and lysine, but pediatric amino acid solutions are lower in methionine than standard solutions. Dose recommendations for oral or intravenous supplementation of carnitine vary from 15 to 70 mmol/kg/day (2–11 mg/kg/day). Doses 10–30 times this level in neonates may result in impaired growth. Although carnitine is not routinely added to PN solutions at this time, it is available for use. Patients at highest risk of carnitine depletion include very-low-birth-weight infants without an exogenous source of carnitine and patients receiving chronic dialysis therapy for end-stage renal disease. Laboratory indicators for carnitine supplementation may include hypertriglyeridemia, hypoglycemia, and low serum carnitine.[108]

VITAMINS

Recommendations for vitamin administration are given in Table 25–9. Recommendations for term infants and children up to 11 years of age were established by the Nutrition Advisory Group of the American Medical Association in 1975.[111] They are based on the 1974 Recommended Dietary Allowances (RDAs), which are guidelines for enteral nutrient intake (Appendix K). Recommendations for adolescents are based on guidelines for adults. Vitamin requirements of premature infants may vary from those of term infants, due to the immaturity of enzyme systems and renal function. Current recommendations are based on numerous studies and extrapolations from term infant data.[63] The vitamin content of MVI Pediatric for Infusion and MVI-12 Multivitamin Infusion (Astra USA, Inc.) are compared with the current vitamin dose recommendations in Table 25–9.

Studies have shown the Food and Drug Administration's current dose recommendations to produce serum levels at or above the reference range for α-tocopherol, 25-hydroxycholecalciferol, thiamin, riboflavin, niacin, pyridoxine, folate, pantothenic acid, cyanocobalamin, and biotin.[112,113] There are no reports of toxic vitamin levels using these recommended doses.

Levels of several vitamins may decrease over time in parenteral nutrient admixtures, due to light degradation, decomposition in the presence of bisulfite (an antioxidant additive) or varying pH, and adsorbence to plastic or glass. For these reasons, it is recommended that multivitamins be added to parenteral nutrient solutions immediately prior to administration, excessive light exposure (direct sunlight or phototherapy light) be avoided, and administration of these admixtures be completed within 24 hours.

MINERALS

Magnesium

Magnesium deficiency is identified by decreased serum levels. Hypomagnesemia may be seen in protein-calorie malnutrition, chronic malabsorption, proximal jejunal resection, ileostomy, cystic fibrosis, neonatal hepatitis, congenital biliary atresia, DiGeorge's syndrome, infants born to diabetic mothers, during chronic diuretic therapy, or during chemotherapy.[10] If seizures occur, repletion dose is 0.2 mEq/kg, given intramuscularly or intravenously every 6 hours until symptoms subside. Blood pressure should be monitored with intravenous magnesium repletion, because hypotension may occur.[42]

Table 25–9 Recommendations for Pediatric Parenteral Daily Vitamin Dosage

Age (in years)	*A* *IU*	*D* *IU*	*E* *mg*	*K* *μg*	*C* *mg*	*B1* *mg*	*B2* *mg*	*B3* *mg*	*B6* *mg*	*B12* *μg*	*FA* *μg*	*PA* *mg*	*biotin* *μg*
Preterm infants (≤ 2.5 kg) (dose per kg)*	1700	160	2.8	80	25	0.35	0.15	6.8	0.18	0.3	56	2	6
MVI Pediatric† (40% dose/kg)*	920	160	2.8	80	32	0.48	0.56	6.8	0.4	0.4	56	2	8
Preterm infants (>2,5 kg) (dose per day)	700–1500	40–160	2–4	6–10	35–50	0.3–0.8	0.4–0.9	5–12	0.3–0.7	0.3–0.7	40–90	2–5	6–13
Term infants, children 1–11 (dose per day)	2300	400	5–7	200	80	1.2	1.4	17	1.0	1.0	140	5	20
MVI Pediatric† (1 dose)	2300	400	7	200	80	1.2	1.4	17	1.0	1.0	140	5	20
Adolescents (dose per day)	3300	200	10	150–700	100	3.0	3.6	40	4.0	5.0	400	15	60
MVI-12 Multivitamin† (1 dose)	3300	200	10	‡	100	3.0	3.6	40	4.0	5.0	400	15	60

Note: A = retinol, D = cholecalciferol, E = α-tocopherol, K = phytonadione, B1= thiamin, B2 = riboflavin, B3= niacin, B6 = pyridoxine, B12 = cyanocobalamin, FA = folic acid, PA = pantothenic acid

* maximum dose not to exceed 1 full dose

† Pediatric MVI = Pediatric parenteral multivitamin, Astra USA. Inc., 50 Otis Street, Westboro, MA 01581-4500.

‡ vitamin K is not included in adult parenteral multivitamin preparations, but can be given separately 1–5 mg/week intramuscularly

Data from references 4, 63, 65, 105 and product literature.

Parenteral doses of 0.5 mEq/kg/day may be needed to allow adequate retention for premature infants, though general dose recommendations for all other infants and children are 0.25–1.0 mEq/kg/day of magnesium, with a maximum allowable dose of 25 mEq/day.[42,69,101] Upper-range doses may be needed during rapid growth phases, diuretic therapy, or chronic malabsorption. Lower-range doses may be indicated if renal function is impaired. Magnesium is added to parenteral admixtures as magnesium sulfate (50% $MgSO_4$), which contains 4.1 mEq (49.3 mg) of magnesium per milliliter. Excessive doses may cause central nervous system depression and hypotonia.[63]

Calcium

Calcium deficiency is not usually identified by low serum levels. If calcium intake is insufficient, serum calcium is maintained at the expense of bone stores in most infants and children.[63] Hypocalcemia is most common during the neonatal period, particularly in premature infants, due to their relatively low calcium stores and inappropriately low parathyroid hormone levels. This initial hypocalcemia usually resolves within the first few days of life when treated with intravenous administration of calcium 1–2 mEq/kg/day.[77]

Nutrition recommendations for parenteral calcium administration to prematurely born infants are generally 50–90 mg/kg/day (which is 1.3–2.3 mmol/kg/day or 2.5–4.5 mEq/kg/day).[63,105,114,115] Most published sources empirically recommend 10–50 mg/kg/day (which is 0.25–1.3 mmol/kg/day or 0.5–2.0 mEq/kg/day) for all other ages[37] (see Table 25–2). Calcium should be administered over 24 hours because parenteral calcium administered chronically as bolus doses over 20 minutes to 1 hour has been associated with hypercalcemia and hypercalciuria.[116,117] Nephrolithiasis and hypercalciuria have been associated with furosemide therapy and inadequate phosphorus intake.[114,118] Older children receiving cyclic PN may have greater urinary losses of calcium.[119]

Calcium gluconate is generally the additive of choice, though there is some concern about aluminum contamination, especially at higher doses.[120] Solutions that deliver 15–30 mcg aluminum/kg/day may result in tissue loading and are considered unsafe.[63,121] Calcium gluconate 10% contains 100 mg of calcium gluconate per milliliter, which provides approximately 0.5 mEq, 0.25 mmol, or 10 mg of elemental calcium per milliliter.

Phosphorus

Phosphorus depletion has been reported in infants and children. It is characterized by hypercalciuria (at least 4 mg/kg/day of calcium), hypophosphatemia (serum levels less than 4 mg/dL), and undetectable levels of urinary phosphorus excretion.[63,122,123] Parenteral repletion of phosphorus may be accomplished by an initial dose of 5–9 mg/kg (0.15–0.3 mmol/kg), given over 6 hours. Excessive phosphorus administration may cause hyperphosphatemia, hypocalcemia, and secondary hyperparathyroidism.[63]

Recommendations for parenteral administration of phosphorus to infants and children are given in Table 25–2. Doses for phosphorus are often given in proportion to calcium as 1:1 molar ratio or 1.3:1 calcium/phosphorus ratio by weight.[63] Phosphorus is added to parenteral nutrient solutions as potassium or sodium phosphate salts. Potassium phosphate contains 93 mg (3 mmol) of phosphorus and 4.4 mEq of potassium per milliliter. Sodium phosphate contains 93 mg (3 mmol) of phosphorus and 4 mEq of sodium per milliliter.

The greatest difficulty in providing adequate calcium and phosphorus parenterally is their relative insolubility in the same admixture, limited further by increasing pH and temperature. Alternating calcium and phosphorus administration results in adverse effects of alternating elevations of serum and urinary excretion of calcium and phosphorus.[124] Recommendations for compounding to minimize precipitation usually include adding phosphate salts early in the process and calcium salts late (but before the lipid emulsion in 3-in-1 admixtures).[89,125] Adherence to compounding protocol is particularly important when lipid is present, because precipitates are more difficult to identify, due to the opacity of the admixture. The addition of L-cysteine increases mineral solubility, and the use of calcium glycerophosphate or monobasic phosphate formulations may also improve solubility.[38] Solubility studies and guidelines for simultaneous administration of calcium and phosphorus have been published for various amino acid products.[124–127] Filters are recommended to prevent precipitate delivery if they occur—a 1.2-micron air-eliminating filter for lipid-containing admixtures and a 0.22-micron air-eliminating filter for non–lipid-containing admixtures.[125] The higher doses of minerals needed for young infants are given through central intravenous access to prevent vascular damage and tissue sloughs. Separate administration of lipid may be needed to allow higher concentrations of calcium and phosphorus for prematurely born infants.

Trace Minerals

Recommendations for daily parenteral doses are given in Table 25–2.[63,128] Zinc, copper, chromium, manganese, selenium, and iodine are available singly or in combination for use in PN admixtures. Neither clinical nor biochemical deficiency of molybdenum or iodine with PN has been reported in the literature, and they are generally not included in PN admixtures. Transdermal absorption of iodine from cleansing or disinfecting solutions or ointments may be an adequate source of iodine.[129] Fluorine is not added because its role in human nutrition is limited primarily to dental health and may be of greater benefit when administered topically once teeth have erupted, around 6 months of age.[64]

Very low-birth-weight infants and infants and children with protein-calorie malnutrition, thermal injury, neoplasms, chronic diarrhea, enterocutaneous fistulas, or bile salt malabsorption are at greatest risk for developing trace element deficiency.[130–133] Zinc supplementation without copper supplementation may interfere with copper metabolism.[132] Copper doses are reduced or eliminated, and manganese is withheld for infants and children who develop cholestatic jaundice because these minerals are excreted primarily through bile, and their accumulation is potentially hepatotoxic.[42,131,133] To prevent the occurrence of copper deficiency when copper intake is reduced or eliminated, regular monitoring of serum copper and/or ceruloplasmin may be indicated. Selenium and molybdenum are not generally used when PN is required for only a short period of time. Selenium may be present as a trace contaminant in parenteral dextrose solutions in amounts up to 0.9 mg/dL of solution. Parenteral selenium toxicity has not been reported, though lower doses may be indicated when renal function is impaired.[63]

Iron deficiency is probably the most common trace mineral deficiency. It manifests as microcytic hypochromic anemia and is characterized by low serum hemoglobin and ferritin levels, low hematocrit, and low percentage of transferrin saturation. Infants and children at risk for iron deficiency include those who are prematurely born, chronically ill, protein-calorie malnourished, have significant unreplaced blood loss, or who receive unsupplemented PN for long periods of time.

There is some controversy over whether iron should be routinely included in PN therapy. Intramuscular injections of iron are not recommended in the small, prematurely born infant or the protein-calorie malnourished patient, due to small muscle mass and increased risk of sarcoma at the site of injection.[134] Anaphylaxis has been reported in some patients with administration of iron dextran.[135] Several authors report that iron may be safely given daily in PN admixtures or in bolus doses given intravenously over 2–3 hours weekly or monthly.[134–137] Often, iron is given parenterally only in treatment of iron deficiency anemia.

Although standard iron dose recommendations for prematurely born infants are 0.2 mg/kg/day,[63,138] trials of recombinant erythropoietin have used iron supplements of 1 mg/kg/day without evidence of harmful side effects, though these are short-term studies.[139,140] Iron toxicity may be difficult to ascertain because iron is quickly stored in hepatic tissue, and serum iron levels may not reflect overload. Excess iron may also increase risk of gram-negative septicemia and increase antioxidant requirements. These risks do not preclude use of standard doses of parenteral iron, but higher doses must be used with caution beyond 4 weeks' duration.[63] Iron doses of 0.1 mg/kg/day up to 1 mg/day total dose are recommended for term infants and children.

Iron dextran is available as the source of iron for parenteral use. Guidelines for dosage and administration of iron dextran in treatment of iron deficiency are given in the manufacturer's package insert.

PATIENT MONITORING

A comprehensive monitoring program for infants and children receiving PN includes evaluation of laboratory measurements of metabolic and electrolyte status (see Table 25–4), anthropometric measurements (see Table 25–10), intake and output measurements, and physical examination (see Table 25–11). Baseline and regularly scheduled laboratory measurements allow timely identification of metabolic complications and assessment of nutritional adequacy. Metabolic complications that may occur during pediatric nutritional support are summarized in Table 25–5. Laboratory values obtained are compared with neonatal and/or pediatric norms, which are often different from adult norms (see Chapter 2). Laboratory monitoring protocols may vary from one setting to another but should take into consideration smaller blood volumes in pediatric patients, using microtechniques whenever possible and avoiding unnecessary blood work. For patients on long-term PN, the need and frequency for some tests can be reevaluated once a stable regimen has been established.

Suggested physical monitoring is given in Table 25–11. Temperature instability, apnea and bradycardia, and increased respirations and pulse may be early signs of sepsis in the pediatric patient. Records of intake provide documen-

Table 25–10 Growth Parameters Monitored During Pediatric Parenteral Nutrition

Parameter	*Frequency*
Weight	Daily (neonates up to 1 month corrected age) Weekly (1–6 months corrected age) Monthly (infants > 6 months corrected age, children)
Length or Height	Weekly (infants < 6 months corrected age) Monthly (infants > 6 months corrected age) Every 3 months (ages 1–3) Every 6 months (ages 4–18)
Head Circumference	Weekly (infants < 6 months corrected age) Monthly (infants > 6 months corrected age) Every 3 months (ages 1–3)
Body Composition Triceps Skinfold Arm Muscle Area	As clinically indicated; comparison against established norms is more useful in children > 3 years than in younger children.

tation that actual administration equals planned intake. Documentation of output establishes a basis for evaluation of fluid balance, as does evaluation of skin turgor and the presence of edema. Insertion sites are monitored for redness, swelling, leaking, or other signs of infection or infiltration. Changes in behavior and/or mental status may precede other signs of sepsis or fluid and electrolyte imbalance.

PSYCHOSOCIAL ISSUES

Eating is basic to life. Parents feed their infants and children. When normal feeding is replaced with PN, parents may feel helpless or useless. An infant or child of any age may feel frustrated at not being able to eat. Older children may have fears or insecurities about body function or body image. The ability of an infant or child and their family to accept and adapt to PN depends on the presenting diagnosis, the acuity or chronicity of the disease or condition, the duration and complexity of the hospitalization, the duration of nutrition support therapy, and the physical and emotional development of the infant or child.[141] When long-term or home PN is needed, the stability of the family unit and their financial, physical, and emotional resources are important factors as well.

Keeping the family informed, providing consistent support through a social worker, care manager, and/or primary nurse, and involving the family and child (appropriately for age and level of understanding) in the actual care activities can empower the family and child to meet some of their own needs and to lessen their feelings of helplessness. Family involvement is crucial in preparing a family for successful home PN.

Members of the hospital-based multidisciplinary team, including the physician, nurse, dietitian, pharmacist, social worker, and developmental specialist must plan a program of home PN that is feasible, given the resources of the family and the community. Resources that support success of home PN are listed in Table 25–12. Education of family members must take into account their readiness and ability to learn. Assessment of learning includes measuring the family's ability to repeat instructions accurately or to demonstrate techniques. Communication with home health care providers is essential for continuity of care.

The technical nature of PN must not overshadow the infant or child and their de-

Table 25–11 Clinical Monitoring During Pediatric Parenteral Nutrition

Clinical Parameter	*Initial*	*Stable*
Temperature Pulse/Respirations	Hourly, then every 4–8 hr	Daily or as indicated
Intake	Hourly, then every 4–8 hr	Daily
Output	Hourly, then every 4 to 8 hr	As indicated
Administration system	Hourly, then every 4–8 hr	Daily
Infusion site/dressing	Hourly, then every 4–8 hr	Daily
Mental status, behavioral status, edema, skin turgor	Every 4–8 hr	Daily or as indicated

Table 25–12 Resources that Support Successful Home Parenteral Nutrition

Environment	Grounded electrical outlets; backup electricity, either battery, generator, or power company priority when there is loss of power
	Lack of physical barriers to maneuvering equipment or storing supplies
	Refrigeration to store adequate supplies of solutions
	Reliable telephone service
	Convenient and safe water supply and hand-washing facilities
Medical support	Convenient and reliable home health care agency for nursing care, ongoing nutritional assessment, supplies, laboratory assessment
	Local physician experienced and amenable to home parenteral nutrition
	Responsive local community emergency care, both ambulance and local emergency room
Family characteristics	At least two responsible adults are competent to provide all care associated with home parenteral nutrition; extended family support
	All children (both the patient and siblings, particularly small children) are protected from harm associated with home parenteral nutrition, such as needle sticks, damage to catheter, tubing, or other equipment, removal of catheter, etc.
Financial	Adequate medical insurance coverage with certified medical necessity for home parenteral nutrition
Attitude	Family and patient must see home parenteral nutrition as having a positive influence on the life of the child
	Respect for risks and safety issues associated with parenteral nutrition
	Ability and willingness to comply with medical plan and techniques

velopmental progress. Occupational and physical therapists, speech pathologists, and child life and/or developmental specialists ensure that the hospital setting is modified as much as possible to support the normal development of the child on PN.

For the neonate whose feedings are limited or who is unable to take oral feedings, pleasant oral stimulation, nonnutritive sucking, and other sensory stimulation is needed to support normal oral development. Prolonged, early oral deprivation can lead to increased oral sensitivity and abnormal tongue movements that can adversely influence the development of future speech patterns.[142] Eating is such a basic, essential function that many parents, particularly the mother, may feel responsible for their infant's problems and may suffer loss of self-esteem or have feelings of inadequacy at being unable to perform the simple caregiving task of feeding. Health care professionals can enhance parents' involvement in "feeding" the PN-dependent infant by encouraging them to hold, cuddle, and offer other forms of oral stimulation during "normal" feeding times. When possible, the infant on PN should be offered some type of oral feeding, if only in very small amounts. If totally deprived of oral sustenance, the introduction of oral feedings may be met with gagging, vomiting, swallowing difficulties, or other signs of feeding aversion.

Infants use their mouths to explore much of their environment. Sucking on fingers or toys can be encouraged to help infants experience and develop trust in their environment. Other types of tactile and visual stimulation can be provided to distract infants from manipulating or chewing on tubes and equipment. Creative ways to protect equipment and maintain safety should be used, rather than physical restraint. Clothing that covers the catheter insertion site and tubing helps prevent pulling and manipulation of equipment and allows a less limited exploration of the environment.

Toddlers present many challenges to the safe delivery of PN. These challenges may include temperament, mobility, and the development of other normal milestones, such as toileting. Creative strategies to allow toddlers some control and independence in their environment can promote autonomy and lessen the negative impact of hospitalization or home PN on normal development. Providing clothes, toys, and photographs from home, sibling visits, and a high level of parent involvement can help the young child deal with the fear of painful procedures, the strange hospital environment, separation from loved ones, and feelings that the illness is a punishment for being naughty. A backpack that contains solution, pump, and tubing in fastened compartments can allow mobility and prevent toddlers from handling equipment, but it allows parents easy access for managing PN. Nocturnal cyclic PN may reduce interference with developmental needs.

The school-aged child who is frequently hospitalized and requires PN needs to maintain involvement in school and with friends, to have some conformity with peers in appearance, and to have as much control over personal issues as possible. In-hospital teachers or private tutors may be needed to maintain educational progress. Choices for the child are offered whenever possible, including selection of the type and placement of the CVC and assisting with dressing changes. An established routine that allows the child to accomplish as many aspects of care as possible is important to avoid feelings of inferiority and to prevent excessive dependency. During home PN, children are encouraged to resume as many normal school and play activities as their clinical condition allows.

Although the technical aspects of PN in the adolescent may be easier to manage, other issues may present greater challenges. With greater intellectual and social sophistication, the adolescent may have concerns, fears, and/or anxiety regarding many issues, such as loss of control, altered body image or appearance, peer acceptance or isolation, dependence on technology, technical failures or malfunctions, health and life expectancy, ability to participate in sports and other peer group activities, financial issues, and the effects on other family members. Sleep disturbances may occur, due to anxiety or frequent urination that occurs with nocturnal fluid administration. Many of these issues may cause anger or depression and lead to poor compliance with the therapeutic regimen.

Backpacks or vests designed to hold PN solutions and equipment may be used to maximize mobility and to minimize changes in physical appearance. Nocturnal cyclic PN circumvents changes in appearance during the day and places less limitation on activities with peers. Other strategies to improve compliance with the PN regimen include: (1) providing information using appropriate terminology for age and educational level, (2) encouraging active participation in decision making and management of PN, and (3) providing psychologic counseling when needed.

REIMBURSEMENT

In response to rapidly escalating health care costs starting in the mid-1970s, reimbursement strategies have been dramatically changing. Parenteral nutrition is a complex and expensive therapy. Costs include nutrient solutions; technical equipment, such as catheters, tubing, and automated pumps; laboratory monitoring; and health care providers, such as physicians, nurses, dietitians, pharmacists, and developmental therapists. Though PN administered at home may generate fewer costs, it is still expensive.

In efforts to contain health care costs, many third-party payers have developed regulations that restrict who can be reimbursed and what is reimbursed, and they place a capitation on reimbursement for PN.[143] Parenteral nutrition provided in the hospital may be considered part of "room and board" because nutrition/feeding is considered a basic need. Because PN is not a directly reimbursed service, reimbursement often depends on the assigned primary diagnosis or specific diagnosis-related group (DRG), or comorbid condition (CC). DRGs or CCs that include the presence of malnutrition or nonfunctioning GI tract with malabsorption are often required, particularly in the home setting. Medical necessity for PN must be justified by the prescribing physician at initiation of therapy and periodically throughout the course of therapy. Even then, reimbursement is usually less than 100%, which leaves the family (or supplemental insurance) with the remaining costs.

Health care providers who prescribe and/or monitor PN should keep abreast of changes in regulations governing reimbursement. Documentation is needed regarding effectiveness and outcomes with PN in terms of costs and benefits from length of hospital stay and complication rates to quality of life and functional status. If PN yields no perceived benefit, it is not needed, and those who provide it will not be reimbursed. Constant efforts must be employed to control costs, whether exploring effective but less expensive modalities of care or designing clinical pathways or standardized policies that maximize the effectiveness of PN.

REFERENCES

1. Steinhorn DM. Nutrition in the PICU: Who needs it? Guidelines for nutritional support of critically ill children. In: Green TP, Zucher AR, eds. *Current Concepts in Pediatric Critical Care.* Chicago: Society of Critical Care Medicine; 1996:77–86.
2. Archer S, Burnett R, Fischer J. Current uses and abuses of total parenteral nutrition. In: *Advances in Surgery.* Chicago: Mosby-Year Book; 1996:29:165–189.
3. Chellis MJ, Sanders SV, Webster H, et al. Early enteral feeding in the pediatric intensive care unit. *J Parenter Enter Nutr.* 1996;20:71–73.
4. Teitelbaum DH, Coran AG. Perioperative nutritional support in pediatrics. *Nutrition.* 1998;14:130.
5. Davis A. Pediatrics. In: Matarese LE, Gottschlich MM, eds. *Contemporary Nutrition Support Practice.* Philadelphia: WB Saunders Co; 1998:349–351.
6. Fisher G, Opper F. An interdisciplinary nutrition support team improves quality of care in a teaching hospital. *J Am Diet Assoc.* 1996;96:176.
7. Fisher A, Poole R, Machie R, et al. Clinical pathway for pediatric parenteral nutrition. *Nutr Clin Pract.* 1997;12:76.
8. American Society for Parenteral and Enteral Nutrition. Guidelines for the use of parenteral and enteral nutrition in adult and pediatric patients. *J Parenter Enter Nutr.* 1993;17(suppl):27SA–52SA.
9. Okada A. Clinical indications of parenteral and enteral nutrition support in pediatric patients. *Nutrition.* 1988; 14:116–118.
10. Sondheimer JM, Cadnapaphornchai M, Sontag M, et al. Predicting the duration of dependence on parenteral nutrition after neonatal intestinal resection. *J Pediatr.* 1998;132:80–84.
11. Sitrin MD. Nutrition support in inflammatory bowel disease. *Nutr Clin Pract.* 1992;7:53–60.
12. Polk DB, Hattner JA, Kerner JA Jr. Improved growth and disease activity after intermittent administration of

a defined formula diet in children with Crohn's disease. *J Parenter Enter Nutr*. 1992;16:499–504.

13. Rickard KA, Grosfield JL, Kirksey A, et al. Reversal of protein-energy malnutrition in children during treatment of advanced neoplastic disease. *Ann Surg*. 1979; 190:771.
14. Filler RM, Dietz W, Suskind RM, et al. Parenteral feeding in management of children with cancer. *Cancer*. 1979;43(suppl):2117.
15. Copeland EM, MacFadgen BV, Dudrick SJ. Effect of intravenous hyperalimentation on established delayed hypersensitivity in the the cancer patient. *Ann Surg*. 1976;184:60.
16. Copeland EM, Daly JM, Ota DM, et al. Nutrition, cancer, and intravenous hyperalimentation. *Cancer*. 1979; 43:2108.
17. Andrassy RJ, Chwals WJ. Nutritional support of the pediatric oncology patient. *Nutrition*. 1998;14:124–129.
18. Christensen ML, Hancock ML, Gattuso J, et al. Parenteral nutrition associated with increased infection rate in children with cancer. *Cancer*. 1993;72:2732–2738.
19. Copeman MC. Use of total parenteral nutrition in children with cancer: A review and some recommendations. *Pediatr Hematol Oncol*. 1994;11:463–470.
20. Perl M. TPN and the anorexia nervosa patient. *Nutr Suppl Serv*. 1981;1:13.
21. Pertschuk MJ, Forster J, Buzby G, et al. The treatment of anorexia nervosa with total parenteral nutrition. *Biol Psychiatr*. 1981;16:539.
22. Andrew M, Marzinotto V, Pencharz P, et al. A cross-sectional study of catheter-related thrombosis in children receiving total parenteral nutrition at home. *J Pediatr*. 1995;126:358–363.
23. Chung D, Ziegler M. Central venous catheter access. *Nutrition*. 1988;14:119–123.
24. Chathas MK. Percutaneous central venous catheters in neonates. *J Obstet Gynecol Neonatal Nurs*. 1986;15: 324.
25. Dolcourt JL, Bose CL. Percutaneous insertion of silastic central venous catheters. *Pediatrics*. 1982;70: 484.
26. Goodwin ML. The Seldinger method of PICC insertion. *J Intravenous Nurs*. 1989;12:238.
27. Brown JM. Peripherally inserted central catheters: Use in home care. *J Intravenous Nurs*. 1989;12:144.
28. Yeung CY, Lee HC, Huang FY, Wang CS. Sepsis during total parenteral nutrition: exploration of risk factors and determination of the effectiveness of peripherally inserted central venous catheters. *Pediatr Infect Dis J*. 1998;17:135–142.
29. Chathas MK, Paton JB. Sepsis outcomes in infants and children with central venous catheters: Percutaneous versus surgical insertion. *J Obstet Gynecol Neonatal Nurs*. 1996;25:500–506.
30. Dubois J, Garel L, Tapiero B, et al. Peripherally inserted central catheters in infants and children. *Radiology*. 1997; 204:622–626.
31. Pemberton LB, Lyman B, Lander V, Covinsky J. Sepsis from triple versus single lumen catheters during total parenteral nutrition in surgical or chronically ill patients. *Arch Surg*. 1986;121:591.
32. Yeung C, May J, Hughes R. Infection rate for single lumen versus triple lumen subclavian catheters. *Inf Control Hosp Epidemiol*. 1988;9:154.
33. Hughes CB. A totally implantable central venous system for chemotherapy administration. *NITA*. 1985;8: 523.
34. Storm HM, Young SL, Sandler RH. Development of pediatric and neonatal parenteral nutrition order forms. *Nutr Clin Pract*. 1995;10:54–59.
35. Puangco M, Nguyen H, Sheridan M. Computerized parenteral nutrition ordering optimizes timely nutrition therapy in a neonatal intensive care unit. *J Am Diet Assoc*. 1997;97:258–261.
36. Mirtallo J. Should the use of total nutrient admixtures be limited? *Am J Hosp Pharm*. 1994;51:2831–2836.
37. Neuzil J, Darlow BA, Inder TE, et al. Oxidation of parenteral lipid emulsion by ambient and phototherapy lights: Potential toxicity of routine parenteral feeding. *J Pediatr*. 1995;126(5):785–790.
38. Alwood M, Driscoll D, Sizer T, Ball P. Physicochemical assessment of total nutrient admixture stability and safety: Quantifying the risk. *Nutrition*. 1998;14(2): 166–167.
39. National Advisory Group on Standards and Practice Guidelines for Parenteral Nutrition. Safe practices for parenteral nutrition formulations. *J Parenter Enter Nutr*. 1998;22:49.
40. Driscoll D, Bacon M, Bistrian B. Effects of in-line filtration on lipid particle size distribution in total nutrient admixtures. *J Parenter Enter Nutr*. 1996;20:296–301.
41. Muller MJ. Hepatic complications in parenteral nutrition. *Z Gastroenterol*. 1996;34:36–40.
42. Kerner JA Jr, ed. *Manual of Pediatric Parenteral Nutrition*. New York: John Wiley & Sons; 1983.
43. Nelson WE, Behrman RE, Vaughan VC, eds. *Nelson's Textbook of Pediatrics*. 12th ed. Philadelphia: WB Saunders Co; 1983:231.
44. Lorenz JM, Kleinman LI, Ahmed G, et al. Phases of fluid and electrolyte homeostasis in the extremely low birth weight infant. *Pediatrics*. 1995;96:484.

45. Kerner JA Jr, Sunshine P. Parenteral alimentation. *Semin Perinatol*. 1979;3:417.

46. Oh W, Karechi H. Phototherapy and insensible water loss in the newborn infant. *Am J Dis Child*. 1972; 124:230.

47. Yeh TF, Voora S, Lillien J. Oxygen consumption and insensible water loss in premature infants in single versus double walled incubators. *J Pediatr*. 1980;97:967.

48. Gruskin AB. Fluid therapy in children. *Urol Clin North Am*. 1976;3:277.

49. Stevenson JG. Fluid administration in the association of patent ductus arteriosus complicating respiratory distress syndrome. *J Pediatr*. 1977;90:257.

50. Brown ER, Stark A, Sosenko I, et al. Bronchopulmonary dysplasia: Possible relationship to pulmonary edema. *J Pediatr*. 1978;92:982.

51. Goldman HI. Feeding and necrotizing enterocolitis. *Am J Dis Child*. 1980;134:553.

52. Goldberg RN, Chund D, Goldman SL, et al. The association of rapid volume expansion and intraventricular hemorrhage in the preterm infant. *J Pediatr*. 1980; 96:1060.

53. VanMarter LJ, Leviton A, Allred ENM, et al. Hydration during the first days of life and the risk of bronchopulmonary dysplasia in low birthweight infants. *J Pediatr*. 1990;116:942.

54. Rao M, Koenig E, Li S, et al. Estimation of insensible water loss in low birth weight infants by direct calorimetric measurement of metabolic heat release. *Pediatr Res*. 1989;25:295A.

55. Ford EG. Nutrition support of pediatric patients. *Nutr Clin Pract*. 1996;11:183.

56. Aperia A, Broberger O, Elinder G, Herin P, Zetterstrom R. Postnatal development of renal function in pre-term and full-term infants. *Acta Paediatr Scand*. 1981;70:183.

57. Peters O, Ryan S, Matthew L, et al. Randomised controlled trial of acetate in preterm neonates receiving parenteral nutrition. *Arch Dis Child*. 1997;77:F12.

58. Eunice J, Klavdianou M, Vidyasagar D. Electrolyte problems in neonatal surgical patients. *Clin Perinatol*. 1989;16:219.

59. Groh-Wargo S, Ciaccia A, Moore J. Neonatal metabolic acidosis: effect of chloride from normal saline flushes. *J Parenter Enter Nutr*. 1988;12:159.

60. Tilden SJ, Watkins S, Tong TK, Jeevanandam M. Measured energy expenditure in pediatric intensive care patients. *Am J Dis Child*. 1989;143:490.

61. Lowery GH. *Growth and Development of Children*, 6th ed. Chicago: Year Book Medical Publishers, 1973: 331–332.

62. Heird WC, Kashyap S, Gomez MR. Parenteral alimentation of the neonate. *Semin Perinatol*. 1991;15:493.

63. Greene HL, Hambidge KM, Schanler R, et al. Guidelines for the use of vitamins, trace elements, calcium, magnesium, and phosphorus in infants and children receiving total parenteral nutrition: Report of the Subcommittee on Pediatric Parenteral Nutrient Requirements from the Committee on Clinical Practice Issues of The American Society for Clinical Nutrition. *Am J Clin Nutr*. 1988;48:1324. (Revised in 1990.)

64. Committee on Nutrition, American Academy of Pediatrics. In: Kleinman RE, ed. *Pediatric Nutrition Handbook*. Elk Grove Village, IL: American Academy of Pediatrics; 1998:285–305.

65. Adamkin DH. Total parenteral nutrition. *Neonatal Intensive Care*. 1997;Sept/Oct:24.

66. Chwals WJ. Overfeeding the critically ill child: Fact or fantasy? *New Horizons*. 1994;2:147.

67. Chwals WJ, Lally KP, Woolley MM, et al. Measured energy expenditure in critically ill infants and young children. *J Surg Res*. 1988;44:467.

68. Zlotkin SH, Bryan MH, Anderson GH. Intravenous nitrogen and energy intakes required to duplicate in utero nitrogen accretion in prematurely born human infants. *J Pediatr*. 1981;99:115.

69. Khaldi N, Coran AG, Wesley JR. Guidelines for parenteral nutrition in children. *Nutr Suppl Serv*. 1984; 4:27.

70. Cochran EB, Phelps SJ, Helms RA. Parenteral nutrition in pediatric patients. *Clin Pharm*. 1988;7:351.

71. Sajbel TA, Dutro MP, Radway PR. Use of separate insulin infusions with total parenteral nutrition. *J Parenter Enter Nutr*. 1987;11:97.

72. Groh-Wargo S. Prematurity/low birth weight. In: Lang C, ed. *Nutritional Support in Critical Care*. Gaithersburg, MD: Aspen Publishers; 1987:287.

73. Rubecz I, Mestyan J, Varga P, Klujber L. Energy metabolism, substrate utilization, and nitrogen balance in parenterally fed postoperative neonates and infants. *J Pediatr*. 1981;98:42.

74. Duffy B, Gunn T, Collinge J, et al. The effect of varying protein quality and energy intake on the nitrogen metabolism of parenterally fed very low birth weight (< 1600 g) infants. *Pediatr Res*. 1981;15:1040.

75. Anderson TL, Muttart CR, Bilber MA, et al. A controlled trial of glucose versus glucose and amino acids in premature infants. *J Pediatr*. 1979;94:947.

76. Zlotkin SH, Stallings VA, Pencharz PB. Total parenteral nutrition in children. *Pediatr Clin North Am*. 1985;32:381.

77. Adan D, LaGamma EF, and Browne LE. Nutritional management and the multisystem organ failure/systemic inflammatory response syndrome in critically ill preterm neonates. *Crit Care Clin*. 1995;11:751.

78. Coran AG, Drongowski RA. Studies on the toxicity and efficacy of new amino acid solution in pediatric parenteral nutrition. *J Parenter Enter Nutr*. 1987;11:368.

79. Helms RA, Christensen ML, Mauer EC, Storm MC. Comparison of a pediatric versus standard amino acid formulation in preterm neonates requiring parenteral nutrition. *J Pediatr*. 1987;110:466.

80. Chessex P, Zebiche H, Pineault M, Lepage D, Dallaire L. Effect of amino acid composition of parenteral solutions on nitrogen retention and metabolic response in very-low-birthweight infants. *J Pediatr*. 1985;106: 111.

81. Wu PYK, Edwards N, Storm M. Plasma amino acid pattern in normal term breast-fed infants. *J Pediatr*. 1986;109:347.

82. Lowe DK, Benfell K, Smith RJ, et al. Safety of glutamine-enriched parenteral nutrient solutions in humans. *Am J Clin Nutr*. 1990;52:1101.

83. Lacey JM, Crouch JB, Benfell K, et al. The effects of glutamine-supplemented nutrition in premature infants. *J Paren Enter Nutr*. 1996;20:74.

84. Heird WC. Essentiality of cyst(e)ine for neonates. Clinical and biochemical effects of parenteral cysteine supplementation. In: Kinney JM, Borum PR, eds. *Perspectives in Clinical Nutrition*. Munich, Germany: Urban Schwarzenberg; 1989:275–282.

85. Gaull GE, Sturman JA, Raiha NCR, Sturman JA. Development of mammalian sulfur metabolism. Absence of cystathionase in human fetal tissues. *Pediatr Res*. 1972;6:538.

86. Zlotkin SH, Bryan H, Anderson H. Cysteine supplementation to cysteine-free intravenous feeding regimens in newborn infants. *Am J Clin Nutr*. 1981;34:914.

87. Heird WC, Hay W, Helms RA, Storm MC, Kashyap S, Dell RB. Pediatric parenteral amino acid mixture in low birth weight infants. *Pediatrics*. 1988;81:41.

88. Heird WC, Dell RB, Helms RA, et al. Amino acid mixture designed to maintain normal plasma amino acid patterns in infants and children requiring parenteral nutrition. *Pediatrics*. 1987;80:401.

89. Eggert LD, Rusho WJ, MacKay MW, Chan GM. Calcium and phosphorus compatibility in parenteral nutrition solutions for neonates. *Am J Hosp Pharm*. 1982; 39:49.

90. Battista MA, Price PT, Kalhan SC. Effect of parenteral amino acids on leucine and urea kinetics in preterm infants. *J Pediatr*. 1996;128:130–134.

91. Adamkin DH, McLead R, Marchildon M, et al. Comparison of two neonatal amino acid formulations in preterm infants: Multicenter study. *Pediatr Res*. 1989; 25:283A.

92. Abitbol CL, Holliday MA. Total parenteral nutrition in anuric children. *Clin Nephrol*. 1976;5:153.

93. Holliday MA, Wassner S, Ramirez J. Intravenous nutrition in uremic children with protein-energy malnutrition. *Am J Clin Nutr*. 1978;31:1854.

94. Motil KJ, Harmon WE, Grupe WE. Complications of essential amino acid hyperalimentation in children with acute renal failure. *J Parenter Enter Nutr*. 1980; 4:32.

95. Takala J. Total parenteral nutrition in experimental uremia: Studies of acute and chronic renal failure in the growing rat. *J Parenter Enter Nutr*. 1984;8:427.

96. Helms RA, Phelps SJ, Mauer EC, Christensen ML, Storm MC. Parenteral protein use in liver disease. *Pediatr Res*. 1989;25:115A.

97. Maldonato J, Gil A, Faus MJ, Periago JL, Loscertales M, Molina JA. Differences in the serum amino acid pattern of injured and infected children promoted by two parenteral nutrition solutions. *J Parenter Enter Nutr*. 1989;13:41.

98. Holman RT, Johnson SB, Hatch TF. A case of human linolenic acid deficiency involving neurologic abnormalities. *Am J Clin Nutr*. 1982;35:617.

99. Friedman Z, Danon A, Stahlman MT, et al. Rapid onset of essential fatty acid deficiency in the newborn. *Pediatrics*. 1976;58:640.

100. American Academy of Pediatrics, Committee on Nutrition. Commentary on parenteral nutrition. *Pediatrics*. 1983;71:547.

101. Levy JS, Winters RW, Heird WC. Total parenteral nutrition in pediatric patients. *Pediatr Rev*. 1980;2:99.

102. American Academy of Pediatrics, Committee on Nutrition. Prudent life-style for children: Dietary fat and cholesterol. *Pediatrics*. 1986;78:51.

103. Sapsford A. Energy, carbohydrate, protein, and fat. In: Groh-Wargo S, Thompson M, Cox JH, eds. *Nutritional Care for High-Risk Newborns*. Chicago: Precept Press; 1994;83.

104. Mitton SG. Amino acids and lipid in the total parenteral nutrition for the newborn. *J Pediatr Gastroenterol Nutr*. 1994;18:25–31.

105. Pereira GR. Nutritional care of the extremely premature infant. *Clin Perinatol*. 1995;22:61.

106. American Academy of Pediatrics, Committee on Nutrition. Use of intravenous fat emulsions in pediatric patients. *Pediatrics*. 1981;68:738.

107. Helms RA, Mauer EC, Hay WW Jr, et al. Effect of intravenous L-carnitine on growth parameters and fat metabolism during parenteral nutrition in neonates. *J Parenter Enter Nutr*. 1990;14:448.

108. Borum, P. Carnitine in neonatal nutrition. *J Child Neurol*. 1995;10(suppl 2):S25–S31.

109. Winter SC, Szabo-Aczel S, Curry CJR, et al. Plasma carnitine deficiency: Clinical observations in 51 pediatric patients. *Am J Dis Child*. 1987;141:660.

110. Coran AG, Drongowshi RA, Baker PJ. The metabolic effects of oral L-carnitine administration in infants receiving total parenteral nutrition with fat. *J Pediatr Surg*. 1985;20:758.

111. American Medical Association, Nutrition Advisory Group. Multivitamin preparations for parenteral use. *J Parenter Enter Nutr*. 1979;3:258.

112. Moore MC, Greene HL, Phillips B, et al. Evaluation of a pediatric multiple vitamin preparation for total parenteral nutrition in infants and children. I. Blood levels of water-soluble vitamins. *Pediatrics*. 1986;77:530.

113. Greene HL, Moore MEC, Phillips B, et al. Evaluation of a pediatric multivitamin preparation for total parenteral nutrition. II. Blood levels of vitamins A, D, and E. *Pediatrics*. 1986;77:539.

114. Greer FR, Tsang RC. Calcium and vitamin D metabolism in term and low-birth-weight infants. *Perinatol Neonatol*. 1986;9:14–18.

115. Koo WWK, Tsang RC, Steichen JJ, et al. Parenteral nutrition for infants: Effect of high versus low calcium and phosphorus content. *J Pediatr Gastroenterol Nutr*. 1987;6:96.

116. Changaris DG, Purohit DM, Balentine JD, et al. Brain calcification in severely stressed neonates receiving parenteral calcium. *J Pediatr*. 1984;104:941.

117. Goldsmith MA, Bhatia SS, Kanto AP, et al. Gluconate calcium therapy and neonatal hypercalciuria. *Am J Dis Child*. 1981;135:538.

118. Hufnagle KF, Khan SN, Penn D, et al. Renal calcifications: A complication of long-term furosemide therapy in preterm infants. *Pediatrics*. 1982;70:360.

119. Wood RJ, Bengoa JM, Sitrin MD, Rosenberg IH. Calciuretic effect of cyclic versus continuous total parenteral nutrition. *Am J Clin Nutr*. 1985;41:614.

120. Koo WWK, Kaplan LA, Horn J, Tsang RC, Steichen JJ. Aluminum in parenteral nutrition solution: Sources and possible alternatives. *J Parenter Enter Nutr*. 1986;10:591.

121. Morena A, Dominguez C, Ballabriga A. Aluminum in the neonate related to parenteral nutrition. *Acta Paediatr*. 1994;83:25.

122. Vileisis RA. Effect of phosphorus intake in total parenteral nutrition infusates in premature neonates. *J Pediatr*. 1987;110:586.

123. Aladjem M, Lotan D, Biochis H, et al. Changes in the electrolyte content of serum and urine during total parenteral nutrition. *J Pediatr*. 1980;97:437.

124. Kimura S, Nose O, Seino Y, et al. Effects of alternate and simultaneous administrations of calcium and phosphorus on calcium metabolism in children receiving total parenteral nutrition. *J Parenter Enter Nutr*. 1986;10:513.

125. Department of Health and Human Services. *FDA Safety Alert: Hazards of Precipitation Associated with Parenteral Nutrition*. Rockville, MD: Food and Drug Administration; April 18, 1994.

126. Fitzgerald KA, MacKay MW. Calcium and phosphate solubility in neonatal parenteral nutrient solutions containing trophamine. *Am J Hosp Pharm*. 1986;43:88.

127. Fitzgerald KA, MacKay MW. Calcium and phosphate solubility in neonatal parenteral nutrient solutions containing aminosyn PF. *Am J Hosp Pharm*. 1987;44:1396.

128. Shils ME, Burke AW, Greene HL, et al. Guidelines for essential trace element preparations for parenteral use: A statement by an expert panel. *JAMA*. 1979;241:2051.

129. Pyati SP, Ramamurthy RS, Krauss MT, Pildes RS. Absorption of iodine in the neonate following topical use of povidone iodine. *J Pediatr*. 1977;91:825.

130. Shaw JCL. Trace elements in the fetus and young infant II. Copper, manganese, selenium and chromium. *Am J Dis Child*. 1980;134:74.

131. Triplett WC. Clinical aspects of zinc, copper, manganese, chromium and selenium metabolism. *Nutr Int*. 1985;1:60.

132. American Academy of Pediatrics, Committee on Nutrition. Zinc. *Pediatrics*. 1978;62:408.

133. Reynolds AP, Keily E, Meadows N. Manganese in long term paediatric parenteral nutrition. *Arch Dis Child*. 1994;71:527.

134. Reed MD, Bertino JS, Halpin TC. Use of intravenous iron dextran injection in children receiving total parenteral nutrition. *Am J Dis Child*. 1981;135:829.

135. Seashore JH. Metabolic complications of parenteral nutrition in infants and children. *Surg Clin North Am*. 1980;60:1239.

136. Wan KK, Tsallas G. Dilute iron dextran formulation for addition to parenteral nutrient solutions. *Am J Hosp Pharm*. 1980;37:206.

137. Halpin T, Reed M, Bertino J. Use of intravenous iron dextran in children receiving TPN for nutritional support of inflammatory bowel disease. *J Parenter Enter Nutr*. 1980;4:600.

138. Ehrenkranz RA. Iron requirements of preterm infants. *Nutrition*. 1994;10:77.

139. Ohls RK, Harcum J, Schibler KR, Christensen RD, et al. The effect of erythropoietin on the transfusion requirements of preterm infants weighing 750 grams or less: A randomized, double-blind, placebo-controlled study. *J Pediatr*. 1997;131:661–665.

140. Meyer MP, Haworth C, Meyer JH, et al. A comparison of oral and intravenous iron supplementation in preterm infants receiving recombinant erythropoietin. *J Pediatr*. 1996;129:258.

141. Bastian C, Driscoll R. Enteral tube feeding at home. In: Rombeau JL, Caldwell MD, eds. *Enteral and Tube Feeding*. Philadelphia: WB Saunders Co; 1984:494–512.

142. Illingsworth RS, Lister J. The critical or sensitive period, with special reference to certain feeding problems in infants and children. *Pediatrics*. 1964; 65:849.

143. Nelson JK. Economics of nutrition support. In: Matarese LE, Gottschlich MM, eds. *Contemporary Nutrition Support Practice*. Philadelphia: WB Saunders Co; 1998:643.

Chapter 26

Botanicals in Pediatrics

John Westerdahl

Since the beginning of time, botanicals have played an important part in the diet and well-being of every major culture. The people of the ancient world relied heavily on various herbs for their medicines. Used by both adults and children, many of these plants were their chief therapy, offering comfort and healing during illness and disease. Botanicals were once the conventional medicines used in treating common health problems such as colds, flu, nausea, heart disease, depression, and most other conditions. Written historical records list many medicinal plants in early *materia medica* from ancient China, Babylon, Egypt, India, Greece, and other parts of the world. The ancient Egyptian medical text *Papyrus Ebers*, written in 1550 BC, lists over 800 medicinal formulas using herbs. The Greek physician Hippocrates (468–377 BC), known as the "father of medicine," used herbs extensively with his patients and wrote about their healing benefits. In the first century, another Greek physician, Dioscorides, listed 500 plant medicines in his classic herbal guide, *De Materia Medica*. Many of the currently popular medicinal herbs were once listed in official monographs in the *United States Pharmacopoeia* (USP) and the *National Formulary* (NF) and were used extensively by physicians. Today, some 25% of prescription drugs now marketed in the United States are derived from plants.[1,2]

Table 26–1 lists the botanicals that are currently approved by the US Food and Drug Administration (FDA) as effective over-the-counter drug ingredients. However, herbal supplements in the United States are not regulated by the FDA. From a global perspective, the World Health Organization (WHO) estimates that 80% of the world's population currently relies mainly on traditional medicines, most of which utilize medicinal plants.[3]

During the past several years, the use of herbs and phytomedicines has increased as consumers have become more aware of their uses. This can be attributed to increased published scientific research documenting the therapeutic efficacy of many medicinal herbs and the passing of The Dietary Supplement Health and Education Act of 1994 (DSHEA), which has created a new regulatory framework for dietary supplement products. It allows herbal manufacturers to make truthful, nonmisleading claims about the herb's effect on the structure and function of the body. These claims are required to be accompanied by a disclaimer that states, "This statement has not been evaluated by the Food and Drug Administration. This product is not intended to diagnose, treat, cure, or prevent any disease." It is wise to look for standardized versions with measured amounts of active ingredients as much as possible. Also, people interested in using herbs should seek reputable manufacturers' products and call companies to ascertain the source of their herbs and manufacturing procedures. As a precaution for the child, herbal supplements should not be used by pregnant or nursing women without first consulting a knowledeable physician.

Table 26–1 Botanicals Approved as OTC Drug Ingredients

Herb	*Approved Use*
Aloe (*Aloe ferox*)	Stimulant laxative
Cascara sagrada (*Rhamnus purshiana*)	Stimulant laxative
Peppermint oil (*Mentha piperita*)	Antitussive
Psyllium (*Plantago psyllium*)	Bulk laxative
Red pepper (*Capsicum* spp.)	Counterirritant
Senna (Alexandrian) (*Cassia senna*)	Stimulant laxative
Slippery elm (*Ulmus fulva*)	Demulcent
Witch hazel (*Hamamelis virginiana*)	Astringent

OTC, over-the-counter.

Source: OTC Drug Review Ingredient Status Report, September 1994, Food and Drug Administration, Rockville, Maryland.

GROWTH OF THE HERBAL MARKET

Consumers have shown a growing interest in trying natural alternatives to synthetic drugs that address their health concerns.[4] As a result, the herbal market during the past few years has experienced rapid growth. In 1994, the size of the botanical medicine market had grown to an estimated annual retail sales figure of $1.6 billion,[5] with estimates for 1998 approaching $4 billion in retail sales, as shown in Table 26–2. Table 26–3 identifies the best-selling herbal products sold in the United States in 1997.[6] This marketing information is helpful to the health professional to identify the types of herbs that are being used by many patients today.

With the growing interest in herbs, there is an increasing number of parents using botanical medicines with their children. Several herbal product companies now market phytomedicines especially formulated for children. More and more parents perceive herbal remedies as effective and having actions that are "gentler," with fewer side effects than those of most conventional drugs. In the United States, the majority of doctors and pharmacists recognize that there is a growing consumer interest in herbal medicine, but most of them have little or no knowledge and absolutely no training in this area. Doctors, pharmacists, registered dietitians, and other health care practitioners should know some basic information about herbal products to better assist their patients who use them.

DEFINITIONS

In the world of herbs and phytomedicines, there is some basic nomenclature that the health professional should be familiar with when working with patients who use these preparations. This starts with adequately defining the word *herb*. Depending on the context, the term *herb* can be defined in a few different ways. An herb is defined botanically as "a seed-producing, nonwoody plant that dies down to its roots at the end of its growing season." Others have described an herb simply as "a useful plant." In the culinary arts field, the term *herb* is described as "a vegetable product that is used in cooking to add flavor and/or aroma to foods." However, in the field of herbal medicine, the term *herb* takes on a more medical meaning. Perhaps the most precise and accurate definition of the term *herb* as it pertains to medicinal values is the definition offered by Varro E. Tyler, PhD, ScD, former Dean and Distinguished Professor Emeritus of the School of Pharmacy and Pharmacal Sciences at Purdue

Table 26–2 US Market for Medicinal Botanicals, July 1998: Shown in Million $ (Estimate)

Natural Foods	$ 1207
Multilevel	1050
Mass Market (food, drug, mass merchandise retail)	663
Mail Order	320
Practitioners	270
Tea (all channels)	266
Specialty Shops	90
Total	**$ 3.87 Billion**

Source: Reprinted with permission from *Herbal Gram,* Vol. 44, pp. 33–46, 1998, American Botanical Council.

Table 26–3 Consumer Sales of Herbal Products in the United States as of Calendar Year 1997 (based on total sales of $3.6 billion)

Herb	*Market %*
Echinacea	9
Ginseng	8
Ginkgo	7
Garlic	6
St. John's Wort	6
Goldenseal	4
Saw palmetto	4
Aloe	3
Multiherb products	27
All others	26

Source: Reprinted with permission from *Nutrition Business Journal,* September 1998, San Diego.

University. In his book, *Herbs of Choice: The Therapeutic Use of Phytomedicinals,* Dr. Tyler defines *medicinal herbs* as "crude drugs of vegetable origin utilized for the treatment of disease states, often of a chronic nature, or to attain or maintain a condition of improved health."[7(p.1)] Commercial herbal and phytomedicine preparations are available in several different forms. Some of the key forms are defined as follows:

- *Extract*—An herbal concentrate that contains the phytochemical constituents found in the herb. Extracts are made when the plant constituents are extracted from the plant by physical and/or chemical means.
- *Standardized extract*—An herbal extract that is guaranteed to provide a "standardized" level of a particular phytochemical constituent. In many cases, this phytochemical constituent is considered to be the key active compound.
- *Infusion*—An herbal tea. An herbal extract prepared by steeping dried plant parts in hot water.
- *Decoction*—An herbal extract prepared by putting the plant material (usually hard or woody parts) in water and boiling the water, then allowing it to simmer gently for ex-

tended periods of time. The liquid is then cooled and strained for use.

- *Tinctures*—An herbal extract prepared by mixing the herb with a solvent (usually an alcohol and water mixture) for a specified period of time (hours to days). The solvent extracts phytochemical constituents from the herb. Any remaining solids are removed, and the solution that results is used medicinally. If glycerol is used as the solvent instead of alcohol, the preparation is referred to as a *glycerite*.
- *Glycerites*—An herbal extract, similar to tinctures. However, glycerol is used as the solvent in preparation instead of alcohol. Because they are alcohol-free, glycerites have recently become very popular for use with children.
- *Fluid Extract*—Liquid preparations that usually contain a ratio of one part solvent to one part herb. They are much more concentrated than tinctures, and their alcohol content can vary.
- *Solid Extract*—Solid extracts (also called *powdered extracts*) are made by evaporating all the residual solvent or liquid used during the extraction process.
- *Powder*—A preparation in the form of finely divided sieved herbal particles made from dried and finely milled herbs for use in herbal preparations such as tablets and capsules.
- *Syrups*—Syrups are a water and sugar solution to which flavoring and an herbal extract may be added. They are often used to relieve coughs or to mask the unpleasant flavor of a tincture. Syrups are a popular form of herbal medicine in pediatrics.

THE USE OF HERBS AND PHYTOMEDICINES IN PEDIATRICS

Although herbs have been used for centuries, most controlled clinical trials using herbs have included only adults. The scientific data examining the use of herbs with children are very limited. As a result, herbal medicine experts do not have a consensus of opinion as to the appropriate use of botanicals for children, particularly the very young. Although more conservative experts feel strongly that botanicals should not be used by children under the age of 12 until there is more research in the pediatric population to confirm their safety, other experts have less concern and recommend their use for young children, even infants. Nevertheless, there are growing numbers of parents who are using many herbal products to treat minor illnesses in small children. The concern among many health professionals, however, is the potential hazards of the inappropriate use of herbal preparations by parents treating their children for serious health conditions without the consultation of a pediatrician.

In general, the safety of most responsibly formulated commercial herb products has been well established. However, there are situations in which specific herbs should not be used. If a child has an allergy to a specific herb, it must be avoided. Certain plants in the Asteraceae, Apiaceae, and other plant families possess a high degree of allergenicity with some children. It is advised to observe caution in the consumption of plants classified as ragweeds, especially flowers found in the Asteraceae family, eg, chamomile.

Parents should observe the child who takes an herbal preparation for the first time for several hours for any adverse reactions. Watery, itchy eyes, sneezing, wheezing, coughing, or hives could be signs of allergy. Pediatricians who utilize herbal remedies in their practice recommend to concerned parents of allergy-prone children that they introduce an herb in the same way they would introduce new foods to an infant. The pediatrician's advice is to try only one herb at a time, administered in very small doses.

Herbs should not be given by the parent to a child who is currently taking a medication without first consulting a doctor. The interaction of an herb with medicinal substances should always be considered. Although there are little data available today on herb–drug interactions, some important information in this area is known by the medical profession.

There is debate among herbal medicine experts as to which herbal remedies are safe and appropriate for use by children. In Germany, Commission E, an interdisciplinary expert committee on herbal medicines consisting of physicians, pharmacists, pharmacologists, toxicologists, representatives of the pharmaceutical industry, and lay persons, is responsible for evaluating the scientific data on the safety and efficacy of phytomedicines. Commission E members are appointed by the former German Federal Health Agency (now the Federal Institute for Drugs and Medical Devices) and are assigned the task of preparing monographs on medicinal plants. These monographs are regarded by most experts as the most accurate scientific information available in the world on the safety and efficacy of herbs and phytomedicines. Whereas the monographs describe the medicinal use of herbs primarily for adults, they also identify herbs that are contraindicated for children (Exhibit 26–1).[8] Table 26–4 gives an overview of several of the internal and external uses of many of the medicinal herbs commonly used in pediatrics.

Laxatives and Stimulants

Most herbal medicine experts caution against the use of herbal stimulant laxatives by children under the age of 12. Herbal stimulant laxatives include aloe (*Aloe ferox*), buckthorn bark (*Rhamnus frangula*), cascara sagrada bark (*Rhamnus purshiana*), and senna leaf or pod (*Cassia senna*). Stimulants such as caffeine-containing herbs are also generally contraindicated for young children. Herbs that are classified as stimulants include not only coffee and black and green tea (*Camellia sinensis*), but also cola nut (also called *kola nut*) (*Cola nitida*), guarana (*Paullina cupana*), and maté (*Ilex paraguariensis*). Ma huang (also known as *ephedra herb*) is also a potent stimulant and is contraindicated for young children, except under

Exhibit 26–1 Herbs and Herbal Products Contraindicated for Children According to the German Commission E Monographs

Aloe
Buckthorn bark and berry
Camphor
Cajeput oil
Cascara sagrada bark
Eucalyptus leaf
Eucalyptus oil
Fennel oil
Horseradish
Mint oil (external)
Nasturtium
Peppermint oil (external)
Rhubarb root
Senna leaf and pod
Watercress

Source: M. Blumenthal et al., eds., S. Klein and R.S. Rister, trans., *The Complete German Commission E Monographs: Therapeutic Guide to Herbal Medicines,* © 1998 American Botanical Council and Integrative Medicine Communications.

Table 26–4 Common Herbal Remedies Used in Pediatrics. Clinical efficacy for each of these herbs has not necessarily been established.

HERB *Common and Latin Names*	*HISTORICAL USAGE** *Internal and External Uses*	*Contraindications/Precautions*
Aloe *(Aloe vera)*	External use: wound healing, minor skin irritation, burns	Not recommended internally for pediatrics
Anise *(Pimpinella anisum)*	Internal use: common colds, coughs, bronchitis, indigestion	Rare allergic reactions to anise and its constituent anethole
Bilberry *(Vaccinium myrtillus)*	Internal use: diarrhea	None known
Calendula Flowers *(Calendula officinalis)*	Internal use: inflammation of mouth and pharynx External use: wounds and burns	Rare allergic reactions through frequent skin contact
Catnip *(Nepeta cataria)*	Internal use: nervous disorders, sleep aid, common colds, colic	None known
Chamomile Flowers *(Matricaria chamomilla)*	Internal use: carminative, sleep aid External use: inflammation and irritations of the skin, wounds, burns	Rare allergic reactions
Cherry Bark *(Prunus sp.)*	Internal use: coughs, common colds	None known
Comfrey Leaf (*Symphytum officinale)*	External use: minor wounds, ulcers, inflammations, bruises, and sprains. Used as poultice for skin disorder	Not to be taken internally. Internal use promotes hepatotoxic effects
Echinacea *(Echinacea angustifolia)* (*Echinacea purpurea*)	Internal use: common colds, flu, coughs, bronchitis, fever, immune stimulant External use: wounds, burns	Allergic reactions may occur with some individuals. Not recommended for individuals with autoimmune diseases
Elder Flowers *(Sambucus nigra)*	Internal use: common colds, antiviral, diaphoretic	None known

Table 26–4 continued. Clinical efficacy for each of these herbs has not necessarily been established.

HERB *Common and Latin Names*	*TRADITIONAL USAGE** *Internal and External Uses*	*Contraindications/Precautions*
Eucalyptus *(Eucalyptus globulus)*	Internal use: expectorant, coughs, congestion of the respiratory tract	Nausea, vomiting, and diarrhea may occur after ingestion in rare cases. Eucalyptus preparations should *not* be applied to the face or nose of infants and very young children
Fennel Seed *(Foeniculum vulgare)*	Internal use: carminative, indigestion, coughs, bronchitis gastrointestinal afflictions	Allergic reactions may occur with some individuals.
Garlic *(Allium sativum)*	Internal use: common colds, bronchitis, fever External use: antibacterial, antifungal, ear infections	Intake of large quantities can lead to stomach complaints. Rare allergic reactions
Ginger *(Zingiber officinale)*	Internal use: carminative, antinausea, indigestion	None known
Goldenseal (*Hydrastis canadensis*)	Internal use: common colds, flu, inflammation of mucous membranes External use: antiseptic, antimicrobial, cuts, wounds, ear infections	Internal use can cause nausea, vomiting, diarrhea, and may disrupt intestinal flora. Internal use is not recommended for young children by many experts due to the herb's alkaloid (berberine and hydrastine) content
Hops *(Humulus lupulus)*	Internal use: nervous disorders, sleep aid	Rare allergic reactions
Horehound *(Marrubium vulgare)*	Internal use: coughs, bronchitis	None known
Hyssop *(Hyssopus officinalis)*	Internal use: coughs, common colds	None known
Lemon Balm *(Melissa officinalis)*	Internal use: nervous disorders, sleep aid	None known

continues

Table 26–4 continued. Clinical efficacy for each of these herbs has not necessarily been established.

HERB *Common and Latin Names*	*TRADITIONAL USAGE** *Internal and External Uses*	*Contraindications/Precautions*
Licorice Root *(Glycyrrhiza glabra)*	Internal use: coughs, bronchitis	Prolonged use with high doses may promote hypertension, edema, and hypokalemia
Marshmallow Root *(Althaea officinalis)*	Internal use: coughs, bronchitis, sore throat	None known
Mullein Leaf (*Verbascum thapsus*)	Internal use: coughs, bronchitis, common colds, flu	None known
Oat Straw (*Avena sativa*)	External use: inflammation of the skin, itching	None known
Passion Flower (*Passiflora incarnata*)	Internal use: nervous disorders, sleep aid	None known
Peppermint Leaf (*Mentha piperita*)	Internal use: carminative, indigestion, nausea, gastrointestinal disorders, common colds, cough, bronchitis	Preparations containing peppermint oil should *not* be applied to the face or nose of infants or very young children
Pleurisy Root (*Asclepias tuberosa)*	Internal use: coughs, pleurisy	Excessive amounts can be toxic due to the herb's cardioactive steroid content which can lead to digitalis-like poisonings. High doses can promote vomiting
St. John's Wort (*Hypericum perforatum*)	Internal use: emotional upsets, including anxiety and depressive moods. External use: cuts and abrasions	Safety of internal use with children has not been established. The safety and ethics of the use of herbal antidepressants with children without the consultation of a doctor is questionable Should not be taken by children already taking prescription medications for depression without first consulting a doctor

continues

Table 26–4 continued. Clinical efficacy for each of these herbs has not necessarily been established.

HERB *Common and Latin Names*	*TRADITIONAL USAGE** *Internal and External Uses*	*Contraindications/Precautions*
		May cause sun sensitivity in some individuals.
Thyme (*Thymus vulgarus)*	Internal use: cough, bronchitis, common colds	None known
Valerian Root (*Valeriana officinalis*)	Internal Use: nervous disorders, sleep aid	The safety and ethics of the use of herbal sedatives with children without the consultation of a doctor is questionable

the guidance of a physician, when it is used for treating respiratory conditions. Asian ginseng (*Panax ginseng*) and American ginseng (*Panax quinquefolium*), traditionally regarded as herbal stimulants, are also not recommended for young children by many herbal medicine authorities.

Sedatives and Antidepressants

There are many plants that have traditionally been used for their sedative properties. There is controversy as to whether it is proper or even ethical to administer any sedative to young children without the consultation of a physician. Definitely, this is quite clear in regard to prescription drugs, but naturally derived herbal sedatives have not always been looked at in the same light. Most health authorities would agree that any sedative, herbal or otherwise, should be given to a child only under medical direction. Many herbal medicine experts would agree that strong sedative herbs such as valerian (*Valeriana officinalis*) should not be given to young children. There is no consensus of opinion on the use of some of the other popular traditional sedative herbs for children, despite the fact that many of them have been used with children for centuries. These herbs include catnip (*Nepeta cataria*), German chamomile (*Matricaria recutita*), hops (*Humulus lupulus*), lemon balm (*Melissa officinalis*), and passion flower (*Passiflora incarnata*). St. John's Wort (*Hypericum perforatum*), an herb that has proven efficacy in treating mild and moderate depression in adults, has not been adequately studied for use by children.

Herbs Containing Alkaloids

Many herbal experts have concerns about children's use of herbs that contain powerful alkaloids. One of the alkaloids of concern is berberine. Berberine is a key principal phytochemical constituent found in several of the currently popular herbal products found in natural food and drug stores. Herbs containing berberine include goldenseal root (*Hydrastis canadensis*), Oregon grape root (*Mahonia aquifolium*), and barberry root (*Berberis vulgaris*). Berberine has antibacterial properties. Overuse of herbs containing this and other alkaloids could disrupt the normal flora in a child's gastrointestinal tract.

Alkaloids that affect the central nervous system (caffeine, ephedrine, pseudoephedrine, and others) are generally not recommended for young children except under a doctor's direction.

Traditional Herbal Remedies Used with Infants and Children

For centuries, medicinal herbs have been used with children worldwide, with an apparently good record of safety. Clinical research has shown that many traditional herbal remedies appear to be effective.[9] However, more research is needed to confirm the safety and efficacy of the use of medicinal herbs in pediatric medicine.

Few studies have ever been done with infants using herbal preparations. In 1993, a prospective, randomized, double-blind, placebo-controlled study[10] published in *The Journal of Pediatrics* examined the effects of an herbal tea in treating infantile colic. The tea was made from herbs known to have antispasmodic activity and traditionally used to treat indigestion and colic in infants. The tea contained chamomile (*Matricaria chamomilla*), vervain (*Verbena officinalis*), licorice root (*Glycyrrhiza glabra*), fennel (*Foeniculum vulgare*), and lemon balm (*Melissa officinalis*). The use of the herbal tea eliminated the colic in 19 (57%) of the 33 infants, whereas the placebo was helpful in only 9 (26%) of 35 ($p < 0.01$). The mean colic score was significantly improved in the herbal tea-treated infants. None of the infants in the study experienced any adverse effects from the herbal tea.[10]

There are many other herbs that have been traditionally used in treating childhood illnesses and conditions. Heinz Schilcher, an expert in pharmacognosy at the Institute of Pharmaceutical Biology at Berlin's Independent University and member of the German Commission E, in his book,[11] *Phytotherapy in Paediatrics: Handbook for Physicians and Pharmacists,* points out the value of herbal remedies in pediatrics. He notes that the benefits of many phytomedicines outweigh the risks because they have a relatively good benefit/risk ratio. In European studies, the actions of many combinations of naturally occurring compounds in herbs have been experimentally established and/or clinically confirmed, with minimal or negligible side effects. Other advantages of herbal remedies mentioned by Schilcher are that herbs have gentle medicinal actions, and their common methods of administration (eg, inhalation, baths, ointments, syrups) are particularly appropriate for children. As a result, this can provide for good compliance. He points out that herbal medicines in pediatrics may be used at a preventive level and not just for the use of treating symptoms. Schilcher also notes that, as a general rule, phytomedicines are less expensive than conventional medicines.[11]

Determining Proper Pediatric Dosage for Medicinal Herbs

There is little scientific or even traditional information available on the proper dosage of herbs and phytomedicines in pediatrics. Because most clinical trials using herbs have been with adults, official dosages have been established for only the adult population. The posology in the German Commission E monographs refers to adults. A general pediatric guide used for determining the dosage of phytotherapeutic drugs is one-third of the adult dose (as established in the Commission E monographs) for very young and young children and one-half the adult dose for school-aged children.[11] Two classic pharmacy rules that are traditionally used in determining the dosages for drugs for children are sometimes used by herbal medicine experts as well. These rules are known as *Clark's Rule* and *Young's Rule*. Exhibit 26–2 illustrates how they are calculated.

Because children have lower body weight than adults and they do not have the sufficient development of liver enzymes necessary to metabolize many medications, their dosages of conventional as well as herbal medicines must be reduced. The proper pediatric dosage is best determined by an experienced and trained health professional. In recent years, some herbal

Exhibit 26–2 How to Calculate a Child's Dosage for Herbal Medicines

The following are two classic rules used to calculate the approximate dosage for a child.

Clark's Rule: Divide the child's weight by 150. The example given is for a 50-lb child:

$$\frac{50}{150} = \frac{1}{3} \text{ adult dosage}$$

Young's Rule: Divide the child's age by child's age + 12. The example given is for a 4-year-old child:

$$\frac{4}{4+12} = \frac{4}{16} = \frac{1}{4} \text{ adult dosage}$$

product manufacturers have formulated their preparations for dosage levels appropriate for children.

CONCLUSION

Medicinal herbs have been used in pediatrics since ancient times. Today, there is a growing trend among parents to use botanical and other natural medicines with their children as alternatives to conventional medicines. Increased public awareness of the therapeutic value of certain herbs and an increasing amount of scientific research in this area have led to an explosion in the marketplace of herbal medicine preparations and products. Several leading pharmaceutical companies are now adding herbal medicines to their product lines. Herbal medicine preparations specifically formulated for children are now being sold in natural food stores. Based on current trends, herbal medicine will undoubtedly play a more prominent role in the pediatric medicine of the twenty-first century. As a result, there is an increasing need for pediatricians and other health professionals who work with pediatric patients to gain some basic knowledge about herbal medicine and its potential role in the health care of infants and children. More clinical research is needed to evaluate the safety and efficacy of medicinal herbs in the pediatric population.

REFERENCES

1. Westerdahl J. *Medicinal Herbs: A Vital Reference Guide*. Dallas, TX: Bruce Miller Enterprises; 1998.
2. Principe PP. The economic significance of plants and their constituents as drugs. *Econ Med Plant Res.* 1989;3: 1–17.
3. Farnsworth NR, Akerele O, Bingel AS, Soejarto DD, Guo Z. Medicinal plants in therapy. *Bull World Health Org.* 1985;63:965–981.
4. Eisenberg DM, Kessler RC, Foster C, et al. Unconventional medicine in the United States. *N Engl J Med.* 1993;328:246–252.
5. Brevoort P. The US botanical market: An overview. *HerbalGram.* 1996;36:49–57.
6. Brevoort P. The booming US botanical market: A new overview. *HerbalGram.* 1998;44:33–46.
7. Tyler VE. *Herbs of Choice: The Therapeutic Use of Phytomedicinals*. Binghamton, NY: Pharmaceutical Products Press; 1994.
8. Blumenthal M, Busse WR, Goldberg A, et al, eds. Klein S, Rister RS, translators. *The Complete German Commission E Monographs: Therapeutic Guide to Herbal Medicines*. Austin, TX: American Botanical Council; Boston, MA: Integrative Medicine Communications; 1998.
9. *PDR for Herbal Medicines.* Montvale, NJ: Medical Economics Company, 1998.
10. Weizman Z, Alkrinawi S, Goldfarb D, Bitran C. Efficacy of herbal tea preparation in infantile cholic. *J Pediatr.* 1993;122:650–652.

11. Schilcher H. *Phytotherapy in Pediatrics: Handbook for Physicians and Pharmacists.* Stuttgart, Germany: MedPharm Scientific Publishers; 1997.

RESOURCES

Associations

American Botanical Council
P.O. Box 144345
Austin, TX 78714
Phone (512) 926–4900
www.herbalgram.org

The Herb Research Foundation
1007 Pearl Street, Suite 200
Boulder, CO 80302
Phone: (303) 449–2265

Books and Periodicals

1. *HerbalGram.* American Botanical Council. Austin, TX (see address above).
2. *The Review of Natural Products.* Facts and Comparisons, 111 West Port Plaza, Suite 300, St. Louis, MO 63146.
3. Tyler VE. *Herbs of Choice: The Therapeutic Use of Phytomedicinals.* New York: Pharmaceutical Products Press, 1994.
4. Blumenthal M, Busse WR, Goldberg A, et al: *The Complete German Commission E Monographs: Therapeutic Guide to Herbal Medicines.* American Botanical Council and Integrative Medicine Communications; 1998.
5. *PDR for Herbal Medicines.* Montvale, NJ: Medical Economics Company, 1998.

APPENDIX A

Premature Infant Growth Charts

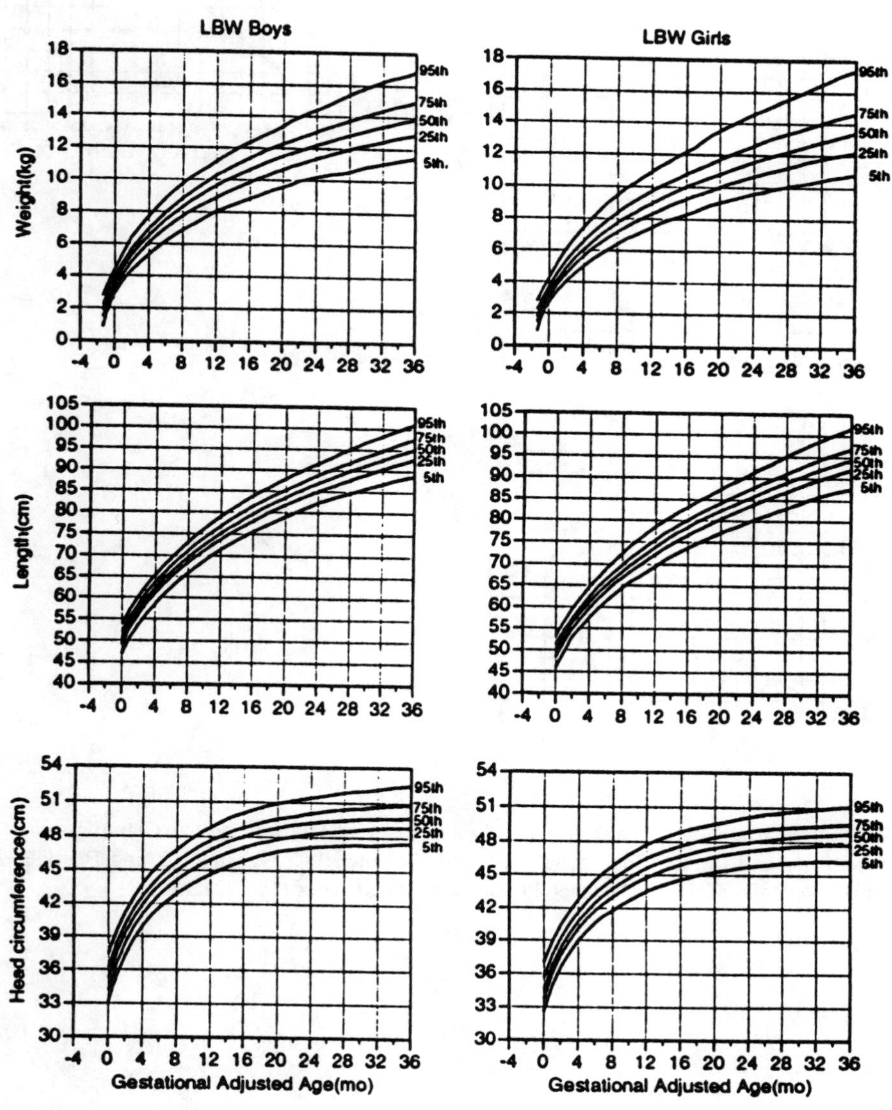

Figure A–1 Selected percentiles for status values of weight, length, and head circumference for very low birth weight (LBW) preterm infants in relation to gestation-adjusted ages. *Source:* Reprinted from S.S. Guo et al., Early Human Development, copyright 1997, pages no. 305–325, with permission from Elsevier Science.

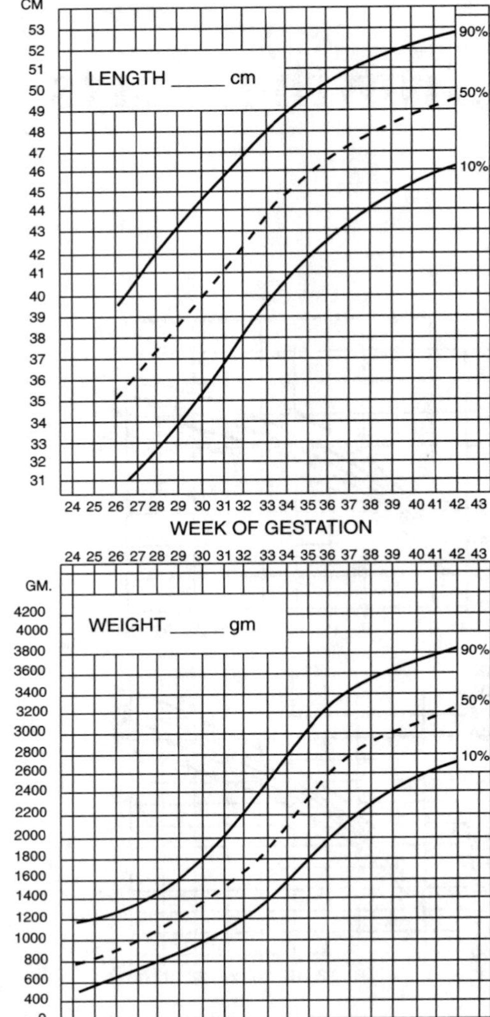

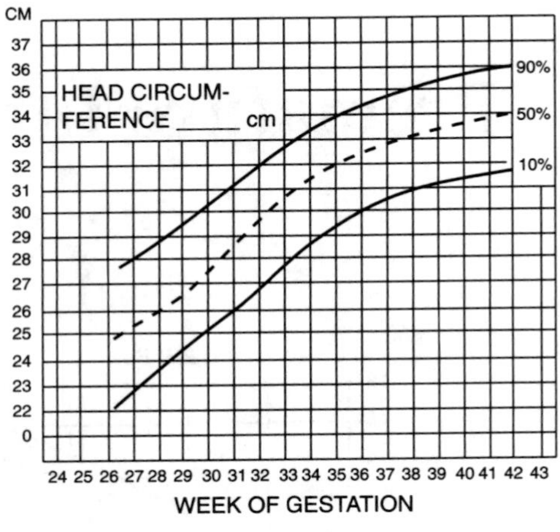

Figure A–2 Intrauterine growth charts. *Source:* Data from Mead Johnson and Co, Classification of newborns based on maturity and intrauterine growth, 1978; Lubchenco LC, Hansman C and Boyd E, *Pediatrics* (1966;37:403); Battaglia FC and Lubchenco LC, *Journal of Pediatrics* (1967;71:159).

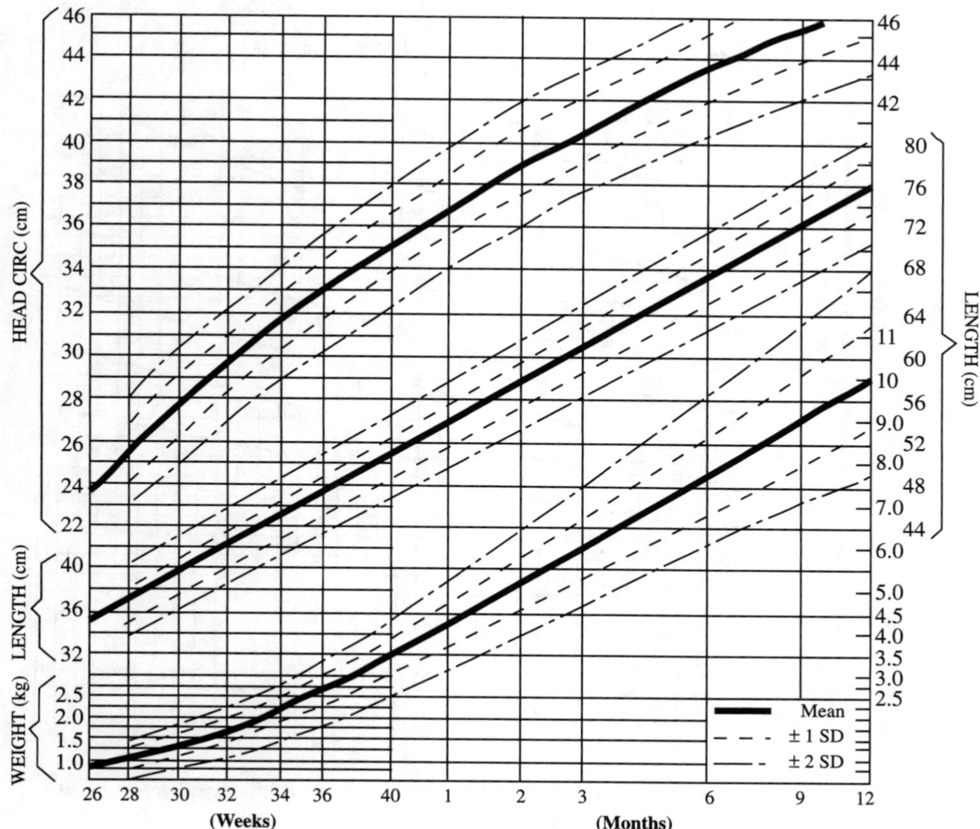

Figure A–3 Growth records for infants birth to 1 year. *Source:* Adapted with permission from SG Babson and GI Benda, Growth graphs for the clinical assessment of infants of varying gestational age, in *Journal of Pediatrics* (1976;89:814–820), copyright © 1976, CV Mosby Co; used with permission of Ross Products Division, Abbott Laboratories, Inc., Columbus, OH 43216.

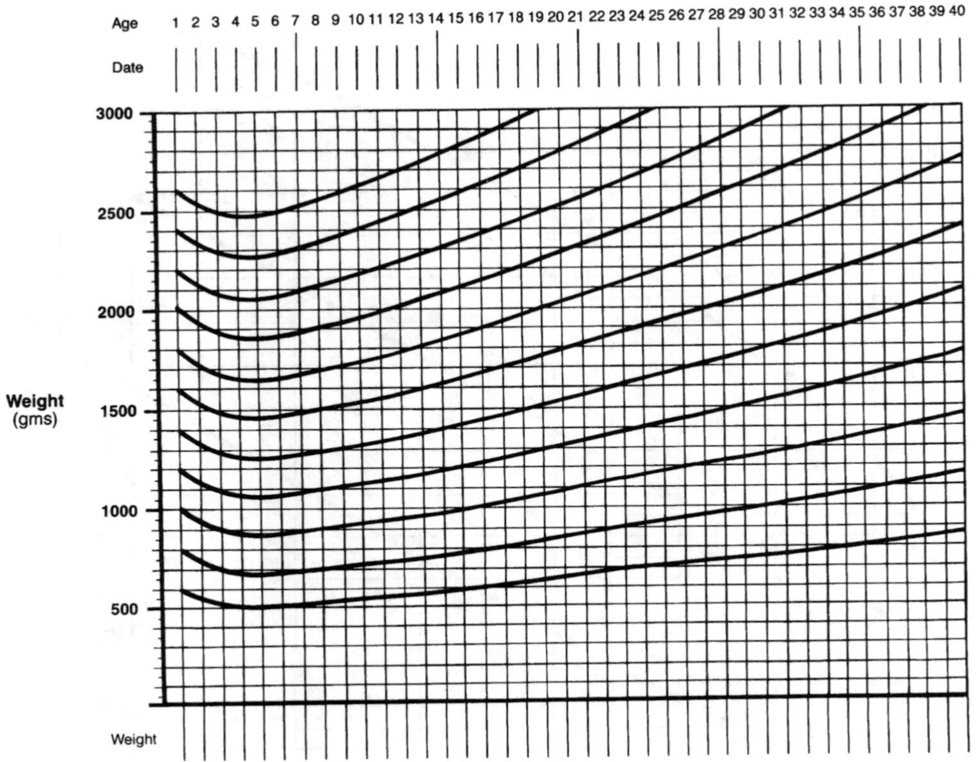

Figure A–4 Premature infant growth grid. *Source:* Reproduced with permission from *Pediatrics,* vol. 79, page 702, 1987.

Appendix B

Incremental Growth Charts

Table B–1 Head circumference of boys: birth to 36 mo of age in 6-mo increments (Fels Longitudinal Study)

	Percentiles of 6-mo increments									
Age at end of interval	*3 (–2 SD)*	*5*	*10 (–1 SD)*	*25*	*50 (mean)*	*75*	*90 (+1 SD)*	*95*	*97 (+2 SD)*	*n*
mo					*cm/6 mo*					
6	5.97 (4.97)	6.21	6.51 (6.83)	7.50	8.58 (8.69)	9.77	10.62 (10.55)	11.13	11.50 (12.41)	263
9	3.58 (3.70)	4.07	4.30 (4.42)	4.67	5.13 (5.14)	5.57	6.02 (5.86)	6.27	6.56 (6.58)	263
12	2.05 (1.74)	2.13	2.40 (2.46)	2.72	3.09 (3.18)	3.54	3.98 (3.90)	4.44	4.68 (4.62)	271
18	0.46 (0.36)	0.61	0.88 (0.95)	1.14	1.51 (1.54)	1.92	2.19 (2.12)	2.47	2.60 (2.71)	270
24	0.03 (–0.08)	0.12	0.38 (0.42)	0.64	0.93 (0.93)	1.18	1.51 (1.43)	1.67	1.96 (1.94)	267
30	0.05 (–0.03)	0.21	0.32 (0.34)	0.52	0.70 (0.71)	0.92	1.07 (1.08)	1.26	1.52 (1.45)	213
36	–0.17 (–0.14)	–0.08	0.12 (0.16)	0.29	0.48 (0.46)	0.62	0.84 (0.76)	0.93	0.98 (1.06)	167

Source: Reprinted with permission from R.N. Baumgartner et al., "Incremental Growth Tables: Supplementary to Previously Published Charts," *The American Journal of Clinical Nutrition* 43, May 1986, pp. 711–722. Copyright © 1986 American Society for Clinical Nutrition.

Table B–2 Head circumference of girls: birth to 36 mo of age in 6-mo increments (Fels Longitudinal Study)

Age at end of interval	*Percentiles of 6-mo increments*									
	3 (–2 SD)	*5*	*10 (–1 SD)*	*25*	*50 (mean)*	*75*	*90 (+1 SD)*	*95*	*97 (+2 SD)*	*n*
mo	*cm/6 mo*									
6	5.53 (5.38)	5.80	6.17 (6.69)	7.14	8.05 (7.99)	8.84	9.48 (9.30)	10.11	10.41 (10.61)	249
9	3.10 (3.31)	3.53	4.03 (4.13)	4.48	4.96 (4.95)	5.40	5.95 (5.77)	6.14	6.44 (6.59)	243
12	1.60 (1.47)	2.08	2.30 (2.28)	2.68	3.12 (3.09)	3.51	3.79 (3.90)	4.02	4.13 (4.72)	252
18	0.34 (0.34)	0.71	0.96 (0.98)	1.34	1.60 (1.63)	1.91	2.34 (2.27)	2.55	2.78 (2.92)	240
24	0.03 (–0.56)	0.26	0.45 (0.23)	0.69	0.95 (1.03)	1.22	1.65 (1.81)	1.94	2.36 (2.61)	236
30	–0.15 (–0.21)	–0.06	0.22 (0.26)	0.50	0.71 (0.74)	0.96	1.23 (1.21)	1.63	1.80 (1.69)	191
36	–0.01 (–0.11)	0.09	0.15 (0.22)	0.34	0.52 (0.54)	0.71	0.94 (0.87)	1.17	1.35 (1.20)	151

Source: Reprinted with permission from R.N. Baumgartner et al., "Incremental Growth Tables: Supplementary to Previously Published Charts," *The American Journal of Clinical Nutrition* 43, May 1986, pp. 711–722.

Table B–3 Recumbent length of boys: birth to 36 mo of age in 6-mo increments (Fels Longitudinal Study)

Age at end of interval	*Percentiles of 6-mo increments*									
	3 (–2 SD)	*5*	*10 (–1 SD)*	*25*	*50 (mean)*	*75*	*90 (+1 SD)*	*95*	*97 (+2 SD)*	*n*
mo					*cm/6 mo*					
6	12.22 (12.00)	12.96	13.71 (14.49)	15.33	17.09 (16.98)	18.57	19.91 (19.47)	20.79	21.70 (21.96)	271
9	8.39 (8.19)	8.90	9.39 (9.72)	10.22	11.08 (11.25)	12.14	13.26 (12.77)	13.93	14.51 (14.30)	265
12	5.89 (5.64)	6.20	6.69 (7.06)	7.55	8.51 (8.48)	9.29	10.14 (9.90)	10.71	10.91 (11.32)	286
18	4.24 (4.03)	4.57	4.99 (5.29)	5.82	6.51 (6.56)	7.31	8.05 (7.82)	8.67	9.02 (9.08)	286
24	3.26 (2.94)	3.58	3.89 (4.17)	4.57	5.40 (5.41)	6.13	6.85 (6.64)	7.39	7.57 (7.88)	280
30	2.84 (2.73)	3.00	3.49 (3.70)	4.00	4.63 (4.67)	5.29	5.77 (5.63)	6.10	6.63 (6.60)	270
36	2.33 (2.23)	2.47	3.02 (3.18)	3.58	4.05 (4.12)	4.66	5.38 (5.07)	5.75	6.01 (6.01)	266

Source: Reprinted with permission from R.N. Baumgartner et al., "Incremental Growth Tables: Supplementary to Previously Published Charts," *The American Journal of Clinical Nutrition* 43, May 1986, pp. 711–722.

Table B–4 Recumbent length of girls: birth to 36 mo of age in 6-mo increments (Fels Longitudinal Study)

Age at end of interval	Percentiles of 6-mo increments									
	3 (−2 SD)	*5*	*10 (−1 SD)*	*25*	*50 (mean)*	*75*	*90 (+1 SD)*	*95*	*97 (+2 SD)*	*n*
mo	*cm/6 mo*									
6	12.00 (11.55)	12.36	13.26 (13.84)	14.51	16.06 (16.13)	17.66	18.85 (18.42)	19.76	20.34 (20.71)	254
9	8.18 (7.92)	8.40	9.10 (9.38)	9.78	10.82 (10.83)	11.77	12.58 (12.29)	13.22	13.53 (13.74)	248
12	5.94 (5.43)	6.20	6.76 (6.99)	7.41	8.49 (8.56)	9.43	10.34 (10.12)	10.87	11.32 (11.69)	263
18	3.94 (4.17)	4.61	5.19 (5.46)	6.00	6.79 (6.76)	7.50	8.15 (8.05)	8.81	9.17 (9.35)	262
24	3.72 (3.41)	4.00	4.40 (4.57)	4.95	5.59 (5.73)	6.45	7.09 (6.89)	7.60	7.87 (8.04)	259
30	2.90 (2.70)	3.19	3.54 (3.71)	4.02	4.66 (4.72)	5.23	6.00 (5.74)	6.39	6.77 (6.75)	245
36	2.54 (2.29)	2.72	2.99 (3.22)	3.62	4.13 (4.16)	4.67	5.25 (5.10)	5.78	6.16 (6.04)	246

Source: Reprinted with permission from R.N. Baumgartner et al., "Incremental Growth Tables: Supplementary to Previously Published Charts," *The American Journal of Clinical Nutrition* 43, May 1986, pp. 711–722. Copyright © 1986 American Society for Clinical Nutrition.

Table B–5 Stature of boys: 3 to 18 yr of age in 6-mo increments (Fels Longitudinal Study)

Age at end of interval	*Percentiles of 6-mo increments*									
	3 (–2 SD)	*5*	*10 (–1 SD)*	*25*	*50 (mean)*	*75*	*90 (+1 SD)*	*95*	*97 (+2 SD)*	*n*
yr	*cm/6 mo*									
3.5	2.54 (2.22)	2.64	2.84 (3.03)	3.36	3.81 (3.84)	4.33	4.72 (4.65)	5.00	5.32 (5.46)	208
4.0	2.14 (2.09)	2.49	2.69 (2.84)	3.11	3.59 (3.60)	4.02	4.41 (4.35)	4.77	4.86 (5.11)	233
4.5	2.27 (2.21)	2.52	2.73 (2.88)	3.05	3.53 (3.55)	4.03	4.40 (4.23)	4.59	4.77 (4.89)	244
5.0	2.08 (2.03)	2.34	2.67 (2.77)	3.05	3.53 (3.50)	3.92	4.41 (4.24)	4.66	4.93 (4.97)	262
5.5	2.25 (2.15)	2.33	2.67 (2.79)	3.02	3.45 (3.43)	3.79	4.20 (4.07)	4.51	4.62 (4.71)	241
6.0	1.99 (2.00)	2.07	2.43 (2.63)	2.93	3.35 (3.30)	3.67	4.10 (3.90)	4.23	4.48 (4.53)	240
6.5	2.00 (1.92)	2.07	2.31 (2.55)	2.76	3.21 (3.19)	3.60	3.96 (3.82)	4.22	4.39 (4.45)	233
7.0	1.99 (1.99)	2.24	2.45 (2.58)	2.70	3.19 (3.17)	3.53	3.93 (3.75)	4.11	4.26 (4.34)	235
7.5	1.83 (1.72)	2.01	2.20 (2.38)	2.62	2.99 (3.03)	3.45	3.88 (3.69)	4.11	4.29 (4.34)	229
8.0	1.69 (1.69)	1.86	2.18 (2.34)	2.51	3.02 (2.98)	3.45	3.75 (3.62)	3.90	4.18 (4.27)	226
8.5	1.80 (1.82)	2.01	2.23 (2.36)	2.59	2.96 (2.90)	3.21	3.56 (3.44)	3.79	3.86 (3.98)	214
9.0	1.77 (1.73)	1.89	2.11 (2.28)	2.45	2.84 (2.83)	3.21	3.52 (3.37)	3.67	3.70 (3.92)	212

continues

Source: Reprinted with permission from R.N. Baumgartner et al., "Incremental Growth Tables: Supplementary to Previously Published Charts," *The American Journal of Clinical Nutrition* 43, May 1986, pp. 711–722.

Table B–5 continued

Age at end of interval	Percentiles of 6-mo increments									n
	3 (–2 SD)	5	10 (–1 SD)	25	50 (mean)	75	90 (+1 SD)	95	97 (+2 SD)	
yr	*cm/6 mo*									
9.5	1.46 (1.43)	1.61	1.83 (2.02)	2.28	2.67 (2.62)	2.96	3.36 (3.22)	3.64	3.75 (3.82)	204
10.0	1.80 (1.56)	1.89	2.06 (2.15)	2.35	2.70 (2.73)	3.06	3.44 (3.31)	3.69	3.91 (3.89)	202
10.5	1.44 (1.30)	1.56	1.83 (1.94)	2.14	2.56 (2.57)	2.93	3.38 (3.20)	3.67	3.94 (3.84)	208
11.0	1.49 (1.31)	1.68	1.87 (1.96)	2.22	2.52 (2.61)	2.96	3.43 (3.26)	3.74	4.11 (3.91)	204
11.5	1.58 (1.22)	1.69	1.86 (1.96)	2.20	2.57 (2.70)	3.06	3.70 (3.44)	4.00	4.18 (4.18)	198
12.0	1.49 (0.99)	1.60	1.86 (1.93)	2.24	2.73 (2.86)	3.27	4.07 (3.79)	4.68	5.01 (4.72)	196
12.5	1.31 (0.67)	1.49	1.83 (1.85)	2.20	2.77 (3.03)	3.53	4.93 (4.20)	5.44	5.83 (5.38)	195
13.0	1.61 (1.05)	1.87	2.10 (2.28)	2.55	3.29 (3.52)	4.45	5.22 (4.75)	5.75	6.06 (5.98)	191
13.5	1.27 (1.26)	1.55	2.19 (2.42)	2.75	3.49 (3.58)	4.41	5.03 (4.74)	5.31	5.55 (5.89)	188
14.0	1.53 (1.49)	1.84	2.15 (2.65)	2.93	4.01 (3.81)	4.64	5.21 (4.97)	5.49	5.71 (6.13)	190
14.5	1.40 (1.00)	1.51	1.75 (2.28)	2.60	3.59 (3.57)	4.54	5.26 (4.85)	5.48	5.63 (6.13)	186
15.0	0.65 (0.67)	0.90	1.42 (1.90)	2.26	3.19 (3.13)	4.01	4.66 (4.36)	5.11	5.22 (5.59)	179
15.5	0.04 (–0.54)	0.32	0.66 (0.87)	1.24	2.05 (2.29)	3.26	4.28 (3.70)	4.66	4.95 (5.12)	178

continues

Table B–5 continued

Age at end of interval	3 (–2 SD)	5	10 (–1 SD)	25	50 (mean)	75	90 (+1 SD)	95	97 (+2 SD)	n
	Percentiles of 6-mo increments									
yr					*cm/6 mo*					
16.0	–0.28 (–0.62)	0.12	0.60 (0.58)	0.94	1.56 (1.78)	2.48	3.57 (2.98)	3.91	4.21 (4.18)	176
16.5	–0.67 (–1.07)	–0.50	0.03 (0.01)	0.44	0.94 (1.08)	1.50	2.44 (2.16)	2.98	3.81 (3.23)	155
17.0	–0.78 (–0.98)	–0.55	–0.16 (–0.04	0.25	0.83 (0.89)	1.33	1.94 (1.83)	2.85	3.24 (2.76)	153
17.5	–0.84 (–1.03)	–0.66	–0.37 (–0.23)	0.12	0.41 (0.57)	1.00	1.43 (1.37)	1.73	2.26 (2.17)	137
18.0	–0.87 (–0.83)	–0.55	–0.33 (–0.24)	–0.03	0.32 (0.36)	0.72	1.01 (0.96)	1.45	1.61 (1.56)	137

Table B–6 Stature of girls: 3 to 18 yr of age in 6-mo increments (Fels Longitudinal Study)

Age at end of interval	Percentiles of 6-mo increments									
	3 (–2 SD)	5	10 (–1 SD)	25	50 (mean)	75	90 (+1 SD)	95	97 (+2 SD)	n
yr	cm/6 mo									
3.5	2.55 (2.31)	2.84	2.98 (3.09)	3.34	3.79 (3.87)	4.33	4.84 (4.65)	5.24	5.52 (5.43)	195
4.0	2.50 (2.37)	2.72	2.91 (3.04)	3.25	3.65 (3.71)	4.09	4.49 (4.38)	4.97	5.21 (5.05)	211
4.5	2.09 (2.07)	2.23	2.71 (2.82)	3.06	3.54 (3.57)	4.05	4.46 (4.31)	4.81	4.99 (5.06)	230
5.0	2.20 (2.06)	2.33	2.52 (2.80)	3.02	3.52 (3.54)	4.03	4.36 (4.27)	4.84	4.89 (5.01)	240
5.5	2.24 (2.08)	2.42	2.57 (2.74)	2.98	3.39 (3.39)	3.79	4.16 (4.05)	4.48	4.55 (4.71)	226
6.0	2.07 (1.99)	2.23	2.46 (2.64)	2.84	3.30 (3.29)	3.75	4.10 (3.95)	4.49	4.62 (4.60)	227
6.5	1.85 (1.76)	1.93	2.20 (2.42)	2.60	3.11 (3.08)	3.49	3.94 (3.74)	4.29	4.35 (4.41)	223
7.0	1.96 (1.86)	2.11	2.36 (2.48)	2.66	3.08 (3.09)	3.50	3.81 (3.71)	3.98	4.17 (4.33)	223
7.5	1.86 (1.81)	1.98	2.23 (2.42)	2.64	3.07 (3.02)	3.39	3.67 (3.63)	4.03	4.14 (4.23)	221
8.0	1.62 (1.64)	1.82	2.17 (2.31)	2.56	3.01 (2.98)	3.35	3.85 (3.65)	4.07	4.20 (4.32)	222
8.5	1.77 (1.58)	1.86	1.99 (2.22)	2.41	2.88 (2.86)	3.27	3.68 (3.50)	3.90	4.09 (4.14)	222
9.0	1.81 (1.70)	1.93	2.13 (2.28)	2.47	2.84 (2.85)	3.22	3.53 (3.43)	3.77	4.08 (4.01)	216

continues

Source: Reprinted with permission from R.N. Baumgartner et al., "Incremental Growth Tables: Supplementary to Previously Published Charts," *The American Journal of Clinical Nutrition* 43, May 1986, pp. 711–722.

Table B–6 continued

Age at end of interval	3 (–2 SD)	5	10 (–1 SD)	25	50 (mean)	75	90 (+1 SD)	95	97 (+2 SD)	n
	Percentiles of 6-mo increments									
yr	*cm/6 mo*									
9.5	1.64 (1.50)	1.78	1.95 (2.16)	2.36	2.80 (2.83)	3.29	3.58 (3.49)	3.92	4.09 (4.16)	219
10.0	1.63 (1.31)	1.70	1.99 (2.11)	2.38	2.91 (2.90)	3.28	3.83 (3.70)	4.38	4.61 (4.49)	220
10.5	1.57 (1.13)	1.64	1.99 (2.07)	2.37	2.82 (3.01)	3.56	4.21 (3.95)	4.70	5.27 (4.90)	212
11.0	1.67 (1.38)	1.87	2.08 (2.27)	2.53	3.06 (3.16)	3.74	4.33 (4.05)	4.76	4.92 (4.94)	203
11.5	1.51 (1.41)	1.84	2.09 (2.38)	2.54	3.34 (3.35)	4.02	4.63 (4.32)	4.84	5.17 (5.29)	202
12.0	1.67 (1.22)	1.60	1.98 (2.25)	2.65	3.32 (3.28)	3.98	4.52 (4.31)	4.86	4.98 (5.34)	196
12.5	0.79 (1.04)	1.11	1.61 (2.07)	2.41	3.19 (3.10)	3.87	4.38 (4.13)	4.58	4.72 (5.16)	186
13.0	0.36 (0.37)	0.52	1.05 (1.52)	1.99	2.76 (2.67)	3.46	4.09 (3.82)	4.21	4.43 (4.97)	185
13.5	0.25 (–0.21)	0.35	0.57 (0.92)	1.20	1.98 (2.05)	2.90	3.56 (3.19)	3.92	4.24 (4.32)	184
14.0	–0.28 (–0.71)	–0.09	0.28 (0.43)	0.78	1.33 (1.58)	2.35	3.11 (2.72)	3.66	4.09 (3.86)	179
14.5	–0.32 (–0.79)	–0.21	0.04 (0.16)	0.47	0.88 (1.11)	1.65	2.77 (2.06)	2.97	3.32 (3.01)	154
15.0	–0.62 (–0.87)	–0.47	–0.16 (–0.04)	0.24	0.68 (0.78)	1.24	1.75 (1.60)	2.33	2.51 (2.43)	150
15.5	–0.88 (–0.88)	–0.67	–0.43 (–0.20)	0.07	0.49 (0.49)	0.83	1.27 (1.17)	1.62	1.91 (1.85)	143

continues

Table B–6 continued

Age at end of interval	Percentiles of 6-mo increments									
	3 (–2 SD)	*5*	*10 (–1 SD)*	*25*	*50 (mean)*	*75*	*90 (+1 SD)*	*95*	*97 (+2 SD)*	*n*
yr	*cm/6 mo*									
16.0	–0.53 (–0.68)	–0.48	–0.33 (–0.13)	0.04	0.46 (0.42)	0.75	1.08 (0.97)	1.42	1.54 (1.52)	139
16.5	–0.66 (–0.70)	–0.61	–0.37 (–0.21)	–0.05	0.23 (0.28)	0.63	0.91 (0.77)	1.02	1.19 (1.25)	132
17.0	–1.14 (–0.94)	–0.84	–0.65 (–0.38)	–0.13	0.19 (0.17)	0.56	0.81 (0.73)	0.94	1.08 (1.29)	133
17.5	–0.81 (–0.97)	–0.74	–0.51 (–0.41)	–0.21	0.04 (0.14)	0.38	0.97 (0.70)	1.25	1.42 (1.26)	126
18.0	–0.80 (–0.91)	–0.78	–0.64 (–0.39)	–0.15	0.09 (0.13)	0.46	0.83 (0.65)	1.05	1.08 (1.17)	123

Table B–7 Weight of boys: birth to 18 yr of age in 6-mo increments (Fels Longitudinal Study)

Age at end of interval	*Percentiles of 6-mo increments* 3 (–2 SD)	5	10 (–1 SD)	25	50 (mean)	75	90 (+1 SD)	95	97 (+2 SD)	*n*
yr	*kg/6 mo*									
0.5	2.90 (2.84)	3.13	3.47 (3.66)	3.91	4.39 (4.47)	5.06	5.51 (5.29)	5.89	6.18 (6.11)	298
0.75	2.18 (1.86)	2.26	2.41 (2.56)	2.73	3.13 (3.26)	3.71	4.20 (3.96)	4.50	4.72 (4.66)	277
1.0	1.20 (0.93)	1.26	1.52 (1.61)	1.81	2.20 (2.28)	2.66	3.13 (2.96)	3.52	3.74 (3.63)	290
1.5	0.48 (0.20)	0.52	0.67 (0.78)	0.99	1.32 (1.36)	1.71	2.03 (1.93)	2.29	2.55 (2.51)	294
2.0	0.38 (0.27)	0.46	0.63 (0.71)	0.86	1.13 (1.15)	1.38	1.65 (1.59)	1.81	2.13 (2.03)	286
2.5	0.25 (0.19)	0.33	0.52 (0.61)	0.77	1.03 (1.03)	1.26	1.54 (1.45)	1.74	1.80 (1.87)	273
3.0	0.28 (0.21)	0.41	0.51 (0.61)	0.73	0.97 (1.00)	1.26	1.52 (1.40)	1.64	1.76 (1.79)	270
3.5	0.19 (0.00)	0.27	0.48 (0.49)	0.71	0.98 (0.99)	1.27	1.54 (1.48)	1.71	1.79 (1.98)	274
4.0	0.24 (0.07)	0.36	0.53 (0.53)	0.70	0.95 (0.98)	1.23	1.46 (1.43)	1.63	1.75 (1.88)	269
4.5	0.25 (0.08)	0.35	0.47 (0.58)	0.73	1.06 (1.07)	1.35	1.67 (1.57)	1.87	2.08 (2.06)	266
5.0	0.14 (–0.07)	0.25	0.48 (0.52)	0.78	1.06 (1.11)	1.38	1.76 (1.71)	2.03	2.21 (2.30)	268
5.5	0.21 (–0.02)	0.38	0.54 (0.59)	0.77	1.16 (1.19)	1.51	1.91 (1.80)	2.20	2.51 (2.40)	244

continues

Source: Reprinted with permission from R.N. Baumgartner et al., "Incremental Growth Tables: Supplementary to Previously Published Charts," *The American Journal of Clinical Nutrition* 43, May 1986, pp. 711–722. Copyright © 1986 American Society for Clinical Nutrition.

Table B–7 continued

Age at end of interval	3 (–2 SD)	5	10 (–1 SD)	25	50 (mean)	75	90 (+1 SD)	95	97 (+2 SD)	n
	Percentiles of 6-mo increments									
yr	*kg/6 mo*									
6.0	0.07 (0.31)	0.24	0.45 (0.46)	0.82	1.18 (1.23)	1.54	2.01 (2.01)	2.23	2.40 (2.78)	243
6.5	0.09 (0.06)	0.21	0.51 (0.65)	0.90	1.16 (1.24)	1.54	2.07 (1.83)	2.34	2.44 (2.42)	232
7.0	0.21 (–0.32)	0.33	0.49 (0.52)	0.88	1.26 (1.37)	1.75	2.25 (2.22)	2.53	3.20 (3.06)	232
7.5	0.13 (–0.30)	0.40	0.60 (0.57)	0.92	1.38 (1.45)	1.79	2.40 (2.33)	2.87	3.29 (3.21)	224
8.0	0.20 (–0.28)	0.34	0.63 (0.66)	1.00	1.52 (1.61)	1.93	2.54 (2.55)	3.23	3.55 (3.50)	221
8.5	–0.10 (–0.49)	0.28	0.45 (0.54)	1.01	1.43 (1.57)	2.07	2.77 (2.60)	3.35	3.86 (3.63)	210
9.0	–0.46 (–0.77)	0.02	0.50 (0.43)	0.95	1.56 (1.64)	2.28	2.95 (2.84)	3.58	3.96 (4.05)	208
9.5	–0.02 (–0.70)	0.21	0.51 (0.50)	0.96	1.54 (1.71)	2.26	3.05 (2.91)	3.60	4.59 (4.12)	201
10.0	0.01 (–0.62)	0.08	0.38 (0.59)	1.18	1.70 (1.80)	2.38	3.14 (3.01)	3.92	4.36 (4.22)	199
10.5	–0.18 (–0.83)	0.22	0.56 (0.53)	1.09	1.61 (1.90)	2.65	3.63 (3.26)	4.30	4.60 (4.62)	205
11.0	0.15 (–0.47)	0.20	0.53 (0.72)	1.01	1.73 (1.91)	2.46	3.51 (3.10)	4.01	4.50 (4.29)	201
11.5	–0.10 (–0.70)	0.34	0.66 (0.76)	1.24	1.91 (2.22)	3.03	4.33 (3.68)	4.99	5.78 (5.14)	195
12.0	–0.36 (–0.93)	–0.21	0.54 (0.68)	1.30	2.00 (2.29)	3.27	4.24 (3.90)	4.85	5.04 (5.52)	193

continues

Table B–7 continued

Age at end of interval	3 (–2 SD)	5	10 (–1 SD)	25	50 (mean)	75	90 (+1 SD)	95	97 (+2 SD)	n
	Percentiles of 6-mo increments									
yr	*kg/6 mo*									
12.5	–0.39 (–1.03)	–0.01	0.60 (0.77)	1.35	2.45 (2.56)	3.47	4.79 (4.36)	5.36	6.12 (6.15)	192
13.0	0.10 (–0.55)	0.54	0.94 (1.20)	1.71	2.81 (2.95)	3.92	5.29 (4.70)	6.17	6.35 (6.46)	186
13.5	–0.04 (–0.69)	0.37	0.62 (1.19)	1.73	3.06 (3.06)	4.20	5.31 (4.94)	5.81	6.17 (6.81)	183
14.0	–0.61 (–0.59)	–0.06	0.95 (1.35)	2.20	3.33 (3.28)	4.23	5.71 (5.21)	6.56	7.04 (7.15)	187
14.5	–0.70 (–0.39)	–0.06	1.08 (1.58)	2.60	3.67 (3.54)	4.57	5.72 (5.51)	6.41	6.78 (7.47)	183
15.0	–2.99 (–2.08)	–0.72	0.44 (0.46)	1.87	3.24 (3.01)	4.48	5.73 (5.55)	6.34	6.51 (8.09)	176
15.5	–2.17 (–1.83)	–1.25	0.10 (0.41)	1.46	2.59 (2.65)	3.79	5.34 (4.89)	6.26	6.95 (7.12)	176
16.0	–2.58 (–2.49)	–1.36	–0.33 (–0.12)	1.03	2.18 (2.25)	3.54	5.07 (4.62)	6.18	6.92 (6.99)	174
16.5	–2.57 (–2.81)	–1.68	–0.73 (–0.54)	0.45	1.69 (1.73)	2.97	3.85 (4.00)	5.18	6.11 (6.27)	154
17.0	–3.42 (–3.33)	–2.32	–1.63 (–1.07)	–0.17	1.21 (1.19)	2.54	3.57 (3.45)	4.37	5.69 (5.71)	152
17.5	–3.00 (–3.38)	–2.57	–1.21 (–1.02)	–0.00	1.09 (1.35)	2.52	3.99 (3.71)	5.43	6.18 (6.08)	139
18.0	–3.86 (–3.83)	–3.05	–2.04 (–1.44)	–0.58	0.77 (0.94)	2.24	3.82 (3.32)	4.97	6.22 (5.71)	138

Table B–8 Weight of girls: birth to 18 yr of age in 6-mo increments (Fels Longitudinal Study)

	Percentiles of 6-mo increments									
Age at end of interval	*3 (–2 SD)*	*5*	*10 (–1 SD)*	*25*	*50 (mean)*	*75*	*90 (+1 SD)*	*95*	*97 (+2 SD)*	*n*
yr					*kg/6 mo*					
0.5	2.61 (2.48)	2.75	2.96 (3.23)	3.41	4.00 (3.99)	4.54	4.97 (4.74)	5.12	5.31 (5.49)	284
0.75	1.85 (1.70)	1.98	2.21 (2.36)	2.55	3.01 (3.02)	3.46	3.88 (3.69)	4.17	4.26 (4.35)	259
1.0	1.30 (1.06)	1.37	1.51 (1.65)	1.83	2.19 (2.24)	2.59	3.02 (2.82)	3.29	3.40 (3.41)	271
1.5	0.42 (0.31)	0.43	0.68 (0.83)	1.03	1.33 (1.34)	1.63	1.94 (1.85)	2.08	2.18 (2.36)	269
2.0	0.41 (0.28)	0.50	0.61 (0.74)	0.88	1.21 (1.20)	1.45	1.80 (1.66)	1.97	2.18 (2.13)	266
2.5	0.21 (0.06)	0.36	0.51 (0.54)	0.75	0.97 (1.02)	1.27	1.60 (1.51)	1.87	2.09 (1.99)	251
3.0	0.24 (0.10)	0.37	0.48 (0.56)	0.69	1.02 (1.03)	1.31	1.59 (1.50)	1.83	1.98 (1.97)	249
3.5	0.34 (0.20)	0.42	0.55 (0.62)	0.76	1.00 (1.04)	1.29	1.56 (1.46)	1.80	1.92 (1.88)	249
4.0	0.11 (0.11)	0.30	0.50 (0.56)	0.73	0.98 (1.01)	1.26	1.54 (1.46)	1.73	1.84 (1.91)	242
4.5	0.13 (0.03)	0.22	0.43 (0.49)	0.67	0.94 (1.02)	1.29	1.78 (1.55)	1.88	2.14 (2.07)	241
5.0	0.05 (–0.18)	0.26	0.46 (0.46)	0.73	1.03 (1.09)	1.41	1.73 (1.72)	2.14	2.32 (2.36)	241
5.5	0.05 (–0.28)	0.22	0.36 (0.41)	0.68	0.97 (1.11)	1.44	2.06 (1.80)	2.37	2.56 (2.49)	221

continues

Source: Reprinted with permission from R.N. Baumgartner et al., "Incremental Growth Tables: Supplementary to Previously Published Charts," *The American Journal of Clinical Nutrition* 43, May 1986, pp. 711–722.

Table B–8 continued

Age at end of interval	3 (−2 SD)	5	10 (−1 SD)	25	50 (mean)	75	90 (+1 SD)	95	97 (+2 SD)	n
	Percentiles of 6-mo increments									
yr	kg/6 mo									
6.0	0.05 (−0.26)	0.23	0.44 (0.46)	0.78	1.12 (1.18)	1.44	1.97 (1.91)	2.49	2.88 (2.63)	221
6.5	0.18 (−0.25)	0.28	0.48 (0.52)	0.83	1.19 (1.29)	1.63	2.00 (2.06)	2.54	2.95 (2.82)	216
7.0	0.16 (−0.22)	0.28	0.44 (0.52)	0.80	1.18 (1.26)	1.59	2.27 (2.00)	2.52	2.74 (2.74)	216
7.5	0.25 (−0.28)	0.36	0.61 (0.60)	0.95	1.32 (1.48)	1.81	2.47 (2.36)	3.03	3.46 (3.24)	211
8.0	−0.08 (−0.42)	0.14	0.39 (0.53)	0.92	1.36 (1.48)	1.98	2.73 (2.43)	3.21	3.48 (3.38)	212
8.5	0.12 (−0.44)	0.26	0.53 (0.60)	1.00	1.48 (1.63)	2.06	2.87 (2.66)	3.36	4.06 (3.71)	214
9.0	0.14 (−0.29)	0.31	0.62 (0.68)	1.02	1.47 (1.65)	2.20	2.97 (2.61)	3.51	3.83 (3.58)	207
9.5	0.00 (−0.69)	0.37	0.58 (0.57)	1.02	1.53 (1.83)	2.48	3.27 (3.09)	3.90	4.77 (4.35)	209
10.0	−0.10 (−1.09)	0.14	0.44 (0.37)	1.05	1.57 (1.84)	2.36	3.48 (3.31)	4.35	5.05 (4.77)	210
10.5	−0.70 (−0.87)	0.23	0.53 (0.62)	1.17	1.96 (2.12)	2.87	4.04 (3.61)	4.80	5.22 (5.11)	202
11.0	−0.50 (−1.07)	−0.12	0.70 (0.57)	1.28	2.01 (2.22)	3.22	3.94 (3.87)	4.63	5.39 (5.51)	194
11.5	0.05 (−0.56)	0.28	0.88 (0.98)	1.39	2.48 (2.52)	3.44	4.39 (4.10)	4.97	5.78 (5.61)	194
12.0	−0.41 (−0.71)	0.31	0.68 (1.06)	1.68	2.74 (2.82)	3.90	5.11 (4.59)	5.47	5.91 (6.36)	187

continues

Table B–8 continued

Age at end of interval	Percentiles of 6-mo increments									
	3 (–2 SD)	5	10 (–1 SD)	25	50 (mean)	75	90 (+1 SD)	95	97 (+2 SD)	n
yr	*kg/6 mo*									
12.5	–0.42 (–0.67)	–0.09	0.51 (1.00)	1.43	2.76 (2.67)	3.69	4.79 (4.34)	5.63	6.14 (6.01)	177
13.0	–1.53 (–1.76)	–0.78	–0.03 (0.19)	1.40	2.15 (2.15)	3.26	4.15 (4.11)	4.76	5.10 (6.06)	175
13.5	–1.13 (–1.09)	–0.40	0.47 (0.68)	1.28	2.31 (2.45)	3.48	4.64 (4.22)	5.14	5.65 (5.99)	174
14.0	–2.15 (–2.02)	–1.52	–0.61 (–0.12)	0.51	1.83 (1.77)	3.11	4.13 (3.67)	4.61	5.21 (5.57)	169
14.5	–3.90 (–3.10)	–2.15	–1.12 (–0.86)	0.41	1.50 (1.38)	2.51	3.67 (3.62)	3.94	4.82 (5.86)	146
15.0	–3.61 (–3.05)	–1.94	–0.92 (–0.99)	–0.01	1.00 (1.07)	2.33	3.45 (3.13)	3.91	4.85 (5.18)	143
15.5	–2.61 (–2.60)	–2.01	–1.23 (–0.81)	–0.01	0.92 (0.97)	2.00	2.92 (2.76)	3.73	4.35 (4.54)	135
16.0	–3.13 (–3.49)	–2.85	–2.10 (–1.62)	–0.76	0.37 (0.25)	1.27	2.08 (2.11)	2.96	3.58 (3.98)	134
16.5	–3.17 (–2.98)	–2.48	–1.60 (–1.15)	–0.20	0.75 (0.68)	1.66	2.82 (2.52)	3.44	3.88 (4.35)	126
17.0	–3.92 (–3.25)	–2.51	–1.96 (–1.43)	–0.59	0.64 (0.40)	1.46	2.54 (2.22)	3.00	3.70 (4.04)	125
17.5	–2.98 (–3.16)	–2.52	–1.75 (–1.40)	–0.86	0.40 (0.36)	1.32	2.45 (2.12)	3.08	3.52 (3.88)	116
18.0	–3.84 (–3.21)	–3.11	–1.41 (–1.35)	–0.72	0.47 (0.50)	1.55	2.93 (2.35)	3.68	4.24 (4.21)	113

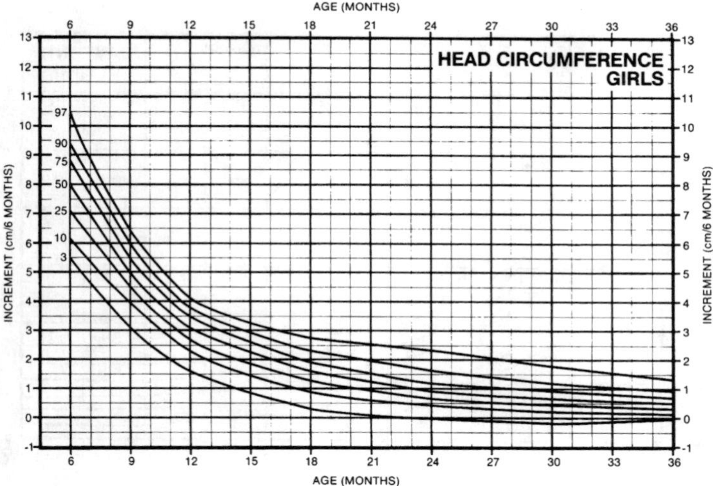

Figure B–9 Incremental growth for head circumference (cm per 6 months) in white girls aged 6–36 months. *Source:* Used with permission of Ross Products Division, Abbott Laboratories, Inc., Columbus, OH 43216. From Ross Growth and Development Programs, © 1981, Ross Products Division, Abbott Laboratories.

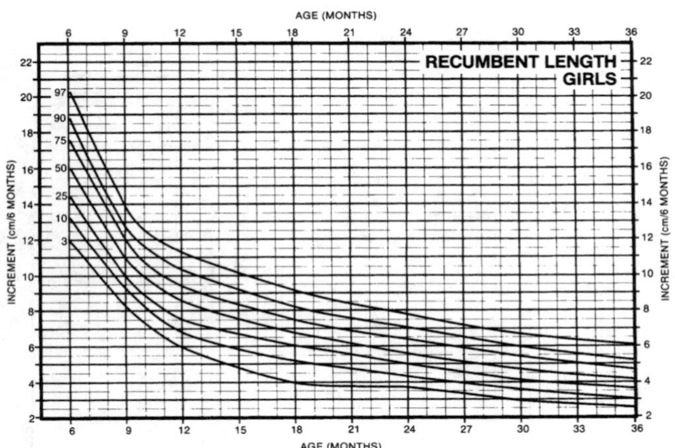

Figure B–10 Incremental growth for recumbent length (cm per 6 months) in white girls aged 6–36 months. *Source:* Used with permission of Ross Products Division, Abbott Laboratories, Inc., Columbus, OH 43216. From Ross Growth and Development Programs, © 1981, Ross Products Division, Abbott Laboratories.

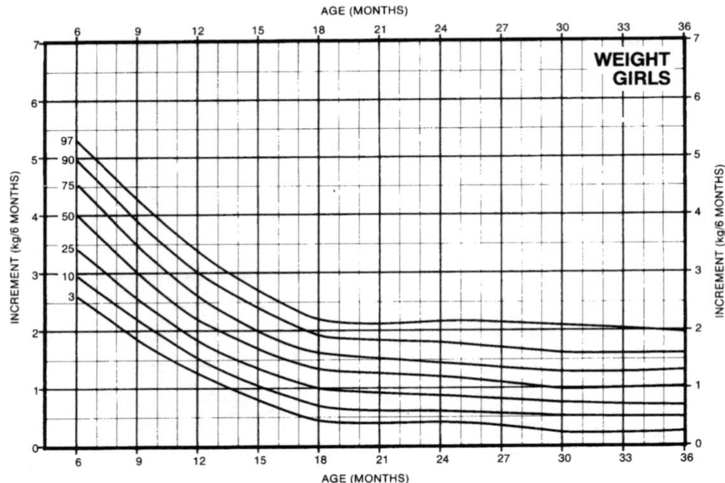

Figure B–11 Incremental growth for weight (kg per 6 months) in white girls aged 6–36 months. *Source:* Used with permission of Ross Products Division, Abbott Laboratories, Inc., Columbus, OH 43216. From Ross Growth and Development Programs, © 1981, Ross Products Division, Abbott Laboratories.

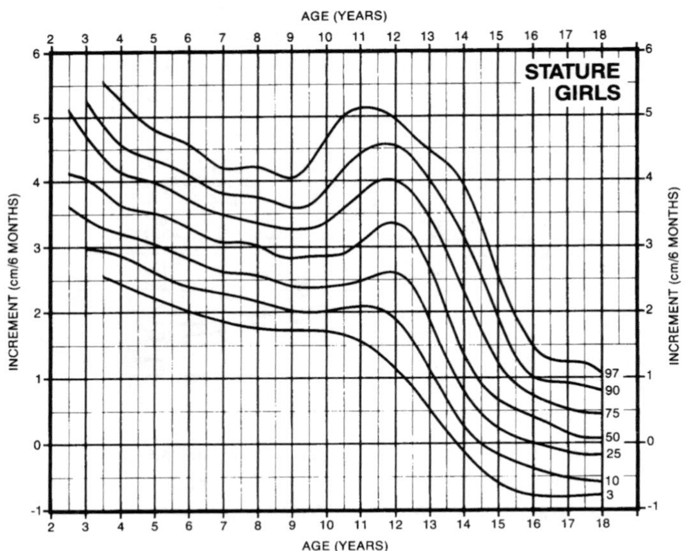

Figure B–12 Incremental growth for stature (cm per 6 months) in white girls aged 2–18 years. *Source:* Used with permission of Ross Products Division, Abbott Laboratories, Inc., Columbus, OH 43216. From Ross Growth and Development Programs, © 1981, Ross Products Division, Abbott Laboratories.

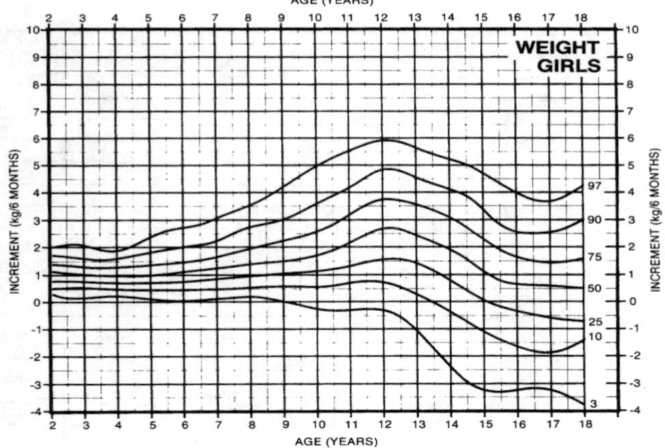

Figure B–13 Incremental growth for weight (kg per 6 months) in white girls aged 2–18 years. *Source:* Used with permission of Ross Products Division, Abbott Laboratories, Inc., Columbus, OH 43216. From Ross Growth and Development Programs, © 1981, Ross Products Division, Abbott Laboratories.

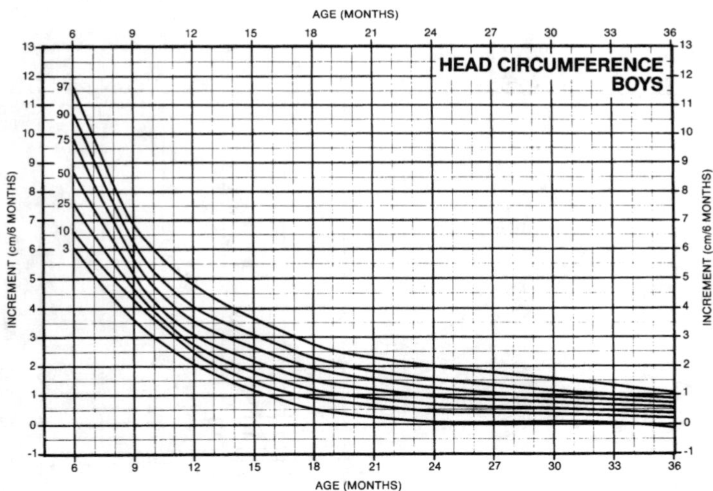

Figure B–14 Incremental growth for head circumference (cm per 6 months) in white boys aged 6–36 months. *Source:* Used with permission of Ross Products Division, Abbott Laboratories, Inc., Columbus, OH 43216. From Ross Growth and Development Programs, © 1981, Ross Products Division, Abbott Laboratories.

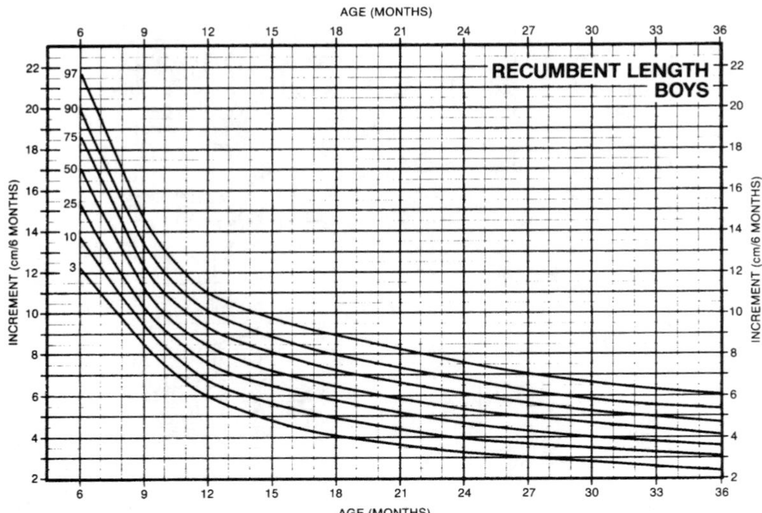

Figure B–15 Incremental growth for recumbent length (cm per 6 months) in white boys aged 6–36 months. *Source:* Used with permission of Ross Products Division, Abbott Laboratories, Inc., Columbus, OH 43216. From Ross Growth and Development Programs, © 1981, Ross Products Division, Abbott Laboratories.

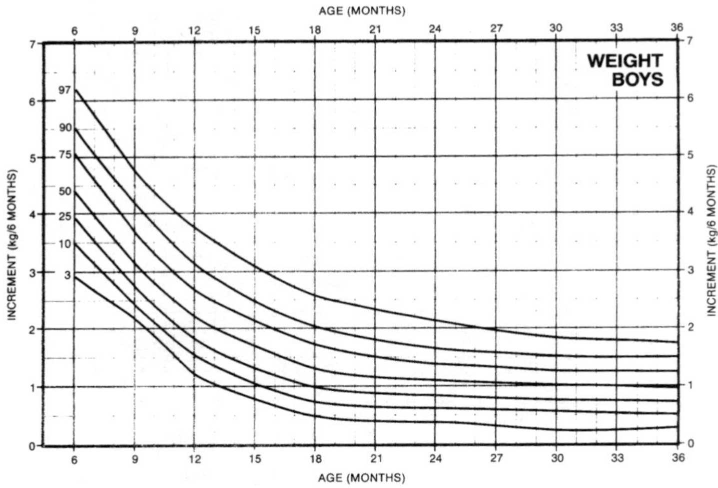

Figure B–16 Incremental growth for weight (kg per 6 months) in white boys aged 6–36 months. *Source:* Used with permission of Ross Products Division, Abbott Laboratories, Inc., Columbus, OH 43216. From Ross Growth and Development Programs, © 1981, Ross Products Division, Abbott Laboratories.

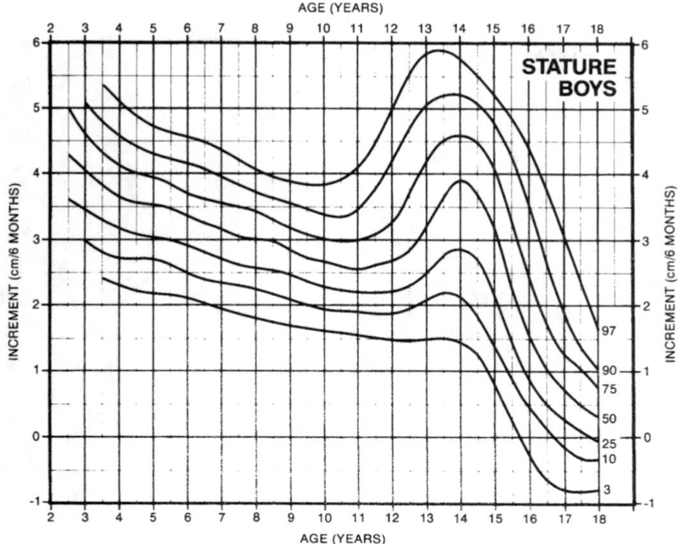

Figure B–17 Incremental growth for stature (cm per 6 months) in white boys aged 2–18 years. *Source:* Used with permission of Ross Products Division, Abbott Laboratories, Inc., Columbus, OH 43216. From Ross Growth and Development Programs, © 1981, Ross Products Division, Abbott Laboratories.

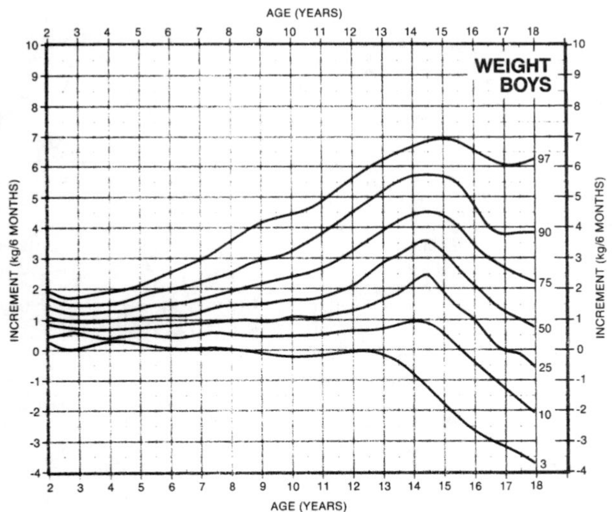

Figure B–18 Incremental growth for weight (kg per 6 months) in white boys aged 2–18 years. *Source:* Used with permission of Ross Products Division, Abbott Laboratories, Inc., Columbus, OH 43216. From Ross Growth and Development Programs, © 1981, Ross Products Division, Abbott Laboratories.

APPENDIX C

Down Syndrome Growth Charts

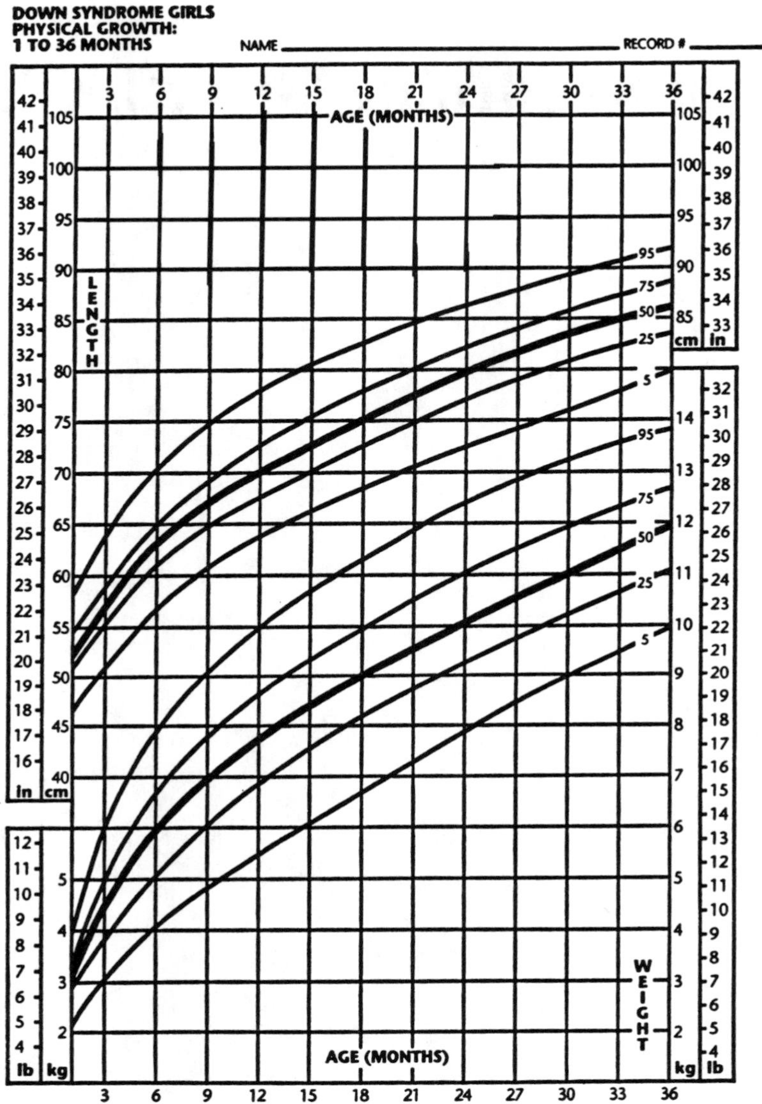

Figure C–1 Down syndrome, length and weight for girls, 1 to 36 months. *Source:* Reprinted with permission from C.C. Crocker et al, Growth Charts for Children with Down Syndrome: 1 Month to 18 Years of Age, *PEDIATRICS,* Vol. 81, pp. 102-110, © 1988, American Academy of Pediatrics.

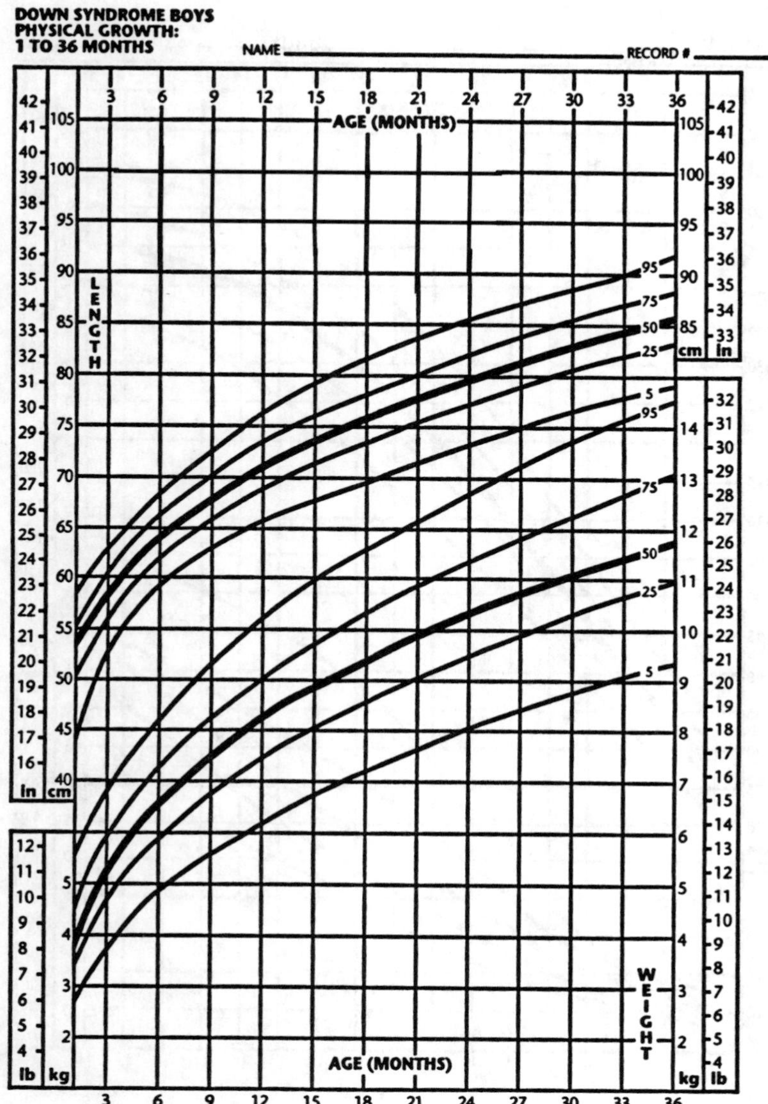

Figure C–2 Down syndrome, length and weight for boys, 1 to 36 months. *Source:* Reprinted with permission from C.C. Crocker et al, Growth Charts for Children with Down Syndrome: 1 Month to 18 Years of Age, *PEDIATRICS,* Vol. 81, pp. 102-110, © 1988, American Academy of Pediatrics.

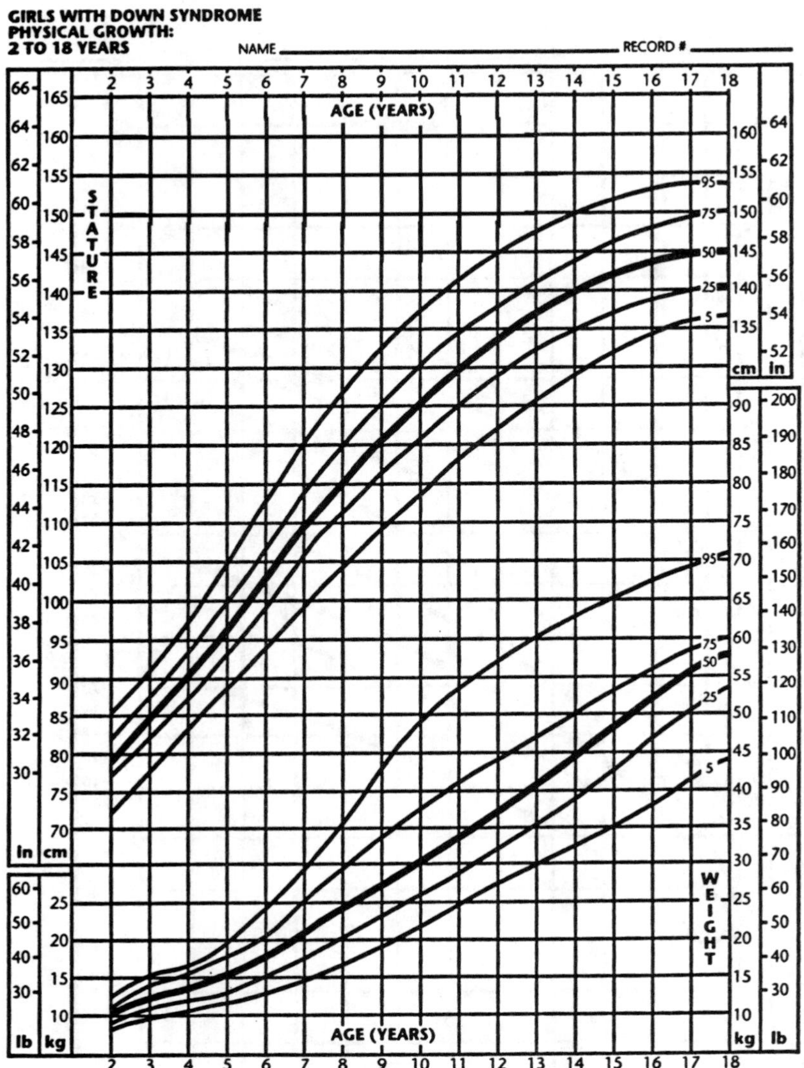

Figure C–3 Down syndrome, height and weight for girls, 2 to 18 years. *Source:* Reprinted with permission from C.C. Crocker et al, Growth Charts for Children with Down Syndrome: 1 Month to 18 Years of Age, *PEDIATRICS,* Vol. 81, pp. 102-110, © 1988, American Academy of Pediatrics.

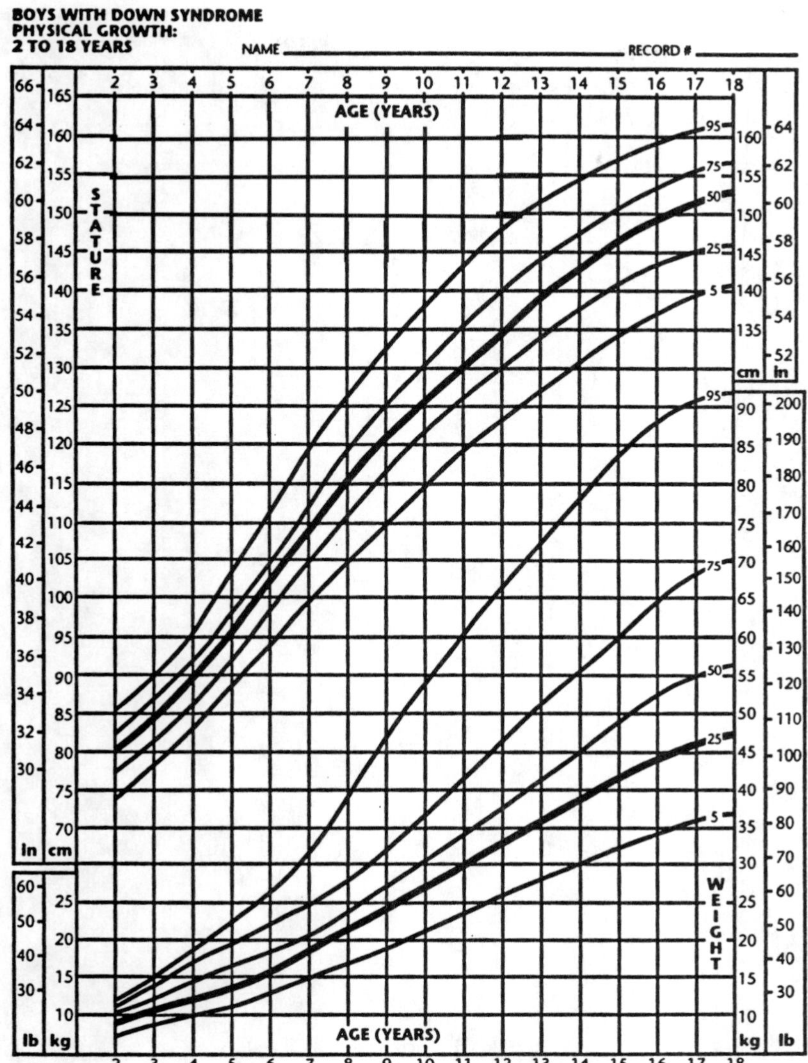

Figure C–4 Down syndrome, height and weight for boys, 2 to 18 years. *Source:* Reprinted with permission from C.C. Crocker et al, Growth Charts for Children with Down Syndrome: 1 Month to 18 Years of Age, *PEDIATRICS,* Vol. 81, pp. 102-110, © 1988, American Academy of Pediatrics.

Appendix D

BMI and Weight Gain Charts

Source: Reprinted from *Supplementary Materials for Nutrition During Pregnancy and Lactation: An Implementation Guide,* Washington, D.C., Food and Nutrition Board, Institute of Medicine, National Academy Press, 1992.

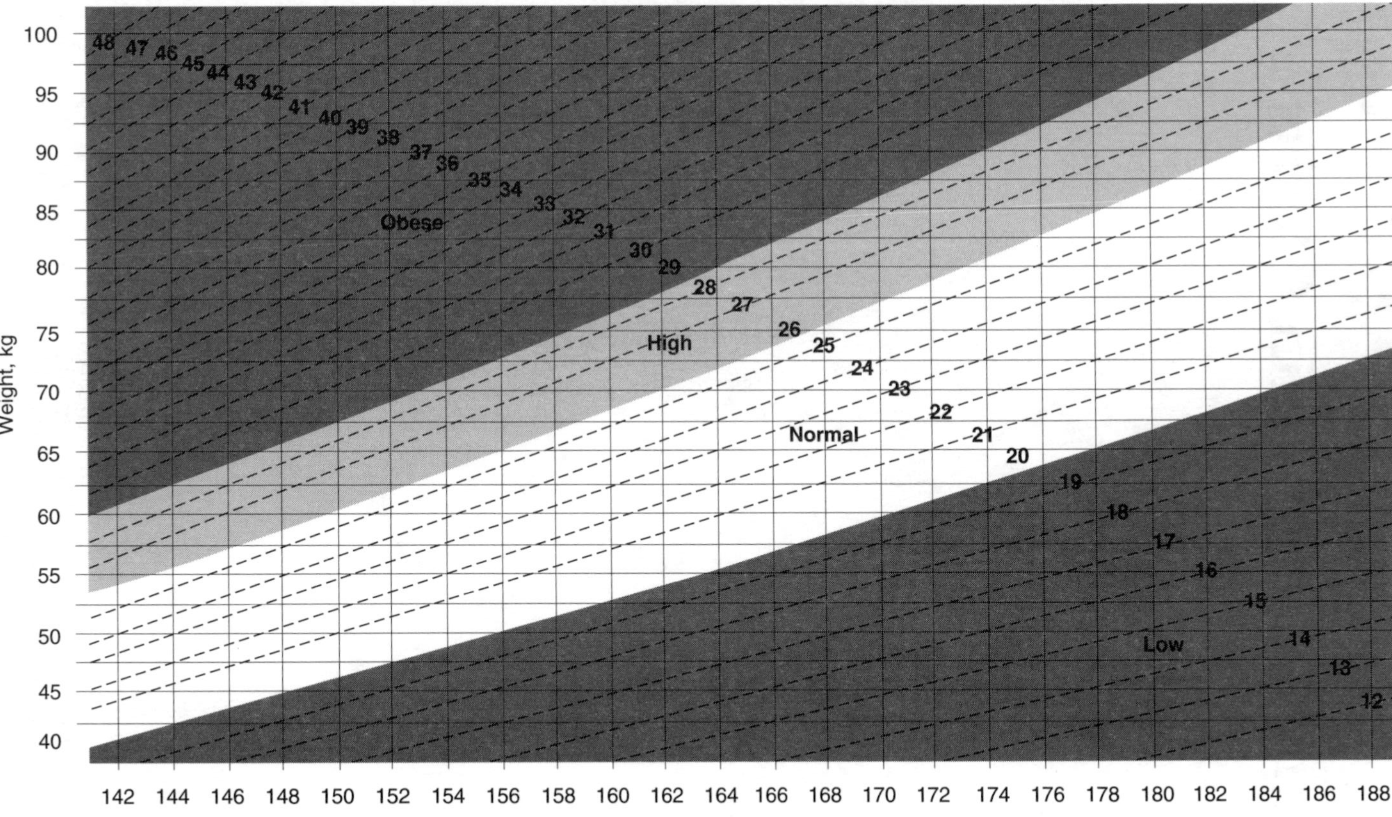

Figure D–1 Chart for Estimating Body Mass Index (BMI) Category and BMI (Metric Units). Directions: To find BMI category (e.g., obese), find the point where the woman's height and weight intersect. To estimate BMI, read the bold number on the dashed line that is closest to this point.

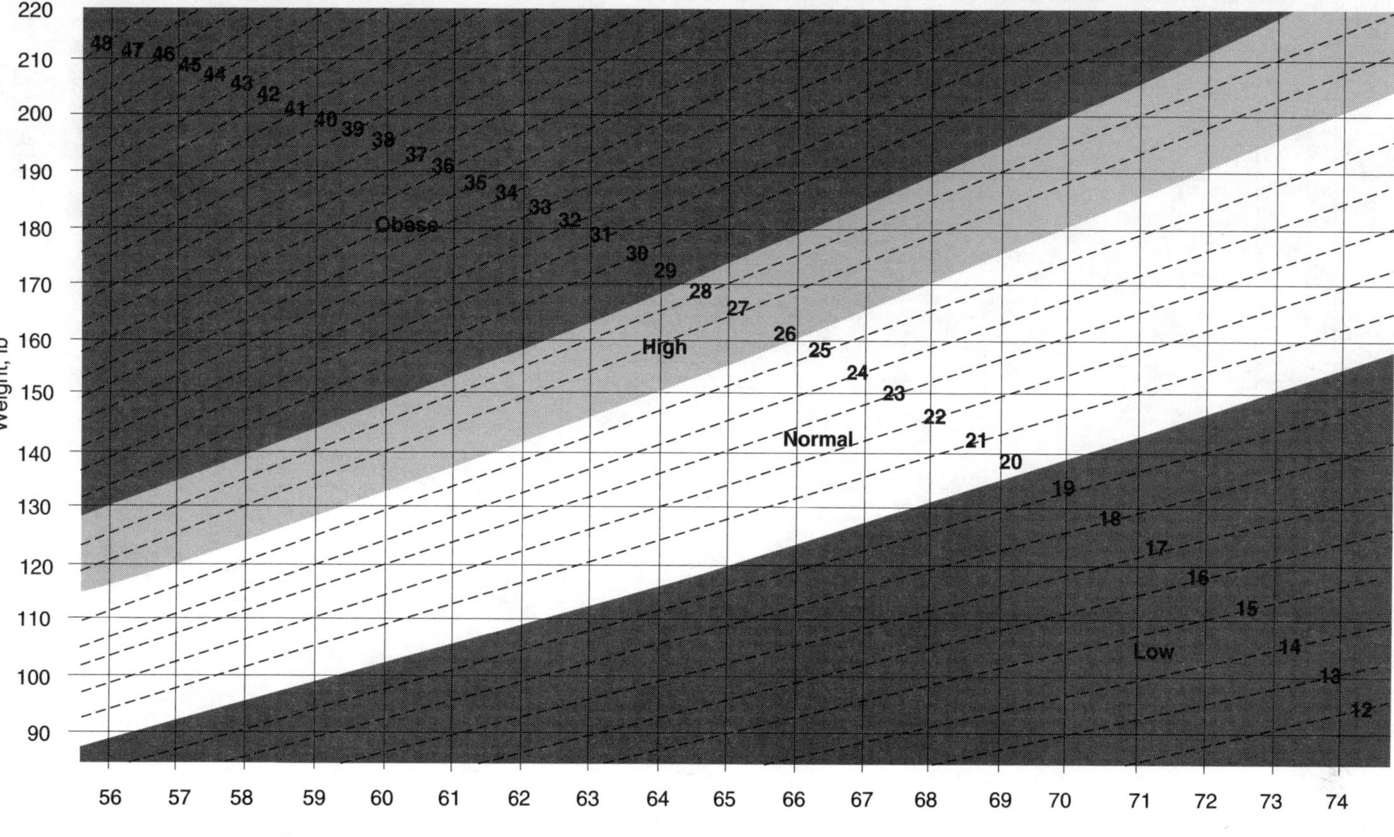

Figure D–2 Chart for Estimating Body Mass Index (BMI) Category and BMI (Pounds and Inches). Directions: To find BMI category (e.g., obese), find the point where the woman's height and weight intersect. To estimate BMI, read the bold number on the dashed line that is closest to this point.

Exhibit D–1 Pound to Kilogram Conversion Chart

lb	kg	lb	kg	lb	kg	lb	kg	lb	kg
85.0	38.6	108.0	49.1	131.0	59.5	154.0	70.0	177.0	80.5
85.5	38.9	108.5	49.3	131.5	59.8	154.5	70.2	177.5	80.7
86.0	39.1	109.0	49.5	132.0	60.0	155.0	70.5	178.0	80.9
86.5	39.3	109.5	49.8	132.5	60.2	155.5	70.7	178.5	81.1
87.0	39.5	110.0	50.0	133.0	60.5	156.0	70.9	179.0	81.4
87.5	39.8	110.5	50.2	133.5	60.7	156.5	71.1	179.5	81.6
88.0	40.0	111.0	50.5	134.0	60.9	157.0	71.4	180.0	81.8
88.5	40.2	111.5	50.7	134.5	61.1	157.5	71.6	180.5	82.0
89.0	40.5	112.0	50.9	135.0	61.4	158.0	71.8	181.0	82.3
89.5	40.7	112.5	51.1	135.5	61.6	158.5	72.0	181.5	82.5
90.0	40.9	113.0	51.4	136.0	61.8	159.0	72.3	182.0	82.7
90.5	41.1	113.5	51.6	136.5	62.0	159.5	72.5	182.5	83.0
91.0	41.4	114.0	51.8	137.0	62.3	160.0	72.7	183.0	83.2
91.5	41.6	114.5	52.0	137.5	62.5	160.5	73.0	183.5	83.4
92.0	41.8	115.0	52.3	138.0	62.7	161.0	73.2	184.0	83.6
92.5	42.0	115.5	52.5	138.5	63.0	161.5	73.4	184.5	83.9
93.0	42.3	116.0	52.7	139.0	63.2	162.0	73.6	185.0	84.1
93.5	42.5	116.5	53.0	139.5	63.4	162.5	73.9	185.5	84.3
94.0	42.7	117.0	53.2	140.0	63.6	163.0	74.1	186.0	84.5
94.5	43.0	117.5	53.4	140.5	63.9	163.5	74.3	186.5	84.8
95.0	43.2	118.0	53.6	141.0	64.1	164.0	74.5	187.0	85.0
95.5	43.4	118.5	53.9	141.5	64.3	164.5	74.8	187.5	85.2
96.0	43.6	119.0	54.1	142.0	64.5	165.0	75.0	188.0	85.5
96.5	43.9	119.5	54.3	142.5	64.8	165.5	75.2	188.5	85.7
97.0	44.1	120.0	54.5	143.0	65.0	166.0	75.5	189.0	85.9
97.5	44.3	120.5	54.8	143.5	65.2	166.5	75.7	189.5	86.1
98.0	44.5	121.0	55.0	144.0	65.5	167.0	75.9	190.0	86.4
98.5	44.8	121.5	55.2	144.5	65.7	167.5	76.1	190.5	86.6
99.0	45.0	122.0	55.5	145.0	65.9	168.0	76.4	191.0	86.8
99.5	45.2	122.5	55.7	145.5	66.1	168.5	76.6	191.5	87.0
100.0	45.5	123.0	55.9	146.0	66.[illegible]	169.0	76.8	192.0	87.3
100.5	45.7	123.5	56.1	146.5	66.6	169.5	77.0	192.5	87.5
101.0	45.9	124.0	56.4	147.0	66.8	170.0	77.3	193.0	87.7
101.5	46.1	124.5	56.6	147.5	67.0	170.5	77.5	193.5	88.0
102.0	46.4	125.0	56.8	148.0	67.3	171.0	77.7	194.0	88.2
102.5	46.6	125.5	57.0	148.5	67.5	171.5	78.0	194.5	88.4
103.0	46.8	126.0	57.3	149.0	67.7	172.0	78.2	195.0	88.6
103.5	47.0	126.5	57.5	149.5	68.0	172.5	78.4	195.5	88.9
104.0	47.3	127.0	57.7	150.0	68.2	173.0	78.6	196.0	89.1
104.5	47.5	127.5	58.0	150.5	68.4	173.5	78.9	196.5	89.3
105.0	47.7	128.0	58.2	151.0	68.6	174.0	79.1	197.0	89.5
105.5	48.0	128.5	58.4	151.5	68.9	174.5	79.3	197.5	89.8
106.0	48.2	129.0	58.6	152.0	69.1	175.0	79.5	198.0	90.0
106.5	48.4	129.5	58.9	152.5	69.3	175.5	79.8	198.5	90.2
107.0	48.6	130.0	59.1	153.0	69.5	176.0	80.0	199.0	90.5
107.5	48.9	130.5	59.3	153.5	69.8	176.5	80.2	199.5	90.7

Exhibit D–2 Sample Prenatal Weight Gain Chart

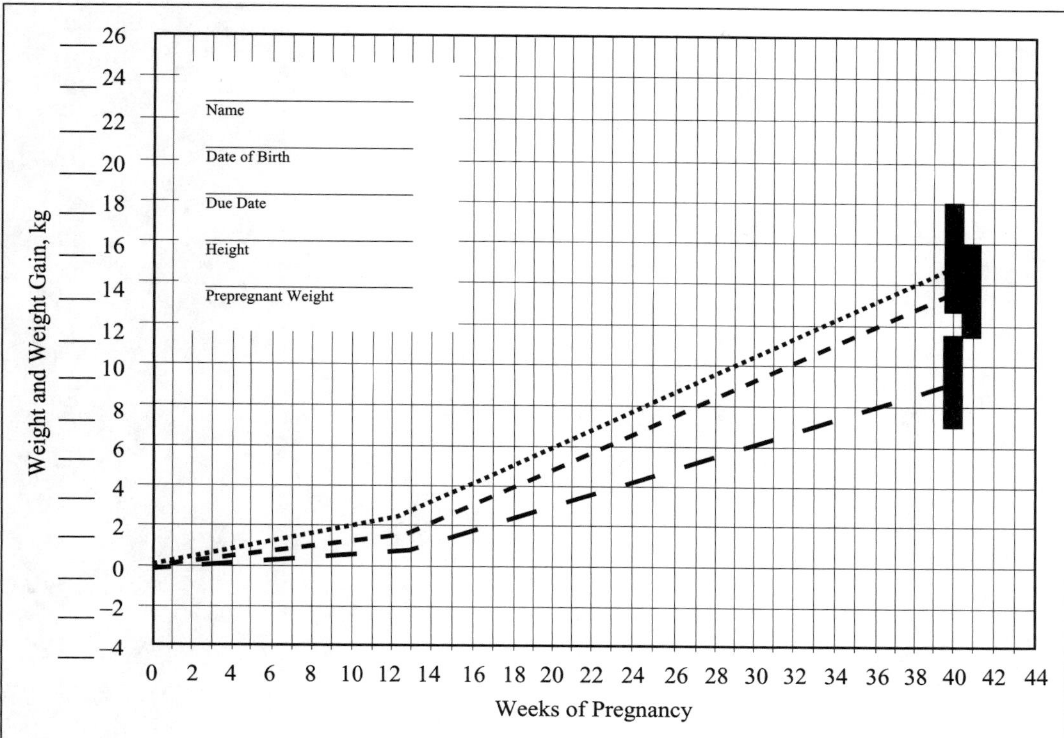

Prepregnancy BMI <19,8 (- - -), Prepregnancy BMI 19.8–26.0 (Normal Body Weight) (– – –), Prepregnancy BMI > 26.0 (— — —)

Weight Record			
Date	Weeks of Gestation	Weight	Notes

APPENDIX E

Body Mass Index for Selected Weights and Statures

Weight		Stature m (in)													
kg	(lb)	1.24 (49)	1.27 (50)	1.30 (51)	1.32 (52)	1.35 (53)	1.37 (54)	1.40 (55)	1.42 (56)	1.45 (57)	1.47 (58)	1.50 (59)	1.52 (60)	1.55 (61)	1.57 (62)
20	(45)	13	13	12	12	11	11	10	10	10	9	9	9	8	
23	(50)	15	14	13	13	12	12	12	11	11	10	10	10	9	9
25	(55)	16	15	15	14	14	13	13	12	12	12	11	11	10	10
27	(60)	18	17	16	16	15	15	14	13	13	13	12	12	11	11
29	(65)	19	18	17	17	16	16	15	15	14	14	13	13	12	12
32	(70)	21	20	19	18	17	17	16	16	15	15	14	14	13	13
34	(75)	22	21	20	20	19	18	17	17	16	16	15	15	14	14
36	(80)	24	22	21	21	20	19	19	18	17	17	16	16	15	15
39	(85)	25	24	23	22	21	21	20	19	18	18	17	17	16	16
41	(90)	27	25	24	23	22	22	21	20	19	19	18	18	17	17
43	(95)	28	27	25	25	24	23	22	21	20	20	19	19	18	17
45	(100)	29	28	27	26	25	24	23	22	22	21	20	20	19	18
48	(105)	31	30	28	27	26	25	24	24	23	22	21	21	20	19
50	(110)	32	31	30	29	27	27	25	25	24	23	22	22	21	20
52	(115)	34	32	31	30	29	28	27	26	25	24	23	23	22	21
54	(120)	35	34	32	31	30	29	28	27	26	25	24	24	23	22
57	(125)	37	35	34	33	31	30	29	28	27	26	25	25	24	23
59	(130)	38	37	35	34	32	31	30	29	28	27	26	26	25	24
61	(135)	40	38	36	35	34	33	31	30	29	28	27	27	25	25
64	(140)	41	39	38	36	35	34	32	31	30	29	28	27	26	26
66	(145)	43	41	39	38	36	35	34	33	31	30	29	28	27	27
68	(150)	44	42	40	39	37	36	35	34	32	31	30	29	28	28
70	(155)	46	44	42	40	39	37	36	35	33	33	31	30	29	29
73	(160)	47	45	43	42	40	39	37	36	35	34	32	31	30	29
77	(170)	50	48	46	44	42	41	39	38	37	36	34	33	32	31
79	(175)	—	49	47	46	44	42	40	39	38	37	35	34	33	32
82	(180)	—	51	48	47	45	44	42	40	39	38	36	35	34	33
84	(185)	—	—	50	48	46	45	43	42	40	39	37	36	35	34
86	(190)	—	—	—	49	47	46	44	43	41	40	39	37	36	35
88	(195)	—	—	—	51	49	47	45	44	42	41	39	38	37	36
91	(200)	—	—	—	—	50	48	46	45	43	42	40	39	38	37
93	(205)	—	—	—	—	—	50	47	46	44	43	41	40	39	38

Weight kg	(lb)	Stature m (in) 1.24 (49)	1.27 (50)	1.30 (51)	1.32 (52)	1.35 (53)	1.37 (54)	1.40 (55)	1.42 (56)	1.45 (57)	1.47 (58)	1.50 (59)	1.52 (60)	1.55 (61)	1.57 (62)
95	(210)	—	—	—	—	—	—	49	47	45	44	42	41	40	39
98	(215)	—	—	—	—	—	—	50	48	46	45	43	42	41	40
100	(220)	—	—	—	—	—	—	—	49	47	46	44	43	42	40
102	(225)	—	—	—	—	—	—	—	51	49	47	45	44	42	41
104	(230)	—	—	—	—	—	—	—	—	50	48	46	45	43	42
107	(235)	—	—	—	—	—	—	—	—	—	49	47	46	44	43
109	(240)	—	—	—	—	—	—	—	—	—	50	48	47	45	44
111	(245)	—	—	—	—	—	—	—	—	—	—	49	48	46	45
113	(250)	—	—	—	—	—	—	—	—	—	—	50	49	47	46
116	(255)	—	—	—	—	—	—	—	—	—	—	—	50	48	47
118	(260)	—	—	—	—	—	—	—	—	—	—	—	—	49	48
120	(265)	—	—	—	—	—	—	—	—	—	—	—	—	50	49
122	(270)	—	—	—	—	—	—	—	—	—	—	—	—	—	50
125	(275)	—	—	—	—	—	—	—	—	—	—	—	—	—	—
127	(280)	—	—	—	—	—	—	—	—	—	—	—	—	—	—
129	(285)	—	—	—	—	—	—	—	—	—	—	—	—	—	—
132	(290)	—	—	—	—	—	—	—	—	—	—	—	—	—	—
134	(295)	—	—	—	—	—	—	—	—	—	—	—	—	—	—
136	(300)	—	—	—	—	—	—	—	—	—	—	—	—	—	—

Source: Reprinted by permission from Guidelines for Adolescent Preventive Services (GAPS), Clinical Evaluation and Management Handbook, © 1995, American Medical Association.

Weight kg	(lb)	Stature m (in) 1.60 (63)	1.63 (64)	1.65 (65)	1.68 (66)	1.70 (67)	1.73 (68)	1.75 (69)	1.78 (70)	1.80 (71)	1.83 (72)	1.85 (73)	1.88 (74)	1.90 (75)	1.93 (76)
20	(45)	9	9	8	—	—	—	—	—	—	—	—	—	—	—
25	(50)	10	9	9	9	—	—	—	—	—	—	—	—	—	—
27	(55)	11	10	10	10	9	9	—	—	—	—	—	—	—	—
29	(65)	12	11	11	10	10	10	10	—	—	—	—	—	—	—
32	(70)	12	12	12	11	11	11	10	10	—	—	—	—	—	—
34	(75)	13	13	12	12	12	11	11	11	10	—	—	—	—	—
36	(80)	14	14	13	13	13	12	12	11	11	11	—	—	—	—
39	(85)	15	15	14	14	13	13	13	12	12	12	11	—	—	—
41	(90)	16	15	15	14	14	14	13	13	13	12	12	12	—	—
43	(95)	17	16	16	15	15	14	14	13	13	13	12	12	—	—
45	(100)	18	17	17	16	16	15	15	14	14	14	13	13	13	12
48	(105)	19	18	17	17	16	16	16	15	15	14	14	13	13	13
50	(110)	19	19	18	18	17	17	16	16	15	15	15	14	14	13
52	(115)	20	20	19	18	18	17	17	16	16	16	15	15	14	14
54	(120)	21	20	20	19	19	18	18	17	17	16	16	15	15	15
57	(125)	22	21	21	20	20	19	19	18	17	17	17	16	16	15
59	(130)	23	22	22	21	20	20	19	19	18	18	17	17	16	16
61	(135)	24	23	22	22	21	20	20	19	19	18	18	17	17	16
64	(140)	25	24	23	22	22	21	21	20	20	19	19	18	18	17
66	(145)	26	25	24	23	23	22	21	21	20	20	19	19	18	18
68	(150)	27	26	25	24	24	23	22	21	21	20	20	19	19	18
70	(155)	27	26	26	25	24	23	23	22	22	21	21	20	19	19
73	(160)	28	27	27	26	25	24	24	23	22	22	21	21	20	19
77	(170)	30	29	28	27	27	26	25	24	24	23	23	22	21	21
79	(175)	31	30	29	28	27	27	26	25	24	24	23	22	22	21
82	(180)	32	31	30	29	28	27	27	26	25	24	24	23	23	22
84	(185)	33	32	31	30	29	28	27	26	26	25	25	24	23	23
86	(190)	34	32	32	31	30	29	28	27	27	26	25	24	24	23
88	(195)	35	33	32	31	31	30	29	28	27	26	26	25	25	24
91	(200)	35	34	33	32	31	30	30	29	28	27	27	26	25	25
93	(205)	36	35	34	33	32	31	30	29	29	28	27	26	26	26

Weight kg	(lb)	Stature m (in) 1.60 (63)	1.63 (64)	1.65 (65)	1.68 (66)	1.70 (67)	1.73 (68)	1.75 (69)	1.78 (70)	1.80 (71)	1.83 (72)	1.85 (73)	1.88 (74)	1.90 (75)	1.93 (76)
95	(210)	37	36	35	34	33	32	31	30	29	28	28	27	26	26
98	(215)	38	37	36	35	34	33	32	31	30	29	28	28	27	26
100	(220)	39	38	37	35	35	33	33	31	31	30	29	28	28	27
102	(225)	40	38	37	36	35	34	33	32	31	30	30	29	28	27
104	(230)	41	39	38	37	36	35	34	33	32	31	30	30	29	28
107	(235)	42	40	39	38	37	36	35	34	33	32	31	30	30	29
109	(240)	43	41	40	39	38	36	36	34	34	33	32	31	30	29
111	(245)	43	42	41	39	38	37	36	35	34	33	32	31	31	30
113	(250)	44	43	42	40	39	38	37	36	35	34	33	32	31	30
116	(255)	45	44	42	41	40	39	38	37	36	35	34	33	32	31
118	(260)	46	44	43	42	41	39	39	37	36	35	34	33	33	32
120	(265)	47	45	44	43	42	40	39	38	37	36	35	34	33	32
122	(270)	48	46	45	43	42	41	40	39	38	37	36	35	34	33
125	(275)	49	47	46	44	43	42	41	39	38	37	36	35	35	33
127	(280)	50	48	47	45	44	42	41	40	39	38	37	36	35	34
129	(285)	50	49	47	46	45	43	42	41	40	39	38	37	36	35
132	(290)	—	50	48	47	46	44	43	42	41	39	38	37	36	35
134	(295)	—	50	49	47	46	45	44	42	41	40	39	38	37	36
136	(300)	—	—	50	48	47	45	44	43	42	41	40	39	38	37

Source: Reprinted by permission from Guidelines for Adolescent Preventive Services (GAPS), Clinical Evaluation and Management Handbook, © 1995, American Medical Association.

Appendix F

Percentiles for Body Mass Index in US Children 5 to 17 Years of Age

Table F–1 Percentiles of BMI for boys 5–17 years of age

Age (yr)	*%ile*	*Asian*	*Black*	*Hispanic*	*White*	*U.S. weighted mean (A)*	*NHANES (B)*	*% Difference**
5	5	13.2	13.7	13.8	13.7	13.7	—	—
	15	14.0	14.4	14.6	14.4	14.4	—	—
	50	15.0	15.5	15.9	15.5	15.6	—	—
	75	15.3	16.2	17.2	16.4	16.5	—	—
	85	15.5	16.8	18.0	17.1	17.2	—	—
	95	17.1	18.1	19.4	18.1	18.3	—	—
6	5	13.3	13.8	13.8	13.8	13.8	12.9	6.7
	15	14.1	14.4	14.7	14.4	14.5	13.4	7.9
	50	15.0	15.5	16.0	15.6	15.6	14.5	7.7
	75	15.5	16.4	17.4	16.6	16.7	—	—
	85	15.7	17.0	18.2	17.3	17.4	16.6	4.5
	95	17.8	18.8	20.2	18.9	19.0	18.0	5.5
7	5	13.5	14.0	14.0	13.9	13.9	13.2	5.6
	15	14.3	14.6	14.9	14.6	14.7	13.9	5.5
	50	15.2	15.8	16.2	15.8	15.8	15.1	4.9
	75	15.8	16.7	17.7	16.9	17.0	—	—
	85	16.1	17.4	18.6	17.7	17.8	17.4	2.1
	95	18.8	19.9	21.2	19.9	20.0	19.2	4.4
8	5	13.7	14.2	14.2	14.1	14.1	13.6	3.9
	15	14.5	14.8	15.1	14.9	14.9	14.3	4.0
	50	15.6	16.1	16.6	16.2	16.2	15.6	3.7
	75	16.4	17.3	18.3	17.5	17.5	—	—
	85	16.9	18.3	19.5	18.6	18.6	18.1	2.7
	95	20.2	21.3	22.7	21.4	21.5	20.3	5.8

Source: Reprinted with permission from B. Rosner et al., Percentiles for Body Mass Index in U.S. Children 5 to 17 Years of Age. *The Journal of Pediatrics,* Vol. 132, pp. 211–222, © 1998, Mosby, Inc.

continues

Table F–1 continued

Age (yr)	*%ile*	*Asian*	*Black*	*Hispanic*	*White*	*U.S. weighted mean (A)*	*NHANES (B)*	*% Difference**
9	5	13.9	14.4	14.4	14.3	14.3	14.0	2.5
	15	14.7	15.1	15.4	15.1	15.1	14.7	2.8
	50	16.0	16.5	17.0	16.6	16.6	16.2	2.7
	75	17.2	18.1	19.1	18.3	18.4	—	—
	85	17.9	19.4	20.7	19.7	19.7	18.9	4.4
	95	21.7	22.9	24.4	23.0	23.1	21.5	7.4
10	5	14.1	14.6	14.7	14.6	14.6	14.4	1.3
	15	15.0	15.4	15.6	15.4	15.4	15.2	1.3
	50	16.6	17.1	17.6	17.1	17.2	16.7	2.8
	75	18.0	19.0	20.0	19.2	19.2	—	—
	85	19.1	20.6	21.9	20.9	20.9	19.6	6.7
	95	23.2	24.4	25.9	24.5	24.6	22.6	8.8
11	5	14.4	14.9	15.0	14.9	14.9	14.8	0.7
	15	15.4	15.8	16.1	15.8	15.8	15.6	1.3
	50	17.1	17.7	18.1	17.7	17.8	17.3	2.7
	75	18.9	19.9	20.9	20.1	20.1	—	—
	85	20.0	21.6	22.9	21.9	21.9	20.4	7.4
	95	24.3	25.5	27.1	25.6	25.7	23.7	8.6
12	5	14.8	15.3	15.4	15.3	15.3	15.2	0.8
	15	16.0	16.3	16.6	16.3	16.3	16.1	1.5
	50	17.8	18.3	18.8	18.4	18.4	17.9	2.8
	75	19.6	20.6	21.7	20.8	20.9	—	—
	85	20.7	22.3	23.6	22.6	22.6	21.1	7.3
	95	25.1	26.3	27.9	26.4	26.5	24.9	6.5
13	5	15.4	15.9	15.9	15.9	15.9	15.7	1.0
	15	16.6	17.0	17.3	17.0	17.0	16.6	2.4
	50	18.4	19.0	19.5	19.1	19.1	18.5	3.2
	75	20.2	21.2	22.3	21.5	21.5	—	—
	85	21.2	22.8	24.2	23.2	23.2	21.9	5.9
	95	25.6	26.9	28.5	27.0	27.1	25.9	4.6
14	5	16.0	16.5	16.6	16.5	16.5	16.2	1.9
	15	17.3	17.7	18.0	17.7	17.7	17.2	2.9
	50	19.2	19.7	20.2	19.8	19.8	19.2	3.2
	75	20.8	21.9	23.0	22.1	22.1	—	—
	85	21.8	23.4	24.8	23.7	23.7	22.8	4.1
	95	26.3	27.6	29.2	27.6	27.8	26.9	3.2
15	5	16.7	17.2	17.3	17.2	17.2	16.6	3.7
	15	18.0	18.3	18.6	18.3	18.4	17.8	3.1
	50	19.9	20.5	21.0	20.5	20.6	19.9	3.3
	75	21.5	22.5	23.6	22.8	22.8	—	—
	85	22.5	24.1	25.6	24.5	24.5	23.6	3.9
	95	27.2	28.5	30.1	28.5	28.7	27.8	3.2

continues

Table F–1 continued

Age (yr)	*%ile*	*Asian*	*Black*	*Hispanic*	*White*	*U.S. weighted mean (A)*	*NHANES (B)*	*% Difference**
16	5	17.3	17.9	18.0	17.9	17.9	17.0	5.1
	15	18.6	18.9	19.2	18.9	19.0	18.3	3.6
	50	20.6	21.2	21.7	21.3	21.3	20.6	3.3
	75	22.2	23.3	24.4	23.6	23.6	—	—
	85	23.4	25.1	26.5	25.4	25.4	24.5	3.9
	95	28.2	29.6	31.2	29.6	29.8	28.5	4.5
17	5	17.8	18.4	18.4	18.3	18.3	17.3	6.0
	15	19.2	19.6	19.9	19.6	19.6	18.7	4.9
	50	21.2	21.7	22.3	21.8	21.8	21.1	3.5
	75	22.9	23.9	25.1	24.2	24.2	—	—
	85	23.8	25.5	27.0	25.9	25.9	25.3	2.3
	95	28.6	29.9	31.6	30.0	30.1	29.3	2.8

*[A – B)/B] × 100%.

Table F–2 Percentiles of BMI for girls 5–17 years of age

Age (yr)	*%ile*	*Asian*	*Black*	*Hispanic*	*White*	*U.S. weighted mean (A)*	*NHANES (B)*	*% Difference**
5	5	13.0	13.3	13.5	13.0	13.1	—	—
	15	13.6	14.0	14.3	13.7	13.8	—	—
	50	14.5	15.4	15.5	14.9	15.1	—	—
	75	15.2	16.6	17.1	15.8	16.1	—	—
	85	15.7	17.7	18.1	16.5	16.9	—	—
	95	16.6	19.8	19.6	18.1	18.5	—	—
6	5	13.3	13.6	13.8	13.3	13.4	12.8	4.9
	15	13.8	14.2	14.5	14.0	14.1	13.4	4.9
	50	14.6	15.5	15.6	15.0	15.2	14.3	6.0
	75	15.5	17.0	17.5	16.1	16.4	—	—
	85	16.1	18.1	18.5	16.9	17.2	16.2	6.5
	95	17.4	20.7	20.5	18.9	19.3	17.5	10.5
7	5	13.4	13.8	13.9	13.5	13.6	13.2	2.8
	15	14.0	14.4	14.7	14.1	14.3	13.8	3.3
	50	14.9	15.8	15.9	15.3	15.4	15.0	2.8
	75	16.1	17.5	18.0	16.7	17.0	—	—
	85	16.7	18.8	19.2	17.6	17.9	17.2	4.3
	95	18.4	21.8	21.6	20.0	20.4	18.9	8.0
8	5	13.5	13.9	14.0	13.5	13.6	13.5	1.0
	15	14.2	14.6	14.9	14 .3	14.4	14.2	1.6
	50	15.3	16.2	16.3	15.7	15.8	15.7	0.7
	75	16.8	18.3	18.8	17.4	17.7	—	—
	85	17.7	19.8	20.2	18.6	18.9	18.2	3.9
	95	19.6	23.1	22.9	21.2	21.7	20.4	6.2
9	5	13.6	14.0	14.1	13.6	13.7	13.9	–1.1
	15	14.4	14.8	15.1	14.5	14.6	14.7	–0.3
	50	15.8	16.7	16.9	16.2	16.4	16.3	0.4
	75	17.7	19.2	19.7	18.3	18.6	—	—
	85	18.8	21.0	21.4	19.7	20.1	19.2	4.6
	95	20.9	24.5	24.3	22.6	23.0	21.8	5.7
10	5	13.9	14.2	14.4	13.9	14.0	14.2	–1.3
	15	14.8	15.2	15.5	14.9	15.0	15.1	–0.4
	50	16.5	17.4	17.6	16.9	17.1	17.0	0.4
	75	18.7	20.2	20.8	19.3	19.6	—	—
	85	20.0	22.3	22.7	21.0	21.4	20.2	5.7
	95	22.4	26.1	25.8	24.1	24.5	23.2	5.8
11	5	14.3	14.7	14.9	14.4	14.5	14.6	–0.8
	15	15.4	15.8	16.1	15.5	15.6	15.5	0.8
	50	17.3	18.3	18.4	17.7	17.9	17.7	1.1
	75	19.7	21.3	21.9	20.4	20.7	—	—
	85	21.2	23.5	24.0	22.2	22.6	21.2	6.5
	95	23.8	27.6	27.4	25.6	26.1	24.6	6.0

continues

Table F–2 continued

Age (yr)	*%ile*	*Asian*	*Black*	*Hispanic*	*White*	*U.S. weighted mean (A)*	*NHANES I (B)*	*% Difference**
12	5	15.0	15.4	15.5	15.0	15.1	15.0	1.0
	15	16.1	16.6	16.9	16.3	16.4	16.0	2.4
	50	18.2	19.2	19.3	18.6	18.8	18.4	2.1
	75	20.7	22.4	22.9	21.4	21.7	—	—
	85	22.2	24.6	25.1	23.2	23.6	22.2	6.4
	95	25.2	29.1	28.9	27.0	27.5	26.0	5.8
13	5	15.8	16.1	16.3	15.8	15.9	15.4	3.3
	15	16.9	17.4	17.7	17.1	17.2	16.4	5.0
	50	19.0	20.0	20.2	19.4	19.6	19.0	3.2
	75	21.5	23.2	23.8	22.2	22.5	—	—
	85	23.0	25.4	25.9	24.0	24.4	23.1	5.6
	95	26.3	30.3	30.0	28.1	28.6	27.1	5.7
14	5	16.5	16.8	17.0	16.5	16.6	15.7	5.8
	15	17.7	18.1	18.5	17.8	18.0	16.8	6.9
	50	19.6	20.7	20.8	20.1	20.2	19.3	4.9
	75	22.1	23.8	24.3	22.8	23.1	—	—
	85	23.5	25.9	26.4	24.5	24.9	23.9	4.2
	95	26.9	31.0	30.7	28.8	29.3	28.0	4.7
15	5	17.0	17.4	17.5	17.0	17.1	16.0	7.0
	15	18.1	18.6	19.0	18.3	18.4	17.2	7.2
	50	20.0	21.1	21.2	20.5	20.6	19.7	4.8
	75	22.3	24.0	24.6	23.1	23.4	—	—
	85	23.8	26.2	26.7	24.8	25.2	24.3	3.7
	95	27.2	31.3	31.0	29.1	29.6	28.5	3.9
16	5	17.2	17.6	17.8	17.3	17.4	16.4	6.1
	15	18.4	18.9	19.2	18.5	18.7	17.5	6.6
	50	20.2	21.3	21.4	20.7	20.9	20.1	3.8
	75	22.5	24.2	24.8	23.2	23.5	—	—
	85	24.0	26.5	27.0	25.1	25.5	24.7	3.1
	95	27.5	31.6	31.4	29.4	29.9	29.1	2.9
17	5	17.5	17.9	18.1	17.6	17.7	16.6	6.6
	15	18.6	19.1	19.5	18.8	18.9	17.8	6.3
	50	20.6	21.6	21.8	21.0	21.2	20.4	4.0
	75	23.0	24.7	25.3	23.7	24.1	—	—
	85	24.5	26.9	27.5	25.5	25.9	25.2	3.0
	95	28.8	33.0	32.8	30.8	31.3	29.7	5.4

*[A – B)/B] × 100%.

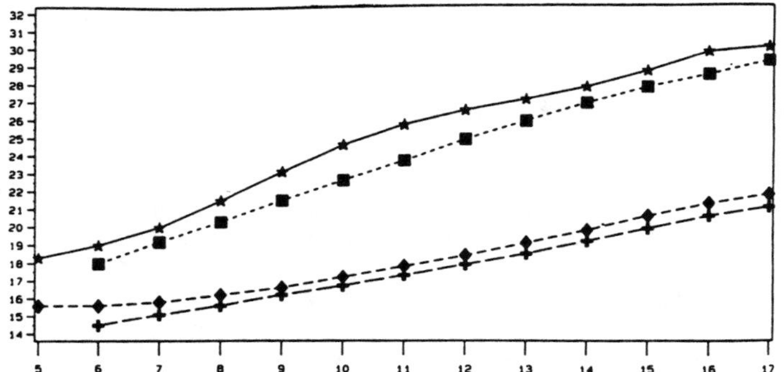

Figure F–1 50th and 95th percentile of body mass index for boys 5–17 years of age. Diamonds denote 50th percentile U.S. weighted values; crosses denote 50th percentile NHANES I values; stars denote 95th percentile U.S. weighted values; squares denote 95th percentile NHANES I values.

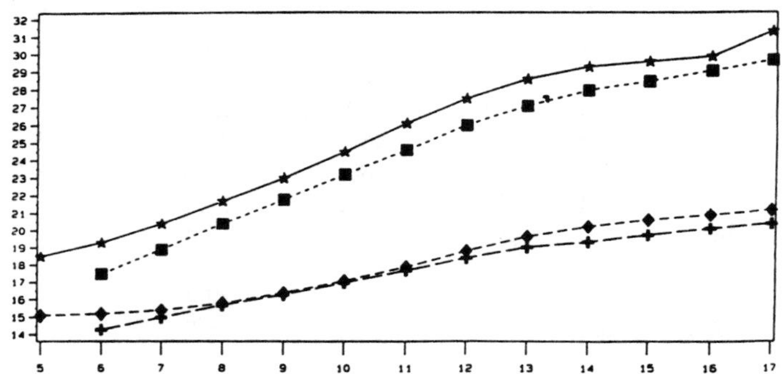

Figure F–2 50th and 95th percentile of body mass index for girls 5–17 years of age. Diamonds denote 50th percentile U.S. weighted values; crosses denote 50th percentile NHANES I values; stars denote 95th percentile U.S. weighted values; squares denote 95th percentile NHANES I values.

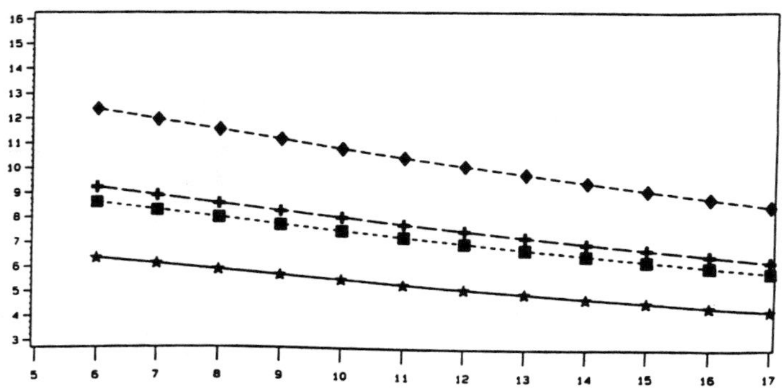

Figure F–3 Percent obese by ethnic group for boys 6–17 years of age. Stars denote Asian subjects; squares denote black subjects; diamonds denote Hispanic subjects; crosses denote white subjects.

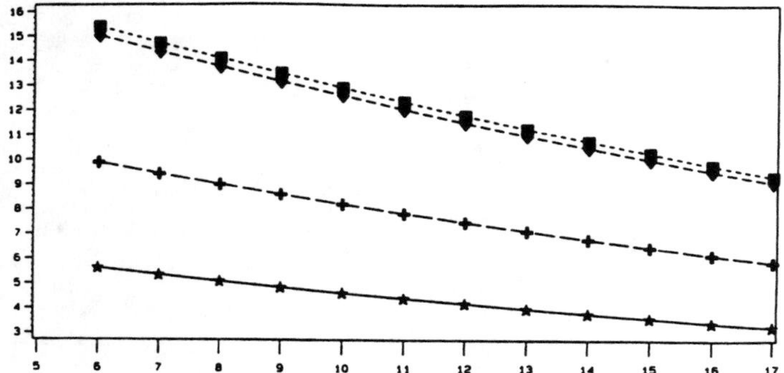

Figure F–4 Percent obese by ethnic group for girls 6–17 years of age. Stars denote Asian subjects; squares denote black subjects; diamonds denote Hispanic subjects; crosses denote white subjects.

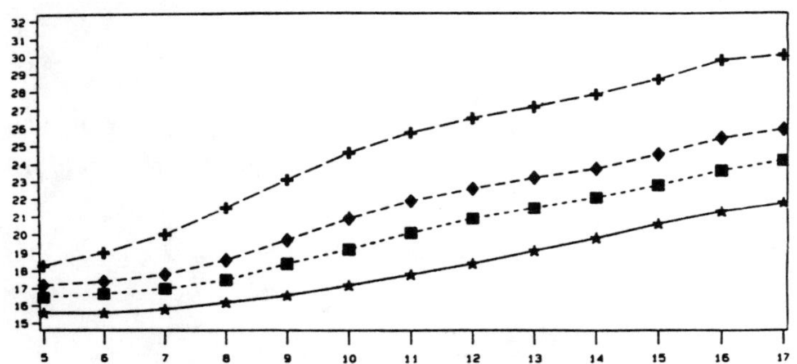

Figure F–5 50th, 75th, 85th, and 95th percentiles of body mass index for boys 5–17 years of age. Stars denote 50th percentile U.S. weighted values; squares denote 75th percentile U.S. weighted values; diamonds denote 85th percentile U.S. weighted values; crosses denote 95th percentile U.S. weighted values.

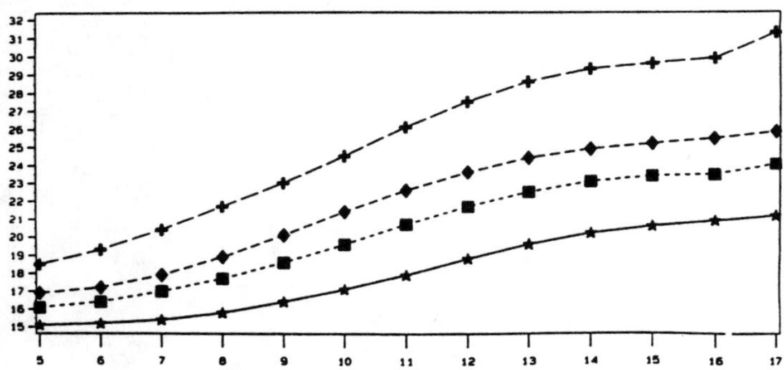

Figure F–6 50th, 75th, 85th, and 95th percentiles of body mass index for girls 5–17 years of age. Stars denote 50th percentile U.S. weighted values; squares denote 75th percentile U.S. weighted values; diamonds denote 85th percentile U.S. weighted values; crosses denote 95th percentile U.S. weighted values.

Appendix G

Nomograms

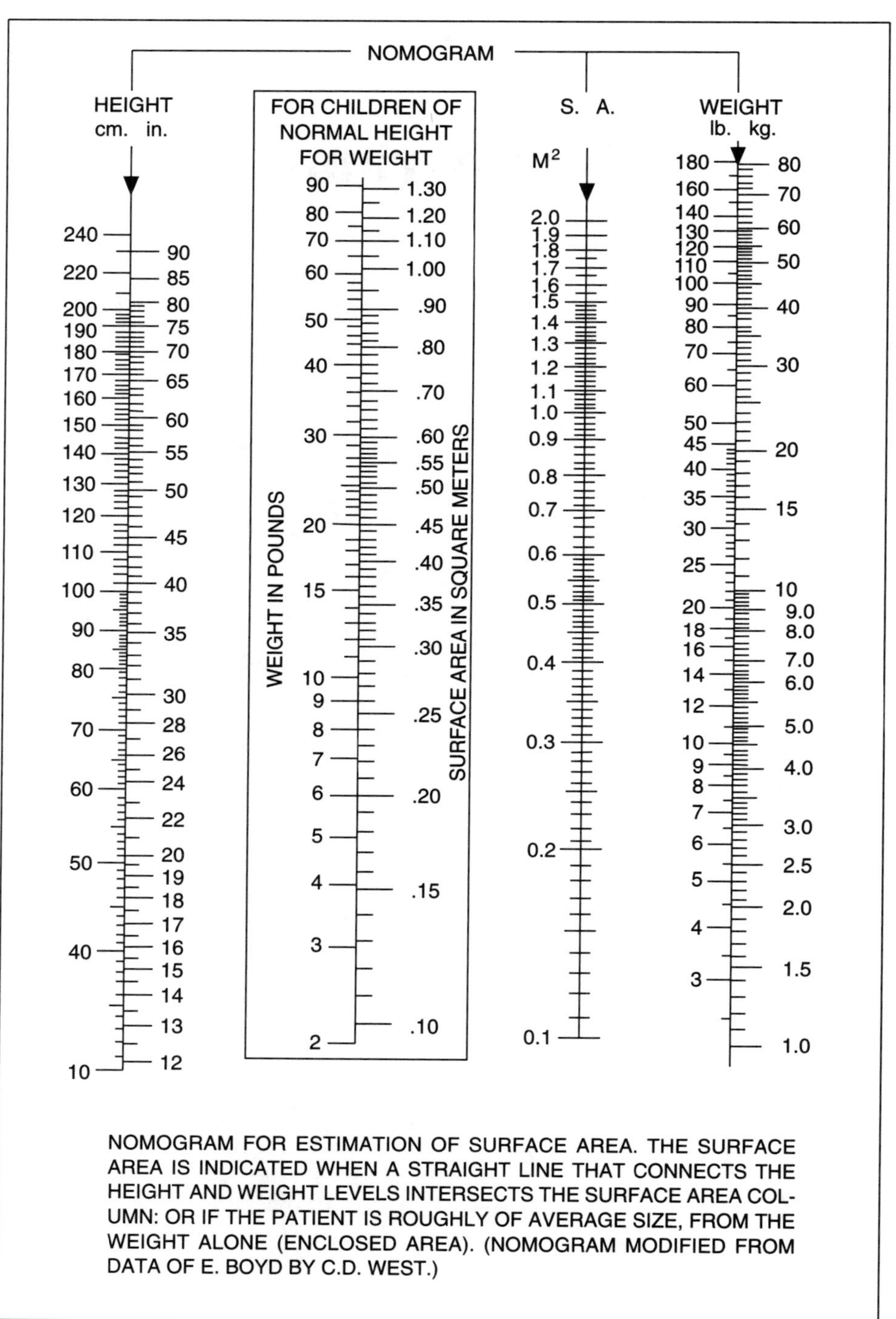

Figure G–1 Nomogram for estimation of surface area. *Source:* Reprinted from *Nelson's Textbook of Medicine,* ed 13 (p 1521) by RE Behrman and VC Vaughan (eds) with permission of WB Saunders, © 1987.

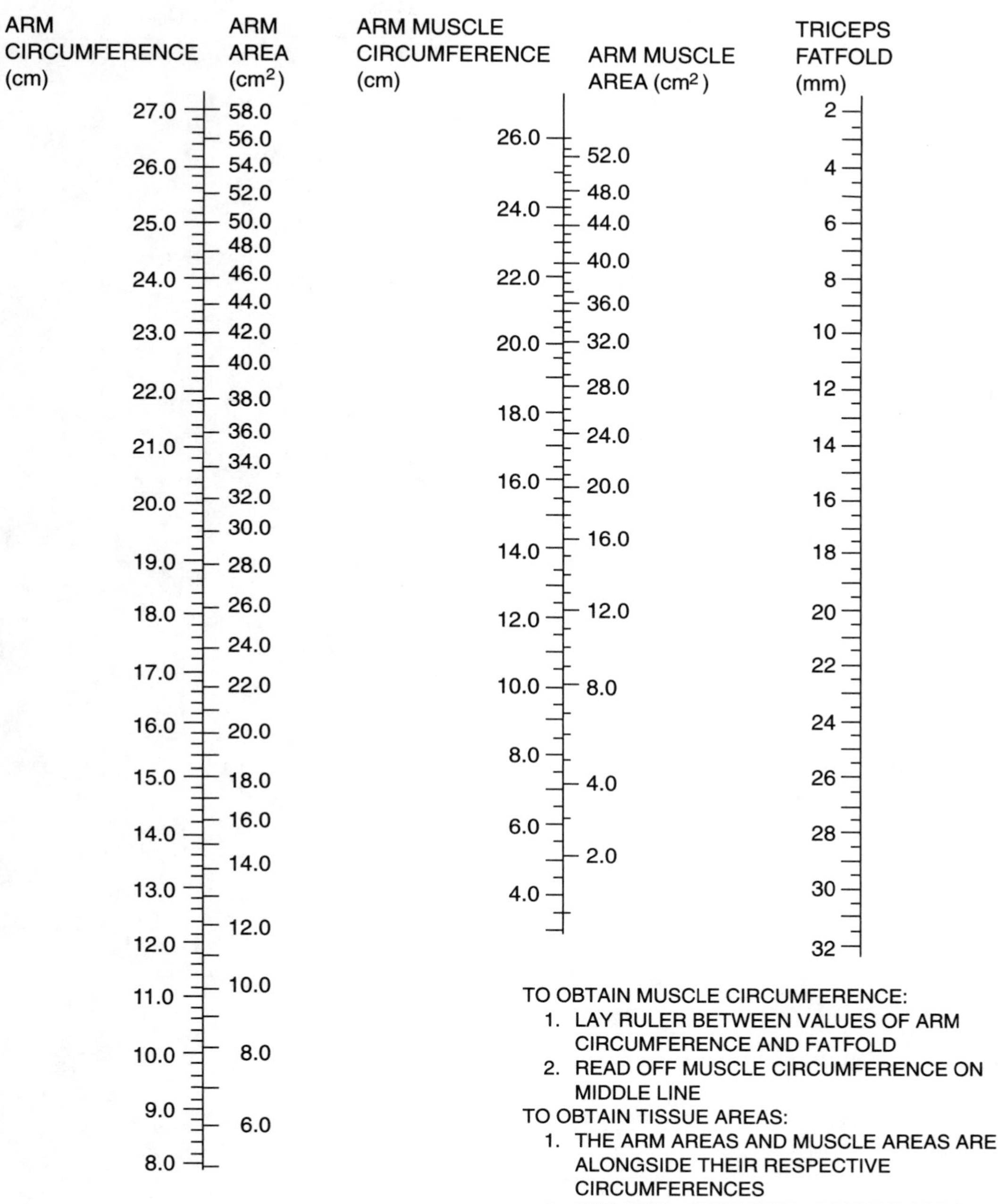

Figure G–2 Arm anthropometry nomogram for children. *Source:* Reprinted with permission from JM Gurney and DB Jeliffe, Arm anthropometry in nutritional assessment: nomogram for rapid calculation of muscle circumference and cross-sectional muscle and fat areas, in *American Journal of Clinical Nutrition* (1973;26:912–915). Copyright © 1973, American Society for Clinical Nutrition.

APPENDIX H

Arm and Skinfold Measurements

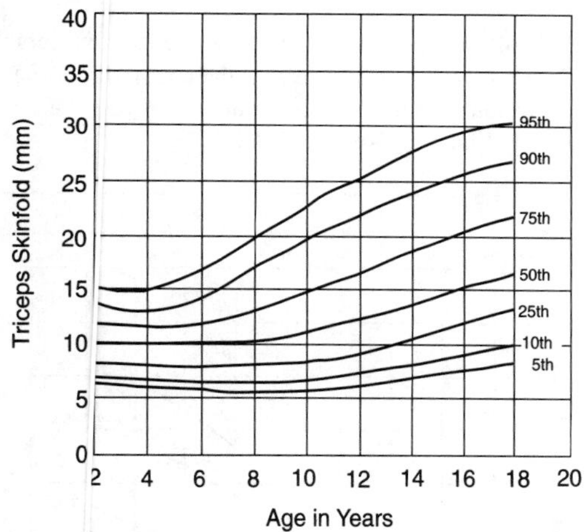

Figure H–1 Smoothed percentiles of triceps skinfold for girls aged 2–18 years, by age: United States, 1963–1965, 1966–1970, 1971–1974. *Source:* Reprinted from Basic data on anthropometric measurements and angular measurements of the hip and knee joints for selected age groups 1–74 years of age, by CL Johnson, R Fulwood, S Abraham, and JD Bryner. DHHS Publication No. (PHS) 81-1669.

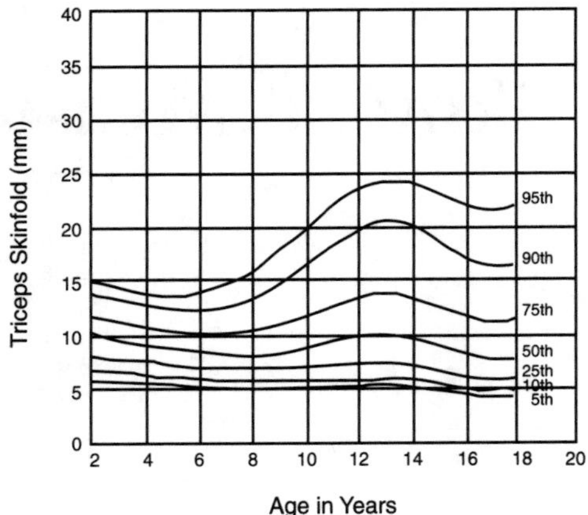

Figure H–2 Smoothed percentiles of triceps skinfold for boys aged 2–18 years, by age: United States, 1963–1965, 1966–1970, 1971–1974. *Source:* Reprinted from Basic data on anthropometric measurements and angular measurements of the hip and knee joints for selected age groups 1–74 years of age, by CL Johnson, R Fulwood, S Abraham, and JD Bryner. DHHS Publication No. (PHS) 81-1669.

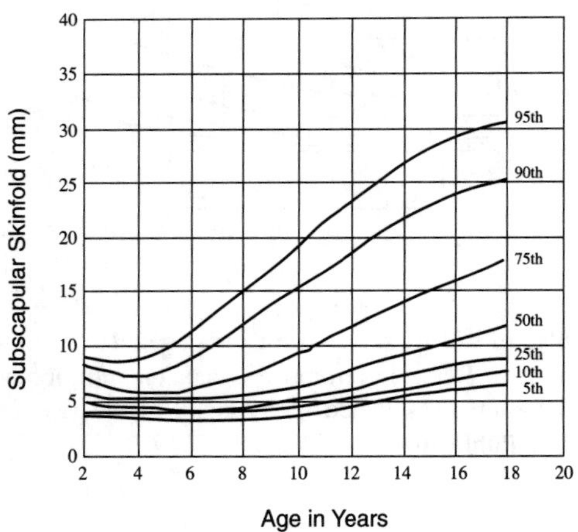

Figure H–3 Smoothed percentiles of subscapular skinfold for girls aged 2–18 years, by age: United States, 1963–1965, 1966–1970, 1971–1974. *Source:* Reprinted from Basic data on anthropometric measurements and angular measurements of the hip and knee joints for selected age groups 1–74 years of age, by CL Johnson, R Fulwood, S Abraham, and JD Bryner. DHHS Publication No. (PHS) 81-1669.

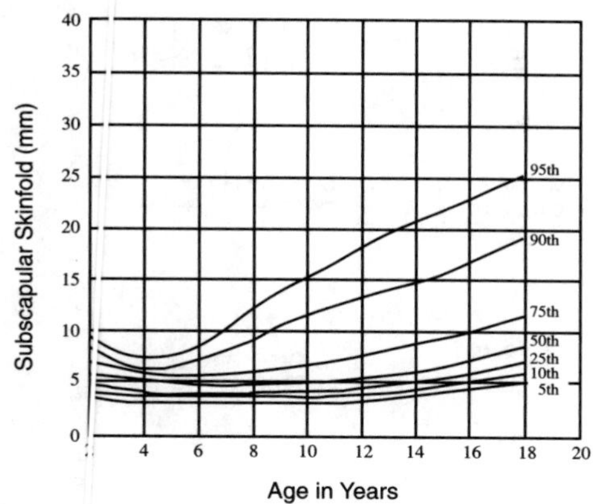

Figure H–4 Smoothed percentiles of subscapular skinfold for boys aged 2–18 years, by age: United States, 1963–1965, 1966–1970, 1971–1974. *Source:* Reprinted from Basic data on anthropometric measurements and angular measurements of the hip and knee joints for selected age groups 1–74 years of age, by CL Johnson, R Fulwood, S Abraham, and JD Bryner. DHHS Publication No. (PHS) 81-1669.

Table H–1 Observed Means, Standard Deviations, and Smoothed Percentile Values of Triceps Skinfold (mm) by Sex and Age for Infants 7–13 Months Old

				Percentile						
Age (months)	*n*	*Mean*	*SD*	*5th*	*10th*	*25th*	*50th*	*75th*	*90th*	*95th*
Males										
7	45	9.2	3.1	—	5.9	7.1	7.5	8.0	11.0	—
8	80	8.8	2.2	5.0	5.9	7.2	8.4	9.2	11.1	11.8
9	95	8.8	2.1	5.2	5.8	7.2	8.6	9.6	11.1	12.1
10	124	9.3	2.3	5.4	6.2	7.4	8.6	9.7	10.8	12.6
11	103	9.3	3.1	5.6	6.8	7.6	8.8	10.3	13.3	15.0
12	68	10.0	3.5	5.6	7.0	7.6	9.3	10.3	13.1	15.9
13	30	9.5	2.5	—	—	—	9.5	—	—	—
Females										
7	46	8.2	2.5	—	3.0	5.2	7.5	9.0	11.0	—
8	88	8.6	2.7	3.0	3.5	5.5	7.5	9.3	10.8	12.0
9	109	8.4	2.5	3.7	4.2	5.6	7.5	9.2	10.8	12.0
10	120	8.7	2.3	3.9	4.6	5.8	7.7	9.5	11.1	13.3
11	95	9.4	3.5	4.4	5.0	6.0	8.3	9.7	11.1	13.8
12	70	9.2	2.7	5.2	5.4	6.4	8.9	10.2	11.1	12.3
13	27	9.5	1.9	—	—	—	9.2	—	—	—

Source: Reprinted with permission from AS Ryan and GA Martinez, Physical growth of infants 7 to 13 months of age: results from a national survey, in *American Journal of Physical Anthropology* (1987;73:449), Copyright © 1987, Wiley-Liss, Inc., a subsidiary of John Wiley & Sons, Inc..

Table H–2 Percentiles for Triceps Skinfold for Whites of the United States Health and Nutrition Examination Survey I of 1971–1974

Age Group	*n*	*5*	*10*	*25*	*50*	*75*	*90*	*95*	*n*	*5*	*10*	*25*	*50*	*75*	*90*	*95*
	Triceps Skinfold Percentiles (mm²)															
	Males								Females							
1–1.9	228	6	7	8	10	12	14	16	204	6	7	8	10	12	14	16
2–2.9	223	6	7	8	10	12	14	15	208	6	8	9	10	12	15	16
3–3.9	220	6	7	8	10	11	14	15	208	7	8	9	11	12	14	15
4–4.9	230	6	6	8	9	11	12	14	208	7	8	8	10	12	14	16
5–5.9	214	6	6	8	9	11	14	15	219	6	7	8	10	12	15	18
6–6.9	117	5	6	7	8	10	13	16	118	6	6	8	10	12	14	16
7–7.9	122	5	6	7	9	12	15	17	126	6	7	9	11	13	16	18
8–8.9	117	5	6	7	8	10	13	16	118	6	8	9	12	15	18	24
9–9.9	121	6	6	7	10	13	17	18	125	8	8	10	13	16	20	22
10–10.9	146	6	6	8	10	14	18	21	152	7	8	10	12	17	23	27
11–11.9	122	6	6	8	11	16	20	24	117	7	8	10	13	18	24	28
12–12.9	153	6	6	8	11	14	22	28	129	8	9	11	14	18	23	27
13–13.9	134	5	5	7	10	14	22	26	151	8	8	12	15	21	26	30
14–14.9	131	4	5	7	9	14	21	24	141	9	10	13	16	21	26	28
15–15.9	128	4	5	6	8	11	18	24	117	8	10	12	17	21	25	32
16–16.9	131	4	5	6	8	12	16	22	142	10	12	15	18	22	26	31
17–17.9	133	5	5	6	8	12	16	19	114	10	12	13	19	24	30	37
18–18.9	91	4	5	6	9	13	20	24	109	10	12	15	18	22	26	30
19–24.9	531	4	5	7	10	15	20	22	1060	10	11	14	18	24	30	34
25–34.9	971	5	6	8	12	16	20	24	1987	10	12	16	21	27	34	37
35–44.9	806	5	6	8	12	16	20	23	1614	12	14	18	23	29	35	38
45–54.9	898	6	6	8	12	15	20	25	1047	12	16	20	25	30	36	40
55–64.9	734	5	6	8	11	14	19	22	809	12	16	20	25	31	36	38
65–74.9	1503	4	6	8	11	15	19	22	1670	12	14	18	24	29	34	36

Source: Reprinted with permission from AR Frisancho, New norms of upper limb fat and muscle areas for assessment of nutritional status, in *American Journal of Clinical Nutrition* (1981;34:2540–2545), Copyright © 1981, American Society for Clinical Nutrition.

Table H–3 Percentiles of Upper Arm Circumference (mm) and Estimated Upper Arm Muscle Circumference (mm) for Whites of the United States Health and Nutrition Examination Survey I of 1971–1974

	Males													
	Arm Circumference (mm)							*Arm Muscle Circumference (mm)*						
Age Group	*5*	*10*	*25*	*50*	*75*	*90*	*95*	*5*	*10*	*25*	*50*	*75*	*90*	*95*
1–1.9	142	146	150	159	170	176	183	110	113	119	127	135	144	147
2–2.9	141	145	153	162	170	178	185	111	114	122	130	140	146	150
3–3.9	150	153	160	167	175	184	190	117	123	131	137	143	148	153
4–4.9	149	154	162	171	180	186	192	123	126	133	141	148	156	159
5–5.9	153	160	167	175	185	195	204	128	133	140	147	154	162	169
6–6.9	155	159	167	179	188	209	228	131	135	142	151	161	170	177
7–7.9	162	167	177	187	201	223	230	137	139	151	160	168	177	190
8–8.9	162	170	177	190	202	220	245	140	145	154	162	170	182	187
9–9.9	175	178	187	200	217	249	257	151	154	161	170	183	196	202
10–10.9	181	184	196	210	231	262	274	156	160	166	180	191	209	221
11–11.9	186	190	202	223	244	261	280	159	165	173	183	195	205	230
12–12.9	193	200	214	232	254	282	303	167	171	182	195	210	223	241
13–13.9	194	211	228	247	263	286	301	172	179	196	211	226	238	245
14–14.9	220	226	237	253	283	303	322	189	199	212	223	240	260	264
15–15.9	222	229	244	264	284	311	320	199	204	218	237	254	266	272
16–16.9	244	248	262	278	303	324	343	213	225	234	249	269	287	296
17–17.9	246	253	267	285	308	336	347	224	231	245	258	273	294	312
18–18.9	245	260	276	297	321	353	379	226	237	252	264	283	298	324
19–24.9	262	272	288	308	331	355	372	238	245	257	273	289	309	321
25–34.9	271	282	300	319	342	362	375	243	250	264	279	298	314	326
35–44.9	278	287	305	326	345	363	374	247	255	269	286	302	318	327
45–54.9	267	281	301	322	342	362	376	239	249	265	281	300	315	326
55–64.9	258	273	296	317	336	355	369	236	245	260	278	295	310	320
65–74.9	248	263	285	307	325	344	355	223	235	251	268	284	298	306

continues

Table H–3 continued

Age Group	Females: Arm Circumference (mm) 5	10	25	50	75	90	95	Arm Muscle Circumference (mm) 5	10	25	50	75	90	95
1–1.9	138	142	148	156	164	172	177	105	111	117	124	132	139	143
2–2.9	142	145	152	160	167	176	184	111	114	119	126	133	142	147
3–3.9	143	150	158	167	175	183	189	113	119	124	132	140	146	152
4–4.9	149	154	160	169	177	184	191	115	121	128	136	144	152	157
5–5.9	153	157	165	175	185	203	211	125	128	134	142	151	159	165
6–6.9	156	162	170	176	187	204	211	130	133	138	145	154	166	171
7–7.9	164	167	174	183	199	216	231	129	135	142	151	160	171	176
8–8.9	168	172	183	195	214	247	261	138	140	151	160	171	183	194
9–9.9	178	182	194	211	224	251	260	147	150	158	167	180	194	198
10–10.9	174	182	193	210	228	251	265	148	150	159	170	180	190	197
11–11.9	185	194	208	224	248	276	303	150	158	171	181	196	217	223
12–12.9	194	203	216	237	256	282	294	162	166	180	191	201	214	220
13–13.9	202	211	223	243	271	301	338	169	175	183	198	211	226	240
14–14.9	214	223	237	252	272	304	322	174	179	190	201	216	232	247
15–15.9	208	221	239	254	279	300	322	175	178	189	202	215	228	244
16–16.9	218	224	241	258	283	318	334	170	180	190	202	216	234	249
17–17.9	220	227	241	264	295	324	350	175	183	194	205	221	239	257
18–18.9	222	227	241	258	281	312	325	174	179	191	202	215	237	245
19–24.9	221	230	247	265	290	319	345	179	185	195	207	221	236	249
25–34.9	233	240	256	277	304	342	368	183	188	199	212	228	246	264
35–44.9	241	251	267	290	317	356	378	186	192	205	218	236	257	272
45–54.9	242	256	274	299	328	362	384	187	193	206	220	238	260	274
55–64.9	243	257	280	303	335	367	385	187	196	209	225	244	266	280
65–74.9	240	252	274	299	326	356	373	185	195	208	225	244	264	279

Source: Reprinted with permission from AR Frisancho, New norms of upper limb fat and muscle areas for assessment of nutritional status, in *American Journal of Clinical Nutrition* (1981;34:2540–2545), Copyright © 1981, American Society for Clinical Nutrition, Inc.

Table H–4 Percentiles for Estimates of Upper Arm Fat Area (mm^2) and Upper Arm Muscle Area (mm^2) for Whites of the United States Health and Nutrition Examination Survey I of 1971–1974

	Males													
	Arm Muscle Area Percentiles (mm^2)							*Arm Fat Area Percentiles (mm^2)*						
Age Group	*5*	*10*	*25*	*50*	*75*	*90*	*95*	*5*	*10*	*25*	*50*	*75*	*90*	*95*
1–1.9	956	1014	1133	1278	1447	1644	1720	452	486	590	741	895	1036	1176
2–2.9	973	1040	1190	1345	1557	1690	1787	434	504	578	737	871	1044	1148
3–3.9	1095	1201	1357	1484	1618	1750	1853	464	519	590	736	868	1071	1151
4–4.9	1207	1264	1408	1579	1747	1926	2008	428	494	598	722	859	989	1085
5–5.9	1298	1411	1550	1720	1884	2089	2285	446	488	582	713	914	1176	1299
6–6.9	1360	1447	1605	1815	2056	2297	2493	371	446	539	678	896	1115	1519
7–7.9	1497	1548	1808	2027	2246	2494	2886	423	473	574	758	1011	1393	1511
8–8.9	1550	1664	1895	2089	2296	2628	2788	410	460	588	725	1003	1248	1558
9–9.9	1811	1884	2067	2288	2657	3053	3257	485	527	635	859	1252	1864	2081
10–10.9	1930	2027	2182	2575	2903	3486	3882	523	543	738	982	1376	1906	2609
11–11.9	2016	2156	2382	2670	3022	3359	4226	536	595	754	1148	1710	2348	2574
12–12.9	2216	2339	2649	3022	3496	3968	4640	554	650	874	1172	1558	2536	3580
13–13.9	2363	2546	3044	3553	4081	4502	4794	475	570	812	1096	1702	2744	3322
14–14.9	2830	3147	3586	3963	4575	5368	5530	453	563	786	1082	1608	2746	3508
15–15.9	3138	3317	3788	4481	5134	5631	5900	521	595	690	931	1423	2434	3100
16–16.9	3625	4044	4352	4951	5753	6576	6980	542	593	844	1078	1746	2280	3041
17–17.9	3998	4252	4777	5286	5950	6886	7726	598	698	827	1096	1636	2407	2888
18–18.9	4070	4481	5066	5552	6374	7067	8355	560	665	860	1264	1947	3302	3928
19–24.9	4508	4777	5274	5913	6660	7606	8200	594	743	963	1406	2231	3098	3652
25–34.9	4694	4963	5541	6214	7067	7847	8436	675	831	1174	1752	2459	3246	3786
35–44.9	4844	5181	5740	6490	7265	8034	8488	703	851	1310	1792	2463	3098	3624
45–54.9	4546	4946	5589	6297	7142	7918	8458	749	922	1254	1741	2359	3245	3928
55–64.9	4422	4783	5381	6144	6919	7670	8149	658	839	1166	1645	2236	2976	3466
65–74.9	3973	4411	5031	5716	6432	7074	7453	573	753	1122	1621	2199	2876	3327

continues

Table H–4 continued

Age Group	Females: Arm Muscle Area Percentiles (mm^2) 5	10	25	50	75	90	95	Arm Fat Area Percentiles (mm^2) 5	10	25	50	75	90	95
1–1.9	885	973	1084	1221	1378	1535	1621	401	466	578	706	847	1022	1140
2–2.9	973	1029	1119	1269	1405	1595	1727	469	526	642	747	894	1061	1173
3–3.9	1014	1133	1227	1396	1563	1690	1846	473	529	656	822	967	1106	1158
4–4.9	1058	1171	1313	1475	1644	1832	1958	490	541	654	766	907	1109	1236
5–5.9	1238	1301	1432	1598	1825	2012	2159	470	529	647	812	991	1330	1536
6–6.9	1354	1414	1513	1683	1877	2162	2323	464	508	638	827	1009	1263	1436
7–7.9	1330	1441	1602	1815	2045	2332	2469	491	560	706	920	1135	1407	1644
8–8.9	1513	1566	1808	2034	2327	2657	2996	527	634	769	1042	1383	1872	2482
9–9.9	1723	1788	1976	2227	2571	2987	3112	642	690	933	1219	1584	2171	2524
10–10.9	1740	1784	2019	2296	2583	2873	3093	616	702	842	1141	1608	2500	3005
11–11.9	1784	1987	2316	2612	3071	3739	3953	707	802	1015	1301	1942	2730	3690
12–12.9	2092	2182	2579	2904	3225	3655	3847	782	854	1090	1511	2056	2666	3369
13–13.9	2269	2426	2657	3130	3529	4081	4568	726	838	1219	1625	2374	3272	4150
14–14.9	2418	2562	2874	3220	3704	4294	4850	981	1043	1423	1818	2403	3250	3765
15–15.9	2426	2518	2847	3248	3689	4123	4756	839	1126	1396	1886	2544	3093	4195
16–16.9	2308	2567	2865	3248	3718	4353	4946	1126	1351	1663	2006	2598	3374	4236
17–17.9	2442	2674	2996	3336	3883	4552	5251	1042	1267	1463	2104	2977	3864	5159
18–18.9	2398	2538	2917	3243	3694	4461	4767	1003	1230	1616	2104	2617	3508	3733
19–24.9	2538	2728	3026	3406	3877	4439	4940	1046	1198	1596	2166	2959	4050	4896
25–34.9	2661	2826	3148	3573	4138	4806	5541	1173	1399	1841	2548	3512	4690	5560
35–44.9	2750	2948	3359	3783	4428	5240	5877	1336	1619	2158	2898	3932	5093	5847
45–54.9	2784	2956	3378	3858	4520	5375	5964	1459	1803	2447	3244	4229	5416	6140
55–64.9	2784	3063	3477	4045	4750	5632	6247	1345	1879	2520	3369	4360	5276	6152
65–74.9	2737	3018	3444	4019	4739	5566	6214	1363	1681	2266	3063	3943	4914	5530

Source: Reprinted with permission from AR Frisancho, New norms of upper limb fat and muscle areas for assessment of nutritional status, in *American Journal of Clinical Nutrition* (1981;34:2540–2545), Copyright © 1981, American Society for Clinical Nutrition, Inc.

APPENDIX I

Progression of Sexual Development

Pubertal Events Profile—Sequence of Events in Adolescent Development

Pubertal Changes by Sex	*Tanner Stage*†	*Mean Age of Onset in Years*
Females		
Breasts	2	11.2
Pubic hair	2	11.7
Peak velocity of height growth		12
Breasts	3	12.2
Pubic hair	3	12.4
Pubic hair	4	12.9
Breasts	4	13.1
Menarche		13
Pubic hair	5	14.4
Breasts	5	15.3
Males		
Genital	2	11.6
Genital	3	12.9
Pubic hair	2	13.4
Genital	4	13.8
Pubic hair	3	13.9
Peak velocity of height growth		14
Pubic hair	4	14.4
Genital	5	14.9
Pubic hair	5	15.2

† Tanner Stage, or sexual maturity rating: 1. Prepubertal; 2. First visible signs of pubertal change appear; 3. Pubic hair increases and becomes darker and coarser, breasts enlarge, and genitalia lengthen and enlarge; 4. Pubic hair becomes more abundant and coarse, genitalia and breasts increase in size; 5. Adult characteristics visible for breasts, pubic hair, and genitalia.

Source: Reprinted with permission from EJ Gong and BA Spear, Adolescent growth and development: implications for nutritional needs, in *Journal of Nutrition Education* (1988;20:274), copyright © 1988, Society for Nutrition Education.

APPENDIX J

Biochemical Evaluation of Nutritional Status

Test	Specimen	Reference Range	
Albumin	Serum		*g/dl*
		Premature:	3.0–4.2
		Newborn:	3.6–5.4
		Infant:	4.0–5.0
		Thereafter:	3.5–5.0
Calcium, Ionized (iCa)	Serum, plasma or whole blood (heparin)		*mg/dl*
		Cord:	5.0–6.0
		Newborn: 3–24h:	4.3–5.1
		24–48h:	4.0–4.7
		Thereafter:	4.48–4.92
		Or	2.24–2.46 mEq/L
Calcium, total	Serum		*mg/dl*
		Cord:	9.0–11.5
		Newborn: 3–24h:	9.0–10.6
		24–48h:	7.0–12.0
		4–7 day:	9.0–10.9
		Child:	8.8–10.8
		Thereafter:	8.4–10.2
	Urine, 24h	Ca in Diet	*mg/day*
		Ca Free:	5–40
		Low to average:	50–150
		Average (20m/mold):	100–300
B-Carotene	Serum		*µg/dl*
		Infant:	20–70
		Child:	40–130
		Thereafter:	60–200

Source: Adapted with permission from *Nelson's Textbook of Pediatrics,* 13th ed., pp. 1535–1558, © 1989, W.B. Saunders Company.

Test	Specimen	Reference Range	
Ceruloplasmin	Serum		*mg/dl*
		Newborn:	1–30
		6 mo–1 yr:	15–50
		1–12 yr:	30–65
		Thereafter:	14–40
Chloride	Serum or plasma (heparin)		*mmol/L*
		Cord:	96–104
		Newborn:	97–110
		Thereafter:	98–106
	CSF	118–132 mmol/L	
	Urine, 24h		*mmol/day*
		Infant:	2–10
		Child:	15–50
		Thereafter:	110–250
		(varies greatly with Cl intake)	
	Sweat		*mmol/L*
		Normal (homozygote):	0–35
		Marginal:	30–60
		Cystic fibrosis:	60–200
		Increases by 10 mmol/L during lifetime	
Cholesterol, total	Serum or plasma (EDTA or heparin)		*mg/dl*
		Cord:	45–100
		Newborn:	53–135
		Infant:	70–175
		Child:	120–200
		Adolescent:	120–210
		Adult:	140–310
		Recommended (desirable) range for	
		adults:	<200
		adolescents:	<170
Copper	Serum		*µg/dl*
		Birth–6 mo:	20–70
		6 yr:	90–190
		12 yr:	80–160
		Adult, M:	70–240
		F:	80–155
	Erythrocytes (heparin)	90–150 µg/dl	
	Urine (24h)	15–30 µg/day	

Test	*Specimen*	*Reference Range*	
Creatinine			
Jaffe, kinetic or enzymatic	Serum or plasma		*mg/dl*
		Cord:	0.6–1.2
		Newborn:	0.3–1.0
		Infant:	0.2–0.4
		Child:	0.3–0.7
		Adolescent:	0.5–1.0
		Adult, M:	0.6–1.2
		F:	0.5–1.1
	Urine 24h		*mg/kg/day*
		Infant	8–20
		Child:	8–22
		Adolescent:	8–30
		Adult:	14–26
		or:	*mg/day*
		Adult, M:	800–2000
		F:	600–1800
Disaccharide absorption test	Serum		*mg/dl*
		Changes in glucose from fasting value:	
		Normal	>30
		Inconclusive	20–30
		Abnormal:	<20
Erythrocyte count	White blood (EDTA)	*millions of cell/mm³ (μl)*	
		Cord blood:	3.9–5.5
		1–3 d (cap):	4.0–6.6
		1 wk:	3.9–6.3
		2 wk:	3.6–6.2
		1 mo:	3.0–5.4
		2 mo:	2.7–4.9
		3–6 mo:	3.1–4.5
		0.5–2 yr:	3.7–5.3
		2–6 yr	3.9–5.3
		6–12 yr:	4.0–5.2
		12–18 yr, M:	4.5–5.3
		F:	4.1–5.1
		18–49 yr, M:	4.5–5.9
		F:	4.0–5.2
Fat, fecal	Feces, 72 h	Coefficient of fat absorption (%)	
		Infant, breast-fed:	>93
		Infant, formula-fed:	>83
		>1 yr:	≥95

Test	*Specimen*	*Reference Range*		
Fatty acids	Serum or plasma (heparin)	Adults:	8–25 mg/dl	
Nonesterified (Free)		Children and obese adults: <31		
Ferritin	Serum		*ng/ml*	
		Newborn:	25–200	
		1 mo:	200–600	
		2–5 mo:	50–200	
		6 mo–15 yr:	7–140	
		Adult, M:	15–200	
		F:	12–150	
Folate	Serum		*ng/ml*	
		Newborn:	7.0–32	
		Thereafter:	1.8–9	
	Erythrocytes (EDTA)	150–450 ng/ml cells		
Glucose	Serum		*mg/dl*	
		Cord:	45–96	
		Premature:	20–60	
		Neonate:	30–60	
		Newborn, 1 d:	40–60	
		>1 d:	50–90	
		Child:	60–100	
		Adult:	70–105	
Glucose Tolerance Test Serum (GTT) Oral Dose: Adult: 75 g Child: 1.75 g/kg of ideal weight up to maximum of 75 g			*mg/dl*	
			Normal	*Diabetic*
		Fasting:	70–105	>115
		60 min:	120–170	>200
		90 min:	100–140	>200
		120 min:	70–120	>140
Growth Hormone (hGH) (Somatotropin)	Serum or plasma (EDTA, heparin) fasting at rest		*ng/ml*	
		Cord:	10–50	
		Newborn:	10–40	
		Child:	<5	
		Adult, M:	<5	
		F:	<8	

Test	*Specimen*	*Reference Range*		
HDL-Cholesterol (HDLC)	Serum or plasma (EDTA)		*mg/dl*	
			Male	*Female*
		Mean	45	55
		Range		
		Cord blood:	5–50	5–50
		0–12 yr:	30–65	30–65
		15–19 yr:	30–65	30–70
		20–29 yr:	30–70	30–75
		30–39 yr:	30–70	30–80
		40+ yr.	30–70	30–85
		Values for blacks—20 mg/dl higher		
Hematocrit	Whole blood (EDTA)	*% of packed red cells (V red cells/V whole blood × 100)*		
Calculated from MCV and RBC (electronic displacement or laser)		1 d (cap):	48–69	
		2 d:	48–75	
		3 d:	44–72	
		2 mo:	28–42	
		6–12 yr:	35–45	
		12–18 yr, M:	37–49	
		F:	36–46	
		18–49 yr, M:	41–53	
		F:	36–46	
Hemoglobin (Hb)	Whole blood (EDTA)		*g/dl*	
		1–3 day (cap):	14.5–22.5	
		2 mo:	9.0–14.0	
		6–12 yr:	11.5–15.5	
		12–18 yr, M:	13.0–16.0	
		F:	12.0–16.0	
		18–49 yr, M:	13.5–17.5	
		F:	12.0–16.0	
	Serum or plasma (heparin, ACD)	< 10 mg/dl < 3 mg/dl with butterfly set-up and 18 g needle		
	Urine, fresh random	Negative		
Hemoglobin, glycosated	Whole blood (heparin, EDTA, or oxalate)			
Electrophoresis		5.6–7.5% of total Hb		
Column		6.9% of total Hb		
HPLC		HbA_{1a} 1.6% total Hb HbA_{1b} 0.8 HbA_{1c} 3–6		

Test	Specimen	Reference Range		
Iron	Serum		*μg/dl*	
		Newborn:	100–250	
		Infant:	40–100	
		Child:	50–120	
		Thereafter, M:	50–160	
		F:	40–150	
		Intoxicated child:	280–2250	
		Fatally posioned child:	>1800	
Iron-binding capacity total (TIBC)	Serum	Infant:	100–400 μg/dl	
		Thereafter:	250–400	
LDL-Cholesterol (LDLC)	Serum or plasma (EDTA)		*mg/dl*	
			Male	*Female*
		Cord blood:	10–50	10–50
		0–19 yr:	60–140	60–150
		20–29 yr:	60–175	60–160
		30–39 yr:	80–190	70–170
		40–49 yr:	90–205	80–190
		Recommended (desirable range for adults: 65–175 mg/dl		
Lead	Whole blood (heparin)		*μg/dl*	
		Child:	< 30	
		Adult:	< 40	
		Acceptable for industrial exposure:	< 60	
		Toxic:	≥ 100	
	Urine 24 h	< 80 μg/dl		
Mean corpuscular hemoglobin (MHC)	Whole blood (EDTA)		*pg/cell*	
		Birth:	31–37	
		1–3 day (cap):	31–37	
		1 wk–1 mo:	28–40	
		2 mo:	26–34	
		3–6 mo:	25–35	
		0.5–2 yr:	23–31	
		2–6 yr:	23–31	
		6–12 yr:	25–33	
		12–18 yr:	25–35	
		18–49 yr:	26–34	

Test	*Specimen*	*Reference Range*	
Mean corpuscular hemoglobin concentration (EDTA)	Whole blood (EDTA)		*% Hb.cell or g Hb/dl RBC*
		Birth:	30–60
		1–3 (cap):	29–37
		1–2 wk:	28–38
		1–2 mo:	29–37
		3 mo–2 yr:	30–36
		2–18 yr:	31–37
		> 18 yr:	31–37
Mean corpuscular volume	Whole blood (EDTA)		*μm³*
		1–3 day (cap):	95–121
		0.5–2 yr:	70–86
		6–12 yr:	77–95
		12–18 yr, M:	78–98
		F:	78–102
		18–49 yr, M:	80–100
		F:	80–100
Niacin (nicotine acid)	Urine 24 h	0.3–1.5 mg/day	
Phenylalanine	Serum		*mg/dl*
		Premature:	2.0–7.5
		Newborn:	1.2–3.4
		Thereafter:	0.8–1.8
			mg/day
	Urine 24 h	10 day–2 wk:	1–2
		3–12 yr:	4–18
		Thereafter:	trace–17
Phosphatase, Alkaline (p-nitrophenyl phosphatase)	Serum		
SKI method 30ºC			*U/L*
		Infant:	50–155
		Child:	20–150
		Adult:	20–70
Bowers and McComb, 30ºC		25–90 U/L	
Phospholipid, total	Serum or plasma (EDTA)		*mg/dl*
		Newborn:	75–170
		Infant:	100–275
		Child:	180–295
		Adult:	125–275

Test	*Specimen*	*Reference Range*	
Phosphorus, inorganic	Serum		*mg/dl*
		Cord:	3.7–8.1
		Premature (1 wk):	5.4–10.9
		Newborn:	4.3–9.3
		Child:	4.5–6.5
		Thereafter:	3.0–4.5
Potassium	Serum		*mmol/l*
		Newborn:	3.9–5.9
		Infant:	4.1–5.3
		Child:	3.4–4.7
		Thereafter:	3.5–5.1
	Plasma (heparin)	3.5–4.5 mmol/L	
	Urine, 24 h	2.5–125 mmol/day varies with diet	
Prealbumin (PA, tryptophan-rich, thyroxine-binding TBPA) R/D	Serum		*mg/dl*
		Cord:	13
		1 yr:	10
		Maternal:	23
		Adult:	10–40
Protein, total	Serum		*g/dl*
		Premature:	4.3–7.6
		Newborn:	4.6–7.4
		Child:	6.2–8.0
		Adult	
		Recumbent:	6.0–7.8
		0.5 g higher in ambulatory patients	
Electrophoresis			*g/dl*
		Albumin	
		Premature:	3.0–4.2
		Newborn:	3.6–5.4
		Infant:	4.0–5.0
		α_1–Globulin	
		Premature:	0.1–0.5
		Newborn:	0.1–0.3
		Infant:	0.2–0.4
		Thereafter:	0.2–0.3
		α_2–Globulin	
		Premature:	0.3–0.7
		Newborn:	0.5–0.5
		Infant:	0.5–0.8
		Thereafter:	0.4–1.0

Test	*Specimen*	*Reference Range*	
		β–Globulin	
		Premature:	0.3–1.2
		Newborn:	0.2–0.6
		Infant:	0.5–0.8
		Thereafter:	0.5–1.1
		γ–Globin	
		Premature:	0.3–1.4
		Newborn:	0.2–1.0
		Infant:	0.3–1.2
		Thereafter:	0.7–1.2
		Higher in blacks	
Total	Urine, 24 h	1–14 mg/dl 50–80 mg/dl (at rest) < 250 mg/d after intense exercise	
Prothrombin time (PT) one-stage (quick)	Whole blood (Na citrate)	In general: 11–15s (varies with type of thromboplastin) Newborn: prolonged by 2–3s	
Retinol-binding protein (RBP)	Serum plasma		*mg/dl*
		2–10 yr:	2.5–4.5
		16 yr and older, M:	4.5–9.0
		F:	2.5–9.0
Riboflavin (vitamin B_2)	Urine, random, fasting		*µg/g* Creatinine
		1–3 yr:	500–900
		4–6 yr:	300–600
		7–9 yr:	270–500
		10–15 yr:	200–400
		Adult:	80–269
Sodium	Serum or plasma (heparin)		*mmol/L*
		Newborn:	134–146
		Infant:	139–146
		Child:	138–145
		Thereafter:	136–146
	Sweat		10–40
		Cystic fibrosis > 70	

Test	*Specimen*	*Reference Range*		
Somatomedin C	Plasma	Vary with laboratory, e.g., Nichols Institute		
			U/L	
			M	*F*
		0.2 yr:	0.10–0.72	0.10–1.7
		3–5 yr:	0.12–1.5	0.15–2.3
		6–10 yr:	0.19–2.2	0.44–3.6
		11–12 yr:	0.22–3.6	1.50–6.9
		13–14 yr:	0.79–5.5	0.81–7.4
		15–17 yr:	0.76–3.3	0.59–3.1
		18–64 yr:	0.34–1.9	0.45–2.2
		Endocrine Sciences		
		Cord:	0.25–0.66	
		0–1 yr:	0.17–0.62	
		1–5 yr:	0.14–0.94	
		6–12 yr:	0.87–2.06	
		13–17 yr:	1.35–3.00	
		18–25 yr:	0.92–2.06	
		Thereafter:	0.70–2.04	
Thiamine (vitamin B_1)	Serum		*µg/g*	
	Urine, acidify with HCl	0–2.0 µg/dl	creatinine	
		1–3 yr:	176–200	
		4–6 yr:	121–400	
		7–9 yr:	181–350	
		10–12 yr:	181–300	
		13–15 yr:	151–250	
		Thereafter:	66–129	
Transferrin	Serum	Newborn:	130–275 mg/dl	
		Adult:	200–400	
Triglycerides (TG)	Serum, after ≥12 h fast		*mg/dl*	
			Male	Female
		Cord blood:	10–98	10–98
		0–5 yr:	30–86	32–99
		6–11 yr:	31–108	35–114
		12–15 yr:	36–138	41–138
		16–19 yr:	40–163	40–128
		20–29 yr:	44–185	40–128
		Recommended (desirable) levels for adults.		
		Male:	40–160 mg/dl	
		Female:	35–135	

Test	*Specimen*	*Reference Range*	
Tyrosine	Serum		*mg/dl*
		Premature:	7.0–24.0
		Newborn:	1.6–3.7
		Adult:	0.8–1.3
Urea nitrogen	Serum or plasma		*mg/dl*
		Cord:	21–40
		Premature (1 wk):	3–25
		Newborn:	3–12
		Infant/Child:	5–18
		Thereafter:	7–18
Vitamin A	Serum		*μg/dl*
		Newborn:	35–75
		Child:	30–80
		Thereafter:	30–65
Vitamin B_1, see Thiamine			
Vitamin B_2, see Riboflavin			
Vitamin B_6	Plasma (EDTA)	3.6–18 ng/ml	
Vitamin B_{12}	Serum	Newborn:	175–800 pg/ml
		Thereafter:	140–700
Vitamin C	Plasma (oxalate, heparin, or EDTA)	0.6–2.0 mg/dl	
Vitamin D_2, 25 Hydroxy	Plasma (heparin)	Summer:	15–80 ng/ml
		Winter:	14–42
Vitamin D_3, 1,25 Dihydroxy	Serum	25–45 pg/ml	
Vitamin E	Serum	5.0–20 μg/ml	
Zinc	Serum	70–150 μg/dl	

Appendix K

Dietary Reference Intakes and Recommended Dietary Allowances

The tables in this Appendix summarize current information on Dietary Reference Intakes and the Recommended Dietary Allowances. Extensive documentation and explanation of numbers in the tables are provided by the various publications of the Food and Nutrition Board Institute of Medicine, National Academy of Sciences. These are available from the National Academy of Sciences, National Academy Press, 2101 Constitution Avenue, Washington, DC or from the National Academy Press web site at http://www.nap.edu.

Table K–1 Food and Nutrition Board, Institute of Medicine—National Academy of Sciences Dietary Reference Intakes: Recommended Intakes for Individuals

Life-Stage Group	*Calcium (mg/d)*	*Phosphorous (mg/d)*	*Magnesium (mg/d)*	*Vitamin D (μg/d)* [a,b]	*Fluoride (mg/d)*	*Thiamin (mg/d)*
Infants						
0–6 mo	210*	100*	30*	5*	0.01*	0.2*
7–12 mo	270*	275*	75*	5*	0.5*	0.3*
Children						
1–3 yr	500*	**460**	**80**	5*	0.7*	**0.5**
4–8 yr	800*	**500**	**130**	5*	1*	**0.6**
Males						
9–13 yr	1,300*	**1,250**	**240**	5*	2*	**0.9**
14–18 yr	1,300*	**1,250**	**410**	5*	3*	**1.2**
19–30 yr	1,000*	**700**	**400**	5*	4*	**1.2**
31–50 yr	1,000*	**700**	**420**	5*	4*	**1.2**
51–70 yr	1,200*	**700**	**420**	10*	4*	**1.2**
>70 yr	1,200*	**700**	**420**	15*	4*	**1.2**
Females						
9–13 yr	1,300*	**1,250**	**240**	5*	2*	**0.9**
14–18 yr	1,300*	**1,250**	**360**	5*	3*	**1.0**
19–30 yr	1,000*	**700**	**310**	5*	3*	**1.1**
31–50 yr	1,000*	**700**	**320**	5*	3*	**1.1**
51–70 yr	1,200*	**700**	**320**	10*	3*	**1.1**
>70 yr	1,200*	**700**	**320**	15*	3*	**1.1**
Pregnancy						
≤18 yr	1,300*	**1,250**	**400**	5*	3*	**1.4**
19–30 yr	1,000*	**700**	**350**	5*	3*	**1.4**
31–50 yr	1,000*	**700**	**360**	5*	3*	**1.4**
Lactation						
≤18 yr	1,300*	**1,250**	**360**	5*	3*	**1.5**
19–30 yr	1,000*	**700**	**310**	5*	3*	**1.5**
31–50 yr	1,000*	**700**	**320**	5*	3*	**1.5**

NOTE: This table presents Recommended Dietary Allowances (RDAs) in **bold type** and Adequate Intakes (AIs) in ordinary type followed by an asterisk(*). RDAs and AIs may both be used as goals for individual intake. RDAs are set to meet the needs of almost all (97 to 98 percent) individuals in a group. For healthy breastfed infants, the AI is the mean intake. The AI for other life-stage and gender groups is believed to cover needs of all individuals in the group, but lack of data or uncertainty in the data prevent being able to specify with confidence the percentage of individuals covered by this intake.

[a] As cholecalciferol. 1 μg cholecalciferol = 40 IU vitamin D.

[b] In the absence of adequate exposure to sunlight.

[c] As niacin equivalents (NE). 1 mg of niacin = 60 mg of tryptophan; 0–6 months = preformed niacin (not NE).

[d] As dietary folate equivalents (DFE). 1 DFE = 1 μg food folate = 0.6 μg of folic acid (from fortified food or supplement) consumed with food = 0.5 μg of synthetic (supplemental) folic acid taken on an empty stomach.

[e] Although AIs have been set for choline, there are a few data to assess whether a dietary supply of choline is needed at all stages of the life cycle, and it may be that the choline requirement can be met by endogenous synthesis at some of these stages.

[f] Because 10 to 30 percent of older people may malabsorb food-bound B_{12}, it is advisable for those older than 50 years to meet their RDA mainly by consuming foods fortified with B_{12} or a supplement containing B_{12}.

[g] In view of evidence linking folate intake with neural tube defects in the fetus, it is recommended that all women capable of becoming pregnant consume 400 μg of synthetic folic acid from fortified foods and/or supplements in addition to intake of food from folate a varied diet.

[h] It is assumed that women will continue consuming 400 μg of folic acid until their pregnancy is confirmed and they enter prenatal care, which ordinarily occurs after the end of the periconceptional period—the critical time for formation of the neural tube.

Riboflavin (mg/d)	*Niacin (mg/d)* [c]	*Vitamin B_6 (mg/d)*	*Folate (μg/d)* [d]	*Vitamin B_{12} (μg/d)*	*Pantothenic Acid (mg/d)*	*Biotin (μg/d)*	*Choline* [e] *(mg/d)*
0.3*	2*	0.1*	65*	0.4*	1.7*	5*	125*
0.4*	4*	0.3*	80*	0.5*	1.8*	6*	150*
0.5	**6**	**0.5**	**150**	**0.9**	2*	8*	200*
0.6	**8**	**0.6**	**200**	**1.2**	3*	12*	250*
0.9	**12**	**1.0**	**300**	**1.8**	4*	20*	375*
1.3	**16**	**1.3**	**400**	**2.4**	5*	25*	550*
1.3	**16**	**1.3**	**400**	**2.4**	5*	30*	550*
1.3	**16**	**1.3**	**400**	**2.4**	5*	30*	550*
1.3	**16**	**1.7**	**400**	**2.4** [f]	5*	30*	550*
1.3	**16**	**1.7**	**400**	**2.4** [f]	5*	30*	550*
0.9	**12**	**1.0**	**300**	**1.8**	4*	20*	375*
1.0	**14**	**1.2**	**400** [g]	**2.4**	5*	25*	400*
1.1	**14**	**1.3**	**400** [g]	**2.4**	5*	30*	425*
1.1	**14**	**1.3**	**400** [g]	**2.4**	5*	30*	425*
1.1	**14**	**1.5**	**400**	**2.4** [f]	5*	30*	425*
1.1	**14**	**1.5**	**400**	**2.4** [f]	5*	30*	425*
1.4	**18**	**1.9**	**600** [h]	**2.6**	6*	30*	450*
1.4	**18**	**1.9**	**600** [h]	**2.6**	6*	30*	450*
1.4	**18**	**1.9**	**600** [h]	**2.6**	6*	30*	450*
1.6	**17**	**2.0**	**500**	**2.8**	7*	35*	550*
1.6	**17**	**2.0**	**500**	**2.8**	7*	35*	550*
1.6	**17**	**2.0**	**500**	**2.8**	7*	35*	550*

Table K–2 Recommended Daily Dietary Allowances, Revised 1989*

Category	Age (years) or Condition	Weight† (kg)	Weight† (lb)	Height† (cm)	Height† (in)	Protein (g)	*Fat-Soluble Vitamins* Vitamin A (μg re)‡	Vitamin D (μg)§	Vitamin E (mg α-te)‖	Vitamin K (μg)
Infants	0.0–0.5	6	13	60	24	13	375	7.5	3	5
	0.5–1.0	9	20	71	28	14	375	10	4	10
Children	1–3	13	29	90	35	16	400	10	6	15
	4–6	20	44	112	44	24	500	10	7	20
	7–10	28	62	132	52	28	700	10	7	30
Males	11–14	45	99	157	62	45	1,000	10	10	45
	15–18	66	145	176	69	59	1,000	10	10	65
	19–24	72	160	177	70	58	1,000	10	10	70
	25–50	79	174	176	70	63	1,000	5	10	80
	51+	77	170	173	68	63	1,000	5	10	80
Females	11–14	46	101	157	62	46	800	10	8	45
	15–18	55	120	163	64	44	800	10	8	55
	19–24	58	128	164	65	46	800	10	8	60
	25–50	63	138	163	64	50	800	5	8	65
	51+	65	143	160	63	50	800	5	8	65
Pregnant						60	800	10	10	65
Lactating	1st 6 months					65	1,300	10	12	65
	2nd 6 months					62	1,200	10	11	65

* The allowances, expressed as average daily intakes over time, are intended to provide for individual variations among most normal persons as they live in the United States under usual environmental stresses. Diets should be based on a variety of common foods in order to provide other nutrients for which human requirements have been less well defined.

† Weights and heights of Reference Adults are actual medians for the U.S. population of the designated age, as reported by NHANES II. The median weights and heights of those under 19 years of age were taken from Hamill et al. (1979). The use of these figures does not imply that the height-to-weight ratios are ideal.

Table K–2 continued

Water-Soluble Vitamins							*Minerals*						
Vitamin C (mg)	*Thiamine (mg)*	*Riboflavin (mg)*	*Niacin (mg NE)*[#]	*Vitamin B6 (mg)*	*Folate (µg)*	*Vitamin B12 (µg)*	*Calcium (mg)*	*Phosphorus (mg)*	*Magnesium (mg)*	*Iron (mg)*	*Zinc (mg)*	*Iodine (µg)*	*Selenium (µg)*
30	0.3	0.4	5	0.3	25	0.3	400	300	40	6	5	40	10
35	0.4	0.5	6	0.6	35	0.5	600	500	60	10	5	50	15
40	0.7	0.8	9	1.0	50	0.7	800	800	80	10	10	70	20
45	0.9	1.1	12	1.1	75	1.0	800	800	120	10	10	90	20
45	1.0	1.2	13	1.4	100	1.4	800	800	170	10	10	120	30
50	1.3	1.5	17	1.7	150	2.0	1,200	1,200	270	12	15	150	40
60	1.5	1.8	20	2.0	200	2.0	1,200	1,200	400	12	15	150	50
60	1.5	1.7	19	2.0	200	2.0	1,200	1,200	350	10	15	150	70
60	1.5	1.7	19	2.0	200	2.0	800	800	350	10	15	150	70
60	1.2	1.4	15	2.0	200	2.0	800	800	350	10	15	150	70
50	1.1	1.3	15	1.4	150	2.0	1,200	1,200	280	15	12	150	45
60	1.1	1.3	15	1.5	180	2.0	1,200	1,200	300	15	12	150	50
60	1.1	1.3	15	1.6	180	2.0	1,200	1,200	280	15	12	150	55
60	1.1	1.3	15	1.6	180	2.0	800	800	280	15	12	150	55
60	1.0	1.2	13	1.6	180	2.0	800	800	280	10	12	150	55
70	1.5	1.6	17	2.2	400	2.2	1,200	1,200	320	30	15	175	65
95	1.6	1.8	20	2.1	280	2.6	1,200	1,200	355	15	19	200	75
90	1.6	1.7	20	2.1	260	2.6	1,200	1,200	340	15	16	200	75

‡ Retinol equivalents. 1 retinol equivalent = 1 µg retinol or 6 µg β-carotene. See text for calculation of vitamin A activity of diets as retinol equivalents.

§ As cholecalciferol. 10 µg cholecalciferol = 400 IU of vitamin D.

‖ α-Tocopherol equivalents. 1 mg d-α tocopherol = 1 α-TE.

1 NE (niacin equivalent) is equal to 1 mg of niacin or 60 mg of dietary tryptophan.

Source: Reprinted with permission from *Recommended Dietary Allowances*, 10th edition, © 1989 by the National Academy of Sciences. Published by National Academy Press.

Table K–3 Median Heights and Weights and Recommended Energy Intake*

Category	Age (years) or Condition	Weight (kg)	Weight (lb)	Height (cm)	Height (in)	REE[†] (kcal/day)	Average Energy Allowance (kcal)[‡] Multiples of REE	Per kg	Per day[§]
Infants	0.0–0.5	6	13	60	24	320		108	650
	0.5–1.0	9	20	71	28	500		98	850
Children	1–3	13	29	90	35	740		102	1300
	4–6	20	44	112	44	950		90	1800
	7–10	28	62	132	52	1130		70	2000
Males	11–14	45	99	157	62	1440	1.70	55	2500
	15–18	66	145	176	69	1760	1.67	45	3000
	19–24	72	160	177	70	1780	1.67	40	2900
	25–50	79	174	176	70	1800	1.60	37	2900
	51+	77	170	173	68	1530	1.50	30	2300
Females	11–14	46	101	157	62	1310	1.67	47	2200
	15–18	55	120	163	64	1370	1.60	40	2200
	19–24	58	128	164	65	1350	1.60	38	2200
	25–50	63	138	163	64	1380	1.55	36	2200
	51+	65	143	160	63	1280	1.50	30	1900
Pregnant	1st trimester								+0
	2nd trimester								+300
	3rd trimester								+300
Lactating	1st 6 months								+500
	2nd 6 months								+500

* REE, resting energy expenditure.

† Calculations based on World Health Organization equations (1985), then rounded (see reference 26).

‡ In the range of light to moderate activity, the coefficient of variation is ±20%.

§ Figure is rounded.

Source: Reprinted with permission from *Recommended Dietary Allowances,* 10th ed, © 1989 by the National Academy of Sciences. Published by National Academy Press.

Table K–4 Estimated Safe and Adequate Daily Dietary Intakes of Selected Vitamins and Minerals*

		Vitamins		*Trace Elements*†				
Category	*Age (Years)*	*Biotin (μg)*	*Pantothenic Acid (mg)*	*Copper (mg)*	*Manganese (mg)*	*Fluoride (mg)*	*Chromium (μg)*	*Molybdenum (μg)*
Infants	0–0.5	10	2	0.4–0.6	0.3–0.6	0.1–0.5	10–40	15–30
	0.5–1	15	3	0.6–0.7	0.6–1.0	0.2–1.0	20–60	20–40
Children and adolescents	1–3	20	3	0.7–1.0	1.0–1.5	0.5–1.5	20–80	25–50
	4–6	25	3–4	1.0–1.5	1.5–2.0	1.0–2.5	30–120	30–75
	7–10	30	4–5	1.0–2.0	2.0–3.0	1.5–2.5	50–200	50–150
	11+	30–100	4–7	1.5–2.5	2.0–5.0	1.5–2.5	50–200	75–250
Adults		30–100	4–7	1.5–3.0	2.0–5.0	1.5–4.0	50–200	75–250

* Because there is less information on which to base allowances, these figures are not given in the main table of RDA and are provided here in the form of ranges of recommended intakes.

† Since the toxic levels for many trace elements may be only several times usual intakes, the upper levels for the trace elements given in this table should not be habitually exceeded.

Source: Reprinted with permission from *Recommended Dietary Allowances*, 10th edition, © 1989 by the National Academy of Sciences. Published by National Academy Press.

Table K–5 Estimated Sodium, Chloride, and Potassium Minimum Requirements of Healthy Persons

Age	*Weight (kg)**	*Sodium (mg)*,†*	*Chloride (mg)*,†*	*Potassium (mg)‡*
Months				
0–5	4.5	120	180	500
6–11	8.9	200	300	700
Years				
1	11.0	225	350	1,000
2–5	16.0	300	500	1,400
6–9	25.0	400	600	1,600
10–18	50.0	500	750	2,000
>18§	70.0	500	750	2,000

* No allowance has been included for large, prolonged losses from the skin through sweat.

† There is no evidence that higher intakes confer any health benefit.

‡ Desirable intakes of potassium may considerably exceed these values (≈3,500 mg for adults).

§ No allowance included for growth. Values for those below 18 years assume a growth rate at the 50th percentile reported by the National Center for Health Sciences (see reference 36) and averaged for males and females. See reference 24 for information on pregnancy and lactation.

Source: Reprinted with permission from *Recommended Dietary Allowances*, 10th edition, © 1989 by the National Academy of Sciences. Published by National Academy Press.

APPENDIX L

General Guidelines, Daily Values, Food Guide Pyramid, and Conversion Tables

Exhibit L–1 USDA/DHHS Dietary Guidelines for Americans, 1995.

- Eat a variety of foods.
- Balance the food you eat with physical activity—maintain or improve your weight.
- Choose a diet with plenty of grain products, vegetables, and fruits.
- Choose a diet low in fat, saturated fat, and cholesterol.
- Choose a diet moderate in sugars.
- Choose a diet moderate in salt and sodium.
- If you drink alcoholic beverages, do so in moderation.

Source: Nutrition and Your Health: Dietary Guidelines for Americans, fourth edition, Home and Garden Bulletin No. 232, 1995, U.S. Department of Agriculture, U.S. Department of Health and Human Services.

Table L–1 Daily Values (DV) for Nutrition Labeling[1]

Food Component	*Daily Value (DV)*
MANDATORY COMPONENTS OF THE NUTRITION LABEL:	
Total Fat	65 g
Saturated Fat	20 g
Cholesterol	300 mg
Sodium	2,400 mg
Total Carbohydrate	300 mg
Dietary Fiber	25 g
Vitamin A	5,000 IU
Vitamin C	60 mg
Calcium	1,000 mg
Iron	18 mg
Voluntary Components of the Nutrition Label:	
Vitamin D	400 IU
Vitamin E	30 IU
Vitamin K	80 mcg
Thiamin	1.5 mg
Riboflavin	1.7 mg
Niacin	20 mg
Vitamin B-6	2.0 mg
Folic Acid	400 mcg
Vitamin B-12	6.0 mcg
Biotin	300 mcg
Pantothenic Acid	10 mcg
Phosphorus	1,000 mg
Iodine	150 mcg
Magnesium	400 mg
Zinc	15 mg
Selenium	70 mcg
Copper	2.0 mg
Manganese	2.0 mg
Chromium	120 mcg
Molybdenum	75 mcg
Chloride	3,400 mg
Potassium	3,500 mg

[1] Daily Values are based on a caloric intake of 2,000 kcal per day. This listing is for foods for adults and children four or more years of age.

Source: Code of Federal Regulations, Food and Drugs, Title 21, Part 101.0, Nutrition Labeling of Food, The Office of the Federal Register, National Archives and Records Administration, Washington, DC. U.S. Government Printing Office, 1996.

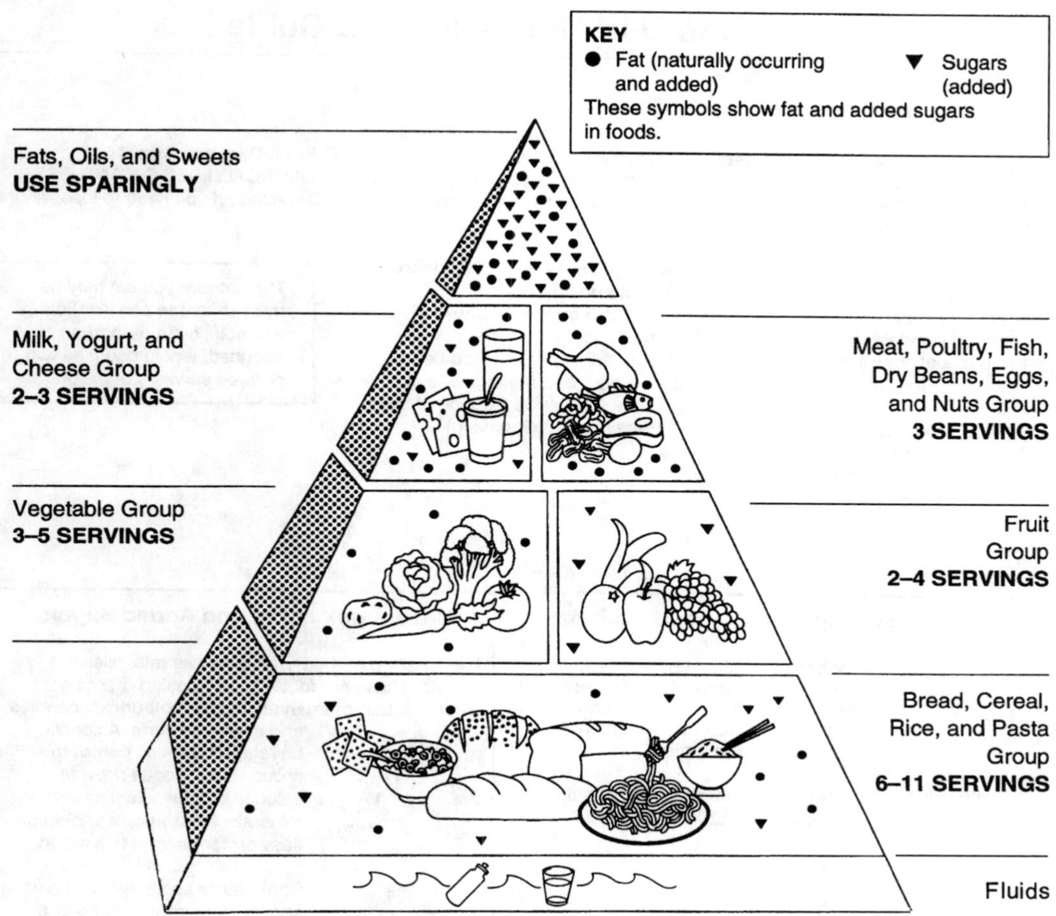

Figure L–1 Food Guide Pyramid, A Guide to Daily Food Choices. *Source:* U.S. Department of Agriculture, U.S. Department of Health and Human Services, 1995. (http://www.nal.usda.gov/fric)

How to Use The Daily Food Guide

What counts as one serving?

Breads, Cereals, Rice, and Pasta
1 slice of bread
1/2 cup of cooked rice or pasta
1/2 cup of cooked cereal
1 ounce of ready-to-eat cereal

Vegetables
1/2 cup of chopped raw or cooked vegetables
1 cup of leafy raw vegetables

Fruits
1 piece of fruit or melon wedge
3/4 cup of juice
1/2 cup of canned fruit
1/4 cup of dried fruit

Milk, Yogurt, and Cheese
1 cup of milk or yogurt
1-1/2 to 2 ounces of cheese

Meat, Poultry, Fish, Dry Beans, Eggs, and Nuts
2-1/2 to 3 ounces of cooked lean meat, poultry, or fish
Count 1/2 cup of cooked beans, or 1 egg, or 2 tablespoons of peanut butter as 1 ounce of lean meat (about 1/3 serving)

Fats, Oils, and Sweets
LIMIT CALORIES FROM THESE especially if you need to lose weight

The amount you eat may be more than one serving. For example, a dinner portion of spaghetti would count as two or three servings of pasta.

How many servings do you need each day?

	Women & some older adults	Children, teen girls, active women, most men	Teen boys & active men
Calorie level*	about 1,600	about 2,200	about 2,800
Bread group	6	9	11
Vegetable group	3	4	5
Fruit group	2	3	4
Milk group	**2-3	**2-3	**2-3
Meat group	2, for a total of 5 ounces	2, for a total of 6 ounces	3 for a total of 7 ounces

*These are the calorie levels if you choose lowfat, lean foods from the 5 major food groups and use foods from the fats, oils, and sweets group sparingly.

**Women who are pregnant or breastfeeding, teen-agers, and young adults to age 24 need 3 servings.

A Closer Look at Fat and Added Sugars

The small tip of the Pyramid shows fats, oils, and sweets. These are foods such as salad dressings, cream, butter, margarine, sugars, soft drinks, candies, and sweet desserts. Alcoholic beverages are also part of this group. These foods provide calories but few vitamins and minerals. Most people should go easy on foods from this group.

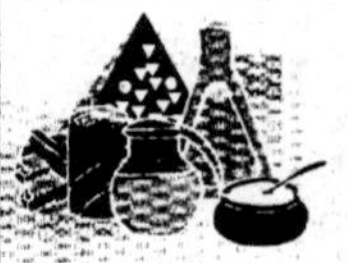

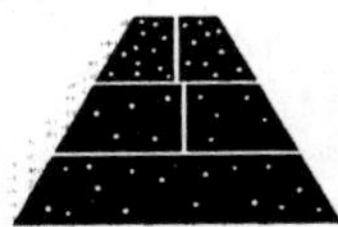

Some fat or sugar symbols are shown in the other food groups. That's to remind you that some foods in these groups can also be high in fat and added sugars, such as cheese or ice cream from the milk group, or french fries from the vegetable group. When choosing foods for a healthful diet, consider the fat and added sugars in your choices from all the food groups, not just fats, oils, and sweets from the Pyramid tip.

Figure L–1 continued. *Source:* U.S. Department of Agriculture, U.S. Department of Health and Human Services, 1995. (http://www.nal.usda.gov/fric)

Exhibit 2–L Conversion tables

Volume

1 t	= 1/3 T	= 16 fl oz	= 4.9 ml
3 t	= 1 T	= 1/2 fl oz	= 14.8 ml
2 T	= 1/8 cup	= 1 fl oz	= 29.6 ml
4 T	= 1/4 cup	= 2 fl oz	= 59.1 ml
5 1/3 T	= 1/3 cup	= 2 2/3 fl oz	= 78.9 ml
8 T	= 1/2 cup	= 4 fl oz	= 118.3 ml
10 2/3 T	= 2/3 cup	= 5 1/3 fl oz	= 157.7 ml
12 T	= 3/4 cup	= 6 fl oz	= 177.4 ml
14 T	= 7/8 cup	= 7 fl oz	= 207.0 ml
16 T	= 1 cup	= 8 fl oz	= 236.6 ml
1 ml	= 0.034 fl oz	= 1 ml	= 0.001 liter
1 liter	= 34 fl oz	= 1000 ml	
1 pint(pt)	=2 cups	= .473 liter	= 473 ml
1 quart (qt)	= 2 pt	= .946 liter	= 946 ml
1 gallon	= 4 qts	= 3.785 liter	= 3785 ml
1 liter	= 1.057 qts	= 0.264 gallon	= 1000 ml

To convert mls to oz divide by 30
to convert oz to mls multipy by 30

Weight

1 gram (g) = 0.035 oz = .001 kg= 1000 mg= 1,000,000 mcg
1 mg = .001 g = 1000 mcg
1 oz = 28.35 g (often rounded to 28 g)
1 lb = 16 oz = 453.59 g = .454 kg
1 kg = 2.21 lb = 1000 g

Length

1 inch = 2.54 centimeters
1 foot = 30.5 centimeters
1 yard = 0.91 meters
1 mile = 1.61 kilometers
1 centimeter = 0.4 inches
1 meter = 3.3 feet
1 meter = 1.1 yard
1 kiltometer = 0.6 miles

To convert inches to centimeters, multiply by 2.54; centimeters to inches, multiply by 0.4

Area

1 square inch = 6.5 square centimeters
1 square foot = 9.29 square meters
1 square yard = 0.84 square meters
1 square centimeter = 0.16 square inches
1 square meter = 1.2 square yards

continues

Exhibit L–2 continued

Heat Measures

1 kilojoule = 0.239 kilocalories
1 kilocalorie = 4.184 kilojoules

Temperatures

Water freezes	0°C	32°F
Room temperature	27°C	72°F
Body temperature	37°C	98.6°F
Water boils	100°C	212°F

To convert Fahrenheit to Celsius (centrigrade), subtract 32, multiply by 5, divide by 9; Celsius (centigrade) to Fahrenheit, multiply by 9, divide by 5, and add 32.

Milliequivalent- milligram conversion table

Mineral element	chemical symbol	atomic weight	Valence
Calcium	Ca	40	2
Choline	Cl	35.4	1
Magnesium	Mg	24.3	2
Phosphorus	P	31	2
Potassium	K	39	1
Sodium	Na	23	1
Sulfate	SO4	96	2
Sulfur	S	32	2
Zinc	Zn	65.4	2

$$\text{Milliequivalents} = \frac{\text{milligrams}}{\text{Atomic weight}} \times \text{valence}$$

1 g. NaCl= 0.4 g Na
(Na+ = 40% of weight of NaCl)
1 g Na+= 2.5g NaCl

Example: convert 1000 mg sodium to MEq of sodium

$\frac{1000}{23} \times 1 = 43$ Meq sodium

To change milliequivalents back to milligrams, multiply the milliequivalents by the atomic weight and divide by the valence.

Example: convert 10 Meq sodium to mg sodium

$\frac{10 \times 23}{1} = 230$ mg sodium

Appendix M

NCHS Growth Charts

GROWTH CHART REVISION UPDATE

The growth charts used since 1977 in private pediatric practice and public health clinics are being revised by the National Center for Health Statistics, Centers for Disease Control and Prevention (NCHS/CDC), to provide a better instrument for evaluating the growth status of infants, children, and adolescents in the United States.

The revisions, scheduled for completion later in 1998, will be based on additional data and improved statistical procedures, to develop smoothed percentile curves. Dissemination of the revised charts is scheduled for 1998–99.

These multipurpose charts have received widespread application:

- as a clinical screening tool for health and nutritional status, to identify and classify children as low length- or stature-for-age, low weight-for-length, -stature or -age, or high weight-for-age, -length or -stature;
- as an educational tool to illustrate, for parents, patterns in their children's size and growth relative to the reference population;
- as an epidemiological tool in nutrition surveillance programs, to categorize and monitor population trends in physical growth.

The charts also have been adapted by the World Health Organization for international use.

The old charts were based on data collected in the NCHS national health examination surveys for children and adolescents ages 2 through 17 years.

The infant charts for birth through age 2 years were based on data from the Fels Research Institute. The Fels data were not ideal, but at the time were considered the best available. The limitations of incorporating the Fels data set were clearly stated with the initial release of the charts.

OLD CHARTS RAISE QUESTIONS

Although the 1977 charts have received diverse and widespread application, a number of concerns also have been raised.

For instance, distributions of birth weights do not match current national data. The Fels percentile values for birth weight were lower than the current national birth weight distributions by approximately 125 gm at the median.

Also, differences between recumbent length and stature in the Fels data set probably are too

---

Note: The NCHS Growth Charts were not available as *Handbook of Pediatric Nutrition,* Second Edition went to press. Check the NCHS website for updates regarding the growth charts. (http://www.cdc.gov/nchswww)

Source: Reproduced by permission of AAP News, vol. 14, no. 9, pp. 1, 8. Copyright 1998.

large. This was due to a systematic overestimation of recumbent length, attributable to measuring procedures used at the Fels Research Institute.

In addition, Fels data from birth to age 3 years were derived mainly from formula-fed infants. During the past two decades, U.S. breastfeeding practices have changed, with approximately one-half of all infants breastfed. Among infants born from 1972 to 1994, approximately one-third breastfed for at least three months or more. Replacing the Fels data for infants with national survey data collected from 1971 to 1994 will better represent the combined growth patterns of breastfed and formula-fed infants.

In the 1977 charts, discontinuities exist between the infant and later curves for recumbent length data from the Fels data set and stature from the NCHS data sets, where the percentile lines for these measures do not exactly join at the usual junction of 24 months. When the transition is made from recumbent length to stature charts (usually at 24 months to 36 months), there appears to be a downward shift in the child's placement on the charts.

Besides this, the smoothed percentiles do not extend beyond the 5th and 95th percentiles. Pediatric endocrinologists have expressed a need for the 3rd and 97th percentiles to better accommodate children growing at the extremes of the distribution.

There also are no weight-for-stature data for most adolescents. Weight-for-stature data are not available beyond approximately age 11½ years for boys and 10 years for girls.

Finally, weight- and stature-for-age charts do not extend beyond 17 completed years of age. Yet pediatricians often evaluate patients' growth and body size through the college years.

To revise the growth charts, NCHS specifically designed the third National Health and Nutrition Examination Survey (NHANES III, 1988–94) to oversample infants and pre-school children ages 2 months through 5 years, allowing for replacement of Fels weight and length data with national survey data for the United States.

CALLING ON THE EXPERTS

Between 1992 and 1997, NCHS conducted workshops to solicit recommendations on the growth chart revision and dissemination process. These workshops focused on content and methodologic issues.

NCHS invited growth and growth chart experts from numerous Federal agencies and academic institutions to provide input based on empirical data. Topics and discussions were diverse and complex.

Recommendations that resulted are summarized broadly here to provide a preview of what may be expected in the revised charts:

- Create revised growth charts representative of infants, children, and adolescents in the United States, after certain exclusions.
- Combine national survey data for all racial/ethnic groups and do not develop ethnic-specific charts. Both current knowledge and expert opinion indicate that all children have a similar genetic potential for growth. Observed racial/ethnic differences in growth appear to be attributable primarily to environmental influences. Furthermore, the national health examination surveys presently do not have adequate samples to create charts specific to all U.S. racial and ethnic groups.
- Exclude preterm, very-low-birth weight (VLBW; < 1,500 gm) infants from birth to age 3 years from the revised charts, because the growth of these infants differs from that of full-term infants of higher birth weight. Special charts, developed previously and published in the scientific literature, will be recommended to track growth in these children.
- Maintain two sets of charts based on age. Infant charts for birth to age 3 years will be constructed from national health examination survey data; the Fels data for weight and length will be eliminated. There will be charts for length-, weight- and head circumference-for-age, and weight-for-length. For

ages 2 through 19 years, charts will be available for stature-, weight- and body mass index-for-age (BMI; kg/m^2). Separate charts for boys and girls will be developed for all variables.

- Extend the charts for children and adolescents 2 additional years to cover adolescents through age 19 years.
- Make the 3rd and 97th percentiles available. Smoothed percentile curves will be available for percentiles 3, 5, 10, 25, 50, 75, 90, 95 and 97.
- Replace the 1977 weight-for-stature charts for prepubescent boys and girls with BMI-for-age charts. BMI has been recommended for evaluating and tracking overweight in children and adolescents. The 85th percentile line will be added to the new BMI charts to help identify children at risk for overweight.
- Pool data from the five national U.S. health examination surveys to achieve stable estimates and maintain precision at the outer percentiles.
- Use additional sources of data to fit the curves at birth. NHANES data begin at age 2 months to age 3 months. To fill the gap from birth to age 3 months, a decision was made to use birth weights derived from national natality data to fit the smoothed percentile lines at birth. Because national survey data are not available for length and weight-for-length at birth, natality data were used from two Midwestern States (Wisconsin and Missouri) that collected birth length data for all births in their States from 1989 through 1994. The shape of these curves will be modeled statistically and verified using published data from the scientific literature.
- Exclude data for NHANES III children and adolescents ages 6 years and over from weight- and BMI-for-age charts. This was prompted after a secular trend toward increasing body weight among children and adolescents, beginning at age 6 years, was documented in the United States between NHANES II (1976–80) and NHANES III (1988–94). This trend, believed to be associated with environmental influences, is not believed to be biologically or medically desirable.

Including the NHANES III children in the revised weight- and BMI-for-age percentile curves elevated the upper percentiles, with significant changes at the 75th percentile and above. This, in turn, had the undesirable effect of raising the outer percentiles, used to characterize overweight. As a result, overweight status would have been clinically underidentified. Therefore, NHANES III children ages 6 years and over, including adolescents, were excluded from the weight-and BMI-for-age charts.

The goal of the NCHS growth chart revision was to develop a single set of reference charts that would satisfy most clinical, epidemiological and research needs and applications to assess body size and monitor growth among U.S. infants, children, and adolescents. For clinical applications with individuals, the growth charts are designed to plot and track anthropometric values to screen for unusual size and growth patterns and to aid in making an overall clinical assessment. As such, these charts are intended to serve as growth references, rather than as growth standards or clinical ideals to be achieved.

AVAILABILITY

Initially, the revised charts will be made available through the Internet on the CDC/NCHS home page. NCHS also has provided financial support to the CDC Epidemiology Program Office to update and enhance the Anthro module in the computer software package known as EpiInfo, where both z-scores and percentiles are available electronically for each chart.

Format options for a hard copy version of the revised charts are being explored in collaboration with other Federal partners, such as CDC National Center for Chronic Disease Prevention and Health Promotion, the Maternal and Child Health Bureau of the Health Resources and Services Administration, and the Food and Nutrition Service of the U.S. Department of Agriculture. More than one format may be available for various clinical applications, although the actual content should not change.

Options also are being considered for additional ancillary products that would contain: background documentation of the revision process; an instruction packet for use of the revised charts, including the calculation and use of the BMI-for-age charts; a detailed reference manual of interpretive guidelines; and related materials that could be distributed electronically on a CD-ROM as well as on the Internet.

Users are encouraged to use the Internet to periodically check the CDC/NCHS home page (http://www.cdc.gov/nchswww/) for announcements and updates regarding dissemination and training materials.

Dr. Kuczmarski, coordinator of the growth chart revision project, is a nutritionist and health statistician at the National Centers for Health Statistics, Centers for Disease Control and Prevention in Hyattsville, Md.

Kuczmarski RJ. Revised growth charts due in late 1998. AAP NEWS, Vol 14, No 9. September 1998.

Index

B

C

D

E

F

G

H

I

J

K

L

M

O

P

Q

R

S

W

Z